LONE-ACTOR TERRORISM

LONE-ACTOR TERRORISM

An Integrated Framework

EDITED BY

JACOB C. HOLZER, MD

Assistant Professor, Clinical and Forensic Psychiatry
Department of Psychiatry, McLean Hospital and MGPO
Harvard Medical School
Boston, MA, USA

ANDREA J. DEW, PHD

Professor of Strategy and Policy, Maritime Irregular Warfare Chair
Department of Strategy and Policy
United States Naval War College
Newport, RI, USA

PATRICIA R. RECUPERO, JD, MD

Clinical Professor of Psychiatry and Human Behavior
Department of Psychiatry and Human Behavior
Warren Alpert Medical School of Brown University
Providence, RI, USA
and

PAUL GILL, PHD

Professor
Department of Security and Crime Science
University College London
London, UK

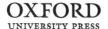

OXFORD
UNIVERSITY PRESS

OXFORD

UNIVERSITY PRESS

Oxford University Press is a department of the University of Oxford. It furthers
the University's objective of excellence in research, scholarship, and education
by publishing worldwide. Oxford is a registered trade mark of Oxford University
Press in the UK and certain other countries.

Published in the United States of America by Oxford University Press
198 Madison Avenue, New York, NY 10016, United States of America.

Names: Holzer, Jacob C., 1955– editor. | Dew, Andrea J., editor. |
Recupero, Patricia R., editor. | Gill, Paul (Lecturer), editor.
Title: Lone-actor terrorism : an integrated framework / edited by Jacob C. Holzer,
Andrea J. Dew, Patricia R. Recupero, and Paul Gill.
Description: New York, NY : Oxford University Press, [2022] |
Includes bibliographical references and index.
Identifiers: LCCN 2021050430 (print) | LCCN 2021050431 (ebook) |
ISBN 9780190929794 (hardback) | ISBN 9780190929817 (epub) |
ISBN 9780190929824 (digital-online)
Subjects: LCSH: Terrorism. | Terrorists. | Terrorism—Risk assessment.
Classification: LCC HV6431 .L655 2022 (print) | LCC HV6431 (ebook) |
DDC 363.325—dc23/eng/20220103
LC record available at https://lccn.loc.gov/2021050430
LC ebook record available at https://lccn.loc.gov/2021050431

DOI: 10.1093/med/9780190929794.001.0001

1 3 5 7 9 8 6 4 2

Printed by Integrated Books International, United States of America

JH: To the honor of having served in the USAF, and to my family,
friends, colleagues, and in memory of my parents.

AD: To my students and military teaching partners—
thank you for the education.

PR: To Samara E. Rainey, with thanks for
all the wisdom and support.

PG: To Noah, Charlie, and Drew.

CONTENTS

FOREWORD

How are people radicalized by extremist groups? Are they drawn in by the lure of violent propaganda or the support of like-minded confederates? Does the path to radicalization satisfy some inner psychological need? Is prior criminality an indicator of future terrorist aspirations?

In the summer of 2014, as the head of the FBI's National Security Branch, my conversations with counterterrorism colleagues focused on what would turn out to be a related question: why were so many subjects of terrorism investigations travelling to Syria? In many cases across the country, we saw budding extremists planning trips, raising money, and traveling to the other side of the world to join the Islamic State of Iraq and Syria, or "ISIS." Over the years we had seen a few ambitious aspiring operatives travel to Pakistan in an effort to join Al Qaeda. But this was different. Scores of western followers—Americans, Canadians, British and Europeans—were joining the Caliphate to fight an apocalyptic battle for the soul of Islam. The siren song of ISIS recruitment was resonating with many people in a new and dangerous way.

We needed to know more about their motivations to better assess the risks presented by these Americans who chose to fight for a foreign terror group. Our analysts compared all the details of their lives that we knew: their backgrounds, educations, socio-economic conditions, experiences with Islam, language capacities, criminal histories, social connections to other targets of investigation, and other factors. I expected there must be some link, some common experience or shared factor that led each of them to terrorist aspirations. When we met to review the preliminary analysis, the team produced a poster-sized composite of the individual photographs of each

target. The poster only clouded our vision. We saw men and women, young and old, white and brown, rich and poor. People with advanced degrees and high school dropouts. People from large cities and remote rural towns. Life-long practitioners of Islam and recent converts. People with no record of trouble in their lives and some with multiple runs through prison. In a single view it revealed the complexity of the problem we faced: we were looking at all of America.

A year later, ISIS changed its strategy and began directing its followers not to travel to Syria, but rather to wage war in their own homelands. With brutally effective propaganda and social media messaging, ISIS dispatched legions of followers to engage in solitary acts of violence around the world, using whatever weapons were at hand. An onslaught of knife attacks, shootings, and vehicle attacks metastasized across Asia, Europe, and the United States. This lone-actor violence continues to this day.

The job of practitioners is to prevent acts of terrorism. At its core this requires a constant assessment of risk, identifying who is most likely to commit an act of terror and when it might happen. Often investigators find themselves looking for the next terrorist in a trove of online monikers whose profiles deliberately conceal every detail. We have an interest not just in the investigator's success, but also in the efficiency and discipline they bring to the work. Lives are saved every time an act of terror is thwarted. But it is also true that innocent lives are disrupted and diverted when the net of investigation is cast too widely. Our shared safety demands that investigators work effectively, while the Constitution demands they do so without trampling on the freedoms we all treasure.

To succeed in this task, our practitioners need the best tools. Primarily, they need the research, analysis, and opinions of experts in fields that shed light on radicalization. *Lone-Actor Terrorism: An Integrated Framework* will be an essential element in that toolbox. With the latest research and theories on indoctrination, social media impact, mental health aspects, linguistic analysis, means, mechanisms, and trends, this text provides a comprehensive understanding of elements that drive lone actors. It is an important evolution in the progress of combating extremist violence—answering counterterror practitioner's questions with the data driven rigor of academic discipline.

Every day, it gets a little bit harder for our law enforcement and intelligence professionals to protect us from extremist violence. Adversaries get smarter—each learning from the other's mistakes. Communications become harder to see and hear—as encryption becomes ubiquitous. Extremist motivations become more fragmented and obtuse—as ideologies and political beliefs morph into grievance driven agendas. Our ability to thrive as a free and fair society increasingly depends on our ability to integrate the best data and research with the front line professionals who keep us safe. This text will serve as a foundation for that integration, a crucial support for that teamwork, and a way to shed light on the dark unknowns of radicalization. Exposing that darkness may enable us to stay one step ahead of the next threat.

The views expressed above are those of Andrew McCabe, FBI, Special Agent (ret.) and former Deputy Director, and not those of the FBI.

FOREWORD

JOHN WYMAN

The world is changing. The threats we face are complex and evolving. Technology has accelerated this change and created challenges that our current system is not well equipped to handle. The systems, processes, and procedures historically used to prevent acts of violence are outdated and insufficient, and there is no tolerance for failure in preventing acts of intended violence. The way we counter and mitigate threats must continually evolve. We must do more. We must adapt.

For the past five years, I have had the privilege of leading the FBI's Behavioral Threat Assessment Center (BTAC) in Quantico, Virginia. BTAC, housed within the FBI's Critical Incident Response Group (CIRG), Behavioral Analysis Unit 1 (BAU1), is a national-level, multidisciplinary and multi-agency threat assessment and threat management task force focused on the prevention of terrorism and acts of targeted violence. BTAC supports our federal, state, and local partners by providing holistic and structured operational support toward mitigating threats and maximizing prevention. Like many of our colleagues in threat management, we were constantly striving to address this most difficult question: why do people move along the pathway to intended violence, and more importantly, what can be done to stop them before they act? Understanding the complexities of why individuals move along the pathway—progressing from thought to action, radicalizing, and mobilizing—is critical to prevention. Effective threat mitigation requires a multidisciplinary, structured, thoughtful, and evidence-based approach. There is a growing body of cutting-edge, empirical research, which should be used to guide our ever-evolving threat mitigation efforts.

Lone-Actor Terrorism: An Integrated Framework consolidates the latest thinking and evidence on these challenging topics, including clinical intervention, historical origins, geographic influences, law enforcement impact, the role of intelligence and military, legal complexities, threat assessment, and potential areas of intervention. The impressive line-up of authors presented within this compendium include some of the world's most respected and renowned experts in this field. Their collective efforts stand impressively side-by-side, and in many cases on the shoulders of, pioneers and innovators who laid the foundation upon which this current research is built. This robust compilation of research should serve as a roadmap for violence prevention practitioners across all levels of government, first responders, and the broad array of stakeholders across communities who play a role in prevention.

One thing is certain: early identification and reporting of concerning behaviors to capable threat management teams is imperative for prevention. A large body of research and operational experience shows that violent actors commit their acts for highly individualized and personal reasons. A wide array of factors, often co-occurring, interrelated, and compounding, contribute to an individual's movement along the pathway to violence. However, even though these individuals move from thought to action for their own reasons, they frequently share similarities in observable and discernable behavior as they move from thought to action. Recognizing these behaviors alone is not sufficient—reporting information to well-trained, well-resourced, and responsible teams of stakeholders is critical to enact and maximize prevention efforts. Law enforcement plays a critical role in this process but so do less traditional partners such as mental health professionals, probation officers, school resource officers, social workers, non-governmental organizations (NGOs), and so on. Effective prevention requires that these non-traditional partners work and train together with law enforcement to understand capabilities and share information prior to a crisis. Too often the training is insufficient or uncoordinated, the resources are lacking, the relationships are dysfunctional or non-existent before crises occur, and information sharing is lacking or unidirectional.

Complicating matters, federal laws related to terrorism were written long ago and they are most effective against actors who are directed and deployed by a centralized foreign adversary. These same laws may be less suited for the reality of homegrown or domestic violent extremism, radicalization, and lone-actor terrorism. In the shadow of this evolution, some states have stepped into the gap and passed legislation which supplements existing federal legislation, but the utility of state efforts may be limited by the challenges of managing classified information, sensitive sources and methods, and the complex cocktail of belief systems contributing to an actor's commitment to violence (including conspiracy theories, involuntary celibacy, racial supremacy, xenophobia, and even reptilian invasions to name a few). The existing legislation—at both federal and state levels—is most effective when addressing individuals who either make overt public threats or regrettably those who have already committed an act of violence. As the threat picture evolves and outpaces the enactment of less-agile legislation, we should not rely solely on law enforcement agencies to be our only line of defense. We must build and amplify the capabilities of all stakeholders to identify persons of concern and to mitigate the threats they pose using methods most appropriate to each underlying, individualized threat.

The limitations of existing criminal legislation are not law enforcement's only challenge in prevention efforts; rather, as currently written, federal law restricts the ability of law enforcement to share threat related information with individuals best positioned to mitigate the threats, such as mental health professionals, medical doctors, family members, school counselors, and other non-law enforcement entities. Limitations on such disclosures are often so restrictive that they challenge the ability of federal law enforcement to share critical information with mental health professionals funded and chartered by the same federal government to help mitigate such threats. Clearly there is opportunity for improvement and society would benefit from careful and thoughtful revisions to these restrictions that balance privacy concerns with the new reality of security and threat management. Regardless of these existing challenges and potential improvements, the reality is and will remain that effective prevention requires early identification and intervention, coordinated with, but often *independent* of, law enforcement.

Many if not most law enforcement officers and other stakeholders dealing with these challenges lack adequate training in threat assessment and threat management principles. As such, these front-line responders (through no fault of their own) are greatly limited in their ability to accurately assess the threats within their communities and to develop and implement effective mitigation strategies. Instead, they must often rely on their own unique professional experience and "gut feel" to address these challenges. This approach, while sometimes effective, is insufficient and lacks the accountability that our communities deserve and demand. Thankfully, the authors of this book have taken a concrete step towards addressing this deficiency by sharing some of the most current, most useful information available.

There have been many outstanding publications in recent years related to the prevention of terrorism and targeted violence, but this important information is often scattered across multiple repositories in a wide array of formats. Finding timely, up-to-date, relevant information is challenging. Thankfully, *Lone-Actor Terrorism: An Integrated Framework* consolidates the latest thinking and research on a wide range of topics, including mental health, variables such as social media, propaganda/rhetoric, ethical issues, law enforcement, intelligence aspects, and forensic assessment. This publication is a valuable resource for anyone working to prevent acts of terrorism or targeted violence. It should serve as such to inform our collective efforts be incorporated into the baseline training for those responsible for terrorism and targeted violence prevention.

Too often, operational lessons learned are not shared between disciplines, e.g. law enforcement, mental health, probation and parole, etc. In addition, academic researchers have a limited optic because important operational learning points are not shared with them. As a result, academic research is often conducted in a vacuum without the input or guidance of operational practitioners and written in a manner that is incongruent with how law enforcement operates—further limiting its utility to law enforcement. Fortunately, the authors have blended lessons that shared osmosis between academia and operations and captured this useful guidance here in this most timely book.

As researchers, we must continue to analyze and assess the evolving threats and the potential solutions. As prevention practitioners, we must continue to apply this new information to our work, broaden our thinking, challenge our preconceived notions and biases, and learn from those outside our disciplines; we must move beyond conclusions based on "gut feel" or "operational experience," and proactively collaborate with our multidisciplinary partners. I am grateful to Drs. Jake Holzer and Paul Gill, as well as the editors and many other authors within this fine publication, for moving us in a direction that deepens our understanding of this priority issue and for doing so with credibility and skill.

The views and opinions, above, are those of John Wyman, FBI, Special Agent (Ret.), and not those of the FBI.

PREFACE

Lone-actor terrorism has unfortunately been on the increase in recent decades, and has appeared to accelerate in recent years. A range of factors, such as the influence of social media, extremist views and ideologies, group influences, availability of weapons, and internal variables, crystallize in certain individuals who may then go on to act violently. This dynamic process is complicated and cannot really be understood from a single perspective. The purpose of this volume is to approach the topic of lone-actor terrorism from different professional vantage points, including clinical, sociological, legal and forensic, ethical, law enforcement, intelligence, and military, in order to develop a broader understanding of the causes and impact on society and potentially lead to an increased ability to reduce risk. A relevant question is why a large number of people may be exposed to various influences and agree with an extremist view but never go on to commit violence, whereas a small segment do go on to commit violence in the name of that ideology. In the development of this volume, co-editors spoke with a large number of people representing different professional areas, including clinical and forensic mental health, law enforcement, the intelligence community, the academic community, members of the uniformed military services, members of the executive branch at the US federal level, and attorneys in national security. A salient theme throughout these discussions is that lone-actor terrorism is fluid regarding definitions, who is included and excluded, types of incidents, types of weapons, influences, etc. There is no uniform approach to the concept of lone-actor terrorism—how to understand it and what to do about it. The goal of this volume is to move in the direction of improved understanding and management.

The book is divided into overlapping sections.

Section I: Introduction, Historical and Case Examples. Chapter 1 provides a broad overview of lone-actor terrorism, addressing definitions, clinical and behavioral variables, roles of rhetoric and social media, legal and forensic issues, and the role of law enforcement, among other topics. Chapter 2 provides an overview of historical aspects involving individuals who acted in different circumstances and times. Chapter 3 discusses a range of disparate case examples based on definitions in the book. A unifying theme in these examples are individuals who act alone or with another, may have been influenced by a larger group, and have associated their actions to an ideology or cause (such as Islamist, right-wing extremist, single issue, or other causes). As will be reviewed in the volume, the associated ideology or cause may be clear, imprecise, or obscure.

Section II: Clinical Aspects. Chapter 4 reviews a limited number of case examples in more detail within a clinical context and discusses various clinical topics which may have bearing on different lone-actor cases. *Chapter 5* discusses the use of psychoactive drugs in some lone-actor terrorism cases. Chapter 6 reviews developmental aspects that may factor into individuals who commit lone-actor terror. Chapter 7 examines the role of psychometrics, the cognitive and psychological assessment in lone-actor terrorism. Chapter 8 discusses research pursuing a better understanding of lone-actor terrorism through the use of language.

Section III: Non-Clinical Professional and Allied Perspectives. Chapter 9 reviews the important concepts of propaganda and rhetoric in relation to lone-actor cases. Chapter 10 discusses lone-actor mass casualty attacks carried out by individuals but inspired by organized groups as a way of examining the nexus between individuals and groups. Chapter 11 provides an important analysis on the growing role of the internet and social media in lone-actor terrorism. Chapter 12 addresses geographical considerations in the United States and Europe between jihadist and right-wing extremist lone-actors. Chapter 13 discusses the diversity of weapons used in attacks, with a focus on, but not limited to, firearms. Chapter 14 discusses the role of forensic mental health assessment in defendants charged in terrorism cases. Chapter 15 addresses ethical issues and complications that can arise in lone-actor cases and raises the importance of considering ethical implications when dealing with specific cases. Chapter 16 reviews two important law enforcement aspects: the first involves collaborative efforts with law enforcement focused on proactive intervention and the second describes a first-hand account of the law enforcement response to a high-profile lone-actor terrorism incident in the United States. Chapter 17 examines the post-9/11 transformation of US counterterrorism policy with a focus on lone-actor terrorism. Chapters 18 and 19 address various legal topics relevant to US and UK national security, respectively. Chapter 20 provides an important discussion about online indoctrination, outlining a model used in cults which may have application in lone-actor terrorism cases. Chapter 21 reviews the topics of hatred and harboring a grievance as drivers in lone-actor incidents and discusses clinical aspects, neurobiology, and hate speech and crimes. Chapter 22 provides an interesting review of comparisons with other groups that result in mass violence or damage to national security, discussing some common and distinguishing variables; these groups include those committing espionage and treason, those committing mass violence without an identified ideology or cause, and school shooting incidents.

Section IV: Aspects of Assessment and Potential Management. Chapter 23 reviews the literature addressing a range of risk factors and discusses the organization of this knowledge base into a framework. Chapter 24 presents a structure for identifying and preempting lone-actors during the formative pre-incident planning phase. Chapter 25 reviews the Terrorist Radicalization Assessment Protocol (TRAP-18) and analyzes a high-profile lone-actor terrorism case using the TRAP-18. Chapter 26 provides an important broad review of threat and risk assessment tools which may have application in lone-actor terrorism cases. The concluding chapter, Chapter 27,

discusses thoughts about risk assessment and intervention and is divided into four parts: (1) an examination of the salient aspects of this volume; (2) a review of contemporary events at the time of writing and their impact on lone-actor terrorism, including the coronavirus pandemic and the January 6, 2021 attack on the US Capitol; (3) a review of various areas discussed in the volume that may provide a context for proactive intervention; and (4) directions for future research.

Due to the nature of this volume—the broad array of topics, the diversity of professions represented, and the range of case examples discussed—there are some inherent limitations and areas to clarify. One important limitation is that much of the content on specific high-profile cases was drawn from open-source news. Efforts were made to use resources that are nationally recognized as reliable and balanced. By definition, content that would be considered classified or legally protected is not included. Due to these issues, accuracy of the content is only as good as the resources used and may not be considered 100% accurate. When clinical material is presented throughout the volume, authors strived to avoid making their own clinical diagnoses; clinical diagnoses discussed in the book originate from or are supported by the references cited. This practice is in keeping with American Psychiatric Association Principles of Medical Ethics as applied to psychiatry in the United States. Another important constraint, as discussed throughout this volume, is related to the multifaceted nature of lone-actor terrorism. In individual chapters, lone-actor cases were identified by name based on the reports found in open news sources. Efforts were made to only cite cases in which the lone actor was found guilty and convicted or had been killed in the index incident. Cases involving individuals pre-trial are identified as "alleged" or reference news reports without inferring guilt. Readers may have differing views of definitions, methods, cases, etc., and may not be in total agreement with the content of this book. That limitation is understood by the authors and editors, with the expectation that the constraints and limitations in this volume will drive further research in understanding and potentially proactively managing the risk of lone-actor terrorism in the United States and internationally.

Jacob C. Holzer, MD
Andrea J. Dew, PhD
Patricia R. Recupero, JD, MD
Paul Gill, PhD

CONTRIBUTORS

Michael Arieli, BA, BS RPh
Director and Founder of Division of
Enforcement MOH Israel (RETIRED) Research
Fellow International Institute For Counter-
Terrorism (ICT)
International Institute For Counter-
Terrorism (ICT)
Reichman University
Herzliya, Israel

Tammy Ayres, PhD, PgDL, MSc, BSc
Associate Professor
Department of Criminology
University of Leicester
Leicester, UK

Terry R. Bard, DD, MAHL, BHL, AB
Lecturer
Department of Psychiatry
Harvard Medical School
Chestnut Hill, MA, USA

Christopher E. Beeler, JD
Assistant United States Attorney
United States Attorney's Office for the Southern
District of California
U.S. Department of Justice
San Diego, CA, USA

Ronnie Berkovitz, PhD
Director Division of Enforcement and Inspection
Ministry of Health
Jerusalem, Israel

Hy Bloom, BA, LLB, MD, FRCPC
Assistant Professor at both institutions
noted below
Medicine (at University of Toronto); Psychiatry
and Behavioural Neurosciences (at McMaster
University)
University of Toronto and McMaster University
Toronto, ON, Canada

Hagit Bonny-Noach, PhD
Senior Lecturer
Department of Criminology
Ariel University
Ariel, Israel

Noémie Bouhana, PhD
Professor
Department of Security and Crime Science
University College London
Cambridge, UK

Douglas Brennan, MD, MPA
Instructor
Department of Psychiatry
Harvard Medical School
University of Colorado
Denver, CO, USA

Philip J. Candilis, MD
Professor
Department of Psychiatry and Behavioral
Sciences George Washington University School
of Medicine Director of Medical Affairs Saint
Elizabeths Hospital
Alexandria, VA, USA

Jon Caven-Atack
Practitioner Scholar
Nottingham, UK

**Mark Concordia, MS, CTM (Association of
Threat Assessment Professionals Certified
Threat Manager)**
Training Manager and Behavioral Threat
Assessment and Management Consultant
Department of Training, Consultant, and
Program Development
AT-RISK International
Chantilly, VA, USA

Emily Corner, BSc (Hons), MSc, PhD
Senior Lecturer
Centre for Social Research and methods
Australian National University
Canberra, Australia

William Costanza, DLS (Doctor of Liberal
Studies)
Adjunct Associate Professor
Security Studies Program, Walsh School of
Foreign Service
Georgetown University
Washington, DC, USA

Eric Y. Drogin, JD, PhD, ABPP
Harvard Medical School
Boston, MA, USA

Theodora Najla Farah
MBE Candidate
Perelman School of Medicine
University of Pennsylvania
Philadelphia, PA, USA

Frank Farnham, MBBS, BSc, FRCPsych
Consultant Forensic Psychiatrist and Honorary
Senior Lecturer
Fixated Threat Assessment Centre
North London Forensic Service
London, UK

Robert P. Granacher, MD, MBAs
Retired, Volunteer Faculty
Department of Psychiatry
University of Kentucky
Lexington, KY, USA

Mark Hamm, PhD
Professor
Department of Criminology
Indiana State University
Terre Haute, IN, USA

Steven Hassan, PhD, MA, MEd, LMHC, NCC
President
Freedom of Mind Resource Center
Newton, MA, USA

Christopher Jasparro, PhD
Jerome Levy Chair of Economic Geography and
National Security
National Security Affairs
United States Naval War College
Newport, RI, USA

Amy Jeffress, JD, Yale Law School
Partner
Arnold & Porter Kaye Scholer LLP
Washington, DC, USA

Bennett Kleinberg, PhD
Assistant Professsor
Department of Methodology & Statistics
Tilburg University
Tilburg, Netherlands

Danielle B. Kushner, MD
Clinical Assistant Professor
Department of Psychiatry
New York University School of Medicine
New York, NY, USA

Suzanne Levi-Sanchez, PhD
Associate Professor
National Security Affairs
US Naval War College
Newport, RI, USA

Stuart Macdonald, BA, PhD
Professor
School of Law
Swansea University
Swansea, UK

Michael Madden, AA
Retired Police Lieutenant
City of San Bernardino Police Department
San Bernardino, CA, USA

Simran Malhotra, BA
Program Manager
Microsoft
Bangalore, India

Karl Mobbs, MD
Supervising Psychiatrist Oregon State
Hospital & DOC
Affiliate Faculty
Oregon Health & Science University
Portland, OR, USA

Nancy P. Moczynski, PhD
Director of Neuropsychology
Department of Psychiatry
Harvard Medical Faculty Physicians at Beth
Israel Deaconess Medical Center
Boston, MA, USA

Alina Poperno, MPH, BPharm, BSc
Pharmacology
National Coordinator
Enforcement and Inspection Division
Ministry of Health
Jerusalem, Israel

Marilyn Price, MD
Assistant Professor of Psychiatry
Newton Center, MA, USA

Samara E. Rainey, BA
Independent Research Consultant
Maple Key Consulting
Willington, CT, USA

J. Reid Meloy, PhD
Clinical Professor of Psychiatry
Department of Psychiatry
Univ of California San Diego
LA Jolla, CA, USA

Phillip J. Resnick, MD
Professor of Psychiatry
Department of Psychiatry
Case Western Reserve University
Cleveland, OH, USA

Allen R. Schiller, PhD
Interim Chief, Neuropsychology / Instructor
Neuropsychology Department / Department of Psychiatry
McLean Hospital / Harvard Medical School
Belmont, MA, USA

Mansi J. Shah, MA
Research Associate
Dare Association, Inc
Framingham, MA, USA

Arya Shah, MD
Department of Psychiatry
Brigham and Women's Hospital/Harvard
Medical School
Boston, MA, USA

Lauren Simpson, BA
Project Coordinator
Department of Psychology
University of Nebraska-Lincoln
Lincoln, NE, USA

Joshua Sinai, PhD
Chair and Professor
Intelligence and Security Studies
Capitol Technology University
Laurel, MD, USA

Jeffrey H. Smith, BS, JD
Senior Counsel
Arnold & Porter, LLP
Washington, DC, USA

Ramón Spaaij, PhD
Professor
Institute for Health and Sport
Victoria University
Melbourne, Australia

Daniel Starr, MA
U.S. Department of State
Malden, MA, USA

Gen Ignatius Tanaka, MD
Assistant Professor
Department of Psychiatry
Oregon Health & Science University
Portland, OR, USA

Emily Threlkeld
Bachelor of Arts in International Affairs;
Bachelor of Science in Psychology
Teacher
Konawaena Middle School
Teach for America
Kealakekua, HI, USA

Isabelle W. J. van der Vegt, PhD
Honorary Research Fellow
UCL
London, UK

Ashley H. VanDercar, MD, JD
Assistant Professor
Case Western Reserve University
Department of Psychiatry
Cleveland, OH, USA

Ryan C. Wagoner, MD
Associate Professor and Vice Chair for Clinical
Services
Department of Psychiatry and Behavioral
Neurosciences
University of South Florida Morsani College of
Medicine
Tampa, FL, USA

Aviv Weinstein, PhD
Full Professor
Department of Behavioral Science
Ariel University
Ariel, Israel

Christopher Winter, BA, MA
PhD Candidate
Institute for Sustainable Industries &
Liveable Cities
Victoria University
Melbourne, Australia

Tian Tian Xin, JD
Associate
Arnold & Porter
Washington, DC, USA

Uri Ben Yaakov, MA
Director of International Relations & Senior
Researcher
The International Institute for Counter-
Terrorism (ICT)
Herzliya, Israel

Reem Zaia, JD, LLM
Lawyer
Gowling WLG (Canada) LLP
Ottawa, ON, Canada

Corri Zoli, PhD
Research Professor
Forensic and National Security Sciences Institute
(FNSSI)
Syracuse University
Syracuse, NY, USA

Olivia Zurek, MD
Instructor in Psychiatry
Department of Psychiatry
Massachusetts General Hospital
Boston, MA, USA

Introduction

Scope of the Problem, Definitions, and Concepts

JACOB C. HOLZER, ANDREA J. DEW,
*PATRICIA R. RECUPERO, AND PAUL GILL**

Contemporary lone-actor terrorism is a complex, multidimensional process, involving different contexts, ideologies, geographic regions, circumstances, drives, individuals, and modes of violence. Despite the complexity behind a violent incident, the outcome unfortunately is quite simple: harm and devastation to victims, families, and society. The purpose of this volume is to explore lone-actor terrorism from different but complementary vantage points. One important focus is on the variability of clinical and forensic mental health concerns. In addition, this volume explores other aspects of lone-actor terrorism, including law enforcement and homeland security, risk and threat assessment, geography, ethical considerations, and legal issues. Lone-actor terrorism does not happen in a vacuum. In the context of a given set of conditions, stressors, and rhetoric, many people will think about acting in some form of opposition, vocalize their disagreement or outrage, protest, and vote in order to effect change. A very small number of individuals, however, think that they have to "take matters in their own hands" and act violently in order to effect change.

DEFINING LONE-ACTOR TERRORISM

Defining terrorism can be challenging. The term is often misunderstood or misinterpreted. On the surface, it can involve individuals or groups with identified goals or ideals who act violently for a defined purpose. Hoffman defines "terrorism" as violence or the threat of violence in pursuit of or in the service of a political goal.[1] There is a rich history of individuals, groups, and states acting within this definition, going back over centuries, a detailed review of which would be beyond the scope of this book. However, patterns of terrorism have evolved in recent history in terms of etiology, context, and means and have included state-sponsored terror, groups associated with anarchism or resistance, the spread of geopolitical groups across various regions, and groups identifying with religious extremism, nationalism, or other causes. While there is a certain "clarity" to groups acting violently for a cause, there has been a more recent proliferation of individual terrorist acts that, in at least some cases, are less clear regarding rationale, motives, and purpose.

The simple definition of a lone-actor terrorist is an individual who commits an act of terrorism on their own, neither part of nor formally directed by an organized group. Although research has shown very few individuals truly act alone, this concept is an important reference because the "lone-actor" individual poses a different threat and requires a response different from those committing terror as part of an organized group.[2] The Merriam-Webster Dictionary refers to a "lone wolf" as a person who prefers to work, act, or live alone, something of a misnomer given that wolves tend to be very social and run in packs.[3] The true "lone wolf" tends to be a rare outcast.[4] For the purposes of this book, the term "lone-actor" will be used in place of "lone-wolf,"

---

* The opinions in this chapter are those of the chapter authors and not that of the U.S. Navy War College or the Department of Defense

"stray-dog," or other designation. James Comey, then director of the FBI, stated before the House Homeland Security Committee in September 2014 that homegrown violent extremists (which can be equated with lone-actor terrorism) present unique challenges in that they do not fit the profile of terrorists linked to a group, their experiences and drives may be unique, they may act on their own, and their motives may be varied.[5] Underscoring the current impact of lone-actor terrorism, FBI Director Christopher Wray, at a Senate Appropriations Committee subcommittee hearing in May 2018, indicated lone-actor terrorism is the FBI's "highest counterterrorism priority at the moment."[6]

For purposes of this book, a lone actor is linked to a radicalized or extremist cause or ideology. The identified causes, ideologies, or beliefs can vary widely across political, extremist religious, geographic, or other spectrums. Two of the cases reviewed in this volume that fit with this standard definition are the 2009 Fort Hood shooting and the 2014 Isla Vista killing spree. The purpose of this approach is to attempt to separate out mass violence events without apparent cause or etiology which may be based on mental illness, emotional anger, or an undefined obscure etiology felt not to be ideologically driven. Some school shootings, the Aurora Colorado movie theater shooting in 2012, and the Germanwings flight 9525 incident may fit into this latter category. Even the attempt to separate groups for definitional purposes may be complicated or ambiguous. The absence or uncertainty of an apparent cause may obscure an underlying different cause. An example of the complicated nature of identifying causation involves the Las Vegas mass shooting in October 2017, where, despite reports that the shooter had expressed anti-government sentiments before the shooting,[7] the investigation was closed without a motive being found.[8]

An important and related issue centers on the relationship of a "hate crime" with lone-actor terrorism and whether these can be considered separate, the same, or partially overlapping crimes. In part, these relationships and definitions depend on one's professional viewpoint. There may be legal distinctions between a hate crime and terrorism, although from an intelligence analysis and law enforcement response position the distinctions may be more academic than practical. Daniel Byman presented a cogent argument that, irrespective of the individuals' political beliefs or agenda, having a goal of mass violence linked to that agenda warrants the designation of terrorism

and would potentially allow for more resources to combat that threat.[9] One could argue that the "emotional" variables of hate, anger, and revenge could potentially apply to a broad spectrum of lone-actor terrorism incidents, whether the targets are military personnel, women, government employees, persons of color, abortion clinic personnel, sexual or gender minorities, or members of the general public. One can potentially refer to the separation of hate crime from lone-actor terrorism as "a distinction without a difference."

An added consideration in defining lone-actor terrorism, for the purposes of this volume, involves the number of participants or assailants. In most cases, there is only one assailant, although in some cases two assailants were identified. Examples of dyad lone-actor terrorist cases include the Tsarnaev brothers involved in the April 2013 Boston Marathon bombing and Syed Farook and Tashfeen Malik in the December 2015 San Bernardino mass shooting. Based on research by one author (JH), in dyad cases there may be an identified "leader" and "follower." In groups of three or more participants, there are potential shifts which occur involving group dynamics, changes in communication, intelligence, planning, fewer mental health issues, and, in the authors' experience, different sociodemographic and psychological backgrounds.[10]

What may appear on the surface to be a lone actor is often someone at least influenced or potentially managed by an organized terror group.[11] For purposes of this volume, individuals receiving face-to-face direct guidance, training, and resources from an organized group would not fall under the "lone-actor terrorist" characterization. However, this underscores the complexity of the relationship between individuals and groups, when someone is truly acting on their own versus to the benefit of a group versus on behalf of a group. Dan Byman refers to this gray area as "lone-ish wolves—wolves who are either acting alone or in very small packs."[12] Subsequent investigation may reveal that an individual who initially appeared to have been radicalized and acting alone or with few others was actually trained and/or formally acting on behalf of a larger organization. One example of this type of case would be Faisal Shahzad, who attempted to detonate a car bomb in Times Square, New York City, in May 2010. Evidence linked the Pakistan Taliban to Shahzad's training, financing, and direction.[13] Another example is that of Richard Reid, who attempted to set off a shoe bomb on an airline flight in December 2001; investigation revealed that he had received training from al-Qaeda after being radicalized.[14]

Carol Flynn discusses criteria which provide a helpful outline for approaching the definitional aspects of lone-actor terrorism, and these will be partially followed in this book: (a) lone-actor terrorists deliberately create and exploit fear through violence or the threat of violence, (b) the lone-actor terrorist is a single person (this volume deviates from this criterion in that we include two-person groups, although exclude larger groups), (c) the lone actor pursues political change linked to an ideology, and (d) no command and control or external support from an organized entity exists (although in this volume there is a recognition that organized groups may influence a lone actor's behavior, particularly through social media).[15]

Although there has been a recent focus on radical Islamist-driven lone-actor violence, the contemporary use of this term is also associated with US far right-wing groups. In the early 1980s, the white supremacist Louis Beam advocated for and popularized the concept of "leaderless resistance" in the United States to describe a strategy of conducting hostilities through small cells of resistance. This strategy was conceptualized earlier by a US intelligence officer in the 1960s as a method to protect CIA-backed operations through the use of small or individual units. It has more recently evolved into a methodology adopted by a large array of groups involving different ideological beliefs.[16] In the 1960s and 1970s, surges in terrorism cases representing extremist geopolitical views (such as the Red Army Faction, the Irish Republican Army, the Popular Front for the Liberation of Palestine, etc.) may have spurred some individuals to act; however, for the most part individuals acted within or formally on behalf of the larger military-like organization. An important reference describing the relationship of organizations within the geopolitical context is David C. Rapoport's approach to the study of terrorism describing four waves of terrorism chronologically.[17]

VARIABLES IN LONE-ACTOR TERRORISM CASES

A unique challenge in understanding lone-actor terrorism involves the wide-ranging nature of the individuals and their reasons for committing violence. Within the context of lone-actor mass violence, several broad groupings are identified based on belief systems and ideologies, including right-wing/ultranationalist views, extremist Islamist, and those taking a position against an identified process or group in society (single issue, e.g., women, the LGBTQ community, development, abortion, etc.). Less commonly found groups include those identifying with other extremist religious or racial orientations or with left-wing political views. An important concept is that, whereas the majority of individuals who identify with one of these groups may agree with the core ideology or foundation of that group and think about acting violently (without actually doing so), a few fringe individuals feel they must take matters into their own hands, thus crossing the line into lone-actor terrorism.

Numerous studies and reports suggest that some individuals who act violently on their ideological beliefs have underlying mental health problems which may factor into their decisional capacity and behavior. Unfortunately, lone-actor terrorism is far more complex than the simple dichotomy of having or not having a psychiatric basis. A more holistic and realistic approach to understanding lone-actor terror involves consideration of numerous other factors, including a propensity for violent behavior, underlying hostility and need for revenge, difficulty with groups and socialization, geography, access to weapons and opportunity, and a willingness to die for a cause. A large proportion of the literature aimed at both professionals and the public has attempted to distinguish "true" politically motivated terror from individuals who commit terror based on internal aberrant reasons.[18] In 2011, President Obama stated "When you've got one person who is deranged or driven by a hateful ideology, they can do a lot of damage, and it's a lot harder to trace those lone wolf operators."[19] Statements at that time led to the understanding of a "false dichotomy" separating terrorists who are rational and act for political gains from those with mental illness who purportedly act on an irrational basis.[20] Numerous case reviews and reports indicate that individual lone-actor terrorists may have a wide range of clinical mental health issues, including personality disorders, mood and psychotic disorders, impulse control disorders, or substance use disorders, yet have been able to engage in an organized, detailed preparation for an attack, which may have a rational motive and basis. As will be reviewed in detail in other chapters of this volume, there may be a common misperception that the presence of a mental health disorder equates with being irrational, consequentially reducing responsibility. In reality, the presence of a mental disorder may or may not impact on current legal competency, but the vast majority of defendants with a diagnosable mental health condition would still be considered criminally responsible when applied against relevant legal tests and standards.

In a study conducted by one author (PG) examining variables related to mental illness and lone-actor terrorism, a number of important findings were revealed: (a) rates of mental illness were significantly greater in the lone-actor sample compared with those belonging to organized groups, (b) there was an association between mental illness in the individual lone actor and a spouse/partner associated with a larger group, (c) there was no association between mental illness and social isolation, (d) those lone actors with mental illness were more likely associated with single-issue ideology rather than extremist religious or political views, and (e) there was no association between the presence of mental illness and prior criminal behavior, but those with mental illness had a strong association with prior violence.[21] Results of this study showed that lone-actor terrorists with a history of mental illness were more likely to engage in specific antecedent events and behaviors, raising important implications for the proactive role of mental health professionals in working with law enforcement and security to help prevent future attacks.

Aside of the issue of mental illness, a range of other variables are important to consider, including personality traits, psychological mechanisms, education, deviant behavior, obsessional thinking, hostility, and the need for revenge. A limiting factor is that much of the research literature reviewing these variables is based on individuals identifying with organized groups or movements, which may or may not have direct application to individual lone actors. One interesting although dated study examining a large number of right-wing militants found numerous common features, including ambivalence toward authority, defective insight, emotional detachment from the consequences of one's actions, destructiveness, low education, and an adherence to a subculture focused on violence and weapons.[22] An important earlier concept stressed the role of narcissism in individuals who commit terrorism—that narcissistic individuals feel superior to others, have volatile self-esteem and interpersonal problems, and are prone to aggression.[23] Although narcissistic traits or personality may play a role in some individual cases, a shift in the literature attempted to explain individual terrorism behavior in terms of group or organizational dynamics and behavior. Numerous studies support findings that mental health issues and maladaptive traits and variables play less of a role in those individuals belonging to larger organized terrorist groups.[20]

Evidence suggests that variables involving education and occupation are also important to consider. Typically, higher levels of education lead to greater occupational opportunities and reduced risk of offending, while lower education results inversely in a higher risk of criminal offending. The lone-actor terrorism group does not follow this trend; studies have revealed two findings: an average higher level of education in the lone-actor group compared with other criminal offending groups, and this higher level of education did not translate into success in employment: more than half of those with at least some college-level education were unemployed at the time of study.[20] However, in many cases, the exposure to the extremist cause occurred within a higher-educational setting.

In a preliminary review by another of this chapter's authors (JH) of high-profile lone-actor terrorism incidents, several common variables were identified among lone-actor cases, although more rigorous research is needed to assess if these variables are statistically meaningful. Variables identified included : (a) mental health issues, including mood disorders, psychosis, alcohol and substance abuse, traumatic brain injury, and personality disorder; (b) a history of undergoing a change or "radicalization" from an earlier period, with resulting isolation or a preoccupation which stood out as atypical or different to those who knew the individual; (c) a context or "triggering event" may have led up to the incident; (d) in some cases there was a history of failing to achieve a personal goal in the military, having an unsuccessful experience in the military, or feigning or posing to be in a military-like organization; (e) in many cases individuals appeared to be bright but existed on the periphery rather than being fully integrated into society; and (f) in many cases there was a pattern of "contradictory" thoughts and beliefs (JH, preliminary research findings).[24] An important review article examined sociodemographic and antecedent behaviors in a large group of lone-actor terrorist cases in which numerous characteristics were described, including education, employment, military experience, criminal activity, and mental health issues. Researchers found that many lone-actor terrorists were socially isolated and engaged in activities with an external group or movement and that true lone-actor terrorist events were rarely unexpected or impulsive.[10]

One significant area of study relates to the use of alcohol and illicit substances, both antecedent to later violence and during the violent event, either alone or in interaction with psychiatric illness. Gill et al. reported in their analysis of antecedent behaviors to lone-actor terrorism that almost a quarter of cases involved a history of substance abuse, although few cases involved drugs or alcohol during the commission of the terrorist act.[10] Use of various illicit substances, however, has been reported in relation to specific lone-actor terrorism incidents. For example, reports indicated that Omar Mateen had used large amounts of anabolic steroids (which are associated with increased irritability and aggression) for years leading up to the Orlando nightclub shooting in 2016.[25,26] The mental health history of Jared Loughner, involved in the Tucson shooting rampage that killed several people and wounded Rep. Gabrielle Giffords, included heavy marijuana use in addition to schizophrenia.[27,28] A review of open source news literature indicates that in individual lone-actor terrorism cases various illicit drugs were used prior to or during an event, including marijuana, cocaine, alcohol, and steroids. An important variable identified in the literature included the potential psychoactive effect of the agents themselves on mood, cognition, and behavior, along with the interplay of the substances with an individual's underlying mental illness. The interplay of mental illness, substances and lone-actor aggression is addressed in more detail within chapters of this volume.

Another variable that has played a predominant role in promoting lone-actor thinking and behavior is the degree of rhetoric in society. Unfortunately, history is replete with examples of how rhetoric may have provided the initiative or motivation to act violently. For instance, Anwar Al-Awlaki, through his sermons, preached themes involving Muslims as victims, the West as the enemy out to humiliate and defeat Muslims, and that jihad was required.[29] Rhetoric can come from various sources, including Islamist, right- and left-wing voices, conservatives and liberals, and those for or against a specific cause. Predating and during the recent administration in the United States, there has been growing concern about rhetoric from various sources fueling right-wing violence.[30] Recent events have displayed an intensification of this concern. Although early reports alluded to Sarah Palin's electoral map with crosshairs over several districts, including Gabrielle Giffords's, as playing a role in the 2011 Tucson shooting, this relationship was considered nebulous, and no direct link between that map or the rhetoric of that time and that shooting was established in later reports.[31,32] Jared Loughner reportedly expressed virulent anti-government ideology, although the extent of influence that political partisanship and rhetoric had on him is unknown.[33]

The multipurpose role of the internet and social media has come under increasing examination as an instrument to communicate rhetoric and hate, as a means for like-minded individuals to connect, and as a process to allow a small number of individuals to plan and operationalize violence. News media outlets and researchers have discussed the role of the internet and social media in fueling hatred and propagating violence in the United States and abroad, sometimes arguing that social media may play an unprecedented role in incitement and provocation.[34,35] A closer examination indicates a more complex relationship between the internet, social media, and individuals prone to lone-actor terrorism than was suspected.[20] For example, the evolution of the internet has not resulted directly in an increase in lone-actor terrorist activity but has played a role in shaping individuals' ideation and behavior prior to the commission of a terrorist attack.[36] The internet provides a platform for those who may be isolated and alienated to increase social activity. Some scholars have argued that so-called lone-actor terrorists for whom social media played a role are not true "lone actors"; other individuals online have often played a role in their radicalization, recruitment, teaching, training, and direction.[37] A person's profile, persona, and behavior on specific platforms can provide insight into their mental state and behavior, potentially providing actionable cues to help prevent a future violent event. An added complexity in understanding the relationship of the internet and social media to lone-actor terrorism is the role of the "dark web," a component of the internet with restricted access that facilitates anonymity, which can be a resource for individuals planning an act of terror. For example, a suspect in a 2018 mosque attack reportedly purchased bomb material on the dark web,[38] and perpetrators of previous attacks have also purchased weapons such as firearms on the dark web (e.g., 2016 Munich mall shooting).[39]

Other important factors related to lone-actor terrorism events include geographical location and mode of violence, both of which have wide variability. The phenomenon of lone-actor terrorism is not unique to the United States or restricted to the use of firearms, but it is on the increase. Using conservative definitions of lone-actor incidents in the United States, a Frontline review in 2016 reported an increase in such incidents as well as in the numbers killed and injured by such incidents; white supremacist ideology was the main inspiration for many lone-actor attacks, although radical Islamist attacks were increasing.[40] Geographic location and weapon choice may have some association, although again there is no simple explanation or equation to understand a lone-actor terrorism incident. Increased firearm access in the United States is only one of several factors in the higher rate of firearm attacks in the United States versus other means (e.g., vehicles, bombs) in other regions. There has been an upswing in firearm usage compared with other weapons in US-based lone-actor terrorism,[40] but there have been numerous examples of non-firearm terrorist incidents in the United States, such as the Boston Marathon bombing and the alleged October 2017 truck attack on a bike path in Manhattan. However, in a review of lone-actor terror incidents in the United States over the past few decades, it appears that firearms and bombs have been the most frequent weapons. There are numerous examples of lone-actor terrorism incidents in countries outside of the United States, including in Canada, and throughout Europe, Africa, Asia, and South America. Outside of the United States, where firearms are less readily accessible, the use of vehicles and construction equipment, bombs and incendiary devices, and knives are more prominent in lone-actor incidents. However, there is not a tight geographic correlation, and numerous incidents of firearm-based lone-actor violence have occurred across the globe.[24]

CLINICAL AND FOREN-SIC ASSESSMENTS

The clinical and forensic mental health assessment of an individual in custody under lone-actor terrorism charges is an important process related to conducting thorough and fair legal proceedings, maintaining ethical standards, and attempting to understand the basis for the incident, motivation, intent, planning, and collaboration with others. As outlined earlier and expanded in the following chapters, various psychiatric issues may arise in individual cases, including personality disorders, major mental illness, substance abuse, and traumatic brain injury. Although clinical mental health issues are a general concern in lone-actor terrorism cases, forensic applications in these cases are

different. In some cases, an individual's mental state and capacity may be sufficiently impaired to warrant evaluation for competence to stand trial and criminal responsibility. A competence-to-stand-trial evaluation is ordered when there is concern about an individual's ability to understand the charges and legal process and to assist in their own defense. Jared Loughner, whom experts diagnosed with schizophrenia, was found incompetent to stand trial after psychiatric assessment revealed bizarre, delusional thoughts and behavioral outbursts.[27] Following treatment, he was later found competent and pled guilty.[41] Following an assassination attempt on then-President Ronald Reagan, the passage of the Insanity Defense Reform Act of 1984[42] made it more difficult to obtain a "not guilty by reason of insanity" (NGRI) verdict. Based on this Act and as described later, at the federal level the burden of proof shifted to the defendant, who needed to prove insanity by clear and convincing evidence.[43] In one of the authors' (JH) experience in forensic psychiatry evaluations, successful insanity defenses—based on severe mental illness resulting in a defendant not knowing the wrongfulness of his acts or being unable to conform his behavior to the requirements of the law—are rare. Cases where the insanity defense was considered or raised but rejected include Lee Boyd Malvo's conviction[44] and the case of Nidal Hasan.[45,46] At the state level, the criteria for a defendant being found NGRI varies, with many states following the M'Naughten or Model Penal Code standards, with burden of proof varying between the state and defendant.[47,48] Most, but not all, lone-actor terrorism cases are tried at the federal level, which follows the stricter criteria that (a) at the time of the offense, due to severe mental illness the defendant was unable to appreciate the nature and quality or wrongfulness of their act, and (b) the defendant has the burden of proving the insanity defense by clear and convincing evidence.[49]

ETHICAL ISSUES

A range of ethical issues can be studied in the context of lone-actor terrorism, such as those related to counterterrorism and proactive law enforcement interventions, and an incident's impact on society. One important consideration is the "dynamic" balance between appropriate law enforcement interventions and surveillance and preserving individual freedoms within society. This balance differs between jurisdictions and over time. For instance, proactive law enforcement measures involving monitoring and restrictions in New York City are, appropriately, more intensive than those found in less densely populated areas. Following an incident, there may be a call for further restrictions and more intensive monitoring, but such measures raise concerns about infringement on individual freedoms of movement, speech, and activity.

Another important area for consideration is the influence of a terror incident and its subsequent media coverage on bias and hate toward a particular group (e.g., ethnic, racial, political, or religious affiliations), particularly if the lone actor belongs to that group. This influence, unfortunately, can have the result of perpetuating violence and intensifying intergroup conflicts and hate. Some lone actors consciously intend to start such an escalation of violent conflict (e.g., David Copeland, Anders Breivik).

Related ethical concerns following terror incidents may concern the appropriate range of free speech in society and access to weapons as covered by constitutional amendments; these issues are the subjects of ongoing controversy. Following mass-casualty incidents involving assault weapons, of which there have been many, some have called for assault weapon bans,[50,51] but legislative approaches to restrict firearm access are often met with intense resistance from lobbyists and others. It is recognized, however, that lone-actor terror incidents in the United States and abroad, as outlined above, have included, in addition to firearms, the use of bombs, knives, and vehicles.

Another important ethical matter is the intensity of media coverage after an incident. One important example of this latter concern was the commentary following the Westminster Bridge vehicle-ramming attack in March 2017. Although the Islamic State in Iraq and al-Sham (ISIS) claimed responsibility for the incident, the subsequent police investigation did not find a formal link between the perpetrator and any terrorist organization.[52] However, for what was an attack of brief duration and limited scope, there was extensive media coverage, raising concerns about the media's role in propagating a terrorist organization's message.[53]

Ethical issues may also arise in research on victims of terrorism. Man-made disasters, including terrorist incidents, have profound effects on victims, first responders and rescue workers, and society, which may impair victims' ability to provide voluntary consent to research, particularly following an incident when victims and families are particularly vulnerable and stressed.[54]

LEGAL ISSUES

Unique challenges to law enforcement and prosecutions exist with regards to lone-actor terrorism, in part because the very nature of a lone actor means a smaller "footprint" to investigate. These challenges were highlighted in a recent review indicating that law enforcement tends to focus on vulnerabilities and liabilities through group interactions, which may limit a preventative approach to lone-actor terrorism; this limitation may be offset by lone actors being poorly trained and operating against lesser targets, thus reducing their threat.[55] The latter part of this statement is debatable however, given the experience of lone-actor terrorist outcomes in recent history. One important focus for law enforcement and counterterrorism is to examine the process from radicalization to violent action. Research has shown that analyzing the speech and correspondence of a lone-actor terrorist (as in the case of Nidal Hasan) can reveal intentions and motivations that could be of critical importance proactively to law enforcement.[56] One model that may have particular relevance in fighting lone-actor terrorism is intelligence-driven law enforcement, in which data and information guide subsequent police operations. The reporting of suspicious activity to law enforcement as intelligence data can have a critical impact on containing threats from self-radicalized terrorism.[57]

Lone-actor terrorism poses an array of legal issues. As outlined earlier, aggressive prosecution of cases is based on a solid foundation of data and evidence, which can be a challenge in cases in which an individual acts with little or no external footprint. An important aspect of lone actors is the relationship to past criminal behavior. Gill reported three types of criminal offenders in a lone-actor sample: individuals with an offense history that was infrequent and minor, those whose offense history was linked to their ideology and activism, and the career prolific criminal offender.[20] Based on a review of the literature, the finding of a relationship between organized terrorism and transnational organized crime, in areas such as human trafficking, firearms, drug trafficking, and money laundering, would be less applicable to lone actors.[58] By definition, collaboration with others for financial or material support to accomplish a political goal moves away from lone-actor terrorism and toward organized terrorism. A wide-ranging legal issue related to lone-actor terrorism is the balance between pursuing aggressive prosecution, avoiding infringement of individual rights and freedoms, and eventual redress to victims of terrorist acts. The Justice Against Sponsors of Terrorism Act (JASTA),[59] which allows victims to sue foreign governments linked to a terrorist attack,[60] would have little application to incidents involving a lone actor. One relevant case involved an Israeli rights group filing a lawsuit against Facebook, claiming the social networking site provided a platform for terrorists to spread incitement and violence. Although the case was dismissed by a New York court, the group plans to appeal.[61]

ASSESSMENT, INTERVENTION, AND PREVENTION

One approach to understanding lone-actor terrorism involves comparing and contrasting lone-actor terrorists as a group with other groups that may serve as "models" regarding variables such as rhetoric and recruitment, motivation, psychological and behavioral mechanisms, and potential interventions. Research by Corner and Gill showed that individuals in the lone-actor group experienced higher rates of mental illness, upcoming life changes, prejudicial victimization, and other stressors.[21] Lone-actor terrorists may be motivated as much by personal grievances as by politics and may have more in common with apolitical mass murderers than with individuals in organized terrorist groups.[21] One example of this "multifactorial" basis to lone-actor motivation is the perpetrator of the Orlando Pulse nightclub shooting in 2016, who was described as being potentially motivated by anguish over his sexual orientation in addition to Islamist ideology.[62]

Two comparison groups which may offer some insight into lone-actor terrorism behavior include individuals at risk for gang recruitment and persons who pose security risks or violate the Espionage Act (high-security risk group). In contrast with the lone-actor terrorism group, persons at risk for gang recruitment have increased delinquency compared with those who do not join a gang and later have increased rates of drug selling, drug use, violent behaviors, and property vandalism compared with non-gang individuals.[63] Delinquency falls to pre-gang levels when the individual leaves the gang. In the high-security risk group, a preliminary review by Holzer and Costanza identified several common variables with lone-actor terrorists.[64] Similar variables between these two groups included a history of psychological or psychiatric symptoms or conditions (although no major mental illness was found in the high-security risk group), a history

of adverse childhood experiences in some, and unfulfilled vocational and social goals. A striking similarity to the lone-actor terrorism group was the finding of a history of some form of conflictual or contradictory views or behaviors.

Of particular relevance is the comparison of lone-actor terrorists and individuals who commit acts of mass violence for less-clear, non-ideological reasons. Unfortunately, recent history is replete with examples of this latter group of individuals, whom the media sometimes labels "terrorists." One area of active study is in examining the relationships between these groups of individuals (i.e., To what degree do these groups overlap?). For purposes of this volume, these groups are considered separately. Examples of the "non-ideological" group include the perpetrators of the 2017 Las Vegas mass shooting, the 2012 Sandy Hook Elementary school shooting, the 2012 Aurora movie theater shooting, and the 2015 Germanwings airline disaster. Two observations in the non-ideological group are the possibility of major mental illness in at least some of the offenders and the lack of a clear motivation for or etiology to the violent act. The motivations of Stephen Paddock, the perpetrator of the 2017 Las Vegas shooting, have remained elusive, although psychological issues may have played a role; variables included the possible influence of his father, having sustained large gambling losses, his family reporting he had accomplished everything he wanted to and was bored, and emotional detachment.[65]

In addition to a clinical assessment of "at-risk" individuals, there are various instruments available to help assess risk of dangerousness, aggression, and mass violence. The Terrorist Radicalization Assessment Protocol-18 (TRAP-18) codes for eight proximal warning behaviors (such as pathway, fixation, identification, and last resort) and ten longer-term distal characteristics (such as personal grievance, ideological framing, failure of sexual pair bonding, and mental disorder).[66] The TRAP-18 provides a means by which professionals can organize data on a person of concern and plan for their risk management.[66] Studies have shown evidence of criterion validity, including usefulness of the instrument across various extremist ideologies (jihadism, ethnic nationalism, and single-issue), ability to discriminate between thwarted and successful attackers, and efficacy in law enforcement, intelligence, and clinical settings.[67] The Historical Clinical Risk Management-20, Version 3 (HCR-20 version 3) instrument[68] is a set of professional guidelines for assessment and management of violence risk. Common applications include forensic and general psychiatric hospital and community settings; the instrument is applicable to adults aged 18 and older who may pose a risk for future violence. The HCR-20 version 3 contains guidelines for the assessment of 20 key violence risk factors and their relevance to the evaluee.[68] The Violence Risk Appraisal Guide (VRAG) is a 12-item instrument that assesses the risk of violent recidivism among men apprehended for criminal violence. The VRAG reliably predicts institutional misconduct and violent recidivism.[69] Threat and risk assessments are reviewed in later chapters.

Consistent with the organization of this volume, the ability to understand and potentially intervene in lone-actor terrorism requires a multifaceted approach. As stressed earlier, lone-actor terrorism presents numerous unique challenges and many potentially interacting variables, including motivations and ideologies (such as extreme right wing, Islamist, and single-issue causes), individual backgrounds (including histories of psychological and psychiatric problems, substance abuse, family dynamics, criminal history, and other psychosocial variables), the influence of rhetoric and use of the internet and social media, access to weapons, and opportunity- or capability-related factors. This inherent complexity lends itself to a multidisciplinary, collaborative effort involving intelligence, law enforcement, homeland security and security services, and clinical professionals, each providing areas of expertise that, when combined, may provide added perspective in understanding this social problem and reducing risk to society. Gill et al. discussed various factors that may be addressed proactively, such as the potential lone actor making his grievances and extremist ideology known to others; engaging in pre-attack behaviors, such as purchasing weapons and scouting potential targets; leaking information about the potential attack to others; and exhibiting new or intensified behavioral symptoms, such as fixating on an issue or expressing a wish to hurt someone.[20] Identification of these and other variables may present opportunities for security and law enforcement professionals to intervene proactively. Additionally, in the clinical context, if an individual with mental health issues is identified as being at risk of imminent harm, an emergency psychiatric hold may allow enough time for the individual to be evaluated and potentially hospitalized. This mechanism can only be applied in situations where there is knowledge of underlying mental illness and violence risk, and precautions are needed to mitigate the potential for abuse. Having mental health professionals embedded in intelligence and law enforcement settings may, in at least some situations, increase the likelihood of proactive intervention in a potential lone-actor terrorism incident.

One interesting and relevant approach in thinking about lone-actor terrorism is the adoption of a public health model. In this paradigm, based on research at the Security Studies Program at Georgetown University's School of Foreign Service, scholars applied the three stages of disease prevention to countering violent extremism. In the public health model, primary prevention includes larger-scale programs like health education and pollution control; secondary prevention focuses on earlier interventions with a population, such as family history and diet; and tertiary prevention involves treatment of an illness. Extension of this model to countering violent extremism could include primary prevention (e.g., increasing community- and population-wide opportunities, including education, occupation, and mental health services), secondary prevention (proactive interventions aimed at the community or early in the course of a potential perpetrator's development), and tertiary interventions (e.g., arrest and prosecution of individuals plotting or after an attack).[62,70]

CONCLUSION

The concept of lone-actor terror is complex and multilayered, involving variables such as clinical mental health, harboring hatred and grievances, geography, modes of violence, the internet and social media, psychosocial factors such as isolation and criminality, and the impact of rhetoric and organizational influence on the individual. An understanding of these various factors may allow a better appreciation of the etiology of this problem and its impact on society. Research into lone-actor terrorism has identified potential areas of proactive intervention that may result in a reduced risk of future incidents.

NOTES AND REFERENCES

1. Hoffman B. *Inside Terrorism – Revised Expanded Edition*, New York: Columbia University Press; 2006.
2. Byman DL. How to hunt a lone-wolf: Countering terrorists who act on their own (op-ed). *Brookings*, 14 Feb 2017. https://www.brookings.edu/opinions/how-to-hunt-a-lone-wolf-countering-terrorists-who-act-on-their-own/

3. "Lone Wolf." *Merriam-Webster Dictionary.* https://www.merriam-webster.com/dictionary/lone%20wolf

4. Perlman M. The origins of the term "lone wolf." *Columbia Journalism Rev.* 13 Oct 2017. https://www.cjr.org/language_corner/the-origins-of-the-term-lone-wolf.php

5. Comey JB. Testimony before the House Homeland Security Committee regarding worldwide threats to the homeland, Washington, DC, 17 Sept 2014. *Worldwide Threats to the Homeland.* https://www.fbi.gov/news/testimony/worldwide-threats-to-the-homeland

6. Hosenball M. U.S. has more than 2,000 probes into potential or suspected terrorists: FBI Director. *Reuters US,* 16 May 2018. https://www.reuters.com/article/us-usa-fbi-wray/u-s-has-more-than-2000-probes-into-potential-or-suspected-terrorists-fbi-director-idUSKCN1IH341

7. SPLC. Las Vegas shooter went on antigovernment rant before massacre: "Sometimes sacrifices have to be made." *Southern Poverty Law Center,* 18 May 2018. https://www.splcenter.org/hatewatch/2018/05/18/las-vegas-shooter-went-antigovernment-rant-massacre-sometimes-sacrifices-have-be-made

8. NPR Law. Las Vegas shooting investigation closed. No motive found. *NPR,* 3 Aug 2018. https://www.npr.org/2018/08/03/635507299/las-vegas-shooting-investigation-closed-no-motive-found

9. Byman D. When to call a terrorist a terrorist. *Foreign Policy,* 27 Oct 2018. https://foreignpolicy.com/2018/10/27/when-to-call-a-terrorist-a-terrorist/

10. Gill P, Horgan J, Deckert P. Bombing alone: Tracing the motivations and antecedent behaviors of lone-actor terrorists. *J Forensic Sci.* 2014;59(2):425–435.

11. Callimachi R. Not "lone wolves" after all: How ISIS guides world's terror plots from afar. *New York Times,* 4 Feb 2017. https://www.nytimes.com/2017/02/04/world/asia/isis-messaging-app-terror-plot.html?_r=0

12. Byman D. Can lone wolves be stopped? *Brookings,* 15 Mar 2018. https://www.brookings.edu/blog/markaz/2017/03/15/can-lone-wolves-be-stopped/

13. Savage C. Holder backs a Miranda limit for terror suspects. *New York Times,* 9 May 2010. https://www.nytimes.com/2010/05/10/us/politics/10holder.html

14. Elliott M. The shoe bomber's world. *Time,* 16 Feb 2002. http://content.time.com/time/world/article/0,8599,203478,00.html

15. Flynn C. *The Lone Wolf Terrorist: Past Lessons, Future Outlook, and Response Strategies.* Arlington VA: Potomac Institute Inter-University Center for Terrorism Studies; 2017. http://www.potomacinstitute.org/images/ICTS/reportlonewolfterrorist.pdf

16. Osnos E. When gun violence meets ideology. *The New Yorker,* 3 Dec 2015. https://www.newyorker.com/news/news-desk/when-gun-violence-meets-ideology

17. Rapoport D. The four waves of modern terrorism. In Ludes JM and Cronin AK, eds., *Attacking Terrorism: Elements of a Grand Strategy.* Washington, DC: Georgetown University Press; 2004:46–73. https://international.ucla.edu/media/files/Rapoport-Four-Waves-of-Modern-Terrorism.pdf

18. Pantucci R. What have we learned about lone wolves from Anders Behring Breivik? *Perspectives on Terrorism.* 2011;5(5–6):27–42.

19. Obama says "lone wolf terrorist" biggest U.S. threat. *Reuters US,* 16 Aug 2011. https://www.reuters.com/article/us-usa-obama-security-idUSTRE77F6XI20110816

20. Gill P. *Lone-Actor Terrorists: A Behavioural Analysis.* London: Routledge; 2016.

21. Corner E, Gill P. A false dichotomy? Mental illness and lone-actor terrorism. *Law Hum Behav.* 2015;39(1):23–34.

22. Ferracuti F, Bruno F. Psychiatric aspects of terrorism in Italy. In Barak-Glantz IL, Huffs CR, eds., *The Mad, the Bad and the Different: Essays in Honor of Simon Dinitz.* Lexington, MA: Heath; 1981:199–213.

23. Hogg M, Vaughan G. *Social Psychology.* London: Pearson Prentice Hall; 2005.

24. Holzer J. Preliminary research.

25. Sullivan K, Wan W. Troubled. Quiet. Macho. Angry. The volatile life of the Orlando shooter. *Washington Post,* 17 Jun 2016. https://www.washingtonpost.com/national/troubled-quiet-macho-angry-the-volatile-life-of-omar-mateen/2016/06/17/15229250-34a6-11e6-8758-d58e76e11b12_story.html

26. Omar Mateen used steroids for years, didn't have HIV autopsy finds. *The Palm Beach Post* (FL) 15 Sept 2016. https://www.palmbeachpost.com/news/omar-mateen-used-steroids-for-years-didn-have-hiv-autopsy-finds/b2tXlB58VaVhfEILg3V0XK/

27. Lacey M. Suspect in shooting of Giffords ruled unfit for trial. *The New York Times,* 25 May 2011. https://www.nytimes.com/2011/05/26/us/26loughner.html

28. Thompson M. How marijuana use aborted Jared Loughner's military career. *Time* (Washington), 10 Jan 2011. http://content.time.com/time/nation/article/0,8599,2041634,00.html

29. Shane S. The enduring influence of Anwar al-Awlaki in the age of the Islamic State. *CTC Sentinel.* 2016(July);9(7):15–19. https://ctc.usma.edu/the-enduring-influence-of-anwar-al-awlaki-in-the-age-of-the-islamic-state/

30. Blessing J, Roberts E. *The Rhetoric of White Supremacist Terror: Assessing the Attribution of Threat.* Syracuse, NY: Institute for National Security and Counterterrorism (INSCT), Syracuse University; Jul 2018. https://securitypolicylaw.syr.edu/wp-content/uploads/2018/07/Blessing_Roberts_Berlin_Report-mwedit070618.pdf

31. Przybyla H. Giffords shooting in Arizona may cool U.S. political rhetoric, hurt Palin. *Bloomberg*, 10 Jan 2011. https://www.bloomberg.com/news/2011-01-09/lawmakers-urge-end-to-political-rhetoric-after-tucson-shootings.html

32. America's lethal politics (editorial). *New York Times*, 14 Jun 2017. https://www.nytimes.com/2017/06/14/opinion/steve-scalise-congress-shot-alexandria-virginia.html

33. Brown CB. Left, right struggle to define Loughner. *Politico.com*, 9 Jan 2011. https://www.politico.com/story/2011/01/left-right-struggle-to-define-loughner-047345

34. Frenkel S, Isaac M, Conger K. On Instagram, 11,696 examples of how hate thrives on social media. *New York Times*, 29 Oct 2018. https://www.nytimes.com/2018/10/29/technology/hate-on-social-media.html

35. Roose K. On Gab, an extremist-friendly site, Pittsburgh shooting suspect aired his hatred in full. *New York Times*, 28 Oct 2018. https://www.nytimes.com/2018/10/28/us/gab-robert-bowers-pittsburgh-synagogue-shootings.html.

36. Hummel ML. Internet terrorism. *Homeland Sec Rev.* 2008;2(2):117–130.

37. Weimann G. Lone wolves in cyberspace. *J Terrorism Res.* 2012;3(2):75–90.

38. Robertson A. "Anti-Islamic" terror suspect "plotted to bomb mosque in name of eight-year-old Manchester Arena victim Saffie-Rose Roussos with kit from dark web." *DailyMail.com*, 7 Nov 2018. https://www.dailymail.co.uk/news/article-6362075/Anti-Islamic-terror-suspect-plotted-bomb-mosque-Manchester-Arena-victim.html

39. Man admits to selling gun used in Munich mall shooting. *The Local*, 28 Aug 2017. https://www.thelocal.de/20170828/man-admits-to-selling-gun-used-in-munich-mall-shooting-spree

40. Worth K. Lone wolf attacks are becoming more common—and more deadly. *Frontline PBS*, 14 Jul 2016. https://www.pbs.org/wgbh/frontline/article/lone-wolf-attacks-are-becoming-more-common-and-more-deadly/

41. Associated Press. Accused Tucson shooter mentally fit, pleads guilty. *CBS News*, 7 Aug 2012. https://www.cbsnews.com/news/accused-tucson-shooter-mentally-fit-pleads-guilty/

42. Insanity Defense Reform Act of 1984, Pub.L.No. 98-473, Title II, Ch. IV (§401 et seq.), Oct. 12, 1984, 98 Stat. 2057 (18 U.S.C. 4241 et seq.).

43. *United States v. Freeman*, 804 F.2d 1574 (11th Cir. 1986).

44. Green F. Is Lee Boyd Malvo, young Beltway Sniper, entitled to a new sentencing? His case will be argued in federal appeals court. *Richmond Times-Dispatch*, 21 Jan 2018. https://www.richmond.com/news/local/government-politics/is-lee-boyd-malvo-young-beltway-sniper-entitled-to-a/article_0993a568-4178-5418-84ad-aa64a31d00a1.html

45. Mears B. Fort Hood shooting jury recommends death penalty for Nidal Hasan. CNN, 29 Aug 2013. https://www.cnn.com/2013/08/28/us/nidal-hasan-sentencing/index.html

46. Brown AK. Atty: Hood suspect may use insanity defense. *Army Times*, 23 Nov 2009.

47. Insanity defense. Legal Information Institute, Cornell Law School. https://www.law.cornell.edu/background/insane/insanity.html

48. The insanity defense among the states. FindLaw, Thomson Reuters, 2020. https://criminal.findlaw.com/criminal-procedure/the-insanity-defense-among-the-states.html

49. 18 U.S. Code §17. Insanity defense. Legal Information Institute, Cornell Law School. https://www.law.cornell.edu/uscode/text/18/17

50. Robinson E. Assault weapons must be banned in America. *Washington Post*, 13 Jun 2016. https://www.washingtonpost.com/opinions/assault-weapons-must-be-banned/2016/06/13/0d6a58f4-3195-11e6-8ff7-7b6c1998b7a0_story.html

51. Rosenwald M. Why banning AR-15s and other assault weapons won't stop mass shootings. *Washington Post*, 16 Jun 2016. https://www.washingtonpost.com/news/local/wp/2016/06/16/why-banning-ar-15s-and-other-assault-weapons-wont-stop-mass-shootings/

52. Sengupta K. Last message left by Westminster attacker Khalid Masood uncovered by security agencies. *The Independent*, 27 Apr 2017. https://www.independent.co.uk/news/uk/crime/last-message-left-by-westminster-attacker-khalid-masood-uncovered-by-security-agencies-a7706561.html

53. Williams L. Reporting on terrorism without spreading terror. *The Ethics Centre*, 11 Apr 2017. http://www.ethics.org.au/on-ethics/blog/april-2017/reporting-on-terrorism-without-spreading-terror

54. Fleischman AR, Wood EB. Ethical issues in research involving victims of terror. *J Urban Health.* 2002;79(3):315–321.

55. Barnes BD. Confronting the one-man wolf pack: Adapting law enforcement and prosecution responses to the threat of lone wolf terrorism. *Boston U L Rev.* 2012;92(5):1613–1662.

56. Zahedzadeh G. Overt attacks and covert thoughts. *Aggress Violent Behav.* 2017;36:1–8. https://www.neuroeconomicstudies.org/images/Articles/Overt_Attacks_and_Covert_Thoughts.pdf

57. Carter JG, Carter DL. Law enforcement intelligence: Implications for self-radicalized terrorism. *Police Pract Res*. 2012;13(2):138–154.

58. Saul B. The legal relationship between terrorism and transnational crime. *Int Crim L Rev*. 2017;17(3):417–452.

59. Pub. L. 114–222 (28 Sept 2016). https://www.congress.gov/114/plaws/publ222/PLAW-114publ222.pdf

60. Redress for victims of terrorism. *Congressional Digest*. 2016(Nov);95(9):1. http://congressionaldigest.com/issue/redress-for-victims-of-terrorism/

61. NY court drops suit against Facebook over Palestinian incitement. *Times of Israel*, 19 May 2017. https://www.timesofisrael.com/ny-court-drops-palestinian-incitment-suit-against-facebook/

62. Connor JC, Flynn CR. E-Notes: What to do about lone wolf terrorism? Examining current trends and prevention strategies. Foreign Policy Research Institute, 26 Nov 2018. https://www.fpri.org/article/2018/11/what-to-do-about-lone-wolf-terrorism-examining-current-trends-and-prevention-strategies/

63. Gordon RA, Lahey BB, Kawai E, Lober R, Stouthamer-Loeber M, Farrington DP. Antisocial behavior and youth gang membership: Selection and socialization. *Criminology*. 2004;42(1):55–87. http://jthomasniu.org/class/781/Assigs/gordon1.pdf

64. Holzer JC, Costanza W. Characteristics in Individuals Who Pose Security Risks. American Academy of Psychiatry and the Law, 47th Annual Meeting, Portland, Oregon, 27 Oct 2016.

65. Elinson Z. One year later, experts dig deeper to find Vegas shooter's motive. *Wall Street Journal*, 30 Sept 2018. https://www.wsj.com/articles/one-year-later-experts-dig-deeper-to-find-vegas-shooters-motive-1538305200

66. Meloy JR. *The TRAP-18 Manual Version 1.0*. Washington, DC: Global Institute of Forensic Research; 2017. https://www.gifrinc.com/trap-18-manual/

67. Meloy JR. The operational development and empirical testing of the Terrorist Radicalization Assessment Protocol (TRAP–18). *J Pers Assess*. 2018;100(5):483–492.

68. Douglas KS, Hart SD, Webster CD, Belfrage H. *HCR-20V3: Assessing Risk of Violence–User Guide*. Burnaby, CAN: Mental Health, Law, and Policy Institute, Simon Fraser University; 2013.

69. Hastings ME, Krishnan S, Tangney JP, Stuewig J. Predictive and incremental validity of the Violence Risk Appraisal Guide scores with male and female jail inmates. *Psychol Assess*. 2011;23(1):174–183.

70. Challgren J, Kenyon T, Kervick L, et al. *Countering Violent Extremism: Applying the Public Health Model*. National Security Critical Issues Task Force (NSCITF), Oct 2016. Washington DC: Georgetown Security Studies Review; 2016.

1

Historical Aspects and Evolution of Lone-Actor Violence

MARK HAMM AND TAMMY AYRES

INTRODUCTION

Scholars generally agree that lone-actor terrorism has, in the words of one authority, "a long and bloody past."[1] There is less consensus about the origins of this curious form of political violence. Where and when did lone-actor terrorism begin? Who was the first lone-actor terrorist? And what does the history of lone-actor terrorism teach us about the current threat? Answers to these questions depend on definitions of lone-actor terrorism used by researchers, their choice of research methods, the nation-states included in a study, and the scope of history considered. Accordingly, scholars have explained the emergence of lone-actor terrorism in various ways.

THE ANARCHIST LONERS

Edwin Bakker and Beatrice de Graaf locate the historical roots of lone-actor terrorism in the nineteenth-century writings of Russian anarchist Makhail Bakunin and his explication of "the propaganda of the deed." In his 1870 essay "Letters to a Frenchman on the Present Crisis" (calling for a general uprising in response to the collapse of the French government during the Franco-Prussian War of 1870), Bakunin announced to the Paris Commune that "we must spread our principles, not with words but with deeds, for this is the most popular, the most potent, and the most irresistible form of propaganda."[2] For Bakunin, the propaganda of the deed was political action meant to be exemplary to others and serve as a catalyst for revolution. Like his contemporary and erstwhile friend Karl Marx, Bakunin envisioned an alliance between the working class and the peasantry with all power given to the grassroots organizations spontaneously created by revolution. France could only be saved, Bakunin argued, by urban workers with "blood in their veins, brains in their heads, energy in their hearts, and if they are not doctrinaires but revolutionaries with doctrines."[2] Over the next 60 years (1878–1934), anarchists across Europe and the United States acted on Bakunin's political theory to shoot and bomb leading statesmen, the bourgeois, and their economic interests. From this revolutionary movement came what Bakker and de Graaf consider to be the original lone-actor terrorist.

Gaetano Bresci (1869–1901) emigrated from Italy to the United States in his late twenties and found work as a silk weaver in Paterson, New Jersey, which had a vibrant Italian American community.[3] Bresci became involved in community politics, which led to his appointment as the founding editor of *La Questione Sociale* (*The Social Question*), an Italian-language anarchist newspaper. Through his contacts with the broadside, Bresci was introduced to the theory of the propaganda of the deed. In 1897, he grew concerned with reports from Italy about trouble with that year's wheat harvest which had increased bread prices across the country. Street demonstrations demanding "bread and work" erupted in the south of Italy. On May 5, 1898, workers in Milan went on strike against the bread prices, leading to the police killing of two protestors. A decorated Italian military leader, General Fiorenzo Bava-Beccaris, was brought in to maintain order with a contingent of 45,000 soldiers at his ready.

On May 7, 60,000 people from the working-class neighborhoods of Milan joined the strike. To quell the uprising, Bava-Beccaris deployed his forces at the city's central square, but they were met with fierce resistance from protestors who fought back with stones and tiles from rooftops. The bread riot continued for two more days. Then, on May 9, the troops used cannon artillery against the protestors, causing a bloodbath. More than 100 demonstrators were killed and over 2,000 were wounded. Once order was restored, King Umberto I of Italy awarded Bava-Beccaris the medal of the Great Cross of Savoy in recognition of his "great service" to Italian institutions "and to civilization." Consequently, King Umberto became a deeply loathed figure in leftist circles.

When news of Bava-Beccaris's award reached Gaetano Bresci in New Jersey, he requested the return of a loan he had made to *La Questione Sociale*, and, with the money, he booked passage back to Italy.

On the evening of July 29, 1900, King Umberto traveled to Monza, near Milan, where he received an honor at the closing of a gymnastics competition. When in public, Umberto's security force demanded that he wear a chainmail armor vest under his shirt, but he refused to do so on this night because of the summer heat. Umberto left the ceremony around 10:30 PM. When he reached his royal carriage and seated himself inside, Bresci emerged from the crowd and shot Umberto four times with a .32-caliber revolver, killing him.

Bresci was tried and convicted of murder, claiming that he had come directly from the United States to avenge the victims of repression during the bread strike and the insult of the award given to Bava-Beccaris. On August 29, 1900, Bresci was sentenced to penal servitude for life. Less than a year later, on May 22, 1901, he was found dead in his prison cell at the age of 31. He was reported to have hanged himself. Yet that did not mark the end of Bresci's influence among anarchists. To the contrary: he became a martyr for the anarchist movement and a catalyst for future acts of terrorism, thereby fulfilling the promise of Bakunin's propaganda of the deed.

American Terrorism

News of Bresci's regicide in Italy soon reached a 28-year-old unemployed Polish American factory worker in Cleveland, Ohio, named Leon Czolgosz (pronounced *Sholl-gosh*).[4] Czolgosz had spent his adult life supporting violent union strikes against Ohio factories that had been crippled by the US economic crash of 1893. Through these experiences, Czolgosz came to believe that there were great injustices in American society which allowed the wealthy to benefit themselves by exploiting the poor. Czolgosz lived with his parents and was constantly at odds with them over their Roman Catholic beliefs. He showed little interest in friendship or romantic relationships

and, by 1901, had become a recluse who spent most of his time in bed reading books on socialism. Czolgosz was introduced to anarchism that same year when he attended a Cleveland speech by the political firebrand Emma Goldman. At the time, Goldman was on record praising the assassination of King Umberto in Italy, declaring in a recent New York speech that the Monarch "was justly put to death by a brave man, who dared to act for the good of his fellow man."[5] It was at this juncture that Czolgosz began reading news reports about Gaetano Bresci's assassination of King Umberto. In justifying his propaganda of the deed, Bresci had told the press that he decided to "take matters into his own hands" for the sake of the common man. Czolgosz would follow suit. He would take matters of injustice into his own hands by assassinating US President William McKinley.

He began by tracking McKinley's scheduled public appearances in the daily newspapers. On August 31, 1901, Czolgosz traveled to Buffalo, New York, the site of the Pan-American Exposition, where President McKinley was scheduled to make such an appearance, and checked into a boarding house where he planned his attack. In his first order of business, Czolgosz went to a local hardware store and paid $4.50 for a silver-plated Iver Johnson .32-caliber revolver—the same model Bresci used against Umberto.[5]

On the afternoon of September 6, Czolgosz went to the exposition armed with his revolver. In his pocket was a neatly folded news clipping about Bresci's assassination of Umberto and six Smith & Wesson bullets. Czolgosz approached McKinley, who was standing in a receiving line greeting the public outside the Temple of Music. Shortly after 4 PM, Czolgosz reached the front of the line holding his gun inside a white handkerchief. McKinley extended his hand, but Czolgosz slapped it aside and shot the President once in the chest and once in the abdomen at point blank range. McKinley died eight days later of an infection that had spread from the bullet wound. Vice President Theodore Roosevelt was sworn in, becoming the youngest president in American history at age 42 and ushering in the Progressive Era. Czolgosz readily admitted to the assassination by later telling police: "I am an anarchist. I killed President McKinley because I done my duty."[5] Forty-five days after the shooting, following his murder conviction in a 1-day trial, Czolgosz was executed in the electric chair at Auburn Prison in upstate New York. However, anarchists were not done with martyring the lone terrorist Gaetano Bresci.

The Anarchist Bombings

Several years after the McKinley assassination, followers of the Italian-born anarchist Luigi Galleani formed the Bresci Circle in New York City in honor of Gaetano Bresci. Luigi Galleani (1861–1931) would do much to mythologize the lone-actor terrorist and, ultimately, transform the landscape of terrorism in America and beyond. Then known as the foremost proponent of the propaganda of the deed in the United States, Galleani was a vehemently radical anarchist who advocated violence to effect change by ridding the world of laws and capitalism. He was imprisoned several times in Europe for leading strikes and demonstrations for workers' rights. Continually investigated by authorities for his political agitation, Galleani fled from Italy to Switzerland to France to Egypt and London before arriving in Paterson, New Jersey, in late 1901, where he became the editor of *La Questione Sociale*, the position once held by Gaetano Bresci. A lawyer by training, Galleani was a skilled polemical writer, a charismatic orator, and a natural-born leader. A follower said of him, "You heard Galleani speak, and you were ready to shoot the first policeman you saw."[6] In the summer of 1902, Galleani led a strike of Paterson silk workers and was shot in the face by police in the process. After fleeing to Canada and recovering from his wound, Galleani returned to the States in 1903, where he established an Italian-language anarchist newspaper, *Cronaca Sovversiva* (*The Subversive Chronicle*), wherein he ran articles celebrating the lives of bombers and assassins as heroes of anarchism, including Gaetano Bresci and Leon Czolgosz.[7] In 1905, Galleani published what may be considered the first underground bomb-making manual called *La Salute é in Voi*! (*Health Is in You!*).[8]

By 1914, the Bresci Circle counted some 600 members who met at homes and grocery stores in New York's East Harlem, in Paterson silk factories, and in the steel mills of Youngstown, Ohio. Among them were the Italian American anarchists Nicola Sacco and Bartolomeo Vanzetti, who would be famously arrested under questionable circumstances in 1920 for the robbery and murder of two shoe store employees in South Braintree, Massachusetts. The Bresci Circle took a step toward the propaganda of the deed in 1915, when two of its members made an unsuccessful attempt to bomb St. Patrick's Cathedral in New York. The group then underwent a notable advancement in their terrorist skills.

In early 1917, to avoid conscription into World War I, Galleani and his core followers (known as Galleanists) moved to Monterrey, Mexico, where they lived communally. Sacco and Venzetti joined Galleani in Mexico along with a financially strapped 33-year-old ex-convict from Boston named Mario Buda. Born in the Romagna region of Northern Italy in 1884, Buda was introduced to anarchism during his teenage years. At age 15, he was jailed for robbery; finding limited employment opportunities upon release, Buda emigrated to the United States in 1907. He could only find menial labor, however, and in 1911 returned to Italy. Two years later, he returned to the United States and found work in a Boston shoe store. Buda met Sacco during a workers' strike in 1913, and, 3 years later, he met Vanzetti who was a follower of Luigi Galleani. In 1916, Buda spent 6 months in a Massachusetts prison for demonstrating against America's intervention in World War I and was paroled shortly before meeting up with the Galleanists in Mexico. Somewhere along the way—most likely through his reading of Galleani's bomb-making manual and discussions with Galleani in Mexico—Buda became experienced in the use of dynamite. Buda is commonly known to historians of the American anarchist movement as its "bombmaker extraordinaire."[9]

Buda returned to the United States in the autumn of 1917, where he is suspected of constructing a bomb made of screws, bolts, jagged shards of metal, and dynamite. On November 24, a 9-year-old girl discovered the bomb alongside the Evangelical Mission Church in Milwaukee. The bomb was intended to be used in retaliation for the recent killing of two local Italian anarchists during a hostile exchange between antiwar Italians and the church's patriotic pastor. The explosive device was taken by two teenage boys to the central police station where it detonated, causing the deaths of nine policemen and a civilian.[6] It would be the largest single loss of police life in America until the terrorist attacks of 9/11. Neither Buda nor anyone else was ever charged with the crime.

In late April 1919, 36 booby trap dynamite-filled bombs were mailed to prominent politicians and appointees across the country, including US Attorney General A. Mitchell Palmer and a Bureau of Investigation field agent once tasked with investigating Galleani and subscribers to his *Cronaca Sovversiva*. While the bombs failed to strike their intended victims, they did blow off the hands of a housekeeper and severely burned a Senator's wife. During the evening of June 2, 1919, within a 90-minute timeframe, mail bombs of extraordinary capacity rocked the homes of judges, businessmen, a mayor, an immigration inspector, and a church in eight major US cities. Each bomb was made of 25 pounds of dynamite wrapped with heavy metal slugs to act as shrapnel. Those targeted included government officials and judges who had sentenced anarchists to prison.[7] Yet again, none of the targeted people was killed, but one bomb took the life of a New York City night watchman.

Unable to secure enough evidence for criminal trials, authorities deported Galleani and eight of his adherents from the United States to Italy in 1919 under the Immigration Act of 1918, which allowed the government to expel foreigners who were involved in subversive activities. Even so, Galleanists have long been suspected of perpetrating the September 16, 1920 Wall Street bombing in New York, killing 38 and wounding more than 200 in the greatest act of American terrorism until the Oklahoma City bombing of 1995. Victims near the JP Morgan building were lifted off the ground, set on fire, and cut to pieces by metal shrapnel. The explosion overturned automobiles and shook skyscrapers three blocks away.[10] Although the crime has never been solved, numerous historians, including the lone-wolf terrorism scholar Jeffrey Simon, convincingly argue that Mario Buda independently committed the bombing as revenge for the recent indictments of his friends Sacco and Vanzetti, both of whom would die in Massachusetts's electric chair at the Charlestown State Prison in 1927.[11]

Summary

Three aspects of these early cases would help to define lone-actor terrorism in the decades ahead. First, even though lone actors are (by most definitions) unaffiliated with a terrorist organization at the time of their attack(s), they may identify or sympathize with extremist groups. These organizations provide ideologies of validation for lone actors and function as communities of radical belief by transferring personal frustrations onto the transgressive "other." As such, the extremist organizations play a vital role in the psychological mechanism of externalization as well as in the formation of ideological belonging. These characteristics of the lone-actor terrorist seem to have special relevance for understanding assassins. In his magisterial survey of nineteenth- and early twentieth-century assassins in Europe and North America, Walter Laqueur concluded that "Inasmuch as the assassins were anarchists—and quite a few were not—they all acted on their own initiative without the knowledge and support of the groups to which they belonged."[12]

Second, lone-actor terrorism often involves a "copycat effect" in terms of tactics, motives, and weaponry. Rather than merely seeking fame for themselves—as is typically the case with non-ideologically motivated mass murderers, for example—lone actors imitate other lone actors to make a political point. Leon Czolgosz may have been content with carrying on his union strikes against Ohio factories were it not for the newspaper articles about Gaetano Bresci's assassination of King Umberto, including the detail that Bresci had used a .32-caliber Iver Johnson revolver in the attack. For Czolgosz, Bresci demonstrated that one person's violence could bring public attention to a political cause. The copycat effect also explains why lone acts of terrorism are so impervious to detection and prevention. Terrorist organizations recruit, radicalize, and direct the actions of their members, making these operations susceptible to law enforcement infiltration and disruption. Lone actors imitate and innovate and answer to no one. Such was the case of Mario Buda. In the lone-terrorist tradition of Bresci and Czolgosz, Buda carried out the first recorded vehicle bombing in history by loading a massive explosive made of 100 pounds of dynamite and 500 pounds of scrap metal into a horse-drawn wagon and parking it on Wall Street.[13] "He then fled the scene, never to be heard from again," as Simon notes.[11]

Finally, and in some ways most importantly, lone-actor terrorism is best understood in a global context. Even by the relatively arcane standards of mass media as it existed between 1898 and 1920, information about anarchist grievances over capital, labor, and perceived injustices efficiently flowed across international borders, ultimately creating common cause among lone terrorists from different cultures with different languages and sociopolitical dynamics. These extremist impulses would crystalize into a pan-ideological form of solo-activated terrorism with the dawning of the Internet Age.

THE IDIOSYNCRATIC LONERS

In the first international study of lone-actor terrorism, Ramón Spaaij identified 88 lone terrorists in the United States, Europe, Canada, and Australia between 1940 and 2010. These terrorists perpetrated a total of 198 attacks, claiming 123 lives and injuring hundreds more in bombings and shootings. Spaaij found that lone-actor terrorism is more prevalent in the United States than in other Western nations; an estimated 40% of the lone attacks occurred in the United States.[14] In a subsequent analysis, Mark Hamm and Ramón Spaaij identified 123 American lone actors responsible for 320 terrorist attacks between 1940 and 2016, killing 256 and injuring nearly 500 with firearms, bombs, vehicles, small aircraft, and biological weapons. Hamm and Spaaij argued that the high rate of lone-actor terrorism in the United States may be attributed to a host of historical factors, including (white) America's tradition of individualism, its gun culture, its foreign policies, the echoes of slavery, the appeal of conspiracy theories, celebrity worship, or what historian Richard Hofstadter called the "paranoid style" in American politics.[15] "The distinguishing thing about the paranoid style," Hofstadter wrote about the American radical right in 1964, "is that the paranoid spokesman sees the fate of conspiracy in apocalyptic terms—he traffics in the birth and death of whole worlds, whole political orders, and whole systems of human values. He is always manning the barricades of civilization. He constantly lives at a turning point."[16] Such social psychological processes created what Hamm and Spaaij believe to be the original lone-actor terrorist.

Over a 16-year period (1940–1956), George Metesky, an unemployed mechanic from Connecticut, planted 33 meticulously assembled pipe bombs, of which 22 exploded, in highly populated areas of New York City, including the Consolidated Edison Building, Grand Central Station, Radio City Music Hall, the New York Public Library, Macy's Department Store, the Empire State Building, and numerous movie theaters. Bombs were also left in subways, phone booths, storage lockers, and public restrooms. Yet Metesky's signature was to insert his bombs into the sliced-open upholstery of movie theater seats. Called the "Mad Bomber" by the New York press, Metesky injured 15 people in the attacks. A contemporaneous news report of one attack claimed that

> A bomb exploded during a showing of *War and Peace* at the Paramount movie palace on Flatbush Avenue, in Brooklyn. At 7:50 PM, a thundering detonation flashed from the orchestra row GG, followed by billows of ashen smoke. Then screams filled the theater—as moviegoers glimpsed faces and scalps scythed open by shrapnel.[17]

Like other lone terrorists who would come later, Metesky's bombings were motivated by a personal frustration combined with a wider but amorphous political agenda. As Jessica Stern helpfully notes, "Lone wolves often come up with their own ideologies that combine personal vendettas with religious or political grievances."[18] Metesky's personal vendetta was against his former employer, the Consolidated Edison company, and was the result of an unsettled workman's compensation claim that left Metesky suffering from tuberculosis. Over time, Metesky's rage against Con Ed became more political as he generalized his grievance to police, politicians, and other organizations that symbolized authority, believing that they had somehow conspired with Con Ed to deprive him of justice. Metesky was 37 years old at the time of his first bombing and 53 at the time of his last. He was single and lived with two older unmarried sisters in Waterbury, a 60-mile drive from New York.[19]

The significance of the Mad Bomber case would turn on Metesky's deliberate broadcasting of his intent to commit terrorism (also known as "signaling"), something that members of a terrorist group would never do. But, for lone terrorists like Metesky who have a grandiose image of themselves, broadcasting intent is crucial to their radicalization because it is based on the terrorists' need to become renowned for their causes. Metesky was, in fact, a prolific broadcaster of terrorist intent. Over the years, he sent more than 100 threatening letters and postcards to reporters, police precincts, private citizens, and Con Ed officials. Metesky even wrote to President Franklin D. Roosevelt after the bombing of Pearl Harbor on December 7, 1941. Ten years later, Metesky began writing letters to newspapers warning of his next bombing. Metesky's letters typically referenced "Con Ed and the others" or "all the liars and cheaters" who had failed to deliver justice in his workman's compensation claim. "I HAVE EXHAUSTED ALL OTHER MEANS," Metesky proclaimed in his customary block-letter style to the *New York Herald Tribune* on October 22, 1951, "I INTEND WITH BOMBS TO CAUSE OTHERS TO CRY OUT FOR *JUSTICE* FOR ME."[19]

By the mid-1950s, hundreds of law enforcement officers and forensic specialists had joined the Mad Bomber investigation, including FBI agents from Washington dispatched by Director J. Edgar Hoover. Their operating assumption was that the bomber was a former Con Ed employee with a grudge against the company. The personnel files of disgruntled or terminated employees were checked and double-checked by investigators, but to no avail. In late 1956, police launched a new investigative strategy whereby portions of the bomber's letters were reprinted in the daily newspapers, and citizens were asked if they could recognize their peculiarities of language. Dr. James Brussel, a criminologist and psychiatrist for the New York State Commission for Mental Hygiene, was assigned to the case and developed a forensics portrait of the bomber, representing the first case of profiling in law enforcement history. Among his conclusions, Brussel theorized that the bomber was a "loner" with no friends, little interest in women, and probably living with an older female relative.

The *New York Times* published Brussel's profile on Christmas Day 1956. The following day, the profile was published in the *New York Journal American*, along with an open letter to the bomber urging him to surrender to police. The bomber immediately replied to the editors, declaring that he would not surrender until he could "BRING THE CON EDISON TO JUSTICE." Later in the letter, the bomber complained about a medical disability, adding that "I CAN STRIKE BACK—EVEN FROM MY GRAVE—FOR THE DASTARDLY ACTS AGAINST ME."[19] This broadcasting of intent led directly to Metesky's capture.

A Con Ed clerk named Alice Kelly had read Brussel's profile and the bomber's reply to the newspaper editors, and she began scouring the company's worker compensation files for employees with a serious health problem, something that police investigators had failed to do. On January 18, 1957, while searching the final batch of claims, Kelly came across a file marked in red with the words "injustice" and "permanent disability"— words that had appeared in Brussel's profile. The marked file was for one George Metesky, an employee from 1929 to 1931, who had been injured in a plant accident on September 5, 1931. Several letters in the file used phrases which also appeared in the bomber's recent letter to the editor, including the term "dastardly acts."[19] Police were notified that afternoon, leading to Metesky's arrest on January 21, 1957.

The main lesson of the Mad Bomber case is that an ordinary citizen—in this instance, the lowly government bureaucrat Alice Kelly—may be well placed to pick up on the broadcasting of violent intent by a potential terrorist and can therefore do something about it. The lesson would resonate down through the years, extending to what is widely considered the archetypical case of lone-actor terrorism.

The Unabomber

Theodore Kaczynski had much in common with George Metesky. Like James Brussel's profile of the Mad Bomber, the FBI profiler James Fitzgerald would theorize that the Unabomber was an unmarried "loner" with no interests in friendship, pop culture, or business. Kaczynski and Meteskey were both meticulous bomb-builders who were patient in carrying out their campaigns of violence. Strategically, they played the long game. Meteskey began his bombing spree in 1940, but, a year later, after America's entry into World War II, he suspended his campaign as a patriotic duty, only to return in March 1950 when he placed an inert bomb in Grand Central Station. Kaczynski ignited more than a dozen bombs at universities and businesses from 1978 to 1987, and then took a 6-year hiatus after being spotted at a bombing scene in Salt Lake City, only to return in June 1993, when he severely wounded a California geneticist with a mail bomb inside his home. Both saw their bombing campaigns end when they were 53 years old. Both manipulated the press and freely provided insights into their motives through extensive writing. There may have been a copycat angle at work: Metesky signed each of his letters with the cypher "*F.P.*" for Fair Play; Kaczynski signed his letters and bombs "*F.C.*" for Freedom Club. Both were unquestionably smart; Kaczynski was a Harvard graduate and a former mathematics professor at the University of California, Berkeley, with an IQ of 167. Indeed, both flummoxed law enforcement officials like they had never been flummoxed before. The Mad Bomber case represented what the New York Police commissioner called "the greatest manhunt in the history of the Police Department." The Unabomber case represented the greatest manhunt in FBI history. And both terrorists suffered from paranoid schizophrenia that went undiagnosed until they were imprisoned for life.[19,20] Accordingly, these cases captured the attention of crime scientists who brought a combined interest in criminology and medicine to bear on the professional study of lone-actor violence.

The year 1995 was a turning point for Theodore Kaczynski. At age 53, he was portrayed in the media as the deadliest serial bomber in world history. For the past 17 years, Kaczynski had mailed or hand-delivered a series of increasingly sophisticated bombs that murdered 2 and injured 23 others in Illinois, Utah, Tennessee, Michigan, Washington State, California, Connecticut, and New Jersey. Targeting university professors and graduate students, technology specialists, and business executives, Kaczynski's bombs propelled shards of nail and wood shrapnel into their bodies, blowing off fingers and arms—blinding, maiming, and killing innocents without mercy. The FBI proved powerless to do anything about it, even though a multiagency Unabomber task force had grown to more than 150 full-time personnel with a dedicated 1-800 tip line offering a $1 million reward for information leading to the Unabomber's arrest. On April 24, 1995, five days after the Oklahoma City bombing, Kaczynski killed his third victim, Gilbert Murray, the president of a timber industry lobbying group, with a mail bomb sent to his Sacramento office. Like the previous attacks, the Murray investigation produced no clues about the Unabomber's identity or motive. This was the FBI's chief conundrum: *Who* was the Unabomber and *why* was he terrorizing Americans? Kaczynski himself would answer those questions through his broadcasting of terrorist intent.

On June 28, 1995, the *San Francisco Chronicle* received a letter from the Unabomber threatening "to blow up an airliner out of Los Angeles International Airport sometime during the next six days."[21] The threat seriously disrupted airline services at LAX and indicated to the FBI that the Unabomber was moving from attacks against lone individuals to a mass casualty event. Yet, later that day, the *New York Times* received a letter from the Unabomber saying that the threat at LAX was a hoax. The hoax was a prelude to a more significant ploy.

On August 2, 1995, Kaczynski mailed letters to the *New York Times* and the *Washington Post* demanding that a 35,000-word essay he had been working on since 1971, entitled *Industrial Society and Its Future* (dubbed the *Unabomber Manifesto* by the FBI), be published verbatim. If this demand was met, said the Unabomber, he would "desist from terrorism."[22] Written on a manual typewriter by Kaczynski at his mountain cabin deep in the Montana wilderness, the *Unabomber Manifesto* advocated revolution against technology as a means of restoring human freedoms that had been "gravely disrupted" by the industrial society. "The world today seems to be going crazy," exclaimed the Unabomber. "This sort of thing is not normal for human societies. There is good reason to believe that primitive man suffered from less stress and frustration and was better satisfied with his way of life than modern man is."[23]

At the recommendation of US Attorney General Janet Reno and FBI Director Louis Freeh, the *Washington Post* and the *New York Times* published the *Unabomber Manifesto* on September 19, 1995, thereby bringing worldwide attention to the Unabomber's provocative complaint about modernism. Among those who read the essay was David Kaczynski, Theodore's brother. Based on the peculiarities of language and the philosophies espoused in the *Manifesto*, David suspected that his brother was the Unabomber. David notified authorities and provided the FBI with details about Kaczynski's whereabouts, which ultimately led to his historic arrest in Montana on April 3, 1996. David Kaczynski was to the Unabomber investigation what Alice Kelly was to the investigation of the Mad Bomber—both challenged a social dynamic known as the "bystander effect," which attempts to explain why people do not intervene when they know violence is about to occur. Moreover, David Kaczynski and Alice Kelly refused to be apathetic bystanders. In today's counterterrorism vernacular, they saw something and said something.

There is a final commonality between these cases which is crucial to understanding the all-important issue of motive in lone-actor terrorism. Kaczynski's political views reflected elements of ecological anarchism and Luddism, which were intricately linked to both his personal resentment over perceived social rejection by organized society and frustration over his inability to establish a relationship with a woman.[14] Metesky's politics hinged on a conspiratorial belief about state authority, which were convolutely tied up in his personal anger against a former employer. As such, the worldviews of Kaczynski and Meteskey do not fit neatly into any of the commonly accepted categories of terrorist ideology such as right-wing racism, Islamic extremism, Black militancy, or anti-abortion absolutism. Instead, terrorists in the tradition of the Unabomber and the Mad Bomber are more accurately conceived as *idiosyncratic loners*.

THE RADICAL RIGHT-WING LONERS

Other scholars advance different views about the origins of lone-actor terrorism. Jeffrey Kaplan contends that this form of terrorism is as old as time itself and "has appeared in every era and in virtually every culture in the world."[24] Kaplan traces the roots of lone-actor terrorism back to the story of Phineas in the Old Testament. In chapter 25 of the Book of Numbers, an Israelite man has an unlawful union with a woman from another tribe and brings down the wrath of God on the Israelites. Phineas slays the couple with a javelin and appeases God, thereby establishing an historical precedent for religious violence. Among fringe elements of the modern racist right in the United States and Israel, Phineas is therefore interpreted as a biblical injunction against race mixing, same-sex marriage, and abortion. This "rabid xenophobia" as Kaplan terms it, led to the founding of the Phineas Priesthood, which counts among its believers such lone-actor terrorists as Larry McQuilliams, who in 2014 fired more than 400 rounds from a long rifle at the federal courthouse in Austin, Texas, before being shot and killed by police.

The eminent terrorism scholar Bruce Hoffman takes a similar position. Recognizing that lone acts of terrorism have been encouraged by the leadership of al-Qaeda and the Islamic State in Iraq and al-Sham (ISIS), Hoffman nevertheless concludes that "the lone wolf strategy has its origins not in the Middle East or with a foreign Muslim terrorist organization but in America and our own variant of far-right violence. It dates, moreover, to the late 1980s."[25] Therefore, lone-actor terrorism begins not with an anarchist, an idiosyncratic loner, or a biblical figure but with the virulent white supremacist Leroy Moody (the only known US lone-actor terrorist of the late 1980s), who committed murder and attempted murder against judges and court personnel in a ruthless bombing campaign across the American South in 1989.[15]

Still other astute observers—including Christopher Hewitt, Paul Gill, and Mathew Feldman—have explained the comparatively high incidence of lone-actor terrorism in the United States in terms of the strategy of leaderless resistance adopted by American right-wing extremists and anti-abortion activists in response to a federal law enforcement crackdown on domestic terrorists during the early 1980s.[1,26,27] *Leaderless resistance* is based on the idea that a terrorist group, no matter how secret or well organized, simply cannot evade law enforcement; hence, terrorism is more readily accomplished by individual actors rather than a group. A decade after the radical right's move to leaderless resistance, FBI agents in San Diego, California, opened an investigation into the criminal activities of a self-proclaimed white supremacist named Alex Curtis. The investigation was dubbed "Operation Lone Wolf" due to Curtis's encouragement of other white supremacists to follow what Curtis referred to as "lone-wolf" activism. As a result of this investigation, the FBI coined the term "lone-wolf terrorism" to describe violence committed by individuals from the far right.

Since the 1990s, loners of the radical right have made significant advances in the lethality of terrorism, much as the anarchists and the Unabomber did in an earlier age, leading to a spectacular rise in political violence across the United States, Europe, and Australia. Fueled by the dark forces of racism, nationalism, and anti-Semitism, this strain of lone-actor terrorism will likely remain an international security threat for decades to come.

THE EVOLUTION OF LONE-ACTOR TERRORISM

More important than answering the question of who the first lone-actor terrorist was is explaining how lone-actor terrorism evolves over time. In this regard, Michel Wieviorka suggests that terrorism cases can be distinguished by their unity with an historical synthesis.[28] For example, research shows that, prior to 9/11, not a single member of the US military was attacked by a lone terrorist. Even during the most turbulent years of protest against the Vietnam War, lone terrorists did not attack military personnel. After 9/11, however, lone-actor terrorists would kill or injure 50 members of the US military. Lone actors would also attack military bases or would be arrested in thwarted attacks against military installations. In every instance, these criminal events were carried out by al-Qaeda or ISIS sympathizers angered over American foreign policy in Muslim lands.[15]

The first such case was Carlos Bledsoe's drive-by shooting at an Army recruiting center in Little Rock, Arkansas, on June 1, 2009, which killed one soldier and injured another. Subsequent attacks included Nidal Hasan's mass shooting at Fort Hood, Texas, on November 5, 2009, which killed 13 soldiers and wounded 30 others in what was then the deadliest terrorist attack against the United States since 9/11 (the shooting was a copycat of the Arkansas attack by Bledsoe 3 months earlier); Naser Jason Abdo's attempted bombing at Fort Hood in 2011 (a copycat of Hasan's attack on Fort Hood); Yonathan Melaku's 2010 shooting spree at military facilities in Washington, DC (also a copycat of Hasan's attack); Khalid Aldawsari's 2010 attempted bombing of the homes of three former US soldiers who were stationed at Iraq's Abu Ghraib prison and the Dallas home of former President George W. Bush; and Mohammad Abdulazeez's 2015 firearm attack on military recruiting centers in Chattanooga, Tennessee, which killed and wounded six unarmed soldiers. In each case, lone jihadists waged terrorist attacks with identical targets, ideological motives, and religious inspiration.[15] Seen through the lens of historical synthesis, then, cases of lone-actor terrorism signify not a mysterious jangle of random occurrences but intelligible actions that form a compelling sociological narrative.

Criminologists have long looked beyond the orbit of criminology for insight into why people turn to crime. As regards lone-actor terrorism, a useful concept is found in the field of botany.[29] A *rhizome* is defined as a continuously horizontal underground plant stem which puts out lateral shoots and adventurous roots deeper into the ground at intervals. A rhizomatic analysis would think about lone-actor terrorism as a deep subterranean social process where law is merely a hypothesis. Strange things grow in dark places. Nourished by a potent emotional mix of terrorist martyring, copycatting, and ideological belonging, the lone-actor phenomenon continuously grows tendrils that spiral and twine their way to ever more dangerous hybrids of violence across time and space, cultures, and technologies.

It was in this dystopian way that, in 2011, the Norwegian terrorist Anders Breivik used the internet to copy and paste entire sections of the 1995 *Unabomber Manifesto* for inclusion in his 1,500-page manifesto entitled *2083: A European Declaration of Independence*, which called for the eradication of all traces of Islamic culture from Europe. Breivik dealt in depth with such foreboding issues as bomb-building, the glories of firing a Ruger semi-automatic rifle, and the infiltration of "the youth camp connected to the largest political party in Norway."[30] E-mailed to some 8,000 European right-wing extremists 90 minutes before he would kill 8 Norwegian politicians and 69 teenage campers, Breivik's manifesto signaled his intent to commit what became the largest massacre in Europe since World War II. Breivik called on others to follow his example.

On March 15, 2019, a heavily armed white supremacist attacked two mosques in Christchurch, New Zealand, indiscriminately killing 51 Muslims at Friday prayers and wounding 50 others. It was terrorism meant for the Internet Age. The Christchurch gunman live-streamed his rampage on Facebook after posting a 74-page manifesto on Twitter saying that he "took true inspiration" from Anders Breivik.

CONCLUSION

Historically, lone-actor terrorism can be traced back to left-wing (anarchist) ideologies, although this is not widely acknowledged or recognized. Instead lone-actor terrorism is more commonly associated with far-right extremism. What is clear, however, is the apparent historical synthesis between incidents of lone-actor terrorism.

A historical through-line can be drawn across paradigmatic cases to show a systematic process of revision, correction, copycatting, adaption, and improvement of lone-actor incidents. Each incident morphs into an increasingly more dangerous hybrid of violence across time, space, culture, and technology to provide *unity with a historical synthesis*. Despite being described as "The New Terrorism of Right-Wing Single Actors,"[31] there is very little that is new about lone-actor terrorism, as highlighted in this chapter. As identified in the preceding discussion, similarities define early lone-actor terrorists; their identification with an extreme group provides ideological validation, there is a copycat effect (e.g., motives, modus operandi, weapons), and the global context sees grievances and perceived injustices disseminated across international borders. However, there is also one commonality omitted from this list that characterizes lone-actor terrorism throughout history and that is *propaganda of the deed*, which is not only true of the lone actors discussed in this chapter, but also those covered in the ensuing chapters of this volume.

Instead of being a new phenomenon, lone-actor terrorism must be seen as a constantly mutating underground rhizome, as a deep subterranean social process that implements propaganda of the deed (or propaganda by deed, *propagande par le fait*), which is fertilized by a potent mix of factors that converge and feed the rhizome, thus creating more dangerous breeds of lone-actor terrorists that we are yet to witness.

NOTES AND REFERENCES
1. Feldman M. Comparative lone wolf terrorism: Toward a heuristic definition. *Democracy and Security.* 2013;9:270–286.
2. Bakunin M. Letters to a Frenchman on the present crisis. In Dolgoff S, ed., *Bakunin on Anarchy.* Quebec: Black Rose Books; 1971:183–217. https://www.marxists.org/reference/archive/bakunin/works/1870/letter-frenchman.htm

3. Jensen R. *The Battle Against Anarchist Terrorism: An International History, 1878–1934*. Cambridge: Cambridge University Press; 2013.

4. Rauchway E. *Murdering McKinley: The Making of Theodore Roosevelt's America*. New York: Hill and Wang; 2004.

5. Miller S. *The President and the Assassin: McKinley, Terrorism, and Empire at the Dawn of the American Century*. New York: Random House; 2013:264, 304.

6. Avich P. *Anarchist Voices: An Oral History of Anarchism in America*. Princeton, NJ: Princeton University Press; 1996:132.

7. Grohsgal L. The anarchist's chronicle. *National Endowment for the Humanities*, 13 Jan 2016; https://www.neh.gov/divisions/preservation/featured-project/the-anarchist's-chronicle

8. Avrich P. *Sacco and Vanzetti: The Anarchist Background*. Princeton, NJ: Princeton University Press; 1991:98.

9. Strang D. *Worse Than the Devil: Anarchists, Clarence Darrow, and Justice in a Time of Terror*. Madison: University of Wisconsin Press; 2016:128.

10. Gage B. *The Day Wall Street Exploded: A Story of America in Its First Age of Terror*. New York: Oxford University Press; 2009.

11. Simon J. *Lone Wolf Terrorism: Understanding the Growing Threat*. Amherst, NY: Prometheus Books; 2013.

12. Laqueur W. *A History of Terrorism*. London: Transaction Publications; 2001:14.

13. Davis M. *Buda's Wagon: A Brief History of the Car Bomb*. New York: Verso; 2007.

14. Spaaij R. *Understanding Lone Wolf Terrorism: Global Patterns, Motivations, and Prevention*. New York: Springer; 2012.

15. Hamm M, Spaaij R. *The Age of Lone Wolf Terrorism*. New York: Columbia University Press; 2017.

16. Hofstadter R. The paranoid style in American politics. *Harper's Magazine*, November 1964; https://harpers.org/archive/1964/11/the-paranoid-style-in-american-politics/

17. Cannell M. Unmasking the Mad Bomber. *Smithsonian Magazine*, April 2017; https://www.smithsonianmag.com/history/unmasking-the-mad-bomber-180962469/

18. Stern J. *Terror in the Name of God: Why Religious Militants Kill*. New York: Ecco; 2003.

19. Greenburg M. *The Mad Bomber of New York: The Extraordinary True Story of the Manhunt that Paralyzed a City*. New York: Union Square Press; 2011.

20. Chase A. *Harvard and the Unabomber: The Education of an American Terrorist*. New York: Norton; 2003.

21. Paddock R, Hubler R. Unabomber threatens LAX flights, then calls it a prank. *Los Angeles Times*, 29 Jun 1995, https://www.latimes.com/archives/la-xpm-1995-06-29-mn-18508-story.html

22. Unabomber sends new warnings. *Los Angeles Times*, 30 Jun 1995, https://www.latimes.com/archives/la-xpm-1995-06-30-mn-18891-story.html

23. *The Unabomber Manifesto: Industrial Society and Its Future*, as delivered to the *New York Times* and *Washington* Post, June 1995, paragraph 45; https://www.washingtonpost.com/wp-srv/national/longterm/unabomber/manifesto.text.htm

24. Kaplan J, Loow H, Malkki L. Introduction to the special issue on lone wolf and autonomous cell terrorism. *Terrorism and Political Violence*. 2014;26(1):1–12.

25. Hoffman, B. Back to the future: The return of violent far-right terrorism in the age of lone wolves. *War on the Rocks*, 2 Apr 2016. https://warontherocks.com/2019/04/back-to-the-future-the-return-of-violent-far-right-terrorism-in-the-age-of-lone-wolves/

26. Hewitt C. *Understanding Terrorism in America: From the Klan to Al Qaeda*. New York: Routledge; 2003.

27. Gill P. *Lone-Actor Terrorism: A Behavioral Analysis*. New York: Routledge; 2015.

28. Wieviorka M. Case studies: History or sociology? In Ragin C, Becker HS, eds., *What Is a Cases? Exploring the Foundations of Social Inquiry*. New York: Cambridge University Press; 1992:159–172.

29. Ferrell J. *Drift: Illicit Mobility and Uncertain Knowledge*. Berkeley: University of California Press; 2018.

30. Seirstad A. *One of Us: The Story of a Massacre in Norway—And Its Aftermath*. New York: Farrar, Straus and Giroux; 2015.

31. Hartleb F. *Lone Wolves: The New Terrorism of Right-Wing Single Actors*. Cham: Springer; 2020.

2

Case Reviews in Lone-Actor Terrorism Incidents

JACOB C. HOLZER, OLIVIA ZUREK, AND LAUREN SIMPSON

INTRODUCTION

This chapter reviews a wide range of individuals who have engaged in lone-actor terrorism and/or mass violence incidents resulting in their prosecutions or deaths. These cases, arranged in alphabetic order, provide an overview of the variance in ideologies, geography, perpetrators, weapons, and intended victims. Each case identifies the perpetrator(s), gives name of the event/location and date, and provides a brief historical background reviewing areas such as development, education, family/home life, and clinical and/or social histories, followed by a brief description of the index incident. For each case, the content for the review was obtained from multiple open source news, as cited in the references. Only clinical information (symptoms, signs, diagnoses) referenced in news sources is used, and the authors do not attempt to make a clinical diagnostic impression for any individual. As open source news information has been used to write this chapter, and no classified or court protected/privileged information is cited, accuracy of the content of this chapter is only as good as the accuracy of the news reports cited. This chapter is not meant to be an all-inclusive, exhaustive review, and most high-profile cases were not included. One purpose of this chapter is to highlight the variability and complexity in ideology and mechanics of lone-actor terrorist offenses. The authors acknowledge that in at least some of the cases cited, the individuals and cases may not fit with the "classic" definition of terrorism. Although most case examples had an identified pre-incident ideology or belief system linked to the violence, in some cases the ideology was not clear or not found in the literature reviewed but was included due to the geopolitical or governmental context of the incident. The concluding section of the chapter lists resources for further case study.

AARON ALEXIS (1979–2013): 2013 WASHINGTON NAVY YARD SHOOTER

Background: Reports indicate that salient features in Aaron Alexis's background include his being upbeat and polite, having an insatiable interest in Thai culture, and that he worshipped at a Buddhist temple, but reports also described someone who had a history of heavy drinking, was at times violent, and had an obsession with firearms. He was described as a devout Buddhist who "carried a gun in his trousers," was prone to violent outbursts, and would spend hours playing violent video games. He was in the US Navy Reserves, and reports indicated he had a "checkered career," marked by repeated run-ins with the military and the law, but he received an honorable discharge in January 2011. He had a criminal history involving an arrest in 2004 for shooting out the tires of a car in what Alexis described as an anger-fueled "blackout." Years later, he spent a short time in jail for disorderly conduct following a disturbance at a nightclub. In 2010, he fired a gun through a ceiling into an upstairs neighbor's apartment after a dispute. Following his time in the Navy, he secured a position as an IT worker with a subcontractor, had access to the Washington Navy Yard, and had during this time experienced serious psychiatric issues, including paranoia, sleep problems, and hearing voices. Although a clear motive or ideology has been difficult to determine, reports indicated that he had multiple frustrations with the US government. These included a sense of not being treated right as a veteran, feeling slighted regarding his salary and benefits, and that he had considered moving out of the United States. In addition, there was evidence to suggest he considered himself a victim of stalking and that he was a targeted individual.

Incident: Two days before the shooting, Alexis practiced shooting at a local range and also bought a shotgun and shells. On the morning of September 16, 2013, Alexis drove to the Washington Navy Yard and walked to the Naval Sea Systems Command headquarters, where he had been working earlier. He was carrying a dissembled shotgun in a bag and went into a bathroom, where he put the shotgun back together. He then went to a higher level that overlooked a crowded atrium and began shooting around cubicles in that area, moving from the atrium overlook area to the stairwell until he was confronted by law enforcement officers and killed.[1-7]

ANDERS BEHRING BREIVIK (1979–): 2011 OSLO AND UTØYA NORWAY

Background: Breivik's parents divorced when he was very young, and, after a custody battle, he lived with his mother but would visit his father as a child. However, news reports indicate that as Breivik's behavior became increasingly difficult as a teenager, he had a falling out with his father. He was described as having had a privileged and international upbringing but held a deep resentment of his father, a diplomat who had supported the Norwegian Labour movement. His diary revealed that he held conflicted thoughts regarding his mother, expressing both fondness and being furious at her for his upbringing. Reports indicate he was teased by friends for living with his mother and not having a girlfriend, and he occasionally wrote about puritanical beliefs. After the attacks, his father reported in an interview that he had not had contact with his son since adolescence, around 1995. During early childhood, Breivik's father reported that while Breivik resided with his mother Norwegian childcare authorities had recommended that he be moved, predating the just mentioned custody battle. Breivik reported in his manifesto that he felt he had had a good relationship with his father and his father's new wife until he was 15 years old. News reports indicate that after Breivik's father remarried for a fourth time, the children from his first marriage were angry with him and wanted to have nothing further to do with him. Breivik reported that his father was not happy with his "graffiti" phase from ages 13 to 16, around the time of increasing strain in his relationship with his father leading to their loss of contact. His father reported that Breivik's spray-painting buildings resulted in police involvement, and he reported Breivik was also shoplifting. One friend described Breivik as

having a "big ego," who would get irritated with people from the Middle East and Asia. Around the mid-2000s, several years before the attacks, Breivik had phoned his father to discuss a business he started in data processing; in his 1,500-page manifesto he later claimed this business was a front to finance his military operations and that he had a multiyear plan to finance his attacks, although the police felt that at least some of this was either delusional, confabulation, or exaggeration. In planning for his 2011 attack, Breivik was an active recipient and participant on far-right websites, and his manifesto provided ideological reasoning for the attack. Asne Seierstad, who has written a book on Breivik, indicated he sought fame and wanted his manifesto widely read, noting that the 2011 attacks were his "book launch," with Breivik essentially referring to the attacks as a marketing operation. In a *New York Times* article, Ms. Seierstad's research uncovered a life full of shame, failures, abuse, and rejections. She described him as more of a danger as a symbol, less of an inspiration in the context of his shortcomings. He had complaints about minor issues once in prison, and notes indicate he was diagnosed by court psychiatrists with a narcissistic personality disorder.

Incident: On July 22, 2011, Breivik engaged in a two-part terrorist attack, first detonating a bomb in a van in Oslo, killing several people, and then shooting 69 people at a youth summer camp on the island of Utøya. Breivik was convicted of terrorism and premeditated murder and sentenced to a relatively lenient 21 years in prison, the maximum under Norwegian law, although news reports indicated that his demeanor and testimony during his trial, where he professed he would have preferred to kill more people, may weigh against his eventual release. An insanity issue was raised by the prosecution during the course of the trial, although he was later found criminally responsible by the court. In court, he introduced himself as the military leader of a resistance movement.[8-18]

ISMAAIYL BRINSLEY (1986–2014): 2014 NYPD OFFICER KILLINGS

Background: Brinsley was born in New York, raised in Atlanta, the youngest of four children, and brought up in a branch of Islam. When he was young, his parents broke up. During childhood he was described as both generous but also as a "handful" who acted out. During adolescence, he moved around a large number of times, drifting between different family members. At age 14, it was reported that he attempted suicide after being sexually abused. Court paperwork indicated he dropped out of high school midway. Into early adulthood, he had run-ins with the police for minor offenses, and reports indicated he was a "name brand thief." He was known to dress and present himself well, and he had a daughter by his early 20s. He used social media to network and look for a place to stay. Reports indicate he had a series of petty crimes and a temper, and he was arrested for making threats to women. He also had a history of depression. He was estranged from his parents, and the police reported he had made a threat against his sister. Despite his temper and run-ins with police, friends reported liking him. He attempted to start clothing businesses that did not work out, and he was the victim of robberies. In the months before the shooting, it was reported that Brinsley was distressed about the deaths of Michael Brown and Eric Garner. Friends thought he had not made threats to the police, however. Sometime during this timeframe, he made a suicide threat. News reports indicated that, rather than his behavior being directed by jihadist beliefs, his thoughts on religion were more muddled and that he may have been hopeless. On the day before the New York Police Department (NYPD) shooting, he shot his former girlfriend outside of Baltimore, then fled to New York.

Incident: Before the shootings, Brinsley had posted on social media his intention of killing police in retribution for the deaths of Michael Brown and Eric Garner, stating "They Take 1 Of Ours . . . Let's Take 2 of Theirs." On December 20, 2014, Baltimore police informed the NYPD of the postings around the same time that Brinsley approached a police car parked in Brooklyn, shooting and killing officers Wenjian Liu and Rafael Ramos, before he fled. He then shot and killed himself.[19-22]

JAMES VON BRUNN (1920–2010): 2009 US HOLOCAUST MEMORIAL SHOOTING

Background: Von Brunn was born in 1920 in St. Louis, Missouri. He graduated from Washington University, in St. Louis, with a degree in journalism in 1943. He was reported to have been the president of the Sigma Alpha Epsilon fraternity and a varsity football player in college. He served as an officer in the US Navy during World War II. After his military service, he moved to New York

City, where he married, had a son, and worked at two major advertising firms. By 1962, he and his family moved to Maryland. He began to get into legal trouble starting in the late 1960s, when he was arrested for driving under the influence following an altercation at a restaurant in 1968. Later that year, he received a 6-month jail sentence for punching a sheriff at the county jail. In 1981, he was arrested for entering the Federal Reserve Board building in Washington, DC, with a shotgun, pistol, and hunting knife and pointing a gun at a security guard. Von Brunn later told police that his actions were politically motivated and that he intended to take the chairman and other members of the Federal Reserve hostage so that he could express his beliefs through the media. He was convicted of attempted kidnapping, burglary, assault, and weapons charges. At his trial, he said that his goal was to "deport all Jews and blacks from the white nations" and that "Jews were the greatest liars that have ever afflicted mankind." He was sentenced up to 11 years in prison in 1983 and was released in 1989. For the next several decades, Von Brunn demonstrated prominent racist and anti-Semitic views and became well-known among white supremacists and hate groups. He had his own website on which he espoused conspiracy theories and anti-Semitic and white supremacist rhetoric. He had been monitored by the Southern Poverty Law Center since 1981. At some point, he worked for Noontide Press, a publishing arm of the anti-Semitic Liberty Lobby and distributor of books on "The Jewish Question." In 1999, Von Brunn self-published a book titled, "Kill the Best Gentiles," which included Holocaust denial conspiracies and praise for Adolf Hitler. He reportedly spoke of having fought for the "wrong side" in World War II. He was described by acquaintances as a "loner, hothead and a man consumed with hatred." He was also thought to be intelligent, and he boasted of being a member of Mensa.

Incident: At 12:44 PM on June 10, 2009, at the age of 88, Von Brunn entered the US Holocaust Memorial Museum and fired a rifle at a security guard. The guard, Stephen T. Johns, was fatally wounded. Other security guards fired back at Von Brunn, wounding him and leading to his apprehension by police. Police later searched his car and found ammunition and a notebook with a list of other possible targets, including the White House, Capitol, and National Cathedral. The notebook also reportedly contained the address of his website and anti-Semitic, Holocaust denial, and anti–President Obama writings. At his apartment, investigators found a rifle, ammunition, a handwritten will, a painting that depicted Hitler and Jesus, and child pornography on his computer. In July 2009, Von Brunn was indicted by a federal grand jury on charges of first-degree murder, committing a hate crime, and gun violations. He died of chronic health problems on January 6, 2010, while incarcerated and awaiting trial.[23-28]

CHRISTOPHER DORNER (1979–2013): 2013 SOUTHERN CALIFORNIA SHOOTINGS AND MANHUNT

Background: Dorner's early life did not portend the later violence he brought to the Los Angeles area. Born in 1979, he and his family moved to California at an early age. He later noted that he was the only black pupil in each of his classes at elementary school and described being racially abused by other students and getting into fights on the playground. He thought of going into law enforcement at an early age, and, as a teenager, he signed up with a police department youth program. After graduating from university in 2001, he entered the US Navy, had combat training, and, in the mid-2000s, applied to join the Los Angeles Police Department while remaining in the Naval Reserve, where he was promoted and received several decorations. It was reported that in contrast with his time in the military, his experience in law enforcement training was not smooth. In a later manifesto he had written, he denied having punched another police recruit. Other reported difficulties included being suspended for discharging a firearm and accounts of his frequently clashing with authority. Other police officers noted warning signs of Dorner's temperament, one observing that his personality did not fit with being in law enforcement. He indicated in the manifesto that he had been racially maltreated by other officers who he felt did not receive adequate punishment for infractions. Dorner reported feeling the police department had worsened with regards to race relations. In 2007, Dorner made an official complaint against a training officer he reported seeing kick a suspect in the head during an arrest. An investigation later concluded the kick did not occur, although the family of the suspect conflicted with this finding. Dorner was charged with making false statements and was criticized for his performance; a disciplinary board later found he had lied, and he was fired from the police, which he took badly. It was reported that the verdict came as a huge

psychological blow and that Dorner attempted unsuccessfully to overturn the decision for years. During that time, it was noted his personal life was unraveling, with one ex-girlfriend writing on the internet that other women should avoid him because of fluctuations in his behaviors, swings from highs to lows. His anger at his mistreatment grew, and he became more isolated. In his manifesto, he signified he had lost his relationships, grew more depressed, felt victimized by the police, and demanded absolution; he indicated that his actions would be drastic and shocking, but a "necessary evil." He signified that his actions were the last resort in an effort to initiate change in the police department and reclaim his name.

Incident: In the first two weeks of February 2013, Dorner engaged in a succession of shootings in several counties in Southern California, resulting in four deaths and three people injured. During this time, Dorner shot and killed the family members of a former police captain who had represented Dorner in a hearing, ambushed and killed a police officer, abandoned his burned-out truck, and led law enforcement on a manhunt in the Big Bear Lake region east of Los Angeles. Officials accused him of domestic terrorism. Following police response to a carjacking, Dorner opened fire, killing another officer. Dorner was found barricaded in a cabin, and, in a standoff, police fired smoke canisters into the cabin, resulting in a fire. News reports indicated that Dorner died of a self-inflicted gunshot wound.[29-36]

JAMES ALEX FIELDS, JR. (1997–): 2017 CHARLOTTESVILLE CAR ATTACK

Background: Fields grew up in Kentucky with his mother, and a former high school teacher of Fields described him as quiet and intelligent, with a fascination with Nazi Germany and Adolph Hitler. A former teacher reported that Fields had confided to him that he had been diagnosed with schizophrenia when younger and prescribed medication for that condition. While in school, a complaint was filed by a teacher about an assignment Fields had turned in, which had indicated his alignment with neo-Nazis. In the year before the attack, Fields and his mother had moved to Ohio, and he had then moved out on his own. News reports indicate that authorities from the sheriff's office and police department responded to his mother's home in Kentucky following 911 calls indicating incidents where Fields was threatening or assaultive to his mother. Reports indicate he was in the

Army for approximately 4 months in 2015, and he worked as a security guard for 2 years. He passed the time playing video games, and the Army later indicated he was released from active duty due to a failure to meet training standards. Following the attack, Field told a judge that he was being treated for various psychiatric conditions, including bipolar disorder and attention deficit hyperactivity disorder (ADHD).

Incident: On August 12, 2017, Fields drove his car into a crowd of people protesting the Unite the Right rally in Charlottesville, Virginia, killing sHeather Heyer and injuring dozens of others. Fields received a life sentence after pleading guilty to federal charges in June 2019, thereby avoiding the death sentence; in July 2019, he received an additional life sentence following a conviction at the state level in Virginia.[37–44]

BARUCH GOLDSTEIN (1956–1994): 1994 HEBRON MASSACRE

Background: Baruch Goldstein was born and raised in New York City in an observant Jewish setting. He attended a religious day school and then medical school, and later became a member of the Jewish Defense League (JDL), founded by Rabbi Meir Kahane. Goldstein immigrated to Israel from the United States in 1983, in his late 20s, and served as a physician in the Israeli Defense Forces (IDF). Following active service, he lived in a Jewish settlement outside of Hebron on the West Bank, working as an emergency physician, where he treated victims of Arab–Israeli violence. He was known to harbor extreme hostile views toward Arabs, even to those who shared his ultranationalist views. It was reported that a year before the massacre he was heard to say that there will come a time when a Jew will kill many Arabs for killing Meir Kahane. As a physician, he eventually refused to treat Palestinians; earlier, as a military physician, it was reported that he may have refused to treat Druze soldiers in the IDF.

Incident: On February 25, 1994, Goldstein, using an automatic weapon, entered the mosque in the Machpela Cave where worshippers attended services during the month of Ramadan. He fired at a large number of the worshippers, killing 29 and wounding numerous others. He was found beaten to death. At his funeral, speakers displayed an extreme view of intolerance, praising Goldstein as the "greatest Jew alive." The massacre resulted in rioting, more deaths, and had an adverse impact diplomatically on the Israeli–Arab peace process. Goldstein was viewed by some settlers as a saint,

and a shrine was established that was forcibly removed by Israel in 1999.[45–50]

NIDAL HASAN (1970–): 2009 FORT HOOD SHOOTING

Background: Nidal Hasan was born in 1970 to parents who had immigrated from the West Bank. The family eventually settled in Roanoke, Virginia, where Nidal and his brothers helped in the family business. He graduated from Virginia Tech, enlisted in the Army, and then entered officer training and was commissioned in 1997. He went on to medical school while in the military, attending the Uniformed Services University of Health Sciences school. After graduation, he completed internship, a residency in psychiatry, and fellowship training. He was described as gentle and kind by neighbors, yet he complained bitterly to people at his mosque about the oppression of Muslims in the military. Reports indicate that he had few friends and was considered a "strange figure" by some at the mosque. Starting in medical school and residency, and in the years leading to the shooting, he grew more vocal about his opposition to the wars in Iraq and Afghanistan, and he struggled in trying to reconcile his being in the military with his religious views. Reports indicate he experienced anti-Islamic harassment, and, among his classmates and peers, he appeared to be isolative, interacting with others to argue why the wars were wrong. While in Washington, he grew closer to Islam, in part prompted by the death of his parents; relatives indicated that he took his parents deaths hard and focused more on Islam. During internship, reports indicated he had been having difficulties that required counseling and extra supervision. By 2004, he grew increasingly unhappy about being in the military and sought information about getting a discharge but was advised that his chances were very slim. He grew increasingly concerned about his prospect of deploying, and he sought advice on counseling young Muslim soldiers who might have objections to the war. In the early 2000s, Hasan attended a mosque in Washington, DC, where Anwar al-Awlaki was the imam for a period of time. Starting in late 2008, Hasan sent al-Awlaki numerous emails, thought to be related to research, although notes indicate that Hasan was deeply engaged in applying religious values to violence.

Incident: On November 5, 2009, Hasan killed 13 people and wounded more than 30 at a military processing center at Fort Hood, Texas. On the day before the shooting, he had acted out of character, saying goodbye to neighbors and giving away possessions before driving to the base on the day of the shootings, smuggling in two guns he had bought with him. In the early afternoon, he opened fire in the center, targeting uniformed soldiers. He later indicated that his mission was to kill as many soldiers as he could to protect Muslims from those soldiers deploying to Afghanistan, and he expressed the wish that he had died in the attack. In January 2011, he was judged sane by a military sanity board, allowing the capital trial to move forward. he was tried and found guilty in 2013 and is on death row.[51-58]

TED KACZYNSKI (1942–): THE UNABOMBER

Background: Kaczynski was born in Chicago to a working-class family; he had one sibling, a younger brother David, who would later play a role in his apprehension. He was considered isolated but excelled academically. Family reported that his early life was marked by his having a social aversion, becoming anxious when friends visited unannounced, and his mother telling his brother "Never abandon Ted, because that's what he fears the most." He skipped a grade in high school and went on to do undergraduate work in math at Harvard, graduating in the early 1960s, before completing graduate studies in math at the University of Michigan. During his years as an undergraduate, he was described as shy, a loner who was brilliant and needed encouragement to engage in discussions with others socially. After completing graduate school at age 25, he became an assistant professor in mathematics at the University of California at Berkeley but resigned 2 years later. Reports indicate that during his time at Harvard as an undergraduate he participated in controversial psychology research, where he was subjected to verbal stress and abuse, which may have had a negative mental and emotional impact on him. After leaving his teaching position, he lived with his parents for 2 years before moving to a cabin he had built in the woods in Montana in 1971. There he lived as a recluse and authored a manifesto entitled "Industrial Society and Its Future," in which he maintained that technology had led humans away from nature and in which he argued for a return to "wild nature." His arguments included an end to all scientific research. By the mid-1970s, Kaczynski was becoming distressed by encroaching real estate and industrial development and began vandalizing construction sites in an effort to disrupt development. By the late 1970s, Kaczynski grew more hostile in letters to his family, and he had made crude and offensive remarks about a female co-worker. It was around this time, in 1978, that he had posted his first mail bomb to a university professor in Chicago, who was mildly injured in the blast. Years later, he would post more letters to family, including a lengthy one to his brother accusing him of "lacking the integrity to lead a pure life."

Incidents: Starting in approximately 1978, Kaczynski engaged in a 17-year series of mail bomb attacks targeting academics, business executives, and others. Three people were killed and 23 injured. The series of attacks continued until 1996, when Kaczynski was caught. The FBI had referenced the nationwide investigation "UNABOM" (for university and airline bomber), with the media dubbing the attacker "the Unabomber," even though Kaczynski's identity was not yet known. Following his first mailing in 1978, he came close to blowing up an American Airlines jet, but the bomb did not detonate. After his manifesto was published, Kaczynski's brother David, with the help of an attorney, was able to assist the FBI in making the connection between the Unabomber and Kaczynski. On April 3, 1996, following authorization of a search warrant for Kaczynski's cabin, the FBI and other officers descended on the compound, where they arrested Kaczynski. He was later indicted by a federal grand jury on multiple counts of illegally transporting, mailing, and using bombs, along with three counts of murder. Although his attorneys wanted to enter a not guilty by reason of insanity plea, he refused and pleaded guilty. He is now serving multiple life sentences without chance of parole at the Supermax prison in Colorado.[59-62]

MIR AIMAL KANSI (KASI) (1964 OR 1967–2002): JANUARY 1993 CIA ENTRANCE SHOOTINGS

Background: Kansi was born in Pakistan, although the year of his birth is unclear. Reports of his early background are limited, with one source indicating that an uncle testified that Kansi was an apolitical loner who talked to himself as a teenager. Teachers described him as solemn, a poor math student, quiet, and shy. One news report described a CIA profile of Kansi as "an underachieving son of a prominent Pakistani family who burned with the desire to make a name for himself." He came to the United States in 1991 and applied for political asylum in the Washington, DC, area before moving in with a roommate in 1993, in Reston,

Virginia. He held a graduate degree in English. News reports indicated that his roommate, Zahed Ahmad Mir, was with Kansi when he bought the assault rifle used in the attack; and Mir later led authorities to suspect Kansi in the attacks.

Incident: On January 25, 1993, Kansi, using an AK-47 assault rifle, fired into cars waiting to turn into the CIA main entrance, killing two CIA employees and wounding three others. At the time of the shooting, Kansi had been working for a courier service and was familiar with the attack area. He fled, resulting in a multiyear manhunt. After the attack, he returned to his family home in Quetta, Pakistan, where he received protection and was smuggled into Afghanistan. He eventually became less guarded and started visiting friends in Pakistan, leading to a joint CIA-FBI operation to lure him back to Pakistan for a surreptitious business meeting that resulted in his capture. He was returned to the United States. Kansi confessed to the slayings during the return flight, saying that he was angry and that he wanted to punish the US government for bombing Iraq, for what he saw as its involvement in the killing of Palestinians, and because the CIA was too deeply involved in the internal affairs of Muslim countries. Protesters in Pakistan said Kansi's actions were understandable. His defense argued that Kansi was brain damaged and mentally ill. He was tried under Virginia state law, found guilty after a 10-day trial in Fairfax County in November 1997, and executed by lethal injection on November 14, 2002, in Virginia. Federal authorities never found any links between Kasi and terrorist organizations.[63–71]

JARED LOUGHNER (1988–): JANUARY 2011 TUCSON SHOOTING

Background: Jared Loughner grew up and lived with his parents in the Tucson, Arizona, area. During his early high school years, he appeared unremarkable and bright, but then appeared to undergo noticeable changes in socializing and how he dressed. Classmates reported that by later high school, he was using various drugs including marijuana, psychedelics, and alcohol. One possible precipitant related to the timing of his downward spiral may have been a breakup with a girlfriend. In 2008, he attempted to join the Army but was rejected after admitting to marijuana use. By the time he attended a local community college, he was reported to be more overtly disturbed; he had disrupted classes frequently and posted online videos that were troubling, leading

to his being suspended and told he would require a mental health clearance in order to return to school. This mental health evaluation and clearance did not appear to occur prior to the shootings. His online videos included statements about mind control, SWAT teams, and the "gold standard." He was reported by media sources as having varied, contradictory views, including right-wing, anti-government, white supremacist, and extreme left-wing, and his readings pointed to a theme of individuals versus the totalitarian state. As indicated later, he was diagnosed with schizophrenia during court-ordered forensic mental health evaluations, and notes indicate that before the shootings he had become increasingly paranoid about the government and developed a hostile obsession with Gabrielle Giffords. He accumulated a number of encounters with law enforcement in the years before the shootings, including drug charges, an altercation, and graffiti. This last incident on the community college campus led law enforcement to take Loughner to see a counselor.

Incident: On January 8, 2011, Loughner shot numerous people at a "Congress on Your Corner" event in Tucson, sponsored by US Representative Gabrielle Giffords. Six people were killed and 13 wounded, including Rep. Giffords, who was shot in the head. He initially pleaded not guilty to all of the charges against him. He was subsequently ordered to undergo a mental health evaluation, where experts reported he experienced delusions, bizarre thoughts, and hallucinations and appeared to suffer from paranoid schizophrenia. He was subsequently found not competent to stand trial. Following treatment, he was found competent to stand trial, and he pleaded guilty to multiple charges in exchange for the government not seeking the death penalty.[72–79]

OMAR MATEEN (1986–2016): 2016 MASS SHOOTING PULSE NIGHTCLUB IN ORLANDO

Background: Omar Mateen was born in 1986, in New York; he moved with his family to Florida around age 5. Reports indicate he had difficulty academically, with low grades and behavioral problems. Around 1999, educators noted problems with conduct and self-discipline and indicated that he had trouble concentrating and was attention-seeking, with below average school performance. He held various jobs while in school and later worked at a gym. He was described as a fitness buff and had a temper. Reports indicated that in an effort to build body mass and muscle, he may have been engaged in long-term steroid use. After graduating community college with an associate's degree in 2006, he worked briefly in corrections and then as a security guard. Following the massacre, law enforcement investigations indicated that Mateen was inspired by foreign terrorist organizations on the internet, although there was no direct link with an organization. His father raised the possibility that his motivation was homophobia, describing an incident where Mateen and his son walked into a public bathroom and saw two men touching each other; Mateen flew into a rage. Reports indicate that, predating the shooting, he was taunted for being Muslim. He evidently responded to these taunts with claims to have ties to other lone-actor terrorists. These responses and expressed interest in radical Islam resulted in FBI investigations but did not show a link to organized terrorism. He was described as "forever aggrieved, not at peace, out of step," one who had made inappropriate jokes about 9/11, spoke casually of killing people who offended him, and had periods of anger that made others feel unsafe.

Incident: In the early morning hours of Sunday, June 12, 2016, Mateen opened fire at the Pulse nightclub in Orlando, Florida, killing 49 people and wounding 53. At the time, it was the deadliest mass shooting in US history. Police attempted to negotiate with Mateen, who had taken hostages during the standoff. After officers were able to breach the inside of the club with explosives, Mateen exchanged gunfire with police and was shot and killed.[80-86]

AHMAD KHAN RAHAMI (1988–): 2016 BOMBINGS IN NEW YORK AND NEW JERSEY

Background: Ahmad Khan Rahami was born in 1988, in Afghanistan, and came to the United States to join family in 1995. He became a naturalized citizen in 2011 and, around that time, attended college. Also in 2011, Rahami married a Pakistani woman while visiting Pakistan; his wife later came to the United States but left before the bombing attacks. Around 2014, Rahami ran into problems with his wife's immigration paperwork and sought help from a US congressman. Reports indicate that, also around 2014, Rahami was involved in a violent domestic dispute in which he stabbed a relative. The family lived above their restaurant in Elizabeth, New Jersey, and had clashes with the community over the

restaurant, at one point filing a lawsuit against the city alleging discrimination and harassment. Customers indicated that Rahami had a "chilling" presence and that he would not talk with them, but just take orders. Rahami made multiple trips to Afghanistan. In 2013, he traveled in Pakistan and Afghanistan for almost a full year, and, in retrospect, investigators wondered if he had been radicalized during that trip even though he was not known as a threat to law enforcement before the attacks.

Incident: In mid-September 2016, Rahami planted bombs in the New York metropolitan area and in New Jersey, three of which exploded, resulting in numerous injuries but no fatalities. The explosive set off in the Chelsea neighborhood of Manhattan was powerful enough to throw a heavy steel dumpster high into the air, injuring numerous people. A pipe bomb went off near a Marine Corps road race in Seaside Heights, New Jersey. Rahami had also planted a pressure-cooker bomb in Chelsea that had not detonated, along with explosive devices at a train station in Elizabeth, New Jersey. The bombings triggered a 2-day manhunt, resulting in a shootout with police in Linden, New Jersey, where Rahami was injured and arrested. It was later reported that he had taken inspiration from Osama bin Laden, and his writings were found to mention the Boston Marathon bombers and Anwar al-Awlaki. He was sentenced to multiple terms of life in prison.[87-92]

ELLIOT RODGER (1991–2014): 2014 ISLA VISTA CALIFORNIA KILLING SPREE

Background: Rodger was a 22-year-old man of Chinese and English descent, born in London; he moved with his family to California during childhood. Reports indicate that during childhood he was shy and was not involved in individual or group sports while growing up, other than riding a skateboard. A comprehensive investigative report indicated he never showed an interest in firearms during adolescence or during adult years and that his family were in disbelief over how he had purchased so many firearms before the attack. When angry, it was reported he would tense up his body and clench his teeth, but not physically act out, get into fights, hurt animals, or damage property. Reports also indicated that he would at times stare off into space and need frequent reassurance. He was reluctant to participate and engage with others in class, although he appeared to respond appropriately to others socially when they sought him out. It was reported that he displayed behaviors consistent with Asperger's syndrome. Much of his social interaction with peers was through playing online video games. He was involved in mental health treatment throughout his adolescence until his death, and reports indicated he was diagnosed with a pervasive development disorder (referred to as an autistic spectrum disorder) and that he suffered from narcissism and anxiety. There are numerous reports of his being bullied during school. In the context of his feeling shy, isolated, and rejected by girls and women during adolescence and in college, he began to share feelings of frustration and rage at having difficulty dating by posting on sites where other young men shared similar feelings, referring to himself as an "involuntary celibate" or "incel." He made a video posting before the attack, referred to as "Elliot Rodger's Retribution," in which he described being forced to endure loneliness, rejection, and unfulfilled desires. He indicated that "I do not know why you girls aren't attracted to me. . . . But I will punish you all for it."

Incident: On May 23, 2014, following a period during which he amassed firearms and ammunition, Rodgers embarked on a premeditated rampage, involving stabbing people, drive-by shootings, and striking people with his car, resulting in six deaths and numerous injuries. He engaged in two gun battles with law enforcement and was wounded before taking his own life.[93–99]

DYLANN ROOF (1994–): 2015 CHARLESTON CHURCH SHOOTING

Background: Dylann Roof was born in 1994, to parents who had earlier divorced, then reconciled for a limited time. He attended multiple schools growing up and helped out neighbors who, it was reported, found him strange; at times he would sit quietly on curbs in his neighborhood. The schools he attended were middle-class and integrated, he had black friends, and it was reported that he came from a respected family, although there were indications of family financial stress during his teenage years. During his earlier school years, he maintained a friendship with someone of mixed race. Once in high school, he appeared to struggle, repeated a grade, and later dropped out. Reports indicate that he then drifted in and out of jobs, engaged in alcohol and illicit drug use, had confrontations with the police, started reading white supremacist websites, and, before the church attack, boasted of wanting to start a race war. It was reported that by age 13 he was

spending money on marijuana. In the months before the church attack, he was noted to be quieter and "emotionless," harbored racist views, and spoke of doing "something big." His racist inclinations were in contrast to his family's beliefs. His confrontations with police included his acting in a threatening manner in a shopping mall, where police searched him and found buprenorphine (Naloxone, Suboxone) on his person, resulting in charges. He was later questioned for loitering by the police, who found rifle parts in his car. He was barred from the mall. Later, he was arrested for trespassing on mall property. In the months before the shooting, he purchased a .45 caliber handgun, although later the FBI would note that there had been a breakdown in the background check system and that the sale should have been blocked due to his earlier admission of drug possession. It was noted that Roof created a website that referenced white-ruled African governments, the confederacy, and Hitler.

Incident: On June 17, 2015, in a racially motivated attack, Roof killed nine people, all African Americans, at the Emanuel African Methodist Episcopal Church in Charleston, South Carolina. During court proceedings, he insisted there was nothing wrong with him psychologically, although a court-appointed psychiatrist indicated several clinical conditions existed, including social anxiety disorder, a mixed substance abuse disorder, a schizoid personality disorder, and depression and a possible autistic spectrum disorder. A significant split existed with his defense team, who had requested a new competency hearing, although he was later found competent to stand trial and able to represent himself. He was found guilty and convicted of all federal charges. In January 2017 he was sentenced to death in federal court. Family and friends of the victims confronted him at the sentencing hearing; some forgave him while others condemned him. In March 2017, he pleaded guilty in state court to avoid a second death sentence. Due to a lack of applicable statutes, the government was unable to charge Roof with terrorist crimes, although it was felt that the Charleston massacre qualified as terrorism under federal law.[100–108]

ERIC ROBERT RUDOLPH (1966–): 1996 OLYMPIC PARK BOMBING

Background: Eric Rudolph was born in 1966 in Florida. His family were described as self-sufficient. During his teenage years in the early 1980s, his father died of cancer. A former state law enforcement agent suggested that Rudolph acted out of anger toward the government, possibly stemming from an earlier issue with the Food and Drug Administration rejecting approval of a cancer treatment Rudolph thought might have helped his father. During high school, Rudolph wrote about his beliefs that the Holocaust was a hoax, and he ultimately dropped out, later earning a GED. He attended college for a limited time before dropping out and enlisting in the US Army in 1987. He was in the Army for approximately 1½ years before being discharged, with reports attributing his discharge to marijuana use. He later worked as a carpenter. Reports indicate that, starting as a teen, he harbored anti-Semitic and racist views, mourned the death of his father, and sought refuge in drugs, the army, racial intolerance, and rage. Rudolph displayed various inconsistencies. Reports indicate that, despite his hostility toward gays, he was close to his brother who had come out as gay. After his capture, although he spoke with local police, he refused to talk with federal authorities.

Incidents: Between 1996 and 1998, motivated by various biases and hatreds, Rudolph set off bombs at various sites around the Atlanta and Birmingham areas, killing two people and injuring hundreds. These bombings included abortion clinics, a lesbian nightclub, and the Atlanta Centennial Olympic Park bombing in 1996 during the Summer Olympics. Following a search lasting 5 years, Rudolph was found and arrested while he searched through a dumpster after surviving in the forests of Appalachia. Rudolph agreed to plead guilty to a series of bombings, including the fatal bombing at the Olympics, in order to avoid the death penalty. He later cited his anti-abortion and anti-homosexual views as motivation for the bombings.[109-114]

JOHN SALVI III (1972–1996): 1994 BROOKLINE, MASSACHUSETTS, REPRODUCTIVE HEALTH CLINIC SHOOTINGS

Background: John Salvi III was born in 1972; he grew up in Massachusetts and Florida. Reports indicated that in school he was determined and outgoing, but that toward his latter teen years, he began to withdraw, his grades declined, his friends withdrew, and he became focused on reading the Bible. He was reported to have had hallucinations during that time. Around the age of 20, he moved out of his parent's house, and it was reported that his behavior became more

extreme. He became reclusive, lived alone for several months in a small apartment, and trained as a hairdresser. At the hairdressing shop, he was reluctant to give his phone number or address to co-workers. It was reported that he got into an argument with a customer. A co-worker described him as a "walking time bomb." A family member described him as a "religious fanatic and someone he felt was bizarre and expressed a dislike for." Some saw him at times as not showing emotion, but then co-workers described him as flying into a rage when he was told he could not cut a client's hair.

Incident: On December 30, 1994, Salvi carried out shootings at two reproductive health clinics in Brookline, Massachusetts, that killed two and wounded five people. His defense team suspected that mental illness played a role in his offenses, a view supported by defense experts who indicated Salvi suffered from paranoid schizophrenia. However, at trial, Salvi was found guilty and sentenced to life in prison. He later committed suicide while in prison.[115-122]

ANDREW JOSEPH STACK III (1956–2010): 2010 AUSTIN ATTACK

Background: Stack grew up in Pennsylvania. He was reportedly orphaned at age 4 after both his parents died in a car accident. He was separated from his two brothers and sister and lived part of his childhood in a Catholic orphanage. He later was sent to the Milton Hershey School, a facility for orphaned boys in Hershey, Pennsylvania. He graduated in 1974 and attended Harrisburg Area Community College from 1975 to 1977, but did not graduate. He moved to California in the early 1980s to pursue a career in software engineering, and he incorporated a company called Prowess Engineering in 1985. Around this time, it is believed that Stack began to have complaints about the IRS and his perceived unconstitutionality of the tax code. He would meet with groups of people to discuss tax code issues and, according to his manifesto, was particularly distressed by tax exemptions granted to religious organizations. In his manifesto, Stack alludes to forming his own "home church" as a means of protest against these exemptions. This endeavor reportedly cost him $40,000 and his retirement savings. In 1986, the federal tax code changed such that technology consultants like Stack could no longer be classified as self-employed workers, thus restricting them from receiving certain tax deductions. After this change, Stack spent thousands of dollars and numerous hours contacting government officials to complain. In 1994, Stack did not file a state tax return. In 2000, the California Franchise Tax Board suspended Stack's company, Prowess. Another company started by Stack in 1995 was suspended in 2004 due to failure to pay $1,153 in state taxes. In 1998, Stack and his first wife divorced. One year later, his ex-wife filed for bankruptcy, citing IRS liabilities totaling nearly $126,000. Stack moved to Austin, Texas, in the early 2000s and started another software company in 2003, but he had difficulty finding consistent work in Austin. Stack was also an avid pilot and musician. He played bass and keyboard in a local band in Austin. Friends of Stack saw no indication of his anger toward the government or the tax code.

Incident: On February 18, 2010, Stack intentionally flew his single-engine Piper Dakota light aircraft into Building I of the Echelon office complex in Austin. The seven-story building housed IRS field offices, among other private businesses. Stack and 68-year-old IRS manager and father of six, Vernon Hunter, were killed in the crash. Thirteen other people were injured. The morning of the crash, Stack posted online a 3,000-word manifesto written over several months in which he outlined his multiple grievances with the government, taxes, and the IRS. Stack ended the manifesto with the statement "Well, Mr. Big Brother I.R.S man, let's try something different, take my pound of flesh and sleep well." He signed the manifesto "Joe Stack (1956–2010)."[123–125]

CONCLUSION

The preceding case examples highlight the wide-ranging variability in lone-actor terrorist backgrounds, ideology and beliefs, methodologies, and choice of target. Despite this variability, this and other chapters in this volume describe various characteristics that at least some individuals appear to have in common. Understanding common traits and patterns may help proactively in the effort to reduce the future risk of a lone-actor terrorism incident. Resources for those interested in pursuing research on lone-actor terrorism incidents and cases are listed here.

- Major news sources including the *New York Times*, *Washington Post*, *LA Times*, *Boston Globe*, CNN, the *Wall Street Journal*, the BBC, NPR, *Frontline*, Foreign Policy, Reuters, the Associated Press, and other major national and international news outlets.
- Publications by organizations including the Brookings Institution, the RAND Corporation, the United Nations, the Southern Poverty Law Center, the International Centre for Counter Terrorism, the Anti-Defamation League, and the Pew Research Center.
- Federal organizations including the National Institute of Justice, the FBI, Homeland Security, and the West Point Combating Terrorism Center.
- Computer assisted research through LexisNexis, Westlaw, Google Scholar, and medical data bases such as Pubmed and OVID.

NOTES AND REFERENCES

AARON ALEXIS

1. McCalmont L. Friend: Alexis wanted to leave U.S. Politico.com, 18 Sep 2013. https://www.politico.com/story/2013/09/aaron-alexis-navy-yard-shooting-096910
2. Allen N, Sherwell P. Washington Navy shootings: Devout Buddhist suspect prone to violent outbursts. *The Telegraph*, 17 Sep 2013. https://www.telegraph.co.uk/news/worldnews/northamerica/usa/10316466/Washington-Navy-shootings-devout-Buddhist-suspect-prone-to-violent-outbursts.html
3. Memmott M. Who was Aaron Alexis? Records offer clues of instability. NPR, 17 Sep 2013. https://www.npr.org/sections/thetwo-way/2013/09/17/223402913/who-was-aaron-alexis-records-friends-offer-confusing-clues
4. Lewis P. Aaron Alexis: Police piece together picture of a man as normal as you or me. *The Guardian*, 20 Sep 2013. https://www.theguardian.com/world/2013/sep/20/aaron-alexis-washington-navy-yard-shooter
5. Aaron Alexis given security clearance to Washington Navy Yard despite recent history of mental illness. National Post and Postmedia Breaking News, 17 Sep 2013. https://nationalpost.com/news/aaron-alexis-given-security-clearance-to-washington-navy-yard-despite-recent-history-of-mental-illness
6. Staff Reports. What happened inside Building 197? *The Washington Post*, 25 Sep 2013. http://www.washingtonpost.com/wp-srv/special/local/navy-yard-shooting/scene-at-building-197/
7. CBS. The Washington Navy Yard shooting, as it happened. CBS News, 31 Oct 2013. https://www.cbsnews.com/news/the-washington-navy-yard-shooting-as-it-happened/

ANDERS BEHRING BREIVIK

8. Allen P. Norway Killer: Father horrified by Anders Behring Breivik killing spree. *The Telegraph*, 24 Jul 2011. https://www.telegraph.co.uk/news/worldnews/europe/norway/8657928/

Norway-Killer-Father-horrified-by-Anders-Behring-Breivik-killing-spree.html

9. Norway killer: Anders Behring Breivik was a "mummy's boy." *The Telegraph*, 25 Jul 2011. https://www.telegraph.co.uk/news/worldnews/europe/norway/8659746/Norway-killer-Anders-Behring-Breivik-was-a-mummys-boy.html

10. Anders Behring Breivik's father: "My son should have taken his own life." *The Telegraph*, 25 Jul 2011. https://www.telegraph.co.uk/news/worldnews/europe/norway/8660397/Anders-Behring-Breiviks-father-My-son-should-have-taken-his-own-life.html

11. Henley J. Anders Behring Breivik trial: The father's story. *The Guardian* US Edition, 13 Apr 2012.   https://www.theguardian.com/world/2012/apr/13/anders-behring-breivik-norway

12. Norwegian mass murder suspect has big ego—friend. *RT*, 23 Jul 2011. https://www.rt.com/news/norwegian-attacks-suspect-friend-exclusive/

13. Taylor M. Norway gunman claims he had nine-year plan to finance attacks. *The Guardian* US Edition, 25 Jul 2011. https://www.theguardian.com/world/2011/jul/25/norway-gunman-attack-funding-claim

14. Fisher M. Terrorist or disturbed loner? Munich attack reveals shifting labels. *New York Times*, 24 Jul 2016. https://www.nytimes.com/2016/07/25/world/europe/terrorist-or-disturbed-loner-munich-attack-reveals-shifting-labels.html

15. Seierstad A. The anatomy of white terror. *New York Times*. Opinion, 18 March 2019. https://www.nytimes.com/2019/03/18/opinion/new-zealand-tarrant-white-supremacist-terror.html

16. Lewis M, Lyall S. Norway mass killer gets the maximum: 21 years. *New York Times*, 24 Aug 2012. https://www.nytimes.com/2012/08/25/world/europe/anders-behring-breivik-murder-trial.html

17. Norway killer Anders Behring Breivik faces victims in court. BBC News, 14 Nov 2011. https://www.bbc.com/news/av/world-europe-15722271/norway-killer-anders-behring-breivik-faces-victims-in-court

18. Anders Behring Breivik: Norway court finds him sane. BBC News, 24 Aug 2012. https://www.bbc.com/news/world-europe-19365616

ISMAAIYL BRINSLEY

19. Mueller B, Baker A. 2 N.Y.P.D. officers killed in Brooklyn ambush: Suspect commits suicide. *New York Times*, 20 Dec 2014. https://www.nytimes.com/2014/12/21/nyregion/two-police-officers-shot-in-their-patrol-car-in-brooklyn.html

20. Barker K, Secret M, Fausset R. Many identities of New York Officers' killer in a life of wrong turns. *New York Times*, 2 Jan 2015. https://www.nytimes.com/2015/01/03/nyregion/ismaaiyl-brinsleys-many-identities-fueled-life-of-wrong-turns.html

21. Holley P. Two New York City police officers are shot and killed in a brazen ambush in Brooklyn. *Washington Post*, 20 Dec 2014. https://www.washingtonpost.com/national/two-new-york-city-police-officers-are-shot-and-killed-in-a-brazen-ambush-in-brooklyn/2014/12/20/2a73f7ae-8898-11e4-9534-f79a23c40e6c_story.html?utm_term=.9ba12d980f3b

22. O'Brien RD, Shallwani P, Calvert S. Ismaaiyl Brinsley led life of trouble before attack. *Wall Street Journal*, 21 Dec 2014. https://www.wsj.com/articles/ismaaiyl-brinsley-suspected-of-shooting-new-york-police-had-criminal-history-ties-to-brooklyn-1419188892

JAMES VON BRUNN

23. Fears D, Fisher M. Holocaust Museum shooting suspect had history of hate, signs of breaking point. *Washington Post*, 11 Jun 2009. http://www.washingtonpost.com/wp-dyn/content/article/2009/06/10/AR2009061003495_3.html?nav=hcmodule&noredirect=on&sid=ST2009061200050

24. Stout D. Museum gunman a longtime foe of government. *New York Times*, 10 Jun 2009. https://www.nytimes.com/2009/06/11/us/11shoot.html?searchResultPosition=7

25. Emery T, Robbing L. Holocaust Museum shooter James von Brunn had history of hate. *Seattle Times*, 12 Jun 2009. https://www.seattletimes.com/nation-world/holocaust-museum-shooter-james-von-brunn-had-history-of-hate/

26. Stein P. Holocaust Museum gunman a WU graduate, University confirms. *Student Life*, 13 Jun 2009.   http://www.studlife.com/news/2009/06/13/holocaust-museum-gunman-a-wu-graduate-university-confirms/

27. Keller L. New evidence shows Holocaust Museum shooter James Von Brunn had long craved attention. SPLC Intelligence Report, 30 Aug 2009.   https://www.splcenter.org/fighting-hate/intelligence-report/2009/new-evidence-shows-holocaust-museum-shooter-james-von-brunn-had-long-craved-attention

28. Ruane ME, Duggan P, Williams C. At a monument of sorrow, a burst of deadly violence. *Washington Post*, 11 Jun 2009. http://www.washingtonpost.com/wp-dyn/content/article/2009/06/10/AR2009061001768.html

CHRISTOPHER DORNER

29. Kelly J. Christopher Dorner: What made a police officer kill? BBC News Los Angeles, 16 Feb 2013. https://www.bbc.com/news/magazine-21476904

30. Mohan G, Schaefer S. Christopher Dorner Manifesto. *LA Times*, 7 Feb 2013. http://documents.latimes.com/christopher-dorner-manifesto/

31. CBS News. Christopher Dorner manhunt: Search for ex-LAPD cop goes on amid Calif. Snowstorm. CBS/AP, 8 Feb 2013. https://www.cbsnews.com/news/christopher-dorner-manhunt-search-for-ex-lapd-cop-goes-on-amid-calif-snowstorm/

32. Vercammen P, Pearson M, Botelho G. Police: 3 dead after ex-copy vows "war" on other police, their families. CNN, 7 Feb 2013. https://www.cnn.com/2013/02/07/us/lapd-attacks/index.html

33. Welch, WM. LAPD: Fugitive ex-cop a "domestic terrorist." *USA Today*, 10 Feb 2013. https://www.usatoday.com/story/news/nation/2013/02/10/ex-cop-manhunt-continues/1906999/

34. CBS Calif. Deputy slain in ex-cop shootout was father of 2. CBS News, 13 Feb 2013. https://www.cbsnews.com/news/calif-deputy-slain-in-ex-cop-shootout-was-father-of-2/

35. CNN. Police: Body found in cabin in hunt for Dorner. CNN Breaking News, 12 Feb 2013. http://news.blogs.cnn.com/2013/02/12/police-checking-reports-that-ex-lapd-officer-dorner-sighted/comment-page-44/

36. Haffner K. Autopsy report confirms suicide for Christopher Dorner. NBC Los Angeles, 3 Oct 2014. https://www.nbclosangeles.com/news/local/Autopsy-Report-Confirms-Suicide-for-Christopher-Dorner-278095681.html

JAMES ALEX FIELDS, JR.

37. Ruiz J. Ohio man charged with murder in fatal car attack on anti-white nationalist march. NPR, The Two-Way, 13 Aug 2017. https://www.npr.org/sections/thetwo-way/2017/08/13/543176250/charlottesville-attack-james-alex-fields-jr

38. Sparling HK, Balmert J, Stinchcomb J. Community: Accused Charlottesville driver James Alex Fields Jr. doesn't represent us. *Cincinnati Enquirer*, 13 Aug 2017. https://www.cincinnati.com/story/news/2017/08/13/maumee-neighbors-shaken-charlottesville-suspect-james-alex-fields-living-nearby/563055001/

39. Strickley B, Brookbank S, Graves C, Mayhew C. 911 calls, records reveal tumultuous past for accused Charlottesville driver, family. *Cincinnati Enquirer*, 15 Aug 2017. https://www.cincinnati.com/story/news/local/northern-ky/2017/08/14/mom-previously-accused-charlottesville-driver-james-alex-fields-jr-beating-her/566078001/

40. Graves C, Pilcher J. Ex-neighbor of James Alex Fields Jr.: "Hope they put him where the sun doesn't shine." *Cincinnati Enquirer*, 13 Aug 2017. https://www.cincinnati.com/story/news/local/northern-ky/2017/08/13/former-classmate-neighbors-fields-seemed-shy-kept-himself/562917001/

41. Hernández AR, Gillum J, Miller ME, Hendrix S. "Very threatening": Mother of Charlottesville suspect James A. Fields called 911 twice. *Washington Post*. 14 Aug 2017. https://www.washingtonpost.com/local/public-safety/judge-denies-bail-for-man-accused-of-ramming-car-into-charlottesville-protesters/2017/08/14/2177a028-80fd-11e7-ab27-1a21a8e006ab_story.html?utm_term=.fe086d65e946

42. Pilcher J. Charlottesville suspect's beliefs were "along the party lines of the neo-Nazi movement," ex-teacher says. *USA Today*, 14 Aug 2017. https://www.usatoday.com/story/news/nation-now/2017/08/13/charlottesville-suspects-views-neo-nazi-ex-teacher/563199001/

43. Associated Press. James Alex Fields' trial in deadly Charlottesville white nationalist rally set to begin. NBC News, 26 Nov 2018. https://www.nbcnews.com/news/us-news/james-alex-fields-trial-deadly-charlottesville-white-nationalist-rally-set-n939991

44. Madani D. James Alex Fields Jr., driver in deadly Charlottesville car attack, gets second life sentence. NBC News, 15 Jul 2019. https://www.nbcnews.com/news/us-news/james-alex-fields-jr-driver-deadly-charlottesville-car-attack-gets-n1030076

BARUCH GOLDSTEIN

45. BBC Home. On this day 25 February 1994: Jewish settler kills 30 at holy site. BBC, 25 Feb 1994. http://news.bbc.co.uk/onthisday/hi/dates/stories/february/25/newsid_4167000/4167929.stm

46. Church GJ. When fury rules. *Time*, 7 Mar 1994. http://content.time.com/time/magazine/article/0,9171,980291,00.html

47. Gurvitz Y. Jewish soldiers refuse to share Seder table with Druze comrades. *+ 972 Magazine*, 8 Apr 2012. https://972mag.com/idf-jewish-soldiers-refuse-to-share-table-with-druze-comrades/40607/

48. Brownfeld AC. Growing intolerance threatens the humane Jewish tradition. Washington Report on Middle East Affairs, Mar 1999. https://www.wrmea.org/1999-march/growing-intolerance-threatens-the-humane-jewish-tradition.html

49. Freishtat S. CIA paper cites Jewish acts of terrorism. Jewish Telegraphic Agency, 26 Aug 2010. https://www.jta.org/2010/08/26/united-states/cia-paper-cites-jewish-acts-of-terrorism

50. Haberman C. West Bank massacre: Israel eases curfew in territories: Ensuing riots deepen pessimism. *New York Times*, 3 Mar 1994. https://www.nytimes.com/1994/03/03/world/west-bank-massacre-israel-eases-curfew-territories-ensuing-riots-deepen.html?scp=1&pagewanted=all

NIDAL HASAN

51. McKinley JC, Dao J. Fort Hood gunman gave signals before his rampage. *New York Times*, 8 Nov 2009. https://www.nytimes.com/2009/11/09/us/09reconstruct.html?pagewanted=all

52. BBC. Profile: Major Nidal Malik Hasan. BBC, 12 Nov 2009. http://news.bbc.co.uk/2/hi/8345944.stm

53. Sherwell P, Spillius A. Fort Hood shooting: Texas army killer linked to September 11 terrorists. *Daily Telegraph*, 7 Nov 2009. https://www.telegraph.co.uk/news/worldnews/northamerica/usa/6521758/Fort-Hood-shooting-Texas-army-killer-linked-to-September-11-terrorists.html

54. Shane S, Dao J. Investigators study tangle of clues on Fort Hood suspect. *New York Times*, 14 Nov 2009. https://www.nytimes.com/2009/11/15/us/15hasan.html?hp

55. Sherwell P, Allen N. Fort Hood shooting inside story of how massacre on military base happened. *The Telegraph*, 7 Nov 2009. https://www.telegraph.co.uk/news/worldnews/northamerica/usa/6521578/Fort-Hood-shooting-inside-story-of-how-massacre-on-military-base-happened.html

56. Fernandez M. Military jury convicts army psychiatrist on all 45 counts in Fort Hood rampage. *New York Times*, 23 Aug 2013. https://www.nytimes.com/2013/08/24/us/fort-hood-shooting-suspect-convicted-on-all-counts.html

57. Christenson S. Hasan ruled sane; faces capital trial. Mysanantonio.com, 26 Jan 2011. https://www.mysanantonio.com/news/military/article/Hasan-ruled-sane-faces-capital-trial-977262.php

58. CBC News. Fort Hood shooter Nidal Hasan sentenced to death. CBC, 28 Aug 2013. https://www.cbc.ca/news/world/fort-hood-shooter-nidal-hasan-sentenced-to-death-1.1391606

TED KACZYNSKI

59. Unabomber (Ted Kaczynski). History.com Editors, 21 Aug 2018. https://www.history.com/topics/crime/unabomber-ted-kaczynski

60. Pilkington E. My brother, the Unabomber. *The Guardian*, 14 Sep 2009. https://www.theguardian.com/world/2009/sep/15/my-brother-the-unabomber

61. Song D. Theodore J. Kaczynski. *Harvard Crimson*, 21 May 2012. https://www.thecrimson.com/article/2012/5/21/ted-kaczynski-unabomber-math/

62. Johnston D. On the suspect's trail: The investigation; long and twisting trail led to Unabom suspect's arrest. *New York Times*, 5 Apr 1996. https://www.nytimes.com/1996/04/05/us/suspect-s-trail-investigation-long-twisting-trail-led-unabom-suspect-s-arrest.html

MIR AIMAL KANSI (KASI)

63. Amal Kasi attacks CIA employees outside Headquarters main gate, killing two people and wounding three. 1/25/93; https://www.cia.gov/legacy/museum/amal-kasi-attacks-cia-employees-outside-headquarters-main-gate/

64. Risen J. Suspect in '93 shooting spree at CIA captured. *LA Times*, 18 Jun 1997. https://www.latimes.com/archives/la-xpm-1997-06-18-mn-4362-story.html

65. Johnston D. How the F.B.I. got its man, half the world away. *New York Times*, 19 Jun 1997. https://www.nytimes.com/1997/06/19/world/how-the-fbi-got-its-man-half-the-world-away.html

66. Serrano RA. Pakistani who killed 2 at CIA is executed. *LA Times*, 15 Nov 2002. https://www.latimes.com/archives/la-xpm-2002-nov-15-na-execute15-story.html

67. FoxNews.com. Pakistani executed for 1993 CIA rampage. 15 Nov 2002; updated 13 Jan 2015. https://www.foxnews.com/story/pakistani-executed-for-1993-cia-rampage

68. Clark Count VA Prosecuting Attorney's Office: MIR AIMAL KASI, 11/15/02. #807. http://www.clarkprosecutor.org/html/death/US/kasi807.htm

69. CNN.com/Law Center. Pakistani man executed for CIA killings. 15 Nov 2002. https://web.archive.org/web/20100323145212/http://archives.cnn.com/2002/LAW/11/14/cia.killings.execution/

70. New York Times. Pakistani defendant pleads not guilty in slayings at C.I.A. 4 Nov 1997. https://www.nytimes.com/1997/11/04/us/pakistani-defendant-pleads-not-guilty-in-slayings-at-cia.html

71. Adams L. Asylum sought by roommate of suspect in CIA shootings. *Washington Post*, 25 Jan 1994. https://www.washingtonpost.com/archive/local/1994/01/25/asylum-sought-by-roommate-of-suspect-in-cia-shootings/11192344-685b-4f9a-9ff3-bffde94e77ea/?utm_term=.c8bf6cd3c283

JARED LOUGHNER

72. Lacey M. Suspect in shooting of Giffords ruled unfit for trial. *New York Times*, 25 May 2011. https://www.nytimes.com/2011/05/26/us/26loughner.html

73. Topping A. Jared Lee Loughner: Army reject with a troubled past. *The Guardian*, 9 Jan 2011. https://www.theguardian.com/world/2011/jan/09/jared-lee-loughner-troubled-past

74. Wagner D. Records detail shooter's agitation before Ariz. rampage. USA Today, 27 Mar 2013; https://www.usatoday.com/story/news/nation/2013/03/27/gabby-giffords-shooting-records/2024589/

75. Jacob J. Who is Jared lee Loughner? *International Business Times,* 10 Jan 2011. https://www.ibtimes.com/who-jared-lee-loughner-253287

76. Potok M. Who is Jared lee Loughner? SPLC Hatewatch, 10 Jan 2011. https://www.splcenter.org/hatewatch/2011/01/09/who-jared-lee-loughner

77. Thompson M. How Jared Loughner changed: The view from his schools. *Time,* 11 Jan 2011. http://content.time.com/time/nation/article/0,8599,2041878,00.html

78. Banfield A, Hooper J, Crews J, Friedman E. Tucson shooting: Jared Loughner stopped for traffic violation hours before shooting. ABC News, 12 Jan 2011. https://abcnews.go.com/US/tucson-shooting-jared-loughner-stopped-authorities-hours-shooting/story?id=12597092

79. CNN Library. Fast Facts: 2011 Tucson shooting. 7 Aug 2012. http://news.blogs.cnn.com/2012/08/07/fast-facts-2011-tuscon-shooting/

OMAR MATEEN

80. Detman G. Omar Mateen had behavioral issues in school, records show. CBS News 12, 16 Jun 2016. https://cbs12.com/news/local/omar-mateen-had-behavioral-issues-in-school-records-show

81. Montgomery B. Before Orlando Massacre, killer Omar Mateen visited parents one last time. *Tampa Bay Times,* 14 Jun 2016. http://www.tampabay.com/news/publicsafety/before-orlando-massacre-killer-omar-mateen-visited-parents-one-last-time/2281507

82. Pilkington E, Roberts D. FBI and Obama confirm Omar Mateen was radicalized on the internet. *The Guardian,* 14 Jun 2016. https://www.theguardian.com/us-news/2016/jun/13/pulse-nightclub-attack-shooter-radicalized-internet-orlando

83. Begley S. Orlando nightclub shooter Omar Mateen was taunted for being Muslim. Time.com, 18 Jul 2016. https://time.com/4411523/orlando-shooting-pulse-nightclub-omar-mateen-muslim/

84. Barry D, Kovaleski SF, Blinder A, Mashal M. "Always agitated. always mad": Omar Mateen, according to those who knew him. *New York Times,* 18 Jun 2016. https://www.nytimes.com/2016/06/19/us/omar-mateen-gunman-orlando-shooting.html

85. Wilber DQ. Orlando gunman was HIV-negative, and probably a long-term steroid user, autopsy shows. *LA Times,* 15 Jul 2016. https://www.latimes.com/nation/la-na-mateen-steroid-hiv-20160715-snap-story.html

86. Stapleton A, Ellis R. Timeline of Orlando nightclub shooting. CNN.com, 17 Jun 2016. https://www.cnn.com/2016/06/12/us/orlando-shooting-timeline/index.html

AHMAD KHAN RAHAMI

87. Shoichet CE, Prokupecz S, Perez E. Ahmad Khan Rahami's wife left US before bombings. CNN, 20 Sep 2016. https://www.cnn.com/2016/09/20/us/ahmad-khan-rahami-wife/

88. Shoichet CE. Ahmad Khan Rahami: What we know about the bombing suspect. CNN, 20 Sep 2016. https://www.cnn.com/2016/09/19/us/ahmad-khan-rahami/index.html

89. Santora M, Goldman A. Ahmad Khan Rahami was inspired by Bin Laden, charges say. *New York Times,* 20 Sep 2016. https://www.nytimes.com/2016/09/21/nyregion/ahmad-khan-rahami-suspect.html

90. Ax J. Accused New York bomber pleads not guilty from hospital bed. Reuters US, 13 Oct 2016. https://www.reuters.com/article/us-usa-attacks-plea-idUSKCN12D2OU

91. Sandoval E, Marcius CR, Rayman G. Cops arrest New Jersey resident Ahmad Khan Rahami, wanted for NYC and N.J. bombings, after he shoots police officer. *NY Daily News,* 20 Sep 2016. http://www.nydailynews.com/new-york/manhattan/man-wanted-nyc-nj-bombings-arrested-shooting-police-officer-article-1.2797960

92. Crimesider Staff. "Chelsea bomber" Ahmad Khan Rahimi gets life in prison for NYC, N.J. blasts. CBS News, 13 Feb 2018. https://www.cbsnews.com/news/chelsea-bomber-ahmad-khan-rahimi-gets-life-in-prison-for-nyc-n-j-blasts/

ELLIOT RODGER

93. Brown B. Santa Barbara County Sheriff's office: Isla Vista mass murder, May 23, 2014. Investigative summary, 18 Feb 2015. https://web.archive.org/web/20150220034256/http://www.sbsheriff.us/documents/ISLAVISTAINVESTIGATIVESUMMARY.pdf

94. Lovett I, Nagourney A. Video rant, then deadly rampage in California town. *New York Times,* 24 May 2014. https://www.nytimes.com/2014/05/25/us/california-drive-by-shooting.html

95. Rodger E. My twisted world: The story of Elliot Rodger. https://www.documentcloud.org/documents/1173808-elliot-rodger-manifesto.html

96. Daily News. Santa Barbara rampage: Stabbing victim identified as Cheng Yuan Hong. *Los Angeles Daily News,* 25 May 2014, updated 28 Aug 2017. https://www.dailynews.com/2014/05/25/santa-barbara-rampage-stabbing-victim-identified-as-cheng-yuan-hong/

97. Medina J. Even in a state with restrictive laws, gunman amassed weapons and ammunition. *New York Times,* 25 May 2014. https://www.nytimes.com/2014/05/26/us/even-in-a-state-with-restrictive-laws-gunman-amassed-weapons-and-ammunition.html

98. CNN Wire. Santa Barbara shooter planned killing spree to exact revenge. Fox 31 and Channel 2 News, 25 May 2014, updated 26 May 2014. https://kdvr.com/2014/05/25/report-deputies-nearly-caught-santa-barbara-shooter-before-his-rampage/

99. White SG, Meloy JR, Mohandie K, Kienlen K. Autism spectrum disorder and violence: Threat assessment issues. *J Threat Assess Manage.* 2017;4(3):144–163.

DYLANN ROOF

100. Robles F, Stewart N. Dylann Roof's past reveals trouble at home and school. *New York Times*, 16 Jul 2015. https://www.nytimes.com/2015/07/17/us/charleston-shooting-dylann-roof-troubled-past.html

101. Blinder A, Sack K. Dylann Roof found guilty in Charleston church massacre. *New York Times*, 15 Dec 2016. https://www.nytimes.com/2016/12/15/us/dylann-roof-trial.html

102. Sack K. Trial documents show Dylann Roof had mental disorders. *New York Times*, 2 Feb 2017. https://www.nytimes.com/2017/02/02/us/dylann-roof-charleston-killing-mental.html

103. Sack K, Blinder A. Anguish, rage and mercy as Dylann Roof is sentenced to death. *New York Times*, 11 Jan 2017. https://www.nytimes.com/2017/01/11/us/dylann-roof-sentencing.html

104. Kinnard M. Dylann Roof to plead guilty to state murder charges, avoiding second death penalty trial. *Chicago Tribune*, 31 Mar 2017. http://www.chicagotribune.com/nation-world/ct-dylann-roof-state-charges-20170331-story.html

105. Levitz J, Kamp J. Charleston shooting suspect Dylan Roof became a loner ini recent years. Wall Street Journal, 6/18/15; https://www.wsj.com/articles/charleston-church-shooting-suspect-dylann-roof-became-a-loner-in-recent-years-1434644808

106. Ball E. The mind of Dylann Roof. *New York Review of Books*, 23 Mar 2017. https://www.nybooks.com/articles/2017/03/23/mind-of-dylann-roof/

107. Norris JJ. Why Dylann Roof is a terrorist under federal law, and why it matters. *Harv J Legis.* 2017;54(1):501–541. https://www.researchgate.net/publication/316218028_Why_Dylann_Roof_is_a_terrorist_under_federal_law_and_why_it_matters

108. Bauerlein V, Levitz J, Kamp J. "Loner" held in Charleston church killings. *Wall Street Journal*, 18 Jun 2015. https://www.wsj.com/articles/charleston-church-shooting-suspect-dylann-roof-in-police-custody-1434642237

ERIC ROBERT RUDOLPH

109. Ross ME. Eric Rudolph's rage was a long time brewing. NBC News, 13 Apr 2005. http://www.nbcnews.com/id/7398701/ns/us_news-crime_and_courts/t/eric-rudolphs-rage-was-long-time-brewing/#.XTdx_zoUmUk

110. Gettleman J, Halbfingerjune DM. Suspect in '96 Olympic bombing and 3 other attacks is caught. *New York Times*, 1 Jun 2003. https://www.nytimes.com/2003/06/01/us/suspect-in-96-olympic-bombing-and-3-other-attacks-is-caught.html

111. Olympic Park bomber Eric Rudolph agrees to plead guilty. History.com, 8 Apr 2005. https://www.history.com/this-day-in-history/olympic-park-bomber-eric-rudolph-agrees-to-plead-guilty

112. CNN Library. Eric Robert Rudolph fast facts. CNN, 4 Sep 2018. https://www.cnn.com/2012/12/06/us/eric-robert-rudolph---fast-facts/index.html

113. FBI information page: Eric Rudolph. https://www.fbi.gov/history/famous-cases/eric-rudolph

114. CNN. Olympic bombing fast facts. CNN, 16 Jul 2018. https://www.cnn.com/2013/09/18/us/olympic-park-bombing-fast-facts/index.html

JOHN SALVI

115. Lemonick MD. An armed fanatic raises the stakes. Time.com, 9 Jan 1995. http://content.time.com/time/magazine/article/0,9171,982287,00.html

116. Golden D, McGrory B. Clinic shooting suspect John Salvi captured. *Boston Globe*, 1 Jan 1995. https://www.bostonglobe.com/metro/1995/01/01/clinic-shooting-suspect-john-salvi-captured/5xfDlnGIUssY3LSnPp5xwO/story.html

117. New York Times News Service. Abortion clinic gunman dies John Salvi, who killed two at Mass. facilities, commits suicide in cell. *Baltimore Sun*, 30 Nov 1996. http://www.baltimoresun.com/news/bs-xpm-1996-11-30-1996335001-story.html

118. Kifner J. Anti-abortion killings: The overview; gunman kills 2 at abortion clinics in Boston suburb. *New York Times*, 31 Dec 1994. https://www.nytimes.com/1994/12/31/us/anti-abortion-killings-overview-gunman-kills-2-abortion-clinics-boston-suburb.html

119. Daly CB. Salvi convicted of murder in shootings. *Washington Post*, 19 Mar 1996. https://www.washingtonpost.com/wp-srv/local/longterm/aron/salvi021996.htm?noredirect=on

120. Koehler R. Murder: The story behind 2 abortion clinic slayings. *LA Times*, 6 Feb 1996. https://www.latimes.com/archives/la-xpm-1996-02-06-ca-32837-story.html

121. Mehren E. Killer of 2 at abortion clinics commits suicide. *LA Times*, 30 Nov 1996. https://www.latimes.com/archives/la-xpm-1996-11-30-mn-4301-story.html

122. Swartz M. Family secret. *The New Yorker*, 9 Nov 1997. https://www.newyorker.com/magazine/1997/11/17/family-secret-2

ANDREW JOSEPH STACK III
123. AP. Friends didn't see pilot's passion for IRS feud. Life on NBS News.com, 18 Feb 2010. http://www.nbcnews.com/id/35469748/ns/us_news-life/t/friends-didnt-see-pilots-passion-irs-feud/#.XP2FxRRKipo

124. Breed AG. Simmering for decades, a Texas engineer's grudge against the IRS explodes into suicidal flight. *LA Times*, 21 Feb 2010. https://web.archive.org/web/20100226191529/http://www.latimes.com/news/nationworld/nation/wire/sns-ap-us-plane-crash-stacks-journey,0,7094353.story?page=1

125. Brick M. Man crashes plane into Texas I.R.S. Office. *New York Times*, 18 Feb 2010. https://www.nytimes.com/2010/02/19/us/19crash.html

3

Clinical Psychiatric and Neuropsychiatric Aspects of Lone-Actor Terrorism

ROBERT P. GRANACHER, JR., DANIELLE B. KUSHNER, AND JACOB C. HOLZER

INTRODUCTION

As reviewed in earlier chapters of this volume, individuals who engage in violence defined as "lone-actor terrorism" vary widely—in background, ideology and the etiological "drive" of their behavior, methodology, and geographic site of the index incident. In addition to these factors, clinical variables are present in at least some cases. These variables include clinical conditions such as schizophrenia, mood and anxiety disorders, personality disorders, traumatic brain injuries, autistic spectrum disorders (ASD) and substance abuse, adjustment difficulties, and psychological trauma and constitute both major/serious mental illness and minor psychiatric or psychological issues. In addition, some reports of cases describe clinical symptoms and experiences that may not meet all the diagnostic criteria for a mental illness. This chapter is divided into two sections: the first section explores a limited number of cases with respect to clinical aspects to highlight the variance in clinical aspects, and the second section reviews different mechanisms, as found in some conditions, which may be relevant in individual cases of lone-actor terrorism. It is important to note that the sections reviewing cases and mechanisms are not meant to imply that these sections are linked (i.e., that the cases reviewed display those mechanisms described). The cases reviewed represent the variance in clinical conditions that may be present. The mechanisms reviewed discuss brain-behavior or psychological processes that may occur in individual lone-actor terrorism cases and may or may not be related to any of the cases described earlier in this chapter.

CLINICAL BACKGROUND

Although this chapter focuses on the relationship of mental illness, mechanisms, and terrorism, the broader medical literature strongly supports the finding that most individuals with psychiatric disorders are not violent. Numerous research studies have shown a complex picture of the relationship between mental illness and violence, with several variables influencing the risk of an individual acting violently, including violence history, substance use, personality disorder, presence of specific psychiatric symptoms, age, gender, and social and personal stressors.[1]

An important concept in this discussion is that the presence of a mental illness in an individual case may or may not have direct relevance to the index incident. In a basic sense, the relationship of an illness to the violent index event may be either causal, associative, or unrelated. A premise of this volume is that it would be very rare to show a causal relationship between illness and a terrorism incident (although a mental illness may play a critical role)—in these rare cases, the individual could be eligible for a "not guilty by reason of insanity" defense (covered in a different chapter). Likewise, it would be very unlikely to actually prove no relationship between mental illness and a terrorism event. It is the author's view that clinical, mental health issues may be one of numerous factors that come together and crystallize in a way that results in an individual moving from "thinking about" acting violently to acting violently. Important *misconceptions* that one needs to be aware of in reviewing this material include (a) the presence of a mental illness means the individual cannot be motivated by an ideological drive, consider and plan out an attack in a thoughtful manner, and carry out that attack in an organized method in order to achieve an end result or goal; (b) that the mental illness "drives" the behavior and incident, in a context that "but for the mental illness, the attack would not have occurred"; and (c) there is a "dichotomy" between lone-actor terrorists who are either mentally ill and the illness is the "primary" driver of behavior and lone-actor terrorists who are psychologically healthy, organized, and driven purely by ideology. In fact, the vast majority of cases encompass individuals with numerous different variables which may play a role in their behavior, including a history of early trauma, domestic violence exposure, substance abuse, maladaptive personality traits, poor academic or occupational functioning, external stressors, past criminality, mental health problems, and/or social isolation or difficulty forming relationships and joining groups. In the right ideological context, with the right triggers, the right social media supports, and the right opportunity, an individual may take it upon himself to act.

A recent study by Corner and Gill[2] revealed that lone actors who were mentally ill were 18.07 times more likely to have a spouse or partner who is involved in a wider movement than those without a history of mental illness. Those with a mental illness were more likely to have a proximate upcoming life change, experienced recent prejudice, and experienced recent and chronic stress. Results of the study support the need to readjust our understanding of terrorism and mental illness in several ways. Their results suggest that there is a stronger association between mental illness and lone-actor terrorists than mental illness in group-based terrorists. This is consistent with the analysis of Gruenewald et al.[3] of extreme right-wing offenders who have caused fatalities in the United States. When Corner and Gill[2] compared lone actors with a history of mental illness to those without, they found that those with a history of mental illness were significantly less likely to have some form of command and control linkage. This research supports the argument that selection effects are at play in the development of terrorism in these lone actors. Other research findings also support the finding of mental illness and selection effects playing a potential role in lone-actor terrorism, although results have been mixed depending on the type of group affiliation. Bijleveld and Hendriks[4] found that lone rapists were significantly more likely to have problematic personality structures than group rapists. Hickle and Roe-Sepowitz,[5] in a study of solo and group

arsonists, found lone juvenile arsonists more often came from unstable homes; experienced school difficulties, behavioral problems, and negative emotions; and expressed suicidal thoughts on a regular basis. Hauffe and Porter[6] suggest differing pathological processes at play between lone and group offenders. Coid et al.[7] found that individuals in gangs collectively demonstrated higher levels of psychiatric morbidity, thus highlighting the complex nature of individuals acting alone versus as part of a group process in the context of criminal and violent behavior.

CASES

Anders Breivik

On the afternoon of July 22, 2011, Anders Breivik killed 77 people in Norway, many of them children and youth, in two separate events. Breivik went through two forensic evaluations. The first concluded he had a psychotic disorder, thus holding him legally *unaccountable*. The first psychiatry examiners concluded that Breivik had schizophrenia, paranoid type.[8] The psychiatrists' report was approved by the Norwegian Board of Forensic Medicine. The second examiners concluded that he had a personality disorder, thus holding him legally *accountable*. In August 2012, the Federal Process of Norway sentenced him to 21 years in prison. If it had been shown that Breivik experienced psychotic symptoms at the time of his crime, then he would have faced trial with a diagnosis of psychosis, and he would not have been regarded as accountable for his actions. In the Norwegian Criminal Procedure Code, when a person exhibits psychotic symptoms associated with a crime, one cannot be attributed *criminal responsibility for action*: "A person is not criminally accountable if psychotic, unconscious, or severely mentally retarded at the time of the crime."[9]

On July 22, 2011, it was a quiet day in Oslo. Breivik detonated a 950-kg fertilizer-based car bomb in the downtown government quarter. This killed eight persons and severely injured nine others. Two hours later, there were reports of gunfire at the summer camp for the Norwegian labor party's youth organization. Breivik had apparently traveled directly from the bomb site to the small island of Utøya, taking a ferry to the island while masquerading as a police officer. He almost immediately started shooting at the approximately 600 persons trapped on the island and killed 69 persons. He used hollow-point expanding ammunition. Survivors reported that he went back to previous victims, shooting them repeatedly, and that several times he persuaded those hidden to come forward by saying he was a policeman. After about 15 minutes of shooting, Breivik called the police stating that he was a commander from the Norwegian Anti-Communist Resistance Movement. Survivors also reported that at times he was laughing and shouting while shooting.[9]

Analysis shortly after Breivik's crime indicates that he was probably acting alone. He was, however, on the periphery of the far right within an anti-Muslin ideological community in Europe with some links and interactions with such groups. He appears to have drawn some ideological sustenance from interactions with these groups, though he seems also to have independently concluded that they were not to be trusted with information, and they did not necessarily share his goals. Other evidence supports that he probably believed he was part of a wider network, but that he did not appear to have much immediate interaction with or knowledge of where these networks were located.[10]

He was evaluated psychiatrically by Drs. Husby and Sórheim. On November 29, 2011, the psychiatrists reported to the court that Breivik was psychotic while planning and implementing his acts and during their evaluation. They later explained during Breivik's trial that this conclusion was based on the central contents of Breivik's thought system. They diagnosed him with paranoid schizophrenia, and some of his most implausible beliefs were regarded as persistent, systematized, bizarre delusions. For instance, one belief that he reported to these examiners was that he was the leader of a Knight's Templar organization, which, according to the Norwegian State Police, did not actually exist.[8] Contents of his delusion also included thoughts that he was a pioneer in a European civil war, and he compared his situation to that of Tsar Nicholas of Russia and Queen Isabella of Spain. He believed it was likely that he could be the new regent in Norway following a coup d'état. He told the psychiatrists that he would decide who should live and who should die in Norway. He believed that several hundred thousand individuals in the Norwegian population supported his deeds. If he became the new regent, he would take the name of Sigurd the Crusader II. The psychiatrists saw these expressions of Breivik as grandiose delusions with bizarre and paranoid qualities that went far beyond conspiracy notions about an Islamist takeover of Europe. They concluded that he had grandiose delusions because of expressions of his own role in this extremist universe. These psychiatrists ultimately concluded that Breivik had schizophrenia, paranoid type,[8] and their report was approved by the Norwegian Board of Forensic Medicine.

Breivik did not want an "insanity defense," and he did not want to evade responsibility or avoid trial. On the contrary, his mass murders were done with the explicit intent of achieving a heavily media-covered trial. The preparations for the trial thus turned into an effort for him to be declared sane, stating he would prefer the death penalty to compulsory treatment.[11]

In January 2013, the Oslo District Court appointed a second pair of psychiatrists for a reevaluation. This was performed in late February to early March 2013, 6 months after the first psychiatric examination. By that time, Breivik had undergone weekly consultations with the prison's psychiatric treatment team since September 2012. He was no longer in isolation, and he had access to the first psychiatric report and to details of the media discussions about his mental health. The core part of the new evaluation was based on the same format as the first evaluation and used the same assessment instruments as the first evaluation, with the exception of the psychiatrists meeting with Breivik separately. An inpatient observation was also performed in the prison by trained psychiatric personnel.[9]

The new evaluator team, along with the observation staff, did not see any signs of gross disorganization or outward signs of auditory hallucinations. They agreed that they were seeing a man with pathological self-aggrandizement. As noted earlier, Breivik had access to the first psychiatric report, and the main difference in his behavior toward the second pair of psychiatrists was that, by this time, he had toned down the importance of the Knights Templar and described himself as a "foot-soldier" doing his duty and suggested that he earlier on had exaggerated his own role.[9] Following the examinations, the new pair of psychiatrists concluded that Breivik's symptoms were due to a severe narcissistic personality disorder combined with pseudologia fantastica (pathological lying).[12] They further concluded that he was not psychotic during their interviews nor at the time of his crimes, thus being legally accountable.

Breivik underwent trial in Oslo District Court from April 16, 2012 to June 22, 2012. In addition to the court-appointed examining psychiatrists, psychiatrists and psychologists were called to testify by Breivik's defense team or by the coordinating counsels for the victims. The verdict was given on August 24, 2012, and, rather extraordinarily for a first-level court verdict, was not appealed. The Court found Breivik accountable and sentenced him to 21 years in preventive custody with a minimum time to serve of 10 years.[9] The Court took as the basis for its verdict the second psychiatric report and the evaluations of other mental health professionals, including witnesses called by Breivik. The Court concluded that Breivik's absurd grandiose notions were non-bizarre and stated that experts on right-wing ideology should have been consulted before deciding that his perceptions of grandeur were culturally implausible.[9] The Court further concluded that Breivik's claim that he knew what others were thinking could as likely be based on his experience as a telephone salesman; his withdrawal and suspiciousness could be a consequence of his terrorist plans; and his odd choice of words could be explained as part of an online war-games/right-wing cultural sphere. The Court concluded that Breivik did not meet International Classification of Disease (ICD-10) criteria for schizophrenia, and defense counsel seemed unaware that he could still meet the *Diagnostic and Statistical Manual of Mental Disorders* (DSM-IV) criteria for schizophrenia.[9]

Melle concludes that the Breivik case shows the importance of the context in which psychiatric evaluations are made.[9] In fact, the Court interpreted diagnostic disagreement, in particular regarding the presence of bizarre delusions, as "differing interpretations of similar observations," ignoring the time difference between the two observations and the different situations in which they took place (particularly Breivik's access to the first psychiatric report before the second psychiatric examination). Melle also noted that some source of confusion might be represented by subtle but relevant differences between ICD-10 and DSM-IV criteria for schizophrenia.[9] Melle discussed an important lesson from the Breivik case: the complexity of forensic evaluations should encourage professionals to be cautious about how they express themselves when taking public positions. In Breivik's case, diagnostic disagreement was front-page news throughout Norway. This conflict added momentum to the newspapers' claims about psychiatric failure, actively supported by persons or groups holding general anti-expert or specific anti-psychiatric views. The central question in the Breivik case was not related to the diagnostic details, but to what it meant not to be accountable due to a mental disorder.[9] The traumatic impact on Norwegian society of Breivik's acts was substantial. The camp where the killings occurred was a meeting place for youth from all over the country, and most knew someone affected by the events.

Nidal Hasan

Nidal Hasan committed the 2009 Fort Hood shooting, killing 13 people and injuring 32 others.[13] Hasan was an Army Medical Corps psychiatrist who was convicted at court martial and unanimously recommended to be dismissed from US military service and sentenced to death. During trial he confessed that radical Islamic beliefs were the motive for the shooting.[14]

Hasan did not have any known history of psychiatric diagnoses or treatment, but there had been concerns regarding his behavior that could be indicative of some underlying pathology. There is no evidence of abuse, bad behavior, or special education as a child, but Hasan was noted to have increasing difficulties following the death of his parents and the 9/11 terror attacks. He struggled in medical school and was granted a leave of absence for family affairs.[15] Subsequently in psychiatric training, colleagues and teachers were reportedly concerned about his job performance and mental health. His behavior was described by various people as "disconnected, aloof, paranoid, belligerent, and schizoid."[16] He reportedly received counseling and extra supervision, but he was not removed from duties or put on probation.[16-18] Family members report that he received anti-Muslim harassment while in the Army following the 9/11 attacks (Hasan was a Muslim). He was also noted to be distressed about his upcoming Army deployment to Afghanistan in the context of his professional hearing of the horrors of war from patients[19] and the potential of joining a war against Islam. Collectively, these factors could have led to underlying emotional instability.

Due to such concerns, during his trial, a psychiatric evaluation was ordered. A military sanity board determined that he did not have a clinical diagnosis when evaluated and was competent to stand trial. Despite concerns regarding the intensity of his religious views, they were not considered delusional according to the psychiatric evaluators.

Ted Kaczynski

The FBI's code name for Kaczynski's case file was UNABOM. These letters denote the targets attacked: UNiversity and Airline BOMbs used in terrorist acts across the United States between 1978 and 1995.[20] Kaczynski's reign of terror lasted nearly 17 years, with his final attack coming only a few days after Timothy McVeigh's assault by explosion on the Alfred P. Murrah federal building in Oklahoma City, Oklahoma.[21]

After years of bombings, the *Washington Post*,[22] on September 22, 1995, published Ted Kaczynski's manifesto "Industrial Society and Its Future." The *Post* article noted that its editors were publishing the text of a 35,000-word manifesto as submitted to the *Washington Post* and the *New York Times* by the serial bomber called the Unabomber. The manifesto appeared in the *Washington Post* as an 8-page supplement that was not part of the news section. The *Washington Post* later published the document with corrections. The original manifesto was sent in to both the *New York Times* and the *Washington Post* in June 1995 by a person calling himself "FC." "FC" was identified by the FBI as the Unabomber. The Attorney General of the United States and the Director of the FBI at the time recommended that this manifesto be published by the newspapers with the hope that someone would recognize the writing style. Ted Kaczynski's brother David recognized the style and took letters and writing samples from his brother to the FBI. The Unabomber was arrested shortly thereafter.

Kaczynski's lawyers were Quin Denver, Judy Clarke, and Gary Sowards. Apparently, they were aware that it would be extremely difficult to convince a jury that Kaczynski was not guilty by reason of insanity, although they felt that his strongest defense would be to allege that his mental status was impaired.[23] Kaczynski considered himself to be sane. He hoped that a trial would be a public forum for an exposition of his anti-technology, Luddite views.[24] Moreover, Kaczynski was deathly afraid that a wrongheaded mental health professional might find him mentally ill; a "sickie" as he put it.[25]

Kaczynski resigned from his position on the mathematics faculty at the University of California at Berkley in 1971 and moved to a one-room cabin in rural Montana. His life has been well chronicled by the *New York Times*.[26] He became convinced that technology was ruining our civilization, and he ultimately began placing bombs around the country from 1978 to 1995. These were alleged to have killed 3 and wounded 23 individuals.

He saw a psychiatrist, David V. Foster. The timeframe is not known and has been assumed to have been after Kaczynski's arrest in April 1996.[24] Dr. Foster published a declaration on his examination of Kaczynski, but he did not give the date of the consultation. Foster stated that the reasons for the consultation were "his oversensitivity to sound, his sleep disturbance, and his fear that his heart might burst from the anxiety of going through his trial."[27] Dr. Foster went on to say: "His paranoia about psychiatrists made it very difficult to broach his psychiatric symptoms with him in a direct way. In fact, early on in our sessions, he looked me in the face and said, 'You are the enemy.'"

Kaczynski also consulted with Karen Bronk Froming, a clinical psychologist.[28] Froming's declaration also does not reveal the dates of the consultations. It is inferred that they occurred after April 1996 because of her statement, "I was asked by the attorneys for Theodore J. Kaczynski to evaluate." Froming also diagnosed Kaczynski with paranoid schizophrenia, consistent with the diagnosis of Dr. Foster.

Kaczynski was arrested in April 1996 and was indicted in June 1996. Kaczynski's lawyers offered a plea bargain in which he would plead guilty to avoid the death sentence. The plea bargain required that he not be committed to a prison psychiatric facility. His counsel served notice that they would allege a mental status defense and would offer expert testimony to back it up. The government requested to have Kaczynski examined by their experts, and the court so ordered, but he refused to submit to another mental examination. At this point, briefs and arguments flowed back and forth. Kaczynski did not get along well with his lawyers and asked for change of counsel, but, on January 7, 1998, he withdrew the request. Judge Burrel, after numerous discussions with Kaczynski in court, finally wrote that he had seen nothing during his contact with him that appeared to be a manifestation of schizophrenia. He stated further, "If anything is present, I cannot detect it."[24] Defense counsel argued to Judge Burrel that Kaczynski's inability to endure presentation of his mental status defense was prima facie evidence of his incompetence. The Judge responded that he had seen no evidence that Kaczynski was incompetent.

Sally Johnson, MD, flew from the US East Coast at the Court's request to examine Kaczynski, as he resided in California at that time.[29] She diagnosed him as suffering from paranoid schizophrenia. On the basis of Dr. Johnson's report, Kaczynski's defense team stipulated he was competent to stand trial. Dr. Johnson obtained a Minnesota Multiphasic Personality Inventory (MMPI-2) on Kaczynski during her examination. As a result of this testing, significant conflict has arisen within the psychological community. Yossef Ben-Porath from Kent State University and author of the most recent version of the MMPI, argued on the misuse of Kaczynski's MMPI, a statement which was published in the *Journal of Personality Assessment*.[30] He described a series of errors of omission and commission, which were identified in an article by Butcher et al. in an effort to criticize the MMPI-2-RF.[31] Ben-Porath summarized Butcher et al.'s description of Kaczynski's MMPI-2 profile and concluded that it was invalid due to a high Fp score. He also criticized that Butcher et al. did not follow-up all the MMPI scores that were discussed, as required to properly interpret the protocol. From the MMPI provided from Dr. Johnson's examination, Ben-Porath noted that it indicated findings of severe mental health problems, paranoia, and delusions. Ben-Porath also argued that Butcher et al. incorrectly claimed that Kaczynski's profile was "very consistent with past research on mass murderers," citing sources that contradicted their claims. Butcher et al. made an extremely strong argument in their self-defense.[31]

Because Ted Kaczynski accepted the plea agreement, the issue of sanity was never determined, and the trial never occurred. He pleaded guilty to 13 federal bombing offenses.[20] He was later sentenced to life in prison without the possibility of parole, and he currently remains within a maximum-security prison in Colorado. He maintains his belief system and continues his prolific writing. Kaczynski has been categorized as a domestic lone-actor terrorist.[32]

Omar Mateen

Omar Mateen, also known as Omar Mir Seddique, orchestrated the Orlando Pulse gay nightclub attack in June 2016, killing 49 people and injuring 53 others. Theories for the motivation behind the crime include Islamic extremist and anti-LGBT beliefs.[33,34] Mr. Mateen was killed by police during the incident.

Mateen was born in New York to parents of Afghan descent. Despite minimal contact with the mental health system, collateral information reported concerns for underlying psychiatric issues. In elementary and middle school, records showed that Mateen displayed aggressive and verbally abusive behavior, struggled academically, and required repeated interventions from teachers and school psychologists. His third-grade teacher described him as being "verbally abusive, rude, aggressive, and [engaging in] much talk about violence."[33] In high school, his disruptive behavior continued, requiring him to attend multiple schools. He was arrested and charged

for battery and disrupting school business after a fight in class and was suspended for terrorist threats, among other infractions.[35,36] Following his graduation from community college, he was noted to have drifted in jobs. He was a recruit for the Florida Department of Corrections. On his application process, he acknowledged previous arrests and use of marijuana and steroids.[37] He was involuntarily dismissed from the program due to failing to pay attention in class and making a threat to bring a gun to school.[38] He later worked with a security firm after completing an MMPI-2 psychological assessment.[39] While on the job, his assignment was changed following threatening statements regarding al-Qaeda that he made toward co-workers.[36]

Mateen's first wife reported to the media that he was "mentally unstable" and that he was physically and verbally abusive. She additionally reported that he was "bipolar" and would "get mad out of nowhere," but no evidence of full manic or bipolar symptoms have been noted in other records or statements, and no previous treatment has been noted.[40] Similar reports of abuse were also noted by his second wife.

Dylann Roof

Dylann Roof was the perpetrator of the 2015 Charleston church shooting in which nine African American parishioners were killed and three were injured. The motive behind the shooting was white extremist and neo-Nazi beliefs that were outlined in his website and manifesto. Roof was convicted and received the death penalty in federal court and life without parole in state court.

Reports indicate Roof had a stressful upbringing, with intrafamily conflict. According to an affidavit filed for his father's divorce, Roof exhibited "obsessive compulsive behavior" during his childhood and was noted to be reportedly obsessive over germs and his haircut.[41] He attended several different schools, eventually dropping out after repeating the ninth grade, but he later earned his GED online. He was noted to have been caught using marijuana in middle school.[42]

In the year prior to the incident, Roof showed increasingly odd behavior. There has been no report of previous mental health treatment, but collateral information showed ongoing concern for underlying psychiatric issues. Co-workers where he worked for two months in 2014–2015 reported that Roof "often spaced or zoned out while working" and would sit by himself, falling asleep anytime he was stationary. Roof reported being isolated and having minimal hobbies or activities. In February 2015, a psychologist reached out to him following a racist Craigslist post. Roof refused his help, stating, "I am in bed, so depressed I cannot get out of bed. My life is wasted. I have no friends even though I am cool. I am going back to sleep."[43] In March–April 2015, he had three encounters with police for loitering or trespassing. During one incident, he was noted to be in possession of buprenorphine (Naloxone, Suboxone) and was charged with a misdemeanor.[43]

Additional concerns for psychiatric symptoms were noted during trial, despite Roof wanting to avoid any mental health defense. Per unsealed court documents, his lawyers requested a competency evaluation due to concerns that Roof focused on nonessential details, had trouble processing multiple sources of information, demonstrated extreme need for predictability, became easily overwhelmed and anxious when things could not be predicted, and had difficulty retaining information when required to focus on multiple things.[44,45] There was also a report of concerns for delusional thoughts regarding a fixed belief that he would eventually be pardoned following a white nationalist takeover of the United States.[46] He was ultimately found fit to proceed twice and was allowed to represent himself at the sentencing phase of his trial. Court documents reported that the court-appointed psychiatrist diagnosed him with "schizoid personality disorder, substance abuse disorder, depression by history, and a possible autistic spectrum disorder" given his history of substance use, recent report of depressed mood, and lack of a social network.[43] Roof's defense team offered evidence for autism at a competency hearing stating that "the defendant's high IQ is compromised by a significant discrepancy between his ability to comprehend and to process information and a poor working memory."[44]

MECHANISMS

The preceding series of cases are meant to highlight the disparate nature of individuals committing mass violence in the context of some identified ideology or cause. In preliminary research by one author (JH) of a large series of high-profile lone-actor terrorists across a spectrum of ideologies, clinical variables were very common and spanned a range of symptoms and diagnoses, including mood disorders, psychotic disorders, substance use, brain injury, personality disorders, development disorders, etc. This section discusses some of the underlying clinical mechanisms which may be seen in lone-actor terrorism cases.

The Neuroscience of Evil

Scholars, for the past few decades, have attempted to classify and define evil, particularly as related to terrorism, yet we remain today with no widely accepted definition. Hervey Cleckley attempted to define evil associated with psychopathy in his classic text, *Mask of Sanity* (1950).[47] Cleckley's book improved our knowledge of the nature of psychopathy, yet not all psychopaths are terrorists or murderers. Social psychiatrist Joel Dimsdale recently completed a 40-year review of records and interviews with principals in the Nuremburg trials.[48] Dr. Dimsdale had access to the Nuremburg archives, the records of the psychiatrists and psychologists who repeatedly interviewed Nazi war criminals, and even Rorschach test interpretations of Nazi defendants. What this astute and lengthy analysis revealed was that most of the Nazi war criminals were not significantly mentally ill. Many could be categorized as malicious, but not necessarily mentally ill.

Stone, a psychiatrist and psychoanalyst, provides psychoanalytic perspectives on evil but also a significant section on recent scientific findings regarding evil.[49] Stone has developed a paradigm for examining personality disorders where psychopathic personality, antisocial personality disorder, sadistic personality, and schizoid personality converge. He opines that there are some cruel and demeaning parents, spouses, and bosses who are sadistic, but who are not necessarily antisocial or psychopathic, or even evil. But acts of evil and murder are often committed by psychopathic-sadistic-schizoid persons.[49]

Raine has conducted an elegant brain study of two different types of murderers: the predatory versus the affective.[50] This is akin to the distinctions made between those who kill methodically and with malice and forethought and those who kill on impulse during some emotional crisis. Positron emission tomography (PET) showed that the more impulsive killers (affective) showed lower prefrontal functioning and heightened subcortical function.[50] This suggested that, for these men, their drives were stronger than their "brakes" (their ability to monitor and inhibit violent ambitions). Predatory killers had prefrontal function that was near normal, though their drive strength was abnormally high, as in the impulsive killers. In other words, predators were more able to plot and scheme successfully, thus lowering their risk of becoming rash and getting caught.[50] Raine, in a later study, used magnetic resonance volumetric imaging to measure the white and gray matter volume in the prefrontal cortex of antisocial men and several control groups.[51] This study rocked the scientific world for those who study psychopathy. The antisocial men showed a substantial (11%) reduction in prefrontal gray matter volume versus controls. This deficit was the first evidence found for structural differences in the brains of antisocial men and helped to explain the low arousal, tendency to boredom, and the need for novelty and thrill-seeking that are well-known characteristics of antisocial and psychopathic men.

It is not clear that the models of neuropsychiatric abnormality found in antisocial persons and psychopaths who have been studied are found in lone-actor terrorists. Neurobiological research application in terrorism is in its infancy. A look at the nature of *acquired sociopathy* may add further to our neuropsychiatric knowledge[52] of those who are involved in evil. In one recent study of vulnerability to violent extremism using functional imaging techniques, Pretus et al. found that research participants in a study design assessing willingness to fight and die for an "in group sacred value" who were believed to be vulnerable to recruitment into violent extremism had significant activity on imaging in the left inferior frontal brain region.[53]

Phineas Gage is the poster child for acquired sociopathy/psychopathy. He fell victim to this acquired disorder while working on the Vermont Railroad in the 1840s. Tamping a dynamite hole caused an explosion, which blew a 3½-foot long iron tamping rod under his left zygomatic facial bone and out the top of his skull and, in the process, harmed the ventromedial prefrontal cortex (vmPFC).[54] This small piece of tissue is found deep in the middle part of the brain, within the prefrontal cortex above the eyes. It is part of a connected pathway brain system (the orbito-fronto-striato-pallidal [OFSP] brain system), which underlies morality.[55] The vmPFC appears to be a critical component of the OFSP pathway, and, in fact, the right-sided component of the vmPFC system is probably more critical than the left-sided component to social conduct, decision-making, and emotional processing.[56] Even though at this time science has not sufficiently studied terrorists to determine the nature of their OFSP and vmPFC, research has shown a significant moral center in normally functioning human beings, and abnormalities in those neuroanatomical areas are found in those with antisocial and psychopathic traits. It is hoped that as science progresses in the future, there may be studies of terrorists that elucidate the functional neuroanatomical correlates of their behaviors.

Alterations in Frontal Brain Systems

A large proportion of persons who join terrorist groups, as well as lone-acting terrorists, have a history of violent behaviors or mental disorders that predated their becoming terrorists. This suggests that brain alterations found to occur in violent perpetrators may also be present in a significant percentage of terrorists. Depending on the subtype of violence (impulsive or instrumental, affective or predatory), deviations in structure or function have been mainly found in prefrontal, orbitofrontal, and insular cortex, as well as in temporolimbic structures (e.g., the amygdala, hippocampus, and parahippocampus). These brain areas are essentially responsible for the control of the archaic neuroneuronal generators of aggression located in the hypothalamus and limbic system. This regional distribution of brain alterations also shows a remarkable overlap and connectivity with those brain regions that are crucial for such prosocial traits as empathy and compassion.[57] Feelings of superiority, dominance, and satisfaction gained by performing violent and terroristic attacks suggests a hedonistic component via an activation of brain reward systems and plays an additional role.

The prefrontal cortex (PFC) subserves decision-making and executive control. It is postulated that the PFC comprises two arbitration systems: (1) a peripheral system comprising premotor/caudal PFC and orbitofrontal regions involved in the selection of actions based on perceptual cues and reward values, respectively, and embedded in behavioral sets associated with external contingencies inferred as being stable; and (2) a core system comprising ventromedial, dorsomedial, lateral, and polar PFC regions involved in superordinate probabilistic reasoning for arbitrating between exploiting/adjusting previously learned behavioral sets and exploring/creating new ones for efficient adaptive behavior in a variable and open-ended environment.[58] This provides a theoretical framework, whereby simple choices (such as those involved in terrorism) use a peripheral PFC system including the lateral premotor and medial orbital frontal cortex. The latter drives the selection of motor responses (such as those involved in carrying an explosive vest) in direct association with stimuli and expected rewards (such as Paradise or an extremist-interpreted reward). The caudal inferior prefrontal cortex has the capacity to abstract multiple stimulus–response and response–outcome associations into action sets. This enables the brain to collectively select multiple associations according to external cues and expected outcomes for carrying out behavioral plans such as an explosion that will kill bystanders but also send the perpetrator to a place of perpetual pleasure.

For those terrorists who meet criteria for antisocial personality disorder (APD), let us not forget that Raine et al. (2000) first showed that the prefrontal gray matter volume in APD persons shows an average 11% reduction in the absence of apparent brain lesions, and this also is associated with reduced autonomic activity during stressors.[51] This explains the calmness often seen during the performance of antisocial acts.

Raine et al. (1998) previously demonstrated, using PET scanning, that predatory murderers had prefrontal functioning with excessively high rates of cortical activity.[50] Their results support the hypothesis that emotional, impulsive murderers who do not plan their attacks are less able to regulate and control aggressive impulses generated from subcortical structures due to deficient prefrontal regulation. It was hypothesized by Raine et al. (1998) that excessive subcortical activity predisposes aggressive behavior, but that while predatory murderers have sufficient prefrontal functioning to regulate these aggressive impulses, when compared to affective murderers, the affective murderers show a reduction in prefrontal control over emotional regulation.[50]

William Casebeer has spent his professional life identifying the neural mechanisms of moral cognition. Like the topics previously mentioned, moral cognition arises in the prefrontal areas of the brain. There is connectivity between limbic areas and the PFC. Research on the role of the PFC and moral judgment has become an important research area in moral cognition, social judgment, and theory of mind (TOM).[59] Our ability to know what others are thinking so that we can interact fruitfully with them is vital. It underlies our ability to empathize with others, judge how they might react in response to our actions, and predict the subjective consequences of our actions for specific features (as in TOM). This ability/capacity—to empathize, judge responses, and predict consequences, appears to be suppressed or absent in the minds of lone-actor terrorists.

Understanding the functional neuroanatomy and connectivity of moral cognition is one thing, but to understand it in terrorists is another. Baez et al.[60] attempted that in a study of the moral judgments and social-cognitive profiles of 66 ex-combatants from a paramilitary terrorist group. Their study found that moral judgment in terrorists is abnormally guided by outcomes rather than by the integration of intentions and outcomes. They also found that moral judgment was the measure that best discriminated between terrorists and non-criminals. As might be expected, the results of this study provide evidence of distorted moral cognition in extreme terrorists. They found that terrorists exhibited a nonstandard pattern, and, unlike non-criminals, they judged attempted harm by focusing on a neutral outcome rather than on the protagonistic negative intention. Similarly, they judged accidental harm by focusing on the negative outcome without considering the neutral intention. This moral judgment pattern resembles that observed in early developmental stages. The authors believe their results suggest that terrorists' moral judgment is characterized by an overreliance on outcomes rather than by the integration of intentions and outcomes. In fact, terrorists judged attempted harm as more permissible and accidental harm as less permissible than did non-criminals. Terrorists from this study considered accidental harm to be more morally wrong than attempted harm. Moreover, the authors concluded that their results support the proposal that terrorists can suppress instinctive and learned moral constraints against harming innocents that arise from such traits as empathy, fairness, and prosociality.[61]

Baez et al. indicate that the results of their study reveal that terrorists judge others' actions by focusing on the outcomes, suggesting that their moral code prioritizes ends over means. Thus, impairments in processing intentions and in integrating them with action outcomes may be one of the key social cognitive factors underlying the cruel acts committed by terrorist paramilitary groups. It is not clear whether the same psychological factors are at play at an individual level.[60]

Mario Mendez (2009) produced a seminal article on the neurobiology of moral behavior.[62] Mendez proffers that morality may be innate to the human brain. Studies reviewed by him indicate a "neuromoral" network for responding to moral dilemmas, centered in the vmPFC and its connections, particularly in the right frontal area of the brain. The neurobiological evidence indicates the existence of automatic "prosocial" mechanisms for identification with others that are part of the moral brain.[62] Terrorists may have either a suspension or an absence of this prosocial mechanism.

In an interesting study of brain lesion localization associated with criminal behavior using lesion network mapping, results showed support for a neurobiological substrate for criminality.

Although the findings are not necessarily specific for terrorism, there is broad application for criminal behavior, and earlier research has reported a high prevalence of distal criminal behavior in lone-actor terrorists.[63] Darby et al. found that these lesion sites were heterogeneous but tended to involve specific brain regions—the medial PFC, the orbitofrontal cortex, and different locations in the bilateral temporal lobes. An important finding was that all the lesion sites were functionally connected to the same neural network of brain regions. Darby et al. indicate that this criminal behavior–associated pattern was unique compared with other neuropsychiatric syndromes and involved regions of the brain identified with morality, value-based decision-making, and TOM, but did not involve brain regions involved in cognition or empathy.[63]

Autism Spectrum Disorders

The core symptoms of autism were first described in 1943, by child psychiatrist Leo Kanner, and in 1944, by pediatrician Hans Asperger.[64,65] Most recently, DSM-5[66] adopted the term *autism spectrum disorder*, focusing on a dyad of symptoms: difficulties in social communication and social interaction and restricted and repetitive behavior, interests, and activities. Previous definitions also included atypical language development as a core criterion, but now this is classified as a co-occurring condition.[66]

The prevalence of ASD has been steadily increasing since the first epidemiological study in the United Kingdom in 1966, partly due to changes in diagnostic criteria, increased recognition of the disorder, and younger age at diagnosis.[67] The US Centers for Disease Control (CDC) estimated that 1 in 59 children were affected in 2018 and that ASD is about four times more common among boys than girls.[68] More than 70% of individuals with autism have co-occurring psychiatric, medical, or developmental conditions. Most commonly, 45% of individuals with autism have intellectual disability. Other common comorbidities include language disorders, attention deficit hyperactivity disorder (ADHD), anxiety, depression, psychosis, and aggressive or self-injurious behaviors, among others.[69] Higher childhood intelligence, communicative phrase speech before 6 years of age, and fewer childhood social impairments predict a better outcome.[70]

Those with high functioning subtypes of autism, previously known as Asperger's disorder, show normal speech and language and average or above average intelligence but atypical development of social reasoning and intuitions. This group, along with all individuals with ASD, is deficient in several social domains, including social reciprocity, developing and maintaining peer relationships, and nonverbal cue use and recognition. They are also noted to be deficient in TOM, the ability to understand and represent the mental states of others.[71]

Recent high-profile violent events have raised concern about the link between ASD and violent crime. Some case reports have suggested an increased violence risk in individuals with ASD compared to the general population, but prevalence studies have provided no conclusive evidence to support this risk.[72] Further research has instead shown a potential risk of aggression rather than criminal behavior in ASD.[73] In review of the case literature, researchers found evidence that several core non-diagnostic features, including TOM deficits, poor emotional regulation, and impaired moral reasoning, may interact to increase the risk of violence in those with ASD and high-functioning subtypes of autism.[71,72] Additionally, it appears that most ASD individuals who commit violent crime also have various co-occurring psychiatric conditions, including obsessive-compulsive disorder, ADHD, conduct disorder, psychosis, depression, and alcohol and drug use disorders.[72,74,75] Psychosis in particular is linked to increased rates of aggression in both autistic and non-autistic samples.[76] Additional associational factors, such as younger age, Asperger's diagnosis, and repetitive behavior, have additionally been associated with violent behavior in autistic individuals.[72] An association with trauma has also been hypothesized.[77]

The current research regarding ASD and violence has produced minimal studies on terrorism in particular. Early terrorism research is beginning to show that lone-actor terrorism, compared to group terrorism, has some association with mental illness and that ASDs have a higher than expected prevalence in lone-actor terrorists than in the general population.[78] Case studies of individuals with autism have been presented that demonstrate the relationship between certain ASD symptoms and terrorist operations and acts. Developing fixated interest in terrorism, a desire to relate to others, and a deficit in being able to critically analyze the beliefs of a social group may be the highest risk factors leading to autistic individuals being used or recruited by terrorists.[79] Further research is needed to fully explore this association.

Personality Disorders

A personality disorder is defined as a way of thinking, feeling, and behaving that deviates from the expectations of the culture, causes distress or problems functioning, and persists over time.[66] A salient feature of personality disorders is impaired self-identity and interpersonal functioning. A clinical diagnosis of personality disorder includes the presence of (a) a persistent, inflexible, pervasive pattern of maladaptive traits; (b) significant distress or impaired functioning; and (c) relative stability and early onset of the pattern.[80] There are several different types of personality disorders, including *antisocial* (a pattern of disregarding the rights of others, not conforming to social norms), borderline (pattern of instability in relationships, intense emotions, poor self-image and impulsivity), *narcissistic* (pattern of need for admiration and lack of empathy for others), *paranoid* (pattern of being suspicious of others), *schizoid* (pattern of detachment from social relationships and expressing little emotion), and *schizotypal* (pattern of being very uncomfortable in close relationships, having distorted thinking and eccentric behavior).[66] These categories are not rigid; some people can have mixed personality disorders, and some people can experience the limited maladaptive traits present in a disorder with less of an impact on day-to-day functioning. Some of the more serious disorders that meet DSM criteria, including antisocial, borderline, and narcissistic, however, have obvious adverse impact on people who experience them and others around them.

The relationship between mental illness and terrorism has been controversial,[81] and earlier research into this relationship may have been limited by poor study design. Research examining the relationship between mental illness and terrorism conducted by lone-actors does in fact support a complex number of variables which may be relevant in this relationship, including clinical variables.[82] One study examined 153 lone-actor terrorists and noted a diverse range of psychiatric disorders, including traumatic brain injury, drug dependence, schizophrenia, delusional disorder, mood and anxiety disorders, dissociative disorder, posttraumatic stress disorder (PTSD), personality disorders, and ASDs. The authors noted that schizophrenia, delusional disorder, and ASDs were more prevalent than in the general population.[83] In a recent study examining mental illness and lone-actor terrorism, the authors reported that the prevalence of mental illness in the lone actor group was within the range of 30% to 50%, co-morbidity of mental illness was prevalent, personality disorders were present as one clinical category, and lone actors rarely had prior contact with mental health services.[84]

In examining the nexus of mental illness and lone-actor terrorism, an important consideration is inclusion of other variables in addition to clinical factors, which together may drive the act of terrorism, including personal historical factors, interpersonal factors, external stressors (i.e., work, finances, relationships), the influence of social media, criminality, access to weapons and the means of committing violence, etc. Trying to draw a straight-line connection between mental illness and terrorism does not take into consideration a myriad of other important variables and influences. Another important consideration is that the presence of mental illness does not portend the lone-actor being irrational and unstable. Corner and Gill discuss that a false dichotomy may exist that categorizes violent individuals as either a rational terrorist or an irrational and unstable individual. They report that the odds of a lone-actor terrorist having a mental illness is 13.49 times higher than the odds of a group actor having a mental illness.[2]

The study of personality traits and disorders in relation to terrorism has been challenging. In 2012, Monahan described that no study to date reported specific personality traits able to distinguish those engaging in terrorism from those who refrain from terrorism.[85] As in the study of other mental disorders and behaviors related to terrorism and mass violence, more recent research examining personality traits underscores that these acts may be based on a complex combination of psychopathology, personal circumstance, and environment.[86] Based on his research, Spaaij described findings, consistent with other reports in the literature, that lone actors tend to have a greater tendency to suffer mental health issues than do individuals involved in group terrorism and that there is a higher likelihood of lone-actors having personality disorders, reporting in a case series that four out of five had a diagnosis of a personality disorder.[87,88] Underscoring the importance of clinical variables in the study of terrorism, the US National Institute of Justice (NIJ) reported that several risk factors or indicators associated with terrorism overlapped with some of the risk factors identified in the Historical Clinical Risk Management-20, Version 3. Although the category of a history of problems with a personality disorder was not identified, possible maladaptive traits were identified, including problems with violence, antisocial behavior, problems with relationships, problems with occupation, and social isolation.[89] Reports of maladaptive personality traits or disorders in relation to lone-actor terrorism cases include John Allen Muhammad,[90] Anders Breivik,[91] Timothy McVeigh,[92,93] Ted Kaczynski,[93] Cesar Sayoc,[94] James T. Hodgkinson,[95] Micah Johnson,[96] Lee Oswald,[97] and David Copeland.[98]

Psychosis

Psychosis is a serious mental health condition individuals experience an altered sense of reality. Psychosis is comprised of a set of symptoms, which can include confused thinking, hallucinations (such as perceived auditory or visual stimuli that do not really exist), and delusions (fixed false beliefs); causes of psychosis include serious psychiatric disorders such as schizophrenia and severe mood disorders, certain substances and medications, and various medical and neurological conditions.[99] Although the medical literature does not show a relationship between psychosis and violence in most patients, and in fact patients who are psychotic or schizophrenic are instead at risk for being victimized, there is a complex relationship between psychosis and violence. Dynamic modifiable risk factors for violence in patients with psychosis include comorbid alcohol and substance abuse, treatment nonadherence, impaired insight, impulsiveness, anger, and hostility, along with adverse experiences (such as being a target of violence).[100] In a study examining serious violence in first-episode psychosis, associated variables included being male, younger, comorbid antisocial personality disorder, and drug use.[101] In this research, three types of delusions were associated with serious violence: those whose content involved being spied on, persecuted, or the object of a conspiracy. Anger due to such threatening delusions was significantly associated with serious violence.[101] Reports have shown a small but significant relation between schizophrenia and violence.[102]

Individual lone-actor terrorism case reports have raised concern for psychosis and schizophrenia in a very limited number of cases (JH research). For example, in the 2018 case of Faisal Hussain, who opened fire in Toronto Canada, killing two and injuring several people, his family later reported that he had struggled with psychosis and depression.[103] Jared Loughner, who killed and wounded numerous people in Tucson, Arizona, including critically wounding Congresswoman Gabrielle Giffords in January 2011, was found to meet criteria for schizophrenia and found incompetent to stand trial during forensic mental health evaluations.[104] News reports describe Aaron Alexis as experiencing psychotic symptoms prior to his attack at the Washington Navy Yard in September 2013.[105,106] David Copeland, convicted of the 1999 London nail bombings, was diagnosed with schizophrenia during his forensic psychiatry evaluations, although this diagnosis was controversial and did not result in a finding of insanity.[98]

As reviewed earlier, it is important to consider the relationship between mental illness and violence in individual cases. Although a person may have a history of psychosis or have active psychotic symptoms at the time of the violent incident, there may or may not be a direct association between the psychosis (or clinical symptoms) and the violent behavior. Possible scenarios include no relationship, an association (such as disinhibition or reduced judgment), or a causal relationship. If in fact a relationship exists, there may still not be a basis, in the legal context, for diminished responsibility or a finding of not guilty by reason of insanity (reviewed elsewhere in this volume chapter 13), which would involve the mental illness having a direct effect on cognition (resulting in lack of capacity to appreciate criminality) or behavior (resulting in being unable to conform conduct to the requirements of the law). Although the literature does not support a direct link between serious mental illness and lone-actor terrorism in most cases, there is stronger support for a link between mental health problems and radicalization,[107] an important element in the development of lone-actor terrorism.

Multivariable

In lone-actor cases, and as supported by the literature,[108,109] a large number of variables come together or crystallize in a specific environment and at the right time to result in a terrorism incident. From a clinical perspective, a prime example of a mass violence incident involving the convergence of multiple variables was the 2012 Kandahar Massacre. On March 11, 2012, Robert Bales killed numerous men, women, and children in villages in Kandahar Province. He pleaded guilty to multiple counts of murder, assault, and attempted murder and was sentenced to life without parole. Although from the perspective of the definition of lone-actor terrorism an underlying ideological cause was not apparent in the literature, a number of distal and proximal variables to this incident are important to consider as an example of how these variables may interact and lead to mass violence. News reports described a wide range of clinical variables in Bale's background and character leading to the incident,[110–117] including (1) a history of aggressive behavior; (2) run-ins with law enforcement; (3) being under financial stress, along with later distress due to his military assignment in Afghanistan; (4) PTSD symptoms; (5) a history of traumatic brain injuries; (6) use of alcohol, sedative-hypnotics, and steroids; and (7) use of the anti-malarial mefloquine. Although issues related to the insanity defense and mitigation are not addressed here, this section is meant to highlight the importance of considering how what appears to be disparate elements or variables may come together to increase the risk of a mass violence incident.

CONCLUSION

This chapter reviews case examples of individual lone-actor terrorism where mental health—clinical psychiatric and psychological issues—may have played a role. It also discusses different underlying mechanisms which may apply in lone-actor cases. A key theme in this chapter is the wide range of clinical symptoms, disorders, and mechanisms that need to be considered in individual cases. As highlighted, major mental illness may be a factor in a limited number of cases, but the presence of some clinical variable or component appears more ubiquitous, and, from a clinical perspective, underlying processes such as brain network dysfunction, a developmental disorder, maladaptive personality, or psychosis are examples of a wide range of mechanisms to consider.

NOTES AND REFERENCES

1. Harvard Mental Health Letter. Mental illness and violence, Jan 2011. https://www.health.harvard.edu/newsletter_article/mental-illness-and-violence
2. Corner E, Gill P. A false dichotomy? Mental illness and lone-actor terrorism. *Law Hum Behav.* 2015;39(1): 23–34.
3. Gruenewald J, Organ J, Freilich JD. Distinguishing "loner" attacks from other domestic extremist violence: A comparison of far-right homicide. Incident and offender characteristics. *Criminol Public Policy.* 2013;12:65–91. doi:10.1111/1745-9133.12009.
4. Bijleveld C, Hendriks J. Juvenile sex offenders: Differences between group and solo offenders. *Psychol Crime Law.* 2003;9:237–245. doi:10.1080/106831602100003568.
5. Hickle KE, Roe-Sepowitz DE. Female juvenile arsonists: An exploratory look at characteristics in solo and group arson offenses. *Legal Criminological Psychol.* 2010;15:385–399. doi:10.1348/135532509X473913.
6. Hauffe S, Porter, L. An interpersonal comparison of lone and group rape offences. *Psychol Crime Law.* 2009; 15(5):469–491. doi:10.1080/10683160802409339.
7. Coid JW, Ullrich S, Keers R, et al. Gang membership, violence, and psychiatric morbidity. *Am J Psychiatry.* 2013;170:985–993. doi:10.1176/appi.ajp.2013.12091188.
8. Bortolotti L, Broome MR, Mameli M. Delusions and responsibility for action: Insights from the Breivik case. *Neuroethics.* 2014;7:377–382. doi:10.1007/s12152-013-9198-4.
9. Melle I. The Breivik case and what psychiatrists can learn from it. *World Psychiatry.* 2013;12(1):16–21.
10. Pantucci R. What have we learned about lone wolves from Anders Behring Breivik? *Perspect Terrorism.* 2011;5(5–6):27–42.
11. BBC News World. Norway massacre: Breivik declared insane. 2011. www.bbc.co.uk
12. Newmark N, Adityanjee KJ. Pseudologia fantastica and factitious disorder: Review of the literature and a case report. *Comprehens Psychiatry.* 1999;40:89–95.
13. McFadden RD. Army doctor held in Ft. Hood rampage. *New York Times*, 5 Nov 2009. https://www.nytimes.com/2009/11/06/us/06forthood.html
14. Allen N. "I am the shooter": US army major Nidal Hasan declares as he faces court martial over Fort Hood massacre. *The Telegraph*, 6 Aug 2013. https://www.telegraph.co.uk/news/worldnews/northamerica/usa/10226875/I-am-the-shooter-US-army-major-Nidal-Hasan-declares-as-he-faces-court-martial-over-Fort-Hood-massacre.html
15. Levin A. Psychiatrist reports inside view of Fort Hood killer's evaluation. *Psychiatric News*, 9 Jun 2016. https://psychnews.psychiatryonline.org/doi/10.1176/appi.pn.2016.6b10
16. Zwerdling D. Walter Reed officials asked: Was Hasan psychotic? National Public Radio, 11 Nov 2009. https://www.npr.org/templates/story/story.php?storyId=120313570
17. Gearan A. Army: Shooting suspect was bound for Afghanistan. *San Diego Union-Tribune*, 6 Nov 2009. https://www.sandiegouniontribune.com/sdut-army-shooting-suspect-was-bound-for-afghanistan-2009nov06-story.html
18. Fort Hood suspect's religion was an issue, family says. CNN, 7 Nov 2009. http://www.cnn.com/2009/CRIME/11/06/fort.hood.suspect.muslim/
19. Dao J. Suspect was "mortified" about deployment. *New York Times*, 5 Nov 2009. https://www.nytimes.com/2009/11/06/us/06suspect.html

20. Kushner H. *Encyclopedia of Terrorism*. Thousand Oaks, CA: Sage;2003.

21. Gall JM. Domestic lone wolf terrorists: An examination of patterns and domestic lone wolf targets, weapons, and ideologies. Dissertation. Fairfax, VA: George Mason University;2014.

22. FC. Industrial society and its future. *Washington Post*. 22 Sep 1995; https://www.washingtonpost.com/wp-srv/national/longterm/unabomber/manifesto.text.htm

23. Jackson DS. At his own request: Is Kaczynski's rejection of his best chance for a defense a result of paranoid schizophrenia: *Time*. 2 Jan, 1998:40.

24. Newman JS. Doctors, lawyers, and the Unabomber. *Montana Law Review*. 1999;60:1–34.

25. Klaidman DK, King P. Suicide mission. *Newsweek*. 19 Jan 1998:22.

26. McFadden RD. Prisoner of rage: A special report: From a child of promise to the Unabomb suspect. *New York Times*, 26 May 1996: $1;1.

27. Declaration of David V. Foster, M.D. n.d. http://unabombertrial.com/documents/dvfoster111797.html

28. Declaration of Karen Bronk Froming, Ph.D. n.d. http://www.unabombertrial.com/documents/froming111797.html

29. Possley M. Doctor says Kaczynski is competent for trial. Chicago Tribune, 1/21/98; https://www.chicagotribune.com/news/ct-xpm-1998-01-21-9801210055-story.html

30. Ben-Porath YS. Uses and misuses of Ted Kaczynski's MMPI. *J Personality Assess*. 2018;40(7):606–613. doi:10.1080/00223891.2018.1468337.

31. Butcher JN, Hass GA, Greene RL, et al. Using the MMPI-2 in forensic assessment: Response to criticism about a case study. *J Personality Assess*. doi:10.1080/00223891.2018.1493488.

32. Turchie T, Puckett K. *Hunting the American Terrorist: The FBI's War on Homegrown Terror*. New York: History Publishing Company; 2007.

33. Perez E, Brown P, Almasy S. Orlando shooting: Killer's behavior had long been an issue. CNN, 6/17/16. https://www.cnn.com/2016/06/17/us/orlando-shooter-omar-mateen/index.html

34. Robles F, Turkewitz J. Was the Orlando gunman gay? The answer continues to elude the F.B.I. *New York Times*, 25 Jun 2016. https://www.nytimes.com/2016/06/26/us/was-the-orlando-gunman-gay-the-answer-continues-to-elude-the-fbi.html

35. Gosk S, Winter T, Connor T. Orlando shooter Omar Mateen arrested as teen for fight, records show. NBC News, 16 June 2016. https://www.nbcnews.com/storyline/orlando-nightclub-massacre/orlando-shooter-omar-mateen-arrested-teen-fight-records-show-n593971

36. Weiss M, Bynum R. Records: Orlando gunman talked about violence in 3rd grade. *Seattle Times*, 17 Jun 2016. https://www.seattletimes.com/nation-world/apnewsbreak-woman-says-nightclub-shooter-stalked-her/

37. Jacobo J. New details emerge about Orlando nightclub shooter Omar Mateen. ABC News, 15 Jun 2016. https://abcnews.go.com/US/details-emerge-orlando-nightclub-shooter-omar-mateen/story?id=39891550

38. Connor T, Winter T. Orlando gunman Omar Mateen talked about bringing gun to training class in 2007. NBC News, 17 Jun 2016. https://www.nbcnews.com/storyline/orlando-nightclub-massacre/orlando-shooter-omar-mateen-talked-about-bringing-gun-training-class-n594786

39. Ovalle D. Orlando shooting sharpens scrutiny on screening of security guards. *Miami Herald*, 25 Jun 2016. https://www.miamiherald.com/news/state/florida/article85868712.html

40. Rothwell J, Alexander H. Orlando shooter Omar Mateen was "mentally unstable wife-beating homophobe." *The Telegraph*, 13 Jun 2016. https://www.telegraph.co.uk/news/2016/06/13/orlando-shooter-omar-mateen-was-mentally-unstable-wife-beating-h/

41. Associated Press. Charleston shooting suspect led troubled life long before radicalization. *The Oregonian*, 27 Jun 2015. https://www.oregonlive.com/today/2015/06/dylann_roof_troubled_life_pave.html

42. Robles F, Stewart N. Dylann Roof's past reveals trouble at home and school. *New York Times*, 16 Jun 2015. https://www.nytimes.com/2015/07/17/us/charleston-shooting-dylann-roof-troubled-past.html

43. Ghansah RK. A most American terrorist: The making of Dylann Roof. *GQ*, 21 Aug 2017. https://www.gq.com/story/dylann-roof-making-of-an-american-terrorist

44. Sack K. Trial documents show Dylann Roof had mental disorders. *New York Times*, 2 Feb 2017. https://www.nytimes.com/2017/02/02/us/dylann-roof-charleston-killing-mental.html

45. McLaughlin EC, Sayers DM. Dylann Roof has mental disorders, attorneys argued. CNN, 2 Feb 2017. https://www.cnn.com/2017/02/02/us/dylann-roof-mental-disorders-competency/index.html

46. Hawes JB, Smith G. Newly released documents show Dylann Roof feared being labeled mentally ill more than he feared death sentence. Death Penalty Information Center, 11 May 2017. https://deathpenaltyinfo.org/node/6762

47. Cleckley HM. *The Mask of Sanity: An Attempt to Clarify Some Issues About the So-Called Psychopathic Personality*. St. Louis, MO: CV Mosby; 1950.

48. Dimsdale JE. *Anatomy of Malice: The Enigma of the Nazi War Criminals*. New Haven, CT: Yale University Press; 2016.

49. Stone MH. *The Anatomy of Evil*. Amherst, NY: Prometheus Books; 2017.

50. Raine A, Meloy JR, Bihrle S, et al. Reduced prefrontal and increased subcortical brain functioning assessed using positron emission tomography in predatory and affective murderers. *Behavi Sci Law.* 1998;16:319–332.

51. Raine A, Lencz T, Bihrle S, et al. Reduced prefrontal gray matter volume and reduced autonomic activity in antisocial personality disorder. *Arch Gen Psychiatry.* 2000;57:119–127.

52. Granacher RP, Fozdar, MA. Acquired psychopathy and the assessment of traumatic brain injury. In Felthous A, Sass H, eds. *International Handbook on Psychopathic Disorders and the Law.* West Sussex, UK: Wiley; 2007:237–250.

53. Petrus C, Hamid N, Sheikh H, et al. Neural and behavioral correlates of sacred values and vulnerability to violent extremism. *Front Psychology.* Dec 2018;9 (2462):1–12.

54. Harlow J. Passage of an iron rod to the head. *Boston Medical and Surgical Journal.* 1848;39:389–393.

55. Braun CM, Léville C, Guimond A. An orbitofrontostriatopallidal pathway for morality: Evidence from post-lesion antisocial and obsessive-compulsive disorder. *Cogn Neuropsychiatry.* 2008;13:296–337.

56. Tranel D, Bechara A, Denburg NL. Asymmetric functional roles of right and left ventromedial prefrontal cortex in social conduct, decision-making, and emotional processing. *Cortex.* 2002;38:589–612.

57. Bogerts B, Schöne M, Braitschuh S. Brain alterations potentially associated with aggression and terrorism. *CNS Spectrums.* 2018;23(2):129–140. doi:10.1017/s1092852917000463. Epub 14 Aug 2017.

58. Domenech P, Koechlin E. Executive control and decision-making in the prefrontal cortex. *Curr Opin Behav Sci.* 2015;1:101–106.

59. Casebeer WD. Moral cognition and its neural constituents. *Nat Rev Neurosci.* 2003;4(10):841–848.

60. Baez S, Herrera E, Garcia AM, et al. Outcome-moral evaluations in terrorists. *Nat Hum Behav.* 2017;1(5):1–8. doi 10.1038/s41562-17-0118.

61. Victoroff J. The mind of the terrorist: A review and critique of psychological approaches. *J Conflict Resolution.* 2005;49:3–42.

62. Mendez MF. The neurobiology of moral behavior: Review and neuropsychiatric implications. *CNS Spectrums.* 2009;14(11):608–620.

63. Darby RR, Horn A, Cushman F, Fox MD. Lesion network localization of criminal behavior. *Proc Natl Acad Sci.* 1/16/18;115(3):601–606.

64. Kanner L. Autistic disturbances of affective contact. *Nerv Child.* 1943;2:217–250.

65. Asperger H. "Autistic psychopathy" in childhood. In Frith U, ed., *Autism and Asperger Syndrome.* Cambridge: Cambridge University Press; 1991:37–92.

66. American Psychiatric Association. *Diagnostic and Statistical Manual of Mental Disorders, Fifth Edition* (DSM-5). 2013. https://www.psychiatry.org/patients-families/personality-disorders/what-are-personality-disorders

67. Elsabbagh M, Divan G, Koh YJ, et al. Global prevalence of autism and other pervasive developmental disorders. *Autism Res.* 2012;5:160–179.

68. Baio J, Wiggins L, Christensen DL, et al. Prevalence of autism spectrum disorder among children aged 8 years: Autism and Developmental Disabilities Monitoring Network, 11 sites, United States, 2014. *MMWR Surveill Summ.* 2018;67(SS-6):1–23. doi:http://dx.doi.org/10.15585/mmwr.ss6706a1External.

69. Lai M, Lombardo MV, Baron-Cohen S. Autism. *Lancet.* 2014;383:896–910.

70. Howlin P, Moss P, Savage S, Rutter M. Social outcomes in mid- to later adulthood among individuals diagnosed with autism and average nonverbal IQ as children. *J Am Acad Child Adolesc Psychiatry.* 2013;52:572–581.

71. Lerner M, Haque OS, Northrup EC, et al. Emerging perspectives on adolescents and young adults with high functioning autism spectrum disorders, violence, and criminal law. *J Am Acad Psychiatry Law.* April 2012;40 (2):177–190.

72. Im D. Template to perpetrate: An update of violence in autism spectrum disorder. *Harv Rev Psychiatry.* 2016;24:14–35.

73. Kanne SM, Mazurek MO. Aggression in children and adolescents with ASD: Prevalence and risk factors. *J Autism Dev Disord.* 2011;41:926–937.

74. Newman SS, Ghaziuddin M. Violent crime in Asperger syndrome: The role of psychiatric comorbidity. *J Autism Dev Disord.* 2008;38:1848–1852.

75. Heeramun R, Magnusson C, Hellner Gumpert C, et al. Autism and convictions for violent crimes: Population-based cohort study in Sweden. *J Am Acad Child Adolesc Psychiatry.* 2017;56(6):491–497.

76. Wachtel LE, Shorter E. Autism plus psychosis: A "one-two punch" risk for tragic violence? *Med Hypotheses.* 2013;81:404–409.

77. Im DS. Trauma as a contributor to violence in autism spectrum disorder. *J Am Acad Psychiatry Law.* 2016;44:184–192.

78. Corner E, Gill P, Mason O. Mental health disorders and the terrorist: A research note probing selection effects and disorder prevalence. *Studies Conflict Terrorism.* 2016;39:560–568.

79. Faccini L, Allely C. Rare instances of individuals with autism supporting or engaging in

terrorism *J Intellect Disabil Offending Behav.* 2017;8:70–82.

80. Skodol A. Overview of personality disorders. *Merck Manual Professional Version*, May 2018. https://www.merckmanuals.com/professional/psychiatric-disorders/personality-disorders/overview-of-personality-disorders

81. Khoshnood A. The correlation between mental disorders and terrorism is weak. *Br J Psych Bull.* 2017 Feb;41(1):56. https://www.ncbi.nlm.nih.gov/pmc/articles/PMC5288096/

82. Corner E, Gill P. The nascent empirical literature on psychopathology and terrorism. *World Psychiatry.* 2018 Jun;17(2):147–148. https://www.ncbi.nlm.nih.gov/pmc/articles/PMC5980584/#wps20547-bib-0003

83. Corner E, Gill P, Mason O. Mental health disorders and the terrorist: A research note probing selection effects and disorder prevalence. *Stud Conflict Terror.* 2016;39:560–568.

84. Rostmeyer KB, Brugh CS, Alexa Katon A, et al. Presence of mental illness among lone actor terrorists. 2018. https://ncsu-las.org/wp-content/uploads/2019/01/Rostmeyer _2018_Symposium_Poster_Final_1543262045.pdf

85. Monahan, J. The individual risk assessment of terrorism. *Psychol Publ Policy Law.* 2012;18:167–205.

86. Corner E, Gill P, Schouten R, Farnham F. Mental disorders, personality traits, and grievance-fueled targeted violence: The evidence base and implications for research and practice. J Personality Assess. 2018;100(5)459–470. doi:10.1080/00223891.2018.1475392.

87. Spaaij R. *Understanding Lone Wolf Terrorism: Global Patterns, Motivations and Prevention.* New York: Springer; 2012

88. Spaaij R. The enigma of lone wolf terrorism: An assessment. *Stud Conflict Terrorism.* 2010;33(9):854–870.

89. Smith AG. National Institute of Justice: Risk factors and indicators associated with radicalization to terrorism in the United States: What research sponsored by the National Institute of Justice tells us. US Department of Justice, Office of Justice Programs, National Institute of Justice, June 2018. https://www.ncjrs.gov/pdffiles1/nij/251789.pdf

90. Teich S. Trends and developments in lone wolf terrorism in the Western world: An analysis of terrorist attacks and attempted attacks by Islamic extremists. International Institute for Counter-Terrorism, Oct 2013. https://i-hls.com/wp-content/uploads/2013/11/Lone-Wolf-Sarah-Teich-2013.pdf

91. Spaaij R. Inside the mind of Anders Breivik: The Norwegian on trial for mass murder. Huffington Post Blog, 13 Jun 2012; https://www.huffingtonpost.co.uk/ram/anders-breivik-psychology-inside-the-mind-of-anders_b_1419343.html

92. Kifner J. McVeighs mind: A special report: Oklahoma bombing suspect: Unraveling of a frayed life. *New York Times*, 31 Dec 1995; https://www.nytimes.com/1995/12/31/us/mcveigh-s-mind-special-report-oklahoma-bombing-suspect-unraveling-frayed-life.html

93. Diamond SA. Terrorism, resentment and the Unabomber. *Psychology Today*, 8 Apr 2008. https://www.psychologytoday.com/us/blog/evil-deeds/200804/terrorism-resentment-and-the-unabomber

94. Spencer T. Rua E. Mail bomb suspect's personality changed radically. AP News, 27 Oct 2018. https://apnews.com/afbae46544cd-430cbaa4a7a325118961

95. Gutowski C, Heinzmann D, Coen J. In Belleville, alleged gunman remembered "as a very irascible, angry little man." *Chicago Tribune*, 15 Jun 2017. https://www.chicagotribune.com/news/breaking/ct-james-hodgkinson-shooter-20170614-story.html

96. Stepansky J, Crane-Newman, Schapiro R. Dallas shooter Micah Xavier Johnson was army reservist in Afghanistan, had massive cache of weapons in his house. *New York Daily News*, 9 July 2016. https://www.nydailynews.com/news/national/dallas-shooter-micah-xavier-johnson-decorated-army-veteran-article-1.2704275

97. Face it: Oswald did it. *The Economist*, 23 Nov 2013. https://www.economist.com/comment/2220158

98. Hopkins N, Hall S. David Copeland: A quiet introvert, obsessed with Hitler and bombs. *The Guardian*, 30 Jun 2000. https://www.theguardian.com/uk/2000/jun/30/uksecurity.sarahhall

99. https://www.healthdirect.gov.au/psychosis

100. Volavka J. Triggering violence in psychosis. *AMA Psychiatry.* 2016;73(8):769–770. doi:10.1001/jamapsychiatry.2016.1348. https://jamanetwork.com/journals/jamapsychiatry/article-abstract/2533650

101. Arehart-Treichel J. Threat delusions linked to violence in first-episode psychosis. *Psychiatric News*, 19 Apr 2013. https://doi.org/10.1176/appi.pn.2013.4b2

102. Silverstein SM, Del Pozzo J, Roché M, et al. Schizophrenia and violence: Realities and recommendations. *Crime Psychol Rev.* 2015; 1(1):21–42. doi:10.1080/23744006.2015.1033154.

103. Callimachi R, Porter C. Toronto shooting rekindles familiar debate: Terrorist? Mentally Ill? Both? *New York Times*, 25 Jul 2018. https://www.nytimes.com/2018/07/25/world/americas/islamic-state-mental-health.html

104. Appelbaum PS. Treatment of incompetent, dangerous criminal defendants: Parsing the law. Psychiatric Serv. 2012;63:630–632. doi:10.1176/appi.ps.2012 00630.

105. Solomon A. An avoidable tragedy: Aaron Alexis and mental illness. *The New Yorker*, 20 Sep 2013. https://www.newyorker.com/news/news-desk/an-avoidable-tragedy-aaron-alexis-and-mental-illness

106. Gabriel T, Goldstein J, Schmidt MS. Suspect's past fell just short of raising alarm. *New York Times*, 17 Sep 2013. https://www.nytimes.com/2013/09/18/us/washington-navy-yard-shootings.html

107. Corner E, Gill P. Is there a nexus between terrorist involvement and mental health in the age of the Islamic State? *CTC Sentinel*. Jan 2017;10(1-10). https://ctc.usma.edu/is-there-a-nexus-between-terrorist-involvement-and-mental-health-in-the-age-of-the-islamic-state/

108. Gruenewald J, Chermak S, Freilich JD. Distinguishing "loner" attacks from other domestic extremist violence: A comparison of far-right homicide. Incident and offender characteristics. *Criminol Publ Policy*. 2013;12(1):65–91.

109. Gill P. *Lone-Actor Terrorists: A Behavioural Analysis*. New York: Routledge; 2015.

110. Michaels J, Dorell O. Killings of civilians threaten Afghanistan mission. *USA Today*, 12 Mar 2012.

111. Dao J. At home, asking how "Our Bobby" became war crime suspect. *New York Times*, 18 Mar 2012; https://www.nytimes.com/2012/03/19/us/sgt-robert-bales-from-small-town-ohio-to-afghanistan.html?ref=todayspaper

112. Flaherty MP, Thompson K, Tate J. Staff Sgt. Robert Bales was found liable in financial fraud. *Washington Post*, 19 Mar 2012; https://www.washingtonpost.com/world/national-security/staff-sgt-robert-bales-was-found-liable-in-financial-fraud/2012/03/19/gIQA4Ni2NS_story.html

113. Raddatz M, Lila M, Schifrin N. Soldier held in Afghan Massacre had brain injury, marital problems. ABC News, 12 Mar 2012. https://www.thesteptoegroup.com/?p=761

114. Schmitt E, Yardley W. Accused G.I. "snapped" under strain, official says. New York Times, 16 Mar 2012. https://archive.nytimes.com/query.nytimes.com/gst/fullpage-9400E4DB173A-F935A25750C0A9649D8B63.html

115. Miller G. A gruesome war crime renews concerns about a malaria drug's psychiatric side effects. *Wired Science*, 15 Aug 2013. https://www.wired.com/2013/08/mefloquine-robert-bales/

116. Vaughan B. Robert Bales speaks: Confessions of America's most notorious war criminal. *GQ*, 21 Oct 2015. https://www.gq.com/story/robert-bales-interview-afghanistan-massacre

117. The Associated Press. Staff Sgt. Robert Bales sentenced to life in prison without chance of parole for Afghanistan massacre that left 16 dead. NY *Daily News*, 23 Aug 2013. https://www.nydailynews.com/news/national/army-staff-sgt-robert-bales-life-no-chance-parole-article-1.1435117

4

Psychoactive Agents and Mental Disorders in Lone-Actor Terrorism

MICHAEL ARIELI, AVIV WEINSTEIN, URI BEN YAAKOV,
RONNIE BERKOVITZ, ALINA POPERNO, HAGIT BONNY-NOACH, AND
ROBERT P. GRANACHER, JR.

INTRODUCTION

Historically, research conducted on the nexus between terror and drugs, known as *narcoterrorism*, has focused mainly on how terrorist groups utilize profits from illegal drug trafficking or how organized crime and drug cartels exploit terrorist tactics to corrupt governments and influence their policies. Terror groups in need of financial resources have found that drug trafficking is exceptionally profitable. According to a report on transnational crime, in 2014, the global drug trafficking market was worth $426 billion to $652 billion.[1] Michael Braun, former Assistant Administrator and Chief of Operations at the US Drug Enforcement Administration (DEA) stated that the DEA had linked 19 of the 43 officially designated foreign terrorist organizations to some aspect of the global drug trade.[2]

Throughout history, combatants in armed conflicts have used psychoactive substances, beginning with the ancient Greeks' use of opium to the tale of the Nizari Ismaili group using hashish and leading to the "national" consumption of methamphetamines by German soldiers in World War II. Psychoactive substances play a role in transforming a peaceful human being into a killer.

Kamienski identified three categories of such psychoactive substances:

1. stimulants (e.g., amphetamines and cocaine)
2. depressants or hypnotics (e.g., alcohol, barbiturates, opium, and opioids)
3. hallucinogens (e.g., atropine, cannabis, mescaline, scopolamine, lysergic acid diethylamide [LSD], and 3,4-methylenedioxymethamphetamine [MDMA], commonly known as ecstasy).[3]

All three categories of drugs have been used at some point in the history of warfare, depending on the time, culture, and accessibility of the substance.

In the modern period, these same substances have been used by "irregular fighting forces" and terrorist groups. Tramadol, an opioid, has been abused by Boko Haram fighters in Nigeria, by both the terrorists themselves and by abducted Nigerian female suicide bombers.[4,5] In the Syrian Civil War, the Islamic State in Iraq and al-Sham (ISIS) and other groups have been accused of consuming stimulants, specifically Captagon, a psychostimulant prescription drug composed of fenethylline.[6] According to the United Nations Office on Drugs and Crime (UNODC), by 1986, fenethylline was banned by most countries. Illegal manufacture of the product has occurred in Lebanon (by Hezbollah), Syria, and other locations. Today, most of the counterfeit Captagon contains not fenethylline but amphetamine, methamphetamine, and other various pharmaceutical products.[7] Captagon is abused by terrorist groups and civilian populations throughout the Middle East and has become the primary drug of abuse in Saudi Arabia.

Within the past decade, both terror groups and lone actors abused psychoactive substances. In such terrorist incidents as the Mumbai attack, wherein the New York Police Department (NYPD) divulged that terrorists abused stimulants and anabolic steroids,[8] and the Berlin Christmas Market attack, in which remnants of both cocaine and cannabis were discovered after the postmortem of Anis Amri,[9] pharmaceuticals have been abused to change the state of consciousness of the assailants. Hence, from Breivik in Oslo to the massacre in Tunis by Seifeddine Rezgui,[10] the concept of pharmacoterrorism has just recently become a topic of interest for researchers.[11]

In contrast to research on pharmacoterrorism, the study of mental illness and terror has extended throughout some 40 years. The various studies of Gill, Corner, Horgan, Borum, Gruenewald, and others are cornerstones regarding mental illness and terror and are relevant regarding abuse of psychoactive substances. Many of the studies conclude that lone-actor terrorists lack a uniform profile.[12] In general, researchers agree that "mental illness" is not the silver bullet or master narrative in terroristic actions but rather one of many variables and risk factors. Another feature of the new research studies stresses the aspect of disaggregation of terrorists and understanding the importance of studying subgroups. There is a consensus among researchers that lone actors, in contrast to group terrorists, have higher rates of mental illness.

Lt. Col. (Res.) Uri Ben Yaakov, Director of Development and Senior Researcher at the International Institute for Counter-Terrorism (ICT) and one of the authors of this chapter, participated in a recent study of lone-actor attackers conducted by Professors Ariel Merari and Boaz Ganor of the ICT, in partnership with the Israel Ministry of Public Security. In the course of the research, they utilized a database of some 700 lone actors and intensely interviewed 45 of these assailants. In an analysis of the 45 interviewees, mental illness was diagnosed in some two-thirds of the sample, and 33–38% expressed suicidal tendencies.[13]

Paul Gill stated, "Psychopathological mechanisms remain systematically unexamined, and there may be grounds to pursue a more concrete understanding of how mental illness and psychological processes influence an individual's participation in and trajectory through terrorist behaviours."[14]

This chapter reveals the relationship between mental illness and psychoactive substances in the context of lone-actor terrorists. This correlation will transcend ideological beliefs, vocational backgrounds, methods of violent terror acts, types of psychoactive substances abused, and mental illnesses. The chapter, via case studies, examines the relationship between such psychoactive substances as cannabis, methamphetamine, and

anabolic androgenic steroids (AAS) poly-drug use, and their interrelationship with mental illness.

In the concluding discussion utilizing the 2019 French legal decision regarding Kobili Traore, we will describe a new challenge for anti-terror experts relating to criminal responsibility, consumption of psychoactive substances, and mental state.

CASE STUDIES: CANNABIS

John Patrick Bedell

Incident

On March 4, 2010, a 36-year-old man identified as John Patrick Bedell shot and wounded two enforcement officers outside the Pentagon Metro station. Bedell, a lone shooter, was killed during the exchange of gunfire.[15]

Motivations and Ideology

Bedell had an academic background in science and engineering and was adept in software programming. He espoused via blog posts, podcasts, YouTube video, and Wikipedia entries controversial surreptitious anti-government theories ranging from the Kennedy assassination, the 9/11 terrorist act, and marijuana laws. Bedell posted numerous times in WeedWiki, an internet site which provided information regarding cannabis products, consumption methods, and policy. He also maintained at least two online blogs, Rothbardix – Technology for liberty and justice, and Information Currency and Information Engineering. Rothbardix advocated and discussed some of the ideas fostered by Murray Newton Rothbard, the ideologue of anarcho-capitalism and libertarianism. In a podcast uploaded to the blog, Bedell stated, "This seizure of the United States government by an international criminal conspiracy is a long-established reality. The murder of the United States President in 1963, the associated murders and institutional subversion, and the manipulation of official inquiries and public opinion, was effected by individuals within organizational structures that play a central role in the United States government up to the present day. The coup regime founded with the murder of President John Kennedy utilizes a number of mechanisms to perpetuate its criminal rule."[16] Bedell's conspiracy and anti-government views are echoed throughout his posts. The following sections in this case study will attempt to determine the extent of the impact of his concurring mental illness and substance abuse had on the formation of these beliefs.

Mental Illness

Bedell had an extensive history of bipolar disorder and previously hospitalized at least three times. In 2006, due to a complaint filed by residents of his apartment complex, Bedell was arrested and criminally charged with cultivation of marijuana and, perhaps indicative of his previous behavior and mental state, resisting/delaying police officers. He pleaded guilty to the charges and, by the court order, on probation attended a drug treatment program. In 2007, while on probation, Bedell was arrested again for instigating an altercation. Bedell claimed that his bipolar disorder was the basis for his behavioral problems. He also displayed a psychiatrist's letter from San Benito County Behavioral Health Department that verified that Bedell had bipolar disorder and had been in treatment since 2004. Bedell's psychiatrist, Dr. J. Michael Nelson, in his letter to the court, verified that Bedell had been diagnosed with a bipolar disorder characterized by depression, anxiety, and mood swings. Nelson alluded to the fact that Bedell's marijuana use was an effort to "self-medicate" and indicated that marijuana could exacerbate Bedell's bipolar symptoms.[17]

Psychoactive Substance Use (Cannabis)

Bedell's extensive use of cannabis is apparent not only from his criminal arrest records and his online expression of concern regarding marijuana laws but also through the written correspondence of his psychiatrist regarding "self-medication." In December 2006, while still on probation and enrolled in the drug court program, Bedell received approval by the San Francisco Department of Public Health to receive medical cannabis for the treatment of chronic insomnia. He posted his approval letter in the WeedWiki site.[18] In February 2010, police in Nevada cited him for driving under the influence, unlawful possession of drug paraphernalia, and possession of marijuana after finding 76 grams of cannabis. Two days before the Pentagon attack, Bedell was due to appear in court.

Michael Adebowale

Incident

On May 22, 2013, in Woolwich, Southeast London, two assailants brutally murdered an off-duty soldier via a vehicle attack and afterward attempted to behead him. The two assailants,

Michael Adebolajo and Michael Adebowale, uttered pro-jihadi statements as the motivation for their attack. Subsequently, they were shot, wounded, and apprehended by enforcement authorities.[19] The two assailants were found guilty of the murder of Lee Rigby and sentenced to life imprisonment.

Motivations and Ideology

Michael Adebowale was a British-born youth of Nigerian descent and raised as a Christian in Southeast London. At the age of 16, he became involved with the Woolwich Boys, a Somali-controlled street gang. In 2008, Adebowale was wounded and witnessed the brutal murder of his friend at the apartment of a known drug dealer. He was diagnosed with posttraumatic stress disorder (PTSD) and received treatment by a psychiatrist. Adebowale converted to Islam in 2009, and the same year was sentenced to prison for drug offenses. Upon release from incarceration, Michael Adebowale completed his radicalization trajectory and appeared in public wearing traditional Islamic dress and attending pro-jihadi demonstrations. Both Adebowale and Adebolajo prayed at mosques where the extremist Imam Shakeel Begg presided. In 2012, Adebowale was known to attend a protest organized by the ISIS supporter Anjem Choudary.

According to a Parliament Intelligence Report, Adebowale had been investigated by MI5 from 2011 until the attack due to his interest in online jihadist sites. The report also revealed that, already in 2010, Adebowale had been in telephone contact with Adebolajo.[20] Hence, besides other essential risk factors, there is no doubt that radicalization into jihadist ideology was incorporated into the motivation by Adebowale to participate in this terrorist act.

Mental Illness

Since 2008, after his traumatic gang-related events, Adebowale not only suffered from PTSD but also had acute attacks of mental illness characterized by delusions and auditory hallucinations.[21] His extensive abuse of "skunk" (high-potency cannabis) contributed to the continuing deterioration of his mental condition. The seriousness of his mental deterioration was later revealed in his trial for the murder of Rigby. His psychiatric impairment led to a trial delay, and he was deemed ineligible to testify in his defense. He suffered from psychotic episodes, including auditory hallucinations, during the whole period of his incarceration. One of the voices talking to him was the attacker from 2008; others with a Nigerian accent "spirits called Djinns" would make him do things and were "playing with him.[22] According to the psychiatrists, his condition was chronic, and he had been suffering from it for a long time. Dr. Phillip Joseph, the forensic psychiatrist for the prosecution, related that Adebowale implied that the spirits, the Djinns, were partly responsible for his actions in the assault but afterward withdrew his claim. According to Dr. Ian Cumming, the psychiatrist who treated Adebowale in Belmarsh Prison, there was a "clear history of psychosis from 2008, post-traumatic anxiety, which had to be considered alongside cannabis misuse."[23] Adebowale was described to the court by psychiatrist Professor Nigel Eastman as falling "into a group that is susceptible to schizophrenia."[24] Moreover, his mental condition was mentioned by the judge as a factor in his sentence of 45 years of imprisonment.[25]

Psychoactive Substance Use (Cannabis)
The media published accounts of both the psychiatrists; court testimonies and of relatives' and acquaintances' depictions of Adebowale's abuse of cannabis. In the trial proceedings, Dr. Neil Boast stated, "His symptoms of psychosis were increased by his heavy use of cannabis and he hears voices speaking in Nigerian accents telling what he is to do next." [24]

Discussion
In this section of the chapter, we described two case studies of lone actors who were under the influence of cannabis, but their cases were complicated by a previous history of mental illness and other risk factors. It is not our contention that the psychoactive substance was the "master narrative explanation" on the pathway to terror, but rather a critical distal factor. Horgan, Gill, Bouhana, Silver, and Corner in 2016 aptly stated, "Background factors mixed with short-term stressors are key to understanding many of the lone extremists."[26] They contend that recent stress and an experienced "tipping point" before radicalization are closely related to various distal risk factors, including mental illness and substance abuse.[26 (p. 33)] We maintain that cannabis, specifically high-potency "skunk," can have a direct and vital influence on the lone actor's mental illness, radicalization process, and, hence, pathway to terror. It is specifically relevant to cases like those of Bedell and Adebowale. Another vivid example of high-potency cannabis influencing a lone-actor's mental illness and pathway to terror is the 2015 attack

at Leytonstone Underground station in London. Muhaydin Mire, influenced by ISIS and other jihadist sources, attempted to behead a passenger at Leytonstone Underground station. During the trial, it was disclosed that, in 2006, Mire was compulsorily hospitalized "when essentially he lost touch with reality."[27] He was diagnosed with paranoid schizophrenia. Dr. Philip Joseph, the consultant forensic psychiatrist, testified that cannabis use made a "significant" contribution to what was "probably" a case of paranoid schizophrenia.[28] The words of Judge Nicholas Hilliard QC underscore this point: "The defendant has himself acknowledged that smoking strong skunk might have affected his mental health." The Judge warned that Mire's mental illness, extremist ideology, and use of cannabis contributed to his posing a danger.[29] Mire was sentenced to life imprisonment with a minimum sentence of 8 years and 6 months; however, due to his mental illness, he was hospitalized in the psychiatric unit at Broadmoor high-security hospital, which also housed Michael Adebowale. Both assailants lived in South London and extensively used skunk.

Cannabis, the illicit "street" drug, is most often found as either the resin (hashish) or as dry herbal material. Pollinated female plants containing floral and foliar material—marijuana in the United States and traditional herbal cannabis in the United Kingdom—were the basis of dry herbal street cannabis products. However, within the past decade herbal cannabis most predominantly appears as sinsemilla, a more potent material whose source is unpollinated female plants. In a comprehensive review of cannabis strength in the United Kingdom in 2016, it was revealed that high-potency "skunk" now has a monopoly over the UK cannabis market. Traditional hashish or marijuana, which contains high amounts of CBD (cannabidiol) that moderates the psychotic effect of tetrahydrocannabinol, has all but disappeared from the illegal cannabis market. In fact, in 2016, 94% of police seizures of cannabis in the United Kingdom were high-potency sinsemilla.[30] Similar to the United Kingdom, high-potency sinsemilla has also overtaken the North American market.[31] Potter and colleagues (2018), in their 2016 analysis of Δ9–tetrahydrocannabinol in sinsemilla samples from United Kingdom police seizures, revealed a median of 14.2% while, "In all but 1 case, the 400 sinsemilla samples were devoid of CBD."[32] The prevalence of high- potency tetrahydrocannabinol in street cannabis products with minimal if any cannabidiol has significant clinical importance.

Di Forti, Marconi, Carra, and colleagues (2015), in their case-control study, researched the possible relationship between frequent use of skunk-like (high-potency) cannabis and psychotic disorders in South London. According to the study, "South London has one of the highest recorded incidence rates of psychosis in the UK."[33] Their investigation concluded that the use of high-potency cannabis (skunk) as compared to low-potency cannabis (hashish) increases the probability of incurring psychosis. Utilizing odds ratios in analyzing the data, they demonstrated that the frequency of use of high-potency cannabis (skunk) increased the imminent danger of experiencing a psychotic event.[33 (p. 236)] Gage, Hickman, and Zammit (2016) state that there is conclusive evidence from epidemiological studies that should warrant a public health warning regarding the link between psychosis and cannabis.[34] Murray and associates not only review the connection between psychosis and cannabis but specifically warn of the risks with high-potency cannabis and confirm a dose-response relationship between the level of use and later psychotic episodes.[35] Volkow, Swanson, Evins, DeLisi, and colleagues (2015) cited, "Longitudinal investigations show a consistent association between adolescent cannabis use and psychosis."[36] The psychotic episodes of Adebowale and Mire and the direct association with their abuse of skunk lead us again to the prominence of substance abuse and mental illness as significant risk factors in the path to violence by lone-actor terrorists.

Bedell had a bipolar illness according to his doctor, which was "characterized by depression, anxiety, mood swings."[37] His physician also expressed that Bedell was relatively symptomless during the periods of taking his prescribed medication, but his "agitation and fearfulness" returned when he fell out of treatment. Bedell's behavioral problems, including his conspiratorial theories and criminal arrests, are related to his mental illness. Cannabis, via "self-medication," contributed to the manifestations of his disease. There is evidence for an association between bipolar disorder and cannabis use.[38] Twenty to fifty percent of bipolar disorder patients endorse some form of cannabis-related problems,[39] with a recent study reporting greater illness severity and treatment noncompliance in chronic cannabis users.[40] Inflated self-esteem or grandiosity, a flight of ideas (the subjective experience that thoughts are racing), and increases in goal-directed activity or psychomotor agitation are among the criteria for a manic episode in bipolar disorder.[41] In one recent review, researchers found a significant relationship between cannabis use and subsequent exacerbation and onset of mania symptoms. A systemic literature review and meta-analysis concluded, "Studies support an association between cannabis use and the exacerbation of manic symptoms in those with previously diagnosed bipolar disorder. Furthermore, a meta-analysis of two studies suggests that cannabis use is associated with an approximately 3-fold (Odds Ratio: 2.97; 95% CI: 1.80–4.90) increased risk for the new onset of manic symptoms."[42]

In Bedell's case, we are aware that his bipolar disorder affected his criminal behavior, and the medical literature claims a probable relationship between use of cannabis and mania. In this specific case, while we are not claiming that cannabis and his mental illness were the mono-casual factors in the terror act, there seems to be evidence that they were prominent risk factors.

CASE STUDIES: STIMULANTS (METHAMPHETAMINE)

Gavin Long

Incident

On July 17, 2016, Gavin Long a 29-year-old ex-Marine anti-police extremist armed with an assault rifle ambushed police officers in Baton Rouge, Louisiana. Three enforcement officers were killed, and three others were wounded in the incident. Long was killed in the exchange of gunfire.[43] In 2016, Daveed Gartenstein-Ross testified to the House Committee on Oversight and Government Reform Subcommittee on National Security, Subcommittee on Government Operations, on the topic of radicalization in the United States and the rise of terrorism. Regarding domestic terrorism, he described the increase of Black nationalist–related acts of terror against the police, citing Gavin Long as an example.[44]

Motivations and Ideology

In 2017, the FBI issued an Intelligence Assessment, "Black Identity Extremists Likely Motivated to Target Law Enforcement Officers." The document claimed that "The FBI assesses it is very likely incidents of alleged police abuse against African Americans since then have continued to feed the resurgence in ideologically motivated, violent criminal activity within the BIE (Black Identity Extremists) movement. The FBI assesses it is very likely some BIEs are influenced by a mix of anti-authoritarian, Moorish sovereign citizen ideology, and BIE ideology."[45] Gavin Long appeared in the document as a "Black Identity Extremist" motivated by the Moorish Sovereign Citizen ideology.

A comprehensive report of the incident by the district attorney reported on Long's extensive use of social media. The document revealed Long's postings on YouTube, including a video from Dallas, Texas, appearing 3 days after five law enforcement officers were ambushed and killed. In the video, Long states that "100% of revolutions, of victims, fighting their oppressors . . . have been successful through fighting back, through bloodshed." He goes on to talk about how he does not believe protesting is ever successful because "revenue and blood are the only thing that gets through to oppressors."[43] [p. 13] Long's affiliation to extremist groups and his acceptance of their ideology as a mode of action are seen as primary motivators in the deadly incident.

Mental Illness

Gavin Long served as a data network specialist in the Marines for 5 years, including 7 months in Iraq, and was honorably discharged in 2010 with the rank of sergeant. In reviewing mental illness problems which may have affected his later radicalization and act of terror, it is imperative to note that, upon discharge, Long received the Marine Corps Good Conduct Medal, Iraq Campaign Medal, Sea Service Deployment Ribbon (third award), Global War on Terrorism Service Medal, National Defense Service Medal, and the Navy Unit Commendation Medal.[46] Hence up, to 2010, Long had served with distinction in the military and had no recorded previous encounters with the police. In 2011, his family noticed changes in his behavior, including anger and aggressiveness. Long complained about sleeping problems and went to a Veterans Affairs healthcare facility.[47]

In reviewing the mental status of Gavin Long, three essential aspects arise.

- *PTSD*: Long told friends and relatives that he suffered from PTSD. In November 2011, the VA Medical Center in Kansas City diagnosed Long with an adjustment disorder with depressed mood.[47] It is important to note that during his PTSD evaluation, the VA cited Long's avoidance of war movies and being "unable to experience tenderness, loving feelings."

It also had a cryptic notation about some "sense of foreshortened future."[47] With this prognosis, the VA informed Long about its mental health clinic and its 24-hour services in the area and issued a prescription for an antidepressant. In July 2016, Micah Xavier Johnson a US soldier who had served in Afghanistan, killed five police officers in Dallas, Texas. Johnson, according to open sources, had suffered symptoms of PTSD. However, records do not indicate that he was ever formally diagnosed as such by the VA medical staff. In 2009, two journalists from the internet site SALON published an expose regarding pressure by the VA not to diagnose PTSD, but instead classify the involved soldier's conditions as "anxiety disorders." The investigating article published the following, "Last year, VoteVets.org and Citizens for Responsibility and Ethics in Washington (CREW) released an e-mail from Norma Perez, a psychologist in Texas, to staff at a Department of Veterans Affairs facility there. In addition to the Army, that department also provides veterans with benefits. 'Given that we are having more and more compensation seeking veterans, I'd like to suggest that you refrain from giving a diagnosis of PTSD straight out,' Perez wrote in the e-mail dated March 20, 2008. She suggested the staff 'consider a diagnosis of Adjustment Disorder.' "[48] According to two National Academy of Science reports published in 2012 and 2013, from 13% to 20% of veterans who had participated in the conflicts in Afghanistan and Iraq suffer from PTSD.[49] Hence, we should question the possible misdiagnosis and mental illness treatment of Gavin Long.

- *Suicide note of Gavin Long*: After Long's terror attack, police discovered a note which some will now call Long's "manifesto" regarding the incident. The manifesto recognized that Long was committing a "horrendous act of violence" but emphasized that "in order to create substantial change within America's police forces and Judicial system," he was obligated to act. In the war between "good and bad cops," Long wrote, "Therefore I must bring the same destruction that bad cops continue to inflict upon my people."[50] Alongside the note/manifesto, police found a printout of Hadith 318 from an Islamic holy book. In the printout, there are references asking forgiveness from Allah and including a prayer passage wherein it states that repeating the prayer and dying on the same day guarantees the person will go to paradise. Hence, the district attorney in his final report concluded that the note indicated premeditated murder and a suicide mission ("suicide by cop").[43 (pp. 14–15)]

- *"Targeted individual"*: Could Gavin Long be designated as a targeted individual, a supposed victim of gang-stalking? In what is now recognized as a worldwide phenomenon and not extensively researched, some individuals allege that they are victims of organized groups which can cause them physical and psychological harm. "Group or gang-stalking" is the commonly used term to describe the incidents, whereas the victim is referred to as the "TI" or targeted individual. Xuan and MacDonald (2019) contend that targeted individuals have embraced social media platforms in order to corroborate their views. They further stated, "Postings to TI groups reflect the pervasive betrayal, isolation, suffering and stress associated with these beliefs."[51]

In one of the initial and significant investigations regarding the topic of targeted individuals, "Stalking was defined as the repeated unwanted intrusion of one person into the life of another in a way that causes anxiety, fear or distress. Intrusions encompassed a range of behaviours involving communications, physical intrusion and impersonation."[52] The authors defined "group" in the study as consisting of at least three perpetrators. The group-stalked cases displayed a significant increase in delusional beliefs as compared to the individually stalked. They also displayed an increased certainty that covert actions were utilized by the stalkers, as well as greater suffering from depression and suicidal thoughts. The research also related that the group-stalked cases expressed increased distrust and aggressiveness.[52 (pp. 608,611)]

Christine M. Sarteschi researched the relationship between group stalking, mass murder, and targeted individuals. Sarteschi stated, "This analysis is guided by the premise that although the majority of those with mental illnesses are not violent, they can be, when they perceive that others are attempting to harm them, or as shown in at least two of the presented cases, when an individual uses violence as a strategy to draw attention to a perceived important injustice."[53] Gavin Long is one of her sample cases. In one of his last blogs before the assault, he claimed to be a targeted individual for at least 11 years. The same source also wrote, "Mr. Long appeared to have latched on to much of the targeted individual belief system, with a fixation on law enforcement officials as his persecutors."[54] Hence, the circumstantial evidence leads us to believe that Long believed and acted like a targeted individual.

In conclusion, perhaps all the factors just listed were factors in defining Long's mental status and aided in his progression to violence.

Psychoactive Substance Use (Stimulant / Methamphetamine)

Gavin Long described himself as a life coach, nutritionist, and personal trainer. Long wrote three books in which he denied the validity of germs causing disease and vociferously objected to the use of prescription drugs. In total contrast to his writing, Long's postmortem toxicology analysis reported that his liver tissue contained traces of methamphetamine.[55] While lacking documented knowledge regarding the extent of Long's abuse of methamphetamine, nevertheless, the fact that he abused it notably within the time frame of the incident—in contrast to his professed lifestyle as a life coach, nutritionist, and personal trainer—is significant in itself.

Discussion

This case involves a lone-actor terrorist, a military veteran with a history of mental illness and under the influence of methamphetamine, who purposely murdered three police officers. There are questions regarding Long's precise mental diagnosis and his history of methamphetamine use.

Methamphetamine is a potent and addicting psychostimulant of the phenethylamine and amphetamine class of psychoactive drugs. It stimulates the release of catecholamines and partially blocks their uptake in the central nervous system. The presence of methamphetamine causes an effect on the predominant dopaminergic, noradrenergic, and serotonergic pathways of the brain. The clinical effects of the drug are affected by dosage, chronic use, and route of administration, all of which are unknown in the case of Long. However, relevant to our case study are some of the psychiatric symptoms experienced by people under the influence of methamphetamine. Clinical symptoms such as euphoria, hyperactivity anxiety, and aggressiveness are possibly present. Methamphetamine-associated psychosis is of significant relevance in perhaps understanding Long's behavior. Cadet and Gold (2017), in clinically describing methamphetamine-induced psychosis, related, "The clinical presentation of methamphetamine-induced psychosis includes delusions of reference and persecutions. Paranoid delusions may be accompanied by violent behavior. Some patients may present with grandiose or jealousy delusions."[56]

Shortly after military service, Gavin Long had been suffering from paranoid symptoms and unexplained mood changes, and he was diagnosed with adjustment disorder with depressed mood. Changes in his behavior, including anger and aggressiveness, were also described by his family. It seems possible that Long was, in reality, struggling with PTSD that was diagnosed otherwise. PTSD symptomatology is a cluster of symptoms that are highly prevalent among methamphetamine users.[57] Studies have demonstrated strong associations between PTSD symptoms and higher rates of aggression.

Gavin Long saw himself as a victim of "gang stalking," which appears to be delusional in basis. People under the influence of methamphetamine also may become suspicious of their friends and family members or think that police officers are stalking them. In one study, individuals who believed themselves to be the victims of group stalking reported more depressive symptoms, posttraumatic symptomatology, and adverse impacts on social and occupational functioning.[52 (p. 601)]

Additionally, Gavin Long was seemingly on a suicide mission during which he committed premeditated murder. In a critical study researching psychiatric symptoms in methamphetamine users, 27% of the large cohort of methamphetamine users reported a suicide attempt in their lifetime.[58]

It is unclear when Long began to use methamphetamine and at what frequency, therefore the causal effect on behavioral changes and psychiatric diagnosis cannot be established. However, we suggest that frustration, anger, persecutory fear, and Long's hatred of police shootings of African American males, when combined with his mental illness, played a role in triggering his violent behavior. In addition

to PTSD symptomatology, the effects of methamphetamine abuse and withdrawal could also act as violence-impelling factors.[57 (pp. 124–125)] Substance abuse and a history of violence have been proved to be prominent factors influencing the likelihood of violent behavior among persons with serious mental illness.[59]

Hence, once again, we are confronted with the importance of not seeking the "master narrative" or a single cause of violent terror acts, but rather of discovering the relationship between many variables and risk factors. However, one cannot underestimate the unique relationship between psychoactive substances, mental illness, and violent lone terror acts.

CASE STUDY: ANABOLIC ANDROGENIC STEROIDS

Khalid Masood

Incident
On March 22, 2017, 52-year-old British-born Khalid Masood killed five people including a police officer and injured 29 in the area of Westminster Bridge, London. Masood initially mounted the pavement at Westminster Bridge in a vehicle-borne terror attack, and, after exiting his vehicle, he fatally stabbed the police officer. In the aftermath, armed police officers shot and killed Masood.[60]

Motivations and Ideology
Adrian Russell Elms, who later was known as Khalid Masood, was born in 1964 in Southeast London. Masood lived in South London, and the family later moved to Tunbridge Wells, Kent. He came from a mixed-race family, in which he had no relationship with his father. In later years, Masood stated that he had experienced blatant racism during his childhood.

According to the official independent assessment of MI5 and police regarding the attacks in London and Manchester, between March and June 2017, Masood had been convicted seven times for various offenses including assault and bodily harm (stabbing). Sometime around 2000, while incarcerated for the stabbing attack, he converted to Islam. According to police intelligence, between 2000 and 2003, Khalid Masood was intensely involved in drug dealing, racketeering, and enforcement.[61] Masood's visits to Saudi Arabia and his association with terrorist subjects were also of interest to MI5. In 2012, MI5 closed his case as a "suspect of interest" after concluding that Masood was not a threat to national security. Interestingly, the intelligence report also related that, in 2013, Masood "expressed contentment that violent actions such as the World Trade Center attacks attracted people to Islam"[61] [(pp. 12–14)] Hence, from an ideological, motivational, and operative standpoint, as appears in the report, Masood held a radical jihadist ideology, researched terrorist literature via the internet, and conducted reconnaissance by himself before the attack. Although he had contact with radical movements, his actions were those of a lone actor motivated at least to some extent by his radical ideology.

Mental Illness

Masood has been described by both family and acquaintances as a violent, angry, and manipulative individual. Dr. James Brock Durham Chisholm, a consultant clinical psychologist, presented a complete postmortem psychological profile of Khalid Masood at the official inquests regarding the Westminster Terror Attack.[62] On September 25, 2018, Chisholm testified that, already in his childhood, Masood had displayed "aggressive and offending behavior." It also noted that Masood's mother had expressed concern regarding his violent behavior. Dr. Chisholm then testified about Masood's lack of empathy and his inability to establish lasting relationships. Reflecting on Masood's controlling and manipulative behavior, Chisholm indicated that it was symptomatic of "longstanding personality difficulties." While rejecting the possibility that Masood had a psychotic disorder, Dr. Chisholm concluded that he most likely had an antisocial personality disorder and also met some of the criteria for narcissistic personality disorder. In concluding his testimony, Dr. Chisholm referred to Masood's radicalization process. In his opinion, Masood was not self-radicalized but was, in essence, an "easy target" to influence. Chisholm also noted that Masood's personal and financial failures, as well as his failure to receive another visa for a trip to Saudi Arabia, were possible triggers in his pathway to the terrorist act.

Psychoactive Substance Use
(Anabolic Androgenic Steroids)

In his earlier years, Khalid Masood was known for his abuse of alcohol, cocaine, and other psychoactive substances. His use of anabolic androgenic steroids (AAS) and aggressive behavior was documented in testimonies at the official inquest by his widow Rohey Hydara and Professor David Cowan.

Hydara testified on September 20, 2018, and described her husband's temperament: "It would get very bad when he was on the steroids. He would rant and complain over every little thing. He was always angry and controlling."[63] She became so concerned that she taped a conversation while he was under the influence. The recordings were played in court and displayed Masood's speech as abusive and incoherent.

On September 25, 2018, professor of pharmaceutical toxicology David Cowan testified regarding Masood's postmortem toxicology analysis. The urine analysis revealed synthetic anabolic steroids, including nandrolone and its metabolites. According to Cowan's testimony, the fact that nandrolone and not just its metabolites were discovered led him to believe that it was administered a short period before Masood's death.[62] [(p. 169)]

Discussion

In our discussion, AAS refers to synthetic pharmaceuticals that are taken orally or injected. They are characterized by their anabolic properties of fat loss and muscle growth. They also have androgenic qualities including beard growth, effects upon secondary sexual characteristics, and a deepening of the voice. According to one estimate, between 2.9 and 4 million Americans between the ages of 13 and 50 have used AAS, and, within this group, approximately 1 million suffered from AAS dependence.[64]

According to the literature and clinical practice, these substances have significant side effects on major organ systems, including cardiovascular, hematologic, hormonal, and metabolic effects. The psychiatric effects are of primary importance to this chapter. An Endocrine Society Scientific Statement in 2014 stated, "In general, these field studies have suggested that some AAS users exhibit hypomanic or manic symptoms during AAS exposure (characterized by irritability, aggressiveness, exaggerated self-confidence, hyperactivity, reckless behavior, and occasional psychotic symptoms) and depressive symptoms during AAS withdrawal (characterized by depressed mood, loss of interest in usual activities, hypersomnia, anorexia, loss of libido, and occasional suicidality)."[65] Importantly, the statement declares that the psychiatric effects seem to be idiosyncratic, and there are extensive variations in individual sensitivity to both androgen excess and withdrawal.[65] [(p. 353)]

Regarding Masood, aggressive and violent behavior characterized his life. Masood's spouse's testimony reflected that this behavior was exacerbated during the use of AAS. The toxicologist surmised, due to the lack of postmortem, verbal, or written evidence of withdrawal symptoms, that Masood was not excessively abusing AAS, despite the spouse's testimony. However, one must consider the potential idiosyncratic and significant variations to androgen excess and withdrawal, as stated in the literature. The use of AAS may have exacerbated Masood's psychiatric symptoms, specifically aggressiveness, exaggerated self-confidence, and reckless behavior.

The suspected use of AAS by lone-actor terrorists has been recorded in recent terror events, as will be evidenced by our analysis of Robert Bales. Anders Behring Breivik's manifesto described the use and "benefits" of the drugs for future terrorists.[66] Omar Mateen, the 2016 Orlando nightclub assailant, and Mohamed Lahouaiej-Bouhlel, the 2016 Nice terrorist, are suspected to have used AAS.[67,68] The official inquest of the 2018 London Bridge attack has also revealed the suspicious use of AAS by the dead terrorists.[69] Cesar Sayoc, the 2018 mail bomb terrorist, is also suspected of chronic administration of AAS.[70] Thus, considering the known psychiatric side effects of AAS misuse, its abuse by potential terrorists becomes a risk factor.

CASE STUDY: POLY-DRUG USE (ALCOHOL, AAS, MEFLOQUINE)

Robert Bales

Incident
In March 2012, in Kandahar Province, Afghanistan, Staff Sergeant Robert Bales opened fire and killed 16 civilians and injured many others. He eventually pleaded guilty in a military court to 16 counts of homicide and other charges and was subsequently sentenced to life imprisonment without eligibility of parole.[71,72]

Motivation
Bales grew up in Norwood, Ohio; played high school football; and was an admired person in the community. After the terror attack on September 11, 2001, he signed up for the military as the "right thing to do."[73]

Bales, an infantry soldier, was on his fourth battle deployment, which included Iraq and Afghanistan, when the incident occurred. During these deployments he participated in many battles, experienced the death of fellow soldiers, and

was injured. In 2002, before his first deployment, he was convicted of assault, fined, and sent to an anger management counseling program. Before his third deployment in Iraq, Bales experienced financial difficulties, and there was speculation regarding complications in his marriage. Upon return from Iraq, Bales requested aid from an Army physician after complaining of headaches and aggressive temper tantrums. He also had been drinking excessively, suffering from insomnia, and expressing paranoiac behavior. He was diagnosed with mild traumatic brain injury (mTBI), conceivably as a result of his exposure to improvised explosive devices (IEDs) or possibly as a result of his activity in high school football. The examination also disclosed that he displayed symptoms of PTSD. Bales was referred to a therapist but discontinued treatment.[74,71] Before his fourth deployment, Bales was disappointed that he did not receive a military promotion and that his next deployment would be Afghanistan and not Germany, Italy, or Hawaii. Preceding the deployment, he underwent an evaluation regarding his TBI, referred to as an automated neuropsychological assessment metrics (ANAM) review. He was declared fit for deployment and sent to Afghanistan.

Bales, seemingly lacking an ideological motivation for his rampage, was a frustrated and angry soldier with personal problems and suffering from mTBI and PTSD symptoms combined with psychoactive substance use. His situation had all the elements of "the perfect storm."

Mental Status
mTBI (concussion) is the "signature wound" of recent conflicts in Iraq and Afghanistan. Researchers estimate that as many as 13– 22% of deployed soldiers report sustaining a concussion during their last deployment.[75] This traumatic injury appears with such symptoms as headaches, fatigue, depression, anxiety, and irritability, as well as impaired cognitive function. Those symptoms are significantly similar to other battlefield maladies such as PTSD and depression. According to one study, soldiers returning from deployments in Iraq and Afghanistan exhibited post PTSD rates of 5–45% depending on the studied population and how PTSD is measured.[76] Relevant to Bales, another article revealed that "Mild traumatic brain injury (i.e., concussion) occurring among soldiers deployed in Iraq is strongly associated with PTSD and physical health problems 3 to 4 months after the soldiers

return home. PTSD and depression are important mediators of the relationship between mild traumatic brain injury and physical health problems."[77] All of these factors complicate the assessment of the pre-deployed soldier. Sadly, even after evaluation, Bales was redeployed despite suffering from the symptoms just cited and a past diagnosis of concussion and possible PTSD.

Psychoactive Substance Use
In 2015, Bales revealed in an interview that about 3 weeks prior to the incident he was using stanozolol, an AAS "because, as he told other soldiers, he wanted to 'get jacked.'" According to Bales, on the evening of the terror event, he took the AAS and sleeping pills and drank six to seven drinks of Jack Daniel's whiskey, which contains 40% alcohol.[74,78]

During his deployments, Bales was taking mefloquine, but it was never recorded in his medical records.

Discussion
The combination of psychoactive substances, including the side effects of mefloquine combined with Bales existing physical and psychological diagnosis, were the significant factors in his violent attack. This situation is problematic, especially regarding the responsibility of the military in effectively evaluating personnel both in pre- and post-deployment. This also pertains to psychoactive substance abuse.

The effects of psychoactive substances on Bales's mental state and actions reiterate the premise of this chapter: namely, that there is an intimate relationship between substance use and mental illness and that together they have a significant effect on the pathway to terror. Whereas in the previous case study of Khalid Masood there was an explicit discussion of the adverse side effects of AAS, this discussion will review the correlation between alcohol consumption and violence. It will then detail the adverse psychiatric effects of mefloquine, including symptoms of psychosis and its specific relevance to Bales.

Researchers have attributed alcohol consumption as the most significant psychotropic factor contributing to aggression. Violent crime and alcohol consumption are significantly related.[79] According to one review and meta-analysis, aggressive behavior regarding combatants is strongly linked with alcohol misuse. It also related that combat veterans diagnosed with PTSD and alcohol dependence displayed significantly more aggressive behavior than those with PTSD alone. While many other factors are evaluated in the review as possible contributors to military personnel violence, the authors emphasize the importance of effective violence screening programs and intervention.[80] Recent research has demonstrated that alcohol consumption combined with "hostile situations or dispositional aggressiveness, alcohol can promote aggressive behavior."[79 (p. 203)] Undoubtedly, this directly relates to Bales. One study, utilizing functional magnetic resonance imaging (fMRI) confirmed the assumption that alcohol-related aggression is related to altered functioning in the prefrontal cortex.[79 (p. 210)] Therefore, we conclude that Bales's ethanol consumption was a possible factor in his aggressive mental state and his subsequent violent incident.

Mefloquine is a quinolone derivative antimalarial drug developed by the US Army. Its approved medical indications, according to the US Food and Drug Administration (FDA), are for the acute treatment and prevention of malaria caused by mefloquine-susceptible mosquitoes *Plasmodium falciparum* and *P. vivax*.[81] The most incriminating evidence regarding the relationship between the Bales incident and mefloquine is disclosed in his petition to the US Supreme Court in May 2018.[82] Whereas the use of mefloquine by Bales is not documented anywhere in his medical records, the legal petition disclosed a secret memorandum issued some 2 months before the incident between the Assistant Secretary of Defense addressed to the Assistant Secretary of the Army. The memorandum stated that "[s]ome deploying Service members have been provided mefloquine for malaria prophylaxis without appropriate documentation in their medical record" and directed that a review of mefloquine prescribing practices be performed in deployed locations.[82 (pp. 5-6)] In 2013, the FDA issued an urgent label change for mefloquine due to the risk of serious psychiatric and nerve side effects. The FDA warned the public that some of the psychiatric symptoms could persist for months or years after mefloquine was discontinued and that the psychiatric side effects could include anxiety, confusion, paranoia, mistrustful, depression, or hallucinations.[83] The petition to the Supreme Court then disclosed affidavits by Dr. Remington Nevin, a globally recognized expert in mefloquine. Nevin's affidavits revealed that, after reviewing Bales's medical records and speaking to him, he was probably exposed to mefloquine in Afghanistan and that it was very likely that Bales had been previously exposed to mefloquine during his tour to Iraq in 2003–2004. Nevin's affidavits declared, "It is likely that Bales did in fact experience visual hallucinations of flashing lights in the region of Alikozai during his guard shift the evening prior to the incident in question" and "that Bales' visual hallucinations of flashing lights were accompanied by paranoia and bizarre, persecutory delusions that these constituted a highly dangerous threat, and that these perceptual disturbances compelled Bales to attack [the compounds]." Nevin's continued that "visual hallucinations, paranoia, persecutory delusions, and subsequent unusual behavior were signs and symptoms of psychosis consistent with a likely severe mental disease or defect at the time of the incident in question" and that these "were a direct result of involuntary intoxication resulting either from his very likely exposure to mefloquine in Iraq, or his likely exposure to mefloquine in Afghanistan, or both."[82 (pp. 15–17)] In conclusion, the premise regarding the relationship between mental illness, psychoactive substances, and lone-actor terror is conclusively displayed in the case of Robert Bales.

BIOLOGY OF PSYCHOAC-TIVE AGENTS AND EARLY LIFE ADVERSITIES

As noted in the abstract for this chapter, the emerging concept of pharmacoterrorism has been introduced in both lone-actor and organized terrorist scenarios. Through case studies, we have examined in depth the use of cannabis and, to a lesser extent, AAS and stimulants by lone-actor terrorists. This section reviews the development of psychosis in early adulthood after exposure to the psychoactive agents described in the case studies, particularly high-potency cannabis. We later explore adult mental illness in those victims of early childhood adversities leading to epigenetic brain changes, particularly antisocial behaviors and substance abuse, and the additive interaction with high-potency cannabis use. Last, this chapter will address the ubiquitous substance of abuse, ethyl alcohol.

Highly Potent Cannabis (Sinsemilla)

In the 1960s, the proportion of THC in commonly used cannabis (marijuana) and resin (hashish) was 3% or less. Subsequently, this began to rise as growers crossbred plants to increase potency. Growers found that preventing pollination increased THC in the product because, in this situation, the female plant converts its energy into producing more cannabinoids rather than seeds.[84] This type of cannabis is referred to as "Sinsemilla," which means "without seed" in Spanish, but it is sometimes colloquially termed "skunk," because of its strong smell.[35] In the United States, the University of Mississippi has a contract with the National Institute on Drug Abuse (NIDA) to, in part, carry out potency monitoring of confiscated marijuana.[85] Their laboratories had documented THC potency changes from approximately 4% in 1995 to greater than 12% in 2014. They attribute the changes to a shift in production from regular marijuana to nondomestic sinsemilla.[31]

It is now well accepted in the scientific community that chronic use of cannabis, particularly in early and late adolescence, markedly increases the risk for psychosis in young adulthood. Recall in the case studies in this chapter that John Patrick Bedell had an extensive use of cannabis. He also had an extensive history of bipolar disorder and was hospitalized at least three times. Michael Adebowale had an extensive abuse history of "skunk," which contributed to his continuing deterioration in mental state. Robert Lewis Dear browsed online cannabis forums. He cultivated marijuana and smoked it as well. Other terrorism actors who engaged in the use of high-potency marijuana or extensive daily use of marijuana later displayed psychosis (as discussed in other cases this chapter).

The concern that cannabis use might induce psychosis is undoubtedly not new. The Scottish psychiatrist T. Clouston visited the Cairo Asylum in the 1890s and noted that 40 out of 253 people in the hospital had insanity attributed to the use of hashish.[86] Moreover, cannabis use and childhood trauma and adversity interact additively to increase the risk of psychotic symptoms.[87] Lone-actor terrorists are more likely to come from adverse social and environmental backgrounds than are group offenders[14 (p. 33),] and the burden of adversity on their brains has not been accounted for in prior terrorist studies. Low socioeconomic status and traumatic stressful events in childhood are associated with common and unique differences in symptoms, neurocognition, and structural and functional brain parameters.[88,89] Thus, the psychotic behavior seen in some lone-actor terrorists likely has a root cause in the additive effects of sinsemilla and early life adversity.

Regular marijuana contains significant cannabidiol (CBD) and sinsemilla does not. CBD is protective against psychosis. Also, research is beginning to demonstrate that many of the individual differences in the development of psychosis after using high-potency marijuana are genetic. The mechanism of an association of psychosis and cannabis appears related to alterations of brain dopamine receptor sensitivity after prolonged high-potency cannabis use.[35]

Methamphetamine

Production and sale of methamphetamine has become one of the primary methods by which terrorists finance their operations. Not only do some terrorists take it themselves for personal use, but it is one of the leading currencies used for the development of revenue to maintain terroristic programs. Money laundering has become a behavior that is widely used by terrorist organizations to finance their programs.[90] Methamphetamine has also been linked directly to the criminal behavior and motivations of some lone-wolf terrorists. One of the best examples was that of Timothy McVeigh, who bombed the Murrah Federal Building in Oklahoma City. Those who have evaluated his behavior noted that, shortly after the Waco, Texas tragedy, McVeigh began using large amounts of methamphetamine. He was serving in the US Army at the time, and he became a drug-addicted lost soldier. It is felt that methamphetamine contributed specifically to the obsession McVeigh developed about bombing the federal building in Oklahoma City. It is ironic that McVeigh's use of crystal methamphetamine was never admitted into evidence or presented at trial. The prosecution believed they had enough evidence to convict McVeigh without getting involved in an insanity plea or an expensive, time-consuming drug evaluation program. Thus, there was no public record made of testimony regarding his methamphetamine use.[91]

The pharmacologic mechanisms of crystal methamphetamine and other methamphetamine products have been fairly well established. Methamphetamine causes the release of the neurotransmitters dopamine, norepinephrine, and serotonin and activates the cardiovascular and central nervous systems. The exact areas of the brain involved in methamphetamine addiction are unknown but probably include dopamine-rich areas such as the striatum and regions that interact with the striatum. At present, there is no therapeutic agent to target dopamine and nondopamine systems. Thus, there are no medications approved for the treatment of relapses in methamphetamine addiction at this time. Data from animals show that a high dose of methamphetamine damages striatal dopamine nerve terminals.[92]

Of relevance to terroristic actions, there is a well-known methamphetamine-associated psychosis. Chronic methamphetamine use profoundly changes brain structures and chemistry. Methamphetamine psychosis seems related to catecholaminergic systems (e.g., dopamine, norepinephrine, serotonin, etc.). We know from studies in schizophrenia and parkinsonism that excess dopamine can often lead to psychosis, and antipsychotic drugs are effective for reducing psychosis in those patients by blocking the effects of dopamine. Human postmortem and imaging studies have consistently shown that chronic methamphetamine use causes a reduction of dopamine transporter density (DAT) in the various dopaminergic systems, including the dorsal striatum, nucleus accumbens, and prefrontal cortex.[93]

There is a recent claim that an analog of methamphetamine was probably used by terrorists in the Paris and Tunis attacks that occurred on November 13, 2015, in Europe. These attacks were the deadliest attacks in France since World War II, and the deadliest attacks in the European Union since the Madrid train bombings in 2004.[11] The product allegedly used by these individuals was speculated to be fenethylline, which acts as a prodrug to amphetamine and theophylline. Its advantage to users is that it does not increase blood pressure to the same extent as amphetamine or methamphetamine, and it can be used by persons who have cardiovascular conditions. It is usually taken orally but can be dissolved into a liquid and injected. However, these claims about the attacks in Paris and Tunis have been widely refuted in follow-up press releases.[94]

It seems clear that methamphetamine plays a major role in terrorism, particularly lone-actor terrorism. Methamphetamine is used by lone-actor terrorists to stimulate themselves, but these individuals run the risk of paranoid thinking, delusional behavior, and psychosis from the drug.

Anabolic Androgenic Steroids

AASs have been linked to a range of problematic behaviors. However, AAS use is sometimes portrayed as more benign than other forms of classical drug abuse. Youngsters enjoy using these drugs in body-building attempts and most of the recent quality studies come from the Nordic countries, which have the highest prevalence of AAS use in the world. In a recent Swedish study,[95] the authors found that, among adolescent boys, AAS use was associated with a significantly higher prevalence of antisocial behavior compared to non-AAS illicit drug users and drug non-users. The study covered 3 years, and the results were consistent across all 3 years, suggesting that the finding is robust. The authors point out that the most important findings contradict the popular view that AAS doping is a "mild" form of substance abuse. On the contrary, young male AAS users appear considerably more antisocial than non-AAS illicit drug users as a whole.

In the Anders Breivik case, as a teenager Breivik was preoccupied with his physical appearance. He worked out frequently, used anabolic steroids, and had cosmetic nose surgery in his early 20s. He even discussed this in his manifesto.[66] Breivik was tried after his massacre of youngsters in Norway at a campground. He was described by the first psychiatrist who examined him as psychotic and was laughing while murdering children. This was also corroborated by eyewitnesses. The prosecution chose not to explore the issue of AAS use because they believed they had sufficient evidence to get a conviction. Thus, the anabolic steroid issue and his apparent psychosis played little role at trial.[96]

With regard to the behavioral changes associated with anabolic steroid use, it is notable that androgen users engage in polypharmacy, often ingesting other hormones such as human growth hormone, thyroid hormone, and insulin, and also use classical drugs of abuse such as cannabis, opioids, and cocaine. The use of androgens can cause hypomania, aggression, or violence in occasional users. These biological effects and psychiatric effects are exaggerated in chronic users. As previously noted, Anders Breivik was charged with killing 77 civilians in Oslo and Utøya, Norway on July 22, 2011. In his 1,500-page manifesto, Breivik details the use of stanozolol (Winstrol) and DBOL, presumably methandrostenolone, in systematic preparation for his terroristic attacks.[66,96]

The psychological effects of AAS are unpredictable. AAS are implicated in cases of violent behavior ("roid rage"), including manslaughter and murder. Polypharmacy with these agents can increase the risk of violent criminality.[97,98]

Ethyl Alcohol

Alcohol is the oldest and most abused substance on our planet. It is the easiest and cheapest mind-altering substance available to all persons, including lone-actor terrorists. Gill[14] has noted its high use among lone-actor terrorists compared with group terrorists. Many lone-actor terrorists come from homes where the father was a binge drinker

and engaged in intimate partner violence toward the mother.[99] Thus, the lone-actor terrorist's background of early life adversity in an abusive home and the resulting epigenetic behavioral changes, combined with the gateway to binge drinking and other substance use, becomes the runway for ideological influences in the personal environment. Father and son are both more likely to be substance abusers.[14] There is emerging evidence that binge drinkers have increased sensitivity to the disinhibiting effects of alcohol.[100] This may explain the link between impulsivity and problem drinking and the impulsivity seen in loners.

Alcohol is a psychoactive drug with relaxant and euphoric effects. Risky drinking patterns for men are defined as consuming more than 14 drinks per week or more than 4 drinks in a single day (bingeing). Neurobehavioral decline is seen in those who have a history of 5 years of drinking 21 or more drinks weekly. There is no one variable that will consistently and completely account for the underpinnings of alcohol-induced brain defects.[101]

Conclusion

Psychoactive substances are defined by the World Health Organization as "substances that, when taken in or administered into one's system, affect mental processes, e.g., cognition or affect." The *Diagnostic and Statistical Manual of Mental Disorders* (DSM-5) defines a mental disorder as a syndrome identified by its dysfunctional clinical disturbances in the cognitive, emotional, and behavioral aspects of an individual. In the course of this chapter, via its case studies and discussions, we have attempted to illustrate the close relationship between mental health and psychoactive substances taken by lone-actor terrorists. In some cases, such as with high-potency cannabis, there is a direct link with psychotic effects, even a dose-response relationship between the level of use and later psychotic episodes. The changing cannabis market to high-potency products as well as its easy accessibility is a significant problem not just for health authorities but also for counter-terror experts. The use of stimulants such as methamphetamine and AAS may exacerbate the manic if not aggressive effects of existing mental illnesses. In the last case study, medical, mental health, and enforcement specialists are confronted with a new multidimensional problem. Previously the relationships among psychoactive substances, mental illness, and terror dealt with the administration or abuse of "traditional" drugs. Bales presents a new challenge: namely, the side effects of prescription drugs. Experts were aware of the misuse of such prescription medications as methylphenidate, fenethylline, synthetic opioids, and benzodiazepines, and others. In Bales's case, the military prescribed the use of mefloquine for a specific medical indication, but its potential for neuropsychiatric side effects had a cumulative effect on his PTSD and eventual substance abuse behavior with alcohol and AAS.

The convergence of criminal liability, psychoactive substances, and mental status was underscored in a landmark decision by the Court of Appeal of Paris in December 2019. In 2017, Kobili Traore, a 29-year-old Muslim man was accused of beating and murdering a 60-year-old Orthodox Jewish woman while chanting verses from the Koran and ranting that she was a demon. Traore had a criminal background, occasionally prayed in a Salafist mosque, and had no notable former psychiatric history. He had been known to abuse cannabis, and toxicological reports after the incident revealed the substance in his body. The accused confessed to the murder and underwent extensive psychiatric examinations. According to various reports, he claimed to have smoked up to 15 cannabis cigarettes per day. In December 2019, the Court of Appeal of Paris upheld a lower court decision that the suspect had a "delusional episode" due to the excessive amount of cannabis he abused. According to Article 122-1 of the Code Pénal he was not criminally responsible for the murder.

Three divergent psychiatric opinions were rendered during the legal hearings. In 2017, Dr. Daniel Zagury, the first psychiatrist to examine Traore, expressed that while undoubtedly cannabis was an important factor regarding the accused's mental state, the fact that he voluntarily consumed the substance did not release him from criminal responsibility. Three psychiatrists gave the second diagnosis, which stated that the accused's "entry into schizophrenia" was unrelated to his consumption of cannabis. They based their conclusion on the "moderate level" of THC in the toxicological examination and the extended length of his delusions.

The third panel of experts confirmed that Traore's "delusional episode" was caused by his excessive cannabis consumption. They were undecided regarding his discernment but leaned toward the opinion that he was not criminally responsible. Two of the psychiatrists summarized that since Traore could not imagine the hallucinogenic effects of his consumption, he was not criminally responsible.[102] The court accepted their analysis. Future criminologists and anti-terror experts will have to grapple with this legal quagmire.

A future concern for experts will be illegal and unregulated consumption of new or novel psychoactive substances (NPS). These are psychoactive substances that mimic the effect of traditional drugs of abuse. They include a multitude of substances including synthetic cannabinoids, cathinone derivatives, psychedelic phenethylamines, novel stimulants, synthetic opioids, psychoactive herbs and plants, and performance-enhancing drugs. The safety profiles and acute and chronic side effects of these drugs are not well documented, if at all. They are easily accessible via the internet and "head shops," hence, with consumption on the increase so are hospitalizations and deaths. Their psychopathological manifestations and their eventual effect on lone actors and mental illness are important areas for future research.

The almost symbiotic relationship between mental illness and psychoactive substances can constitute a significant risk factor in the lone actor's path to terror. We believe that future researches in lone-actor terror must examine the use of psychoactive substances as a potent and dangerous risk factor. In the United Kingdom, as in other places, counter-terror researchers must work with their mental health clinician counterparts. Health officials must also be aware of the path to radicalization and its relation to mental health and substance abuse.

NOTES AND REFERENCES

1. May C. *Transnational Crime and the Developing World*. Washington DC: Global Financial Integrity; 2017:11. https://www.gfintegrity.org/wp-content/uploads/2017/03/Transnational_Crime-final.pdf
2. Braun M. Drug trafficking and Middle Eastern terrorist groups: A growing nexus? Washingtoninstitute.org, 2008. https://www.washingtoninstitute.org/policy-analysis/view/drug-trafficking-and-middle-eastern-terrorist-groups-a-growing-nexus.
3. Kamienski Ł. *Shooting Up: A Short History of Drugs and War*. New York: Oxford University Press; 2016: xix.
4. The drug fuelling death, despair and Boko Haram. BBC News, 2018. https://www.bbc.com/news/world-africa-44306086
5. Laing A. The Boko Haram suicide bomber who survived her deadly mission. *The Telegraph*, 2016. https://www.telegraph.co.uk/news/2016/03/31/the-boko-haram-suicide-bomber-who-survived-her-deadly-mission/

6. Santacroce R, Bosio E, Scioneri V, Mignone M. The new drugs and the sea: The phenomenon of narco-terrorism. *Int J Drug Policy*. 2018;51: 67–68. doi:10.1016/j.drugpo.2017.10.012.

7. AL-Imam A, Santacroce R, Roman-Urrestarazu A, et al. Captagon: Use and trade in the Middle East. *Hum Psychopharmacol*. 2017;32(3):1–8. doi:10.1002/hup.2548.

8. Mumbai attack analysis information as of December 4, 2008 N.Y.P.D. Intelligence Division, 2008. Info.publicintelligence.net. https://info.publicintelligence.net/nypdmumbaireport.pdf

9. Berlin terrorist Amri regularly used cocaine: Autopsy. ANSA.it. 2017. http://www.ansa.it/english/news/2017/03/03/berlin-terrorist-amri-regularly-used-cocaine-autopsy_b80dc04a-192c-4a51-af0c-c0e0c309fb1d.html

10. "Cowardice" delayed Tunisian authorities. BBC News, 2017. https://www.bbc.com/news/uk-38912629

11. Fond G, Howes O. Pharmacoterrorism: The potential role of psychoactive drugs in the Paris and Tunisian attacks. *Psychopharmacology (Berl)*. 2016;233(6):933–935. doi:10.1007/s00213-016-4204-2.

12. Gill P, Horgan J, Deckert P. Bombing alone: Tracing the motivations and antecedent behaviors of lone-actor terrorists. *J Forensic Sci*. 2013;59(2):425–435. doi:10.1111/1556-4029.12312.

13. Ministry of Public Security. Study: Terrorists post info on social media before attacking. Gov. il, 2018. https://www.gov.il/en/Departments/news/study_on_lone_wolf_terror_phenomena_120618

14. Gill P. *Lone-Actor Terrorists: A Behavioural Analysis*. 1st ed. New York: Taylor and Francis. Kindle Edition; 2015:108

15. Incident Summary for GTDID: 201003040016. Start.umd.edu. https://www.start.umd.edu/gtd/search/IncidentSummary.aspx?gtdid=201003040016

16. Bedell J. Rothbardix –Technology for liberty and justice. Rothbardix.blogspot.com, 2006. http://rothbardix.blogspot.com

17. Irving D, Hernandez S. O.C. court filing: Pentagon shooter bipolar. *Orange County Register*, 2010. https://www.ocregister.com/2010/03/07/oc-court-filing-pentagon-shooter-bipolar/

18. Bedell J. JPatrickBedell/JPatrickBedell 2007-01-08 cannabis evidence. WeedWiki, 8 Jan 2007. https://cannabis.wikia.org/wiki/User:JPatrickBedell/JPatrickBedell_2007-01-08_cannabis_evidence.

19. Incident Summary for GTDID: 201305220004. Start.umd.edu, 2013. https://www.start.umd.edu/gtd/search/IncidentSummary.aspx?gtdid=201305220004

20. Intelligence and Security Committee of Parliament. The Intelligence and Security Committee of Parliament Report on the intelligence relating to the murder of Fusilier Lee Rigby. Isc.independent.gov.uk, 2014. http://isc.independent.gov.uk/

21. O'Neill S, Gardham D. Woolwich killers: Lost boys went from drugs and gangs to radical Islam. Thetimes.co.uk, 2013. https://www.thetimes.co.uk/article/woolwich-killers-lost-boys-went-from-drugs-and-gangs-to-radical-islam-g272lxx8fcq?_ga=2.234097433.68036373.1535704409-1434477669.1535366019

22. Dodd V, Howden D. Woolwich murder: What drove two men to kill a soldier in the street? *The Guardian*, 2013. https://www.theguardian.com/uk-news/2013/dec/19/woolwich-murder-soldier-street-adebolajo-radicalised-kenya

23. Whitehead T. Adebowale on path to Islamist extremism after seeing 9/11. Telegraph.co.uk, 2013. https://www.telegraph.co.uk/news/uknews/terrorism-in-the-uk/10518784/Adebowale-on-path-to-Islamist-extremism-after-seeing-911.html

24. Cheston P, Davenport J. Lee Rigby murderer Adebowale "is borderline schizophrenic": Recommended for Broadmoor. *Evening Standard*, 2013. https://www.standard.co.uk/news/crime/lee-rigby-murderer-adebowale-is-borderline-schizophrenic-recommended-for-broadmoor-9015617.html

25. Sentencing remarks of Mr. Justice Sweeney. Judiciary.uk, 2014. https://www.judiciary.uk/wp-content/uploads/JCO/Documents/Judgments/adebolajo-adebowale-sentencing-remarks.pdf

26. Horgan J, Gill P, Bouhana N, Silver J, Corner E. Across the universe? A comparative analysis of violent behavior and radicalization across three offender types with implications for criminal justice training and education. Ncjrs.gov, 2016. https://www.ncjrs.gov/pdffiles1/nij/grants/249937.pdf

27. Dodd V, Addley E. Leytonstone knife attack: Man convicted of attempted murder. *The Guardian*, 2016. https://www.theguardian.com/uk-news/2016/jun/08/leytonstone-knife-attack-man-convicted-of-attempted

28. Dearden L. Leytonstone Tube attacker "thought Tony Blair was his guardian angel." *The Independent*, 2016. https://www.independent.co.uk/news/uk/crime/leytonstone-tube-stabbing-attack-isis-news-latest-sentencing-muhiddin-mire-attempted-murder-tony-a7158841.html

29. Spillett R, Gardham D. Leytonstone knifeman is jailed for life. Mail Online, 2016. https://www.dailymail.co.uk/news/article-3717890/Leytonstone-knifeman-jailed-life.html

30. Survey finds UK cannabis market dominated by high-potency skunk. News and features. Medical Research Council. Mrc.ukri.org, 2018. https://

mrc.ukri.org/news/browse/survey-finds-uk-cannabis-market-dominated-by-high-potency-skunk/.

31. ElSohly M, Mehmedic Z, Foster S, Gon C, Chandra S, Church J. Changes in cannabis potency over the last 2 decades (1995–2014): Analysis of current data in the United States. *Biol Psychiatry*. 2016;79(7):613–619. doi:10.1016/j.biopsych.2016.01.004.

32. Potter D, Hammond K, Tuffnell S, Walker C, Di Forti M. Potency of Δ9-tetrahydrocannabinol and other cannabinoids in cannabis in England in 2016: Implications for public health and pharmacology. *Drug Test Anal*. 2018;10(4):628–635. doi:10.1002/dta.2368.

33. Di Forti M, Marconi A, Carra E et al. Proportion of patients in south London with first-episode psychosis attributable to use of high potency cannabis: A case-control study. *Lancet Psychiatry*. 2015;2(3):233–238. doi:10.1016/s2215-0366(14)00117-5.

34. Gage S, Hickman M, Zammit S. Association between cannabis and psychosis: Epidemiologic evidence. *Biol Psychiatry*. 2016;79(7):549–556. doi:10.1016/j.biopsych.2015.08.001.

35. Murray R, Quigley H, Quattrone D, Englund A, Di Forti M. Traditional marijuana, high-potency cannabis and synthetic cannabinoids: Increasing risk for psychosis. *World Psychiatry*. 2016;15(3):195–204. doi:10.1002/wps.20341.

36. Volkow N, Swanson J, Evins A et al. Effects of cannabis use on human behavior, including cognition, motivation, and psychosis: A review. *JAMA Psychiatry*. 2016;73(3):292. doi:10.1001/jamapsychiatry.2015.3278.

37. Irving D, Hernandez S. O.C. court filing: Pentagon shooter bipolar. *Orange County Register*, 2010. https://www.ocregister.com/2010/03/07/oc-court-filing-pentagon-shooter-bipolar/

38. Agrawal A, Nurnberger J, Lynskey M. Cannabis involvement in individuals with bipolar disorder. *Psychiatry Res*. 2011;185(3):459–461. doi:10.1016/j.psychres.2010.07.007.

39. Cerullo MA, Strakowski SM. The prevalence and significance of substance use disorders in bipolar type I and II disorder. *Subst Abuse Treat Prevent Policy*. 2007;2:29.

40. van Rossum I, Boomsma M, Tenback D, Reed C, van Os J, EMBLEM Advisory Board. Does cannabis use affect treatment outcome in bipolar disorder? A longitudinal analysis. *J Nerv Mental Dis*. 2009;197:35–40.

41. American Psychiatric Association. *Diagnostic and Statistical Manual of Mental Disorders*. 5th ed. Arlington, VA: American Psychiatric Publishing; 2013.

42. Gibbs M, Winsper C, Marwaha S, Gilbert E, Broome M, Singh S. Cannabis use and mania

symptoms: A systematic review and meta-analysis. *J Affect Disord*. 2015;171:39. doi:10.1016/j.jad.2014.09.016.

43. Moore, III H. The final report of the circumstances, the investigation, and the determination of criminal responsibility for the officer involved death of Gavin Long on July 17, 2016. Ebrda.org., 2017. http://www.ebrda.org/ois/Final%20Report/Report%20OIS%20Gavin%20Long.pdf

44. Gartenstein-Ross D. Radicalization in the US and the rise of terrorism. Oversight.house.gov, 2016. https://oversight.house.gov/wp-content/uploads/2016/09/Gartenstein-Ross-Statement-Radicalization-9-14.pdf

45. Black identity extremists likely motivated to target law enforcement officers. Vault.fbi.gov, 2017. https://vault.fbi.gov/black-identity-extremist-bie-intelligence-assessment-august-3-2017/black-identity-extremist-bie-intelligence-assessment-august-3-2017-part-01-of-01.pdf

46. Kansas City Star. The latest on Gavin Long: Shooter killed an officer and a deputy then returned to wounded officer and killed him, police say. kansascity.com, 2016. https://www.kansascity.com/news/local/article90266242.html

47. Hegeman R. VA records: Baton Rouge gunman Gavin Long had mood disorder, not PTSD, wasn't seen as threat. *The Advocate*, 2016. https://www.theadvocate.com/baton_rouge/news/baton_rouge_officer_shooting/article_4c364eb6-6e3b-11e6-a5ec-276c72f8bba0.html

48. Benjamin M, De Yoanna M. "I am under a lot of pressure to not diagnose PTSD." Salon, 2009. https://www.salon.com/2009/04/08/tape/

49. Committee on the Assessment of Ongoing Efforts in the Treatment of Posttraumatic Stress Disorder; Board on the Health of Select Populations; Institute of Medicine. Treatment for Posttraumatic Stress Disorder in Military and Veteran Populations: Final Assessment. Washington (DC): National Academies Press (US); 2014 Jun 17. PMID: 25077185.

50. Read suicide note left by Gavin Eugene Long, gunman in deadly Baton Rouge officer shooting in July 2016. *The Advocate*, 2017. https://www.theadvocate.com/baton_rouge/news/baton_rouge_officer_shooting/article_9748d2c0-5daa-11e7-af6d-ab3966e08d70.html

51. Xuan L, MacDonald A. T120. Examining psychosis in social media: The targeted individuals movement and the potential of pathological echo-chambers. *Schizophr Bull*. 2019;45(Supplement_2):S250–S251. doi:10.1093/schbul/sbz019.400.

52. Sheridan L, James D. Complaints of group-stalking ("gang-stalking"): An exploratory study of their nature and impact on complainants. *J*

Forens Psychiatry Psychol. 2015;26(5):601–623. doi:10.1080/14789949.2015.1054857.

53. Sarteschi C. Mass murder, targeted individuals, and gang-stalking: Exploring the connection. *Violence Gend.* 2018;5(1):45–54. doi:10.1089/vio.2017.0022.

54. The Baton Rouge gunman and "targeted individuals." Nytimes.com, 2016. https://www.nytimes.com/2016/07/20/us/gavin-long-baton-rouge-targeted-individuals.html?action=click&module=RelatedCoverage&pgtype=Article&region=Footer

55. Toxicology Gavin Long. Ebrda.org, 2016. http://www.ebrda.org/ois/Autopsy%20Reports/Gavin%20Long%20Tox_Redacted.pdf

56. Lud Cadet J, Gold M. Methamphetamine-induced psychosis: Who says all drug use is reversible?. Mdedge.com, 2017. https://www.mdedge.com/psychiatry/article/150344/addiction-medicine/methamphetamine-induced-psychosis-who-says-all-drug-use

57. Wahlstrom LC, Scott JP, Tuliao AP, DiLillo D, McChargue DE. Posttraumatic stress disorder symptoms, emotion dysregulation, and aggressive behavior among incarcerated methamphetamine users. *J Dual Diagn.* 2015;11(2):118–127. doi:10.1080/15504263.2015.1025026.

58. Zweben J, Cohen J, Christian D et al. Psychiatric symptoms in methamphetamine users. *Am J Addict.* 2004;13(2):181–190. doi:10.1080/10550490490436055.

59. Elbogen EB, Johnson SC. The intricate link between violence and mental disorder. *Arch Gen Psychiatry.* 2009;66(2):152. doi:10.1001/archgenpsychiatry.2008.537.

60. Hill M. The Westminster Bridge terrorist attack 22nd March 2017 Operation Classific: A report on the use of terrorism legislation. Assets.publishing.service.gov.uk, 2018. https://assets.publishing.service.gov.uk/government/uploads/system/uploads/attachment_data/file/697221/The_WestBridge_Attack_report_Accessible.pdf

61. Anderson D. Attacks in London and Manchester March-June 2017: Independent assessment of MI5 and police internal reviews. Assets.publishing.service.gov.uk, 2017. https://assets.publishing.service.gov.uk/government/uploads/system/uploads/attachment_data/file/664682/Attacks_in_London_and_Manchester_Open_Report.pdf

62. Inquests arising from the deaths in the Westminster Terror Attack of 22 March 2017 Day 11 September 25, 2018. Westminsterbridgeinquests.independent.gov.uk, 2018:46–58. https://westminsterbridgeinquests.independent.gov.uk/wp-content/uploads/2018/09/WI-Day-11-25-September-2018.pdf

63. Inquests arising from the deaths in the Westminster Terror Attack of 22 March 2017 Day 9 September 20, 2018. Westminsterbridgeinquests.independent.gov.uk, 2018:39. https://westminsterbridgeinquests.independent.gov.uk/wp-content/uploads/2018/09/WI-Day-9-20-September-2018.pdf

64. Pope H, Kanayama G, Athey A, Ryan E, Hudson J, Baggish A. The lifetime prevalence of anabolic-androgenic steroid use and dependence in Americans: Current best estimates. *Am J Addict.* 2014;23(4):371–377. doi:10.1111/j.1521-0391.2013.12118.x.

65. Pope H, Wood R, Rogol A, Nyberg F, Bowers L, Bhasin S. Adverse health consequences of performance-enhancing drugs: An Endocrine Society scientific statement. *Endocr Rev.* 2014;35(3):341–375. doi:10.1210/er.2013-1058.

66. Breivik A. 2083: A European Declaration of Independence: Anders Behring Breivik. Internet Archive, 2011. https://archive.org/details/2083_A_European_Declaration_of_Independence

67. Sullivan K, Wan W. Troubled. Quiet. Macho. Angry. The volatile life of the Orlando shooter. *The Independent*, 2016. https://www.independent.co.uk/news/world/americas/omar-mateen-orlando-gay-lgbt-nightclub-shooting-shooter-gunman-what-we-know-florida-a7090301.html

68. Charlton A. Father, dancer, extremist: The multiple lives of the Nice attacker. CBC News, 2016. https://www.cbc.ca/news/world/nice-attacker-details-emerge-1.3692947

69. London Bridge inquests day 15 May 28, 2019. Londonbridgeinquests.independent.gov.uk, 2019. https://londonbridgeinquests.independent.gov.uk/wp-content/uploads/2019/05/LBI-Day-15.pdf

70. Dillon N. Mail bomb suspect Cesar Sayoc was "mentally disturbed," used steroids and cut ties with Democrat mom who's "deeply regretful": Lawyer. Nydailynews.com, 2018. https://www.nydailynews.com/news/ny-news-florida-bombing-suspect-estranged-from-family-20181026-story.html

71. University of Chicago Law School. Robert Bales. Law.uchicago.edu. https://www.law.uchicago.edu/clinics/mandel/mental/combat/bales

72. Incident Summary for GTDID: 201203110028. Start.umd.edu, 2012. https://www.start.umd.edu/gtd/search/IncidentSummary.aspx?gtdid=201203110028

73. Dao J. Robert Bales: From small-town Ohio to Afghanistan. Nytimes.com, 2012. https://www.nytimes.com/2012/03/19/us/sgt-robert-bales-from-small-town-ohio-to-afghanistan.html

74. Vaughan B. Exclusive: America's most notorious war criminal speaks. *GQ*, 2015. https://www.gq.com/story/robert-bales-interview-afghanistan-massacre

75. Coldren R, Russell M, Parish R, Dretsch M, Kelly M. The ANAM lacks utility as a diagnostic or screening tool for concussion more than 10 days following injury. *Mil Med.* 2012;177(2):179–183. doi:10.7205/milmed-d-11-00278.

76. Shen Y, Arkes J, Lester P. Association between baseline psychological attributes and mental health outcomes after soldiers returned from deployment. *BMC Psychol.* 2017;5(1). doi:10.1186/s40359-017-0201-4.

77. Hoge C, McGurk D, Thomas J, Cox A, Engel C, Castro C. Mild traumatic brain injury in US soldiers returning from Iraq. *N Engl J Med.* 2008;358(5):453–463. doi:10.1056/nejmoa072972.

78. Murphy K. (2012). Massacre hearing raises questions. *Sun-Sentinel (Fort Lauderdale, Fla.).*

79. Denson T, Blundell K, Schofield T, Schira M, Krämer U. The neural correlates of alcohol-related aggression. *Cogn Affect Behav Neurosc.* 2018;18(2):203–215. doi:10.3758/s13415-017-0558-0.

80. MacManus D, Rona R, Dickson H, Somaini G, Fear N, Wessely S. Aggressive and violent behavior among military personnel deployed to Iraq and Afghanistan: Prevalence and link with deployment and combat exposure. Epidemiol Rev. 2015;37(1):196–212. doi:10.1093/epirev/mxu006.

81. Mefloquine. FDA approved label. Accessdata.fda. gov, 2013. https://www.accessdata.fda.gov/drug-satfda_docs/label/2009/019591s026s028lbl.pdf

82. In the Supreme Court of the United States Robert Bales, Petitioner, v. United States, Respondent. Supremecourt.gov, 2018. https://www.supremecourt.gov/DocketPDF/17/17-1583/47007/20180516105516057_Bales%20Petition%20for%20E-Filing%205%2016%202018.pdf

83. FDA approves label changes for antimalarial drug mefloquine hydroc. US Food and Drug Administration, 2013. https://www.fda.gov/drugs/drug-safety-and-availability/fda-drug-safety-communication-fda-approves-label-changes-antimalarial-drug-mefloquine-hydrochloride

84. Potter D. A review of the cultivation and processing of cannabis (Cannabis sativa L.) for production of prescription medicines in the UK. *Drug Test Anal.* 2013;6(1-2):31–38. doi:10.1002/dta.1531.

85. Mehmedic Z, Chandra S, Slade D et al. Potency trends of Δ9-THC and other cannabinoids in confiscated cannabis preparations from 1993 to 2008. *J Forensic Sci.* 2010;55(5):1209–1217. doi:10.1111/j.1556-4029.2010.01441.x.

86. Clouston T. The Cairo Asylum. Dr. Warnock on hasheesh insanity. *J Mental Sci.* 1896;42(179):790–795. doi:10.1192/bjp.42.179.790.

87. Harley M, Kelleher I, Clarke M et al. Cannabis use and childhood trauma interact additively to increase the risk of psychotic symptoms in adolescence. *Psychol Med.* 2009;40(10):1627–1634. doi:10.1017/s0033291709991966.

88. Gur R, Moore T, Rosen A et al. Burden of environmental adversity associated with psychopathology, maturation, and brain behavior parameters in youths. *JAMA Psychiatry.* 2019. doi:10.1001/jamapsychiatry.2019.0943.

89. Hackman D, Farah M. Socioeconomic status and the developing brain. *Trends Cogn Sci (Regul Ed).* 2009;13(2):65–73. doi:10.1016/j.tics.2008.11.003.

90. Samantha Maitland Irwin A, Raymond Choo K, Liu L. Modelling of money laundering and terrorism financing typologies. *J Money Laundering Control.* 2012;15(3):316–335. doi:10.1108/13685201211238061.

91. Fetter, Mark Lawson, "The criminal behavior and motivations behind McVeigh's decision to bomb the Murrah Federal Building" (2002). *Theses Digitization Project.* 2251. https://scholarworks.lib.csusb.edu/etd-project/2251

92. Ricaurte G, Seiden L, Schuster C. Further evidence that amphetamines produce long-lasting dopamine neurochemical deficits by destroying dopamine nerve fibers. *Brain Res.* 1984;303(2):359–364. doi:10.1016/0006-8993(84)91221-6.

93. Grant K, LeVan T, Wells S et al. Methamphetamine-associated psychosis. *J Neuroimmune Pharmacol.* 2012;7:113–139. doi:10.107/s11481.011.9288.1.

94. Paris attackers not on drugs, toxicology report finds. France 24, 2016. https://www.france24.com/en/20160105-paris-attackers-not-drugs-toxicology-report-finds-captagon-terrorism-france

95. Hallgren M, Pope Jr H, Kanayama G, Hudson J, Lundin A, Källmén H. Anti-social behaviors associated with anabolic-androgenic steroid use among male adolescents. *Eur Addict Res.* 2015;21(6):321–326. doi:10.1159/000433580.

96. Melle I. The Breivik case and what psychiatrists can learn from it. *World Psychiatry.* 2013;12(1):16–21. doi:10.1002/wps.20002.

97. Kanayama G, Pope H. Illicit use of androgens and other hormones. *Curr Opin Endocrinol Diabetes Obesity.* 2012;19(3):211–219. doi:10.1097/med.0b013e3283524008.

98. Klötz F, Petersson A, Isacson D, Thiblin I. Violent crime and substance abuse: A medico-legal comparison between deceased users of anabolic androgenic steroids and abusers of illicit drugs. *Forensic Sci Int.* 2007;173(1):57–63. doi:10.1016/j.forsciint.2007.01.026.

99. Hines D, Douglas E. Understanding the use of violence among men who sustain intimate terrorism. *Partner Abuse.* 2011;2(3):259–283. doi:10.1891/1946-6560.2.3.259.

100. Marczinski C, Combs S, Fillmore M. Increased sensitivity to the disinhibiting effects of alcohol in binge drinkers. *Psychol Addict Behav.* 2007;21(3): 346–354. doi:10.1037/0893-164x.21.3.346.

101. Oscar-Berman M, Marinković K. Alcohol: Effects on neurobehavioral functions and the brain. *Neuropsychol Rev.* 2007;17(3):239–257. doi:10.1007/s11065-007-9038-6.

102. Couvelaire L. Meurtre de Sarah Halimi: Pas de procès pour le suspect, jugé pénalement irresponsable. Le Monde.fr., 2019. https://www.lemonde.fr/societe/article/2019/12/19/meurtre-de-sarah-halimi-le-suspect-juge-penalement-irresponsable_6023491_3224.html

5

Developmental Aspects of Lone-Actor Terrorists

KARL MOBBS, GEN IGNATIUS TANAKA, AND TERRY R. BARD

INTRODUCTION

Notwithstanding that a person's belief system frames their moral compass, the popular idiom "Hurt people hurt people" captures a common human practice of a need for others to feel that some pivotal life event can explain adverse human actions. Explanatory narratives may well be true in some cases, but the motivation behind making them is often more telling. In the case of the lone-actor terrorist, it should be noted that we are often considering the individual's complex subjective perception of being hurt or wronged since many commit suicide, thus leaving us with little understanding of their actions. It is human nature to create an empathic narrative to explain the actions of others when we assume only damaged humanity can explain such behavior. In those who survive, we may seek to make their actions more palatable with a more charitable post-hoc analysis. In order to avoid such nebulous post-hoc analysis, one should note that this text, in defining the lone-actor terrorist, will focus on perpetrators with clear ideologies behind their tragic actions.

Although life events or trauma are significant in many cases, empathically attributing later actions to life events fails to recognize that most people do not become lone-actor terrorists after tragic events. This chapter seeks to explain, not excuse, the possible factors that lead the lone-actor terrorist down the pathway to destruction. In so doing we recognize there will be unknowns that we are unaware of and that, in analyzing the vast developmental factors leading to rare events, we lack the statistical rigor to buttress the science.

SHADES OF GRAY, LACK OF EVIDENCE, AND HIGH POTENTIAL FOR MISATTRIBUTION

There is no single gene, environment, character, or trigger to explain what operationalizes a lone-actor terrorist. Lone-actor terrorists comprise a diverse group, and no ethical scientific experiment can delineate tipping points to prevent such atrocities. In reality, anecdotes and small sample sizes fuel the dataset for what are increasingly frequent but still rare events. There is also the major confound of terrorist groups, such as the Islamic State of Iraq and al-Sham (ISIS), shifting their modus operandi toward the lone-actor approach.[1] It is a social phenomenon that we will seek to understand developmentally, but one should note that the complexities of human behavior necessarily limit full understanding. For example, a comprehensive developmental analysis may be of little use if someone is radicalized at a latter age, close to the time of action. All such an analysis would accomplish is to identify those prone to radicalism rather than those prone to becoming lone-actor terrorists. Human behavior is complex, and each case carries a unique thumbprint for how misanthropic thoughts morph into real-world tragedies.

MENTAL ILLNESS AND THE LONE-ACTOR TERRORIST

In line with the prior notation about the need to explain lone-actor terrorist actions in some form of disordered development, public figures often seek to attribute lone-actor violence to mental illness. Many research studies have confirmed that treatable mental illness is rarely a factor in such cases. Although some research has found some *indications* of mental illness in up to 35% of cases, the World Health Organizations has estimated the prevalence of mental illness to be 27% of the global population.[2] These numbers are comparable, at best; alongside case analysis, mental illness cannot be considered a major factor. We know beliefs drive behavior, but we can learn more about the pathway to terrorism through delineating contributing factors.

BIOPSYCHOSO-
CIAL APPROACH

Irrespective of the onset, type of grievance, or pathology, how can we best analyze the development of lone actors? We divide this chapter based loosely on a biopsychosocial approach to better understand lone-actor violence. Separating biological, psychological, and social factors is problematic, hence the various following factors will be considered from a broader psychosocial perspective and will overlap. We will look at character makeup that lends itself to impaired social functioning and social ostracism, inclusive of family dynamics. Finally, we will look at the social world, divided into real-world and virtual relationships and influences, ultimately leading to a greater understanding of how misanthropy may evolve into socially destructive action.

THE LONE-ACTOR
TERRORIST ARCHETYPE

In one comprehensive analysis of 119 lone-actor terrorists, researchers found no single identifiable "profile" of a perpetrator. The study noted the following selected characteristics: 96% male, a mean age of 33 but a mode age of 22, 50% were single, 40% were unemployed, and 41% had previous criminal convictions. Interestingly 37% lived alone at the time of their planning or execution of said plan.[3]

In another study, based on analysis of 98 cases, the developmental pathway to becoming a lone-actor terrorist was characterized as follows:

> The study validates a series of commonalities associated with pathways to radicalization for lone wolf terrorists. The radicalization model indicates that lone wolf terrorism begins with a combination of personal and political grievances which form the basis for an affinity with online sympathizers. This is followed by the identification of an enabler, followed by the broadcasting of terrorist intent. The final commonality is a triggering event, or the catalyst for terrorism.[4]

One of the most important questions is what type of ideology drives a lone-actor terrorist. In a European study, looking at 120 cases from 2000–2014,[2] the breakdown of ideology was very informative—right-wing extremists, nationalists, and anti-government actors accounted for 80% of deaths. The breakdown of the subgroups was noteworthy: religiously inspired, 24%; right-wing operators, 28%; and school shooters, 63%.[2]

In a comparison of lone-actor terrorists with common homicides, most lone-actor terrorists attacked "seemingly random victims,"[5] compared to 10% of common homicides. Ninety-six percent of lone-actor terrorists were male, compared to 90% for common homicides. Thirty percent of lone-actor terrorists had a prior history of violence, compared to almost double that number for common homicide.[5]

In summary, the lone-actor terrorist is highly likely to be male, be in the midst of young adulthood, be anti-government, target random victims, and is enabled to nurture a grievance.

BIOLOGICAL FACTORS

Propensity for Violence and Epigenetic, in Utero and Birth Complications, and Head Injuries

In general we know that when one considers development, we must consider the biology or genetics of individuals. However, research shows that we cannot do so in isolation, without considering the environment; research lends itself to "nature through nurture"[6] rather than nature versus nurture. For example, we now know that a diverse environment will lead to more environmental influence on gene expression over purely genetic influence. Biological genetics also presents us with evidence that heritability varies with developmental stage and time: phenotypic expression is a dynamic, time-sensitive process, not static.[7,8] As such, in many ways, we are analyzing a moving target.

Are Epigenetics a Missing Variable?

If one looks at preconception factors, the field of epigenetics has recently shown that trauma can be inherited from prior generations.[7,8] Such a predisposition may be a factor in explaining why we have found it so difficult to analyze an assailant's current life to identify developmental pathways. We do not know what additional preconception factors may unfold over the coming years. Are we missing additional intergenerational factors that may account for the predisposition to violence? Obviously, the counter-argument is easily made that many others with intergenerational trauma do not become lone-actor terrorists. In all fairness, most but not all traits are no more than 50% genetic; as such, the environment must be considered alongside the biological substrate on which the environment acts. It is highly likely that solid analysis involving genetic factors will be informative in the future, but at this time much remains to be learned about gene–environment interplay.

Callous Unemotional Traits, Violence, and Antisocial Personality Disorder

In those afflicted with psychopathy, there is a so-called "warrior gene" that carries a deficiency of monoamine oxidase A. This deficiency is linked to increased risk-taking behavior.[9] Such a deficiency is also present in those afflicted by the genetic disorder *Brunner syndrome*; these individuals exhibit increased violence, hypersexuality, and tendency to commit arson. If one looks specifically at the propensity for violent behavior from a neurodevelopmental perspective, a case can be made that many factors play a role.[10] In one study, antisocial behavior coupled with "callous unemotional traits" in children was 81% heritable.[11] Twin studies show up to 48% heritability for "rule-breaking behavior."[12] Broader rule-breaking behavior with externalized blame was also found to be 80% heritable.[13]

In a Finish study of 749 violent prisoners, offenders were 1.7 times as likely to have low-activity monoamine oxidase A genes.[14] This enzyme deficiency results in a decreased ability to break down certain neurotransmitters, rendering the individual as having a heightened state of stimulation and so being triggered to impulsive violence. Again, this predisposition does not explain lone-action terrorists' actions entirely, as most are able to be planful and purposeful in their actions, but it does explain a major factor in those who are more willing to cross the line and become violent.

There are conflicting data about whether trauma before age 15 is required to activate the warrior gene. Genetics alone cannot explain complex human behavior. Social circumstance tends to push a genetically predisposed subgroup toward violence, but many people with the warrior gene do lead prosocial lives. As a result, we could not expect to eradicate lone-actor violence—or crime for that matter—through screening for callous unemotional traits or genes or developmental trauma.

Prenatal Nutrition and Violence

When considering the environment, the first environment is the womb. In one study exploring biosocial influences on violent behavior, poor nutrition during the perinatal period resulted in higher rates of aggression in children during follow-up at ages 8, 11, and 17.[15] Adriane Raine,

an expert in violence, also noted in an additional study,

> Because low IQ was found to mediate these relationships, these findings are consistent with the notion that poor nutrition results in brain maldevelopment, resulting in impaired neurocognitive functioning and aggressive behavior.[10]

Minor physical habitus abnormalities, acting as proxies for neurological maldevelopment, are also associated with violence. Such imperfections, coupled with a rejecting mother, were associated with a 90% occurrence of violent behavior in adulthood.[10] In addition, maternal prenatal use of alcohol and tobacco, as well as hypoxia at birth, are known to increase the risk of antisocial and violent behavior in adults.[10] A Finish study of 12,058 individuals found that brain injuries during childhood or adolescence conferred a 1.6-fold increased risk for criminal behavior in adulthood.[11]

Neuroscience and the Developing Brain

Lone-actor terrorists are often young men whose emotional immaturity is exacerbated by social isolation. A good example of this pattern is Dylann Roof, the perpetrator of the Charleston church shooting in 2015. During his developing years, he alternated between marijuana and buprenorphine abuse and playing video games after he stopped attending high school, leading to a socially isolated, disconnected life. We now know that the human brain, primarily the frontal lobes, is not fully developed until one reaches the mid-20s.[12] Add in a cocktail of trauma, social isolation, character pathology, and substance use and that development may be further emotionally delayed or stalled. The balance between rational evolved frontal lobes versus emotional limbic responses is worth consideration. The unleashed limbic brain gives rise to unreasonable behavior based on fixed concrete thinking, catastrophizing, premature conclusions, and paranoid perceptions. This emotionally reactive worldview is more consistent with the development of the lone actor. It is also consistent with those suffering from social isolation and societal rejection.

Drug Use

As with many aspects of human behavior, separating factors that influence behavior from those which are common in the general population is complicated by numerous confounding variables. In one study, 21% of lone-actor terrorists had a history of substance abuse.[5] In comparison, data from the US Centers for Disease Control and Prevention (CDC) show that 10% of the general population had used a drug in the prior month.[16] Thus, substance abuse may be a relevant factor in the development of the lone-actor terrorist, but it is only one among many potential influencing factors.

Religious Development

Understanding lone-actor terrorism from a religious developmental perspective remains complex. Many researchers have distinguished between lone-terrorist acts conducted and justified by religious beliefs and lone-terrorist acts having no connection with formal groups. There is a significant difference between these two orientations. For example, the anti-abortion lone actor who attacks a clinic or an obstetrician may claim that religious beliefs justify such action. Conversely, a lone actor who perpetrates a mass shooting in a school or movie theater may endorse a quite different ideology or motivation for the attack. However, the mental health and emotional stability of these two types of lone actors may be similar.

A lone actor's religious convictions may be the result of formal or informal indoctrination programs, such as religious cults or more fundamental religious traditions that view life in doctrinaire, black-and-white terms. Such models often reinterpret or reinvent common social values in order to justify their views and actions.

Conversely, lone actors who act independently from such systems often seem to act out as a result of personal pain, feelings of isolation and displacement, or simply a nebulous void of meaning or ideology. In more general terms, the etiology for their actions may well be more existential. Most appear to have experienced early developmental difficulties. Most are and feel isolated, different, and unable to fit in within more normative social contexts. Such additive responses to a sense of failure in the modern world are often referred to as "globalization of resentment." The problematic behavior of such persons stems from psychological and/or social pain. Although tipping points toward the decision to commit acts of terror may be elusive, a common thread of increasing psychological suffering or desperation typically precedes the violent behavior. The trigger for a violent response to an unbearable situation may have roots in the actor's religious or social upbringing.

Domestic Violence

Although we would characterize the data on this issue as largely anecdotal with regard to lone-actor terrorists, some authors, such as Hadley Freeman of *The Guardian*, have noted the correlation of domestic violence exposure and perpetration in lone-actor terrorists. Freeman cited the cases of Khalid Masood (Westminster attack, 2017), Dylann Roof (Charleston, 2014), Robert Lewis Dear (Colorado, Planned Parenthood, 2015), Mohamed Lahouaiej-Bouhlel (Bastille Day, Nice, France, 2016), and Seung-Hui-Cho (Virginia Tech, 2007) as cases examples.[14] World Health Organization (WHO) data estimate that one-third of women globally experience intimate partner violence. Exposure to such violence is associated with "perpetrating or experiencing violence later in life."[17] Given such a prevalence, exposure to domestic violence is a common developmental variable in lone-actor terrorists; however, such exposure is common in the nonviolent general population as well.

Attachment Style

In assessing any psychopathology, characterological or otherwise, one's attachment style can be vital. Many researchers have identified how childhood attachment style has implications for adult relationships. In the case of lone-actor terrorists, there are many cases that indicate an avoidant or anxious resistant attachment style, with both types being typical of 20% of the adult population.

Those afflicted with an avoidant attachment style tend to put little emphasis on close relationships and have little interest in being dependent on others. In contrast, those with an avoidant-resistant attachment style sense rejection from others if they fail to reciprocate their desire for closeness; they fear rejection and, as a result, scare others away. [18,19] In short, attachment styles may be a factor in determining the lone-actor terrorist's level of engagement, if any, with others. Attachment researchers have found that loneliness is related in part to a lack of confidence in the presence of the caregiver. If the world does not meet one's needs, then connecting to a particular cause or engaging in destruction may provide a sense of purpose and security.

A good example to illustrate some of these points is Timothy McVeigh, the perpetrator of the 1995 Oklahoma City Bombing. According to Dr. John Smith, the psychiatrist who evaluated McVeigh for the defense during his 1995 trial, McVeigh reported being bullied in school and characterized the federal government as "the ultimate bully."[20] He was also reported to have been frightened by witnessing intimate partner violence between his parents.[20] He described his father as "distant and unadventurous."[21] It was noted that his own interpersonal style reflected inadequacies that may have exacerbated his worldview of rejection: "[he] always said the wrong thing to women he was trying to impress."[21] It was noted that, while in the military, he "showed more interest in cleaning his collection of guns than girls or beer."[21]

How does one connect attachment related to action and social deficits? Meloy noted several characteristics of lone-actor terrorists consistent with a less than optimal attachment style. For example, failure to attach in romantic or affiliation relationships was prevalent. Also common were thwarting of occupational goals and general moral outrage fueled by perceived personal grievance. This subgroup experienced rigidity in their thinking and clandestine excitement at their actions—in short, an ideology-framed misanthropic worldview fueled by poor interpersonal connections.[22]

Family Dynamics

In addition to personal attachment, it is believed that a poor attachment style coupled with a hands-off parental approach can lead this subgroup, which is already prone to diversion, to lone-actor terrorism. It could well be that the parental style is a reaction to the child's presentation rather than an individually triggering parental style. As a result of this parental dynamic, this subgroup further socially isolates, creates separate hidden worlds, and sets the archetypal lone-actor terrorist up for sensitivity to social slights.

Triggers and Social Slights

In their social exclusion, lone individuals feel deprived of what they perceive as values to which they are entitled, and form grievances against the government responsible for their unemployment, discrimination and injustices. Their violence is a deviant adaptation to this gap between means and goals.[4]

Being more sensitive to social slights leads this type of lone-actor terrorist to sublimate such slights to a "greater" cause, one which they may or may not have previously identified. In various high-profile cases, the nodal "cause" has been highly variable: anti-technology, anti-abortion,

retribution for US military action, xenophobia, and Islamophobia. It has been proposed that the difference between lone-actor terrorists and common homicide offenders is the use of violence as being expressive versus being instrumental.[5]

Or is it feasible that any connection to a social slight is a cloak for the reality of "murders in search of a cause" and seeking to "botch together a narrative that suits them."[5] To provide a purpose is a means to legitimize their actions.[5]

Personality and Temperament

What character or temperament can we link to lone-actor terrorists? Putting current advances aside, we can say that someone who has a character predisposed to antisocial behavior and asocial tendencies fits many characteristics of a lone-actor terrorist. However, again, many of this same cohort do not revert to terrorism.

If one looks at the behavioral-genetic interactivity on personality development, it is clear that "human personality is based on the accumulated action of a very large number of genes."[18] In other words, one cannot look to specific genetic inheritance to track most traits that may lend to lone-actor terrorist archetypes.

Development of Vulnerable Personality Disorder Traits

As an individual progresses toward independence from their family members, whether they may be advancing to higher education or entering a workforce, they cannot easily rid themselves of the product of parental attachments. This often manifests in the form of personality disorder or disorder traits, defined by the *Diagnostic and Statistical Manual of Mental Disorders* (DSM-5) as inflexible "enduring patterns of inner experience and behavior" that deviate from cultural norms and encompass cognition, affectivity, interpersonal functioning, and impulse control.[23] Such personality traits or disorders can manifest in multiple settings and often lead to "significant distress or disability."[23] As with many vicious cycles, personality disorders or disorder traits begotten of an unhealthy parenting style can predispose one to be increasingly vulnerable to external stressors. Therefore, the model of "self-absorbed parents begets vulnerable self-absorbed children" is sustained despite the passage of time. Such an enduring pattern may partially explain why there is a nearly equal representation of perpetrators older than 40 as younger perpetrators in lone-actor terrorism,[24] reinforcing the DSM-5's definition of personality disorder as an affliction that is both "stable and of long duration."

Personality disorders are widely observed in violent offenders. A Dutch study observed a higher prevalence of personality disorder among matched samples of 275 male and 275 female prison inmates.[25] For females, borderline personality disorder was seen predominantly, whereas in males, antisocial personality disorder and narcissistic personality disorder were seen at higher rates. A report by the FBI cautioned stakeholders to be wary of certain personality traits that may be associated with violence,[26] many of which are consistent with characteristics of personality disorders described in the DSM. Traits of nursing "resentment over real or perceived injustices," being "untrusting and chronically suspicious of others," and having low frustration tolerance are all hallmark traits of paranoid personality disorder.[23,26] Attempting "to con and manipulate others," externalizing blame, and dehumanizing others with lack of empathy are typical traits of antisocial personality disorder.[23,26] Those with an "exaggerated sense of entitlement," a need for attention, and a sense of superiority who present themselves "as smarter, more creative, more talented," as noted in the FBI report, appear to meet clinical traits seen in narcissistic personality disorder as outlined by the DSM-5.[26] The FBI report in no way states that personality disorder equates to one becoming a school shooter, but the listed warning signs largely correlate with symptoms of various personality disorders.[26] Furthermore, Nesser notes that "there have been observed similarities between perpetrators of school massacres and terrorists,"[27] suggesting high utility of the FBI findings in the study of lone-actor terrorists.

Personality Disorder Traits and Maladaptive Coping

Studies demonstrate that those with personality disorders tend to cope with stressors in a maladaptive fashion. In the 119 lone-actor terrorists studied by Gill et al., 32.8% experienced elevated levels of stress, with a major stressor occurring within 1 year of the terrorist attack for 74.3% of those subjects.[28] Some had lost their employment, and many had change of addresses within 6 months prior to the offense.[28] Furthermore, behavioral changes were noted in work performance, religion, physical activities, and "outdoor excursions."[28] These factors indicate a high probability of vulnerability to external stressors, thus demonstrating observable changes in behaviors antecedent to acts of terrorism. Such vulnerability

is consistent with the poor coping skills seen in those with personality disorders. Spaaj noted lone-actor terrorists' poor coping mechanism as their tendency to mix personal frustrations and extremist ideologies that lead to externalization of blame.[29]

Myth of Social Isolation

There appears to be a commonly accepted myth of social isolation among lone-actor terrorists,[24] but this is questioned by multiple studies.[30,31] Studies by Gill et al. note that the vast majority of lone-actor terrorists are not "loners" in a classical sense of the categorization.[28,31] The Countering Lone-Actor Terrorism (CLAT) project has studied 120 perpetrators of lone-actor terrorism within the European Union from 2000 to 2014 and found "28% to be socially isolated, which does not confirm the idea" that the majority of actors are estranged from society.[32] For religiously inspired lone-actor terrorists, many are actively involved in their religious community, with social isolation found in only 9%.[32] Right-wing inspired lone-actor terrorists often find others with similar ideologies through the internet. Potential actors with a single-issue grievance often find niche communities through social media. Hence, through utilization of the internet, many lone-actor terrorists have active virtual interactions. In a strategic publication by the Inter-University Center for Terrorism Studies, Raphaeli notes that "the linkage and symbiotic relationship between the terrorist organizations and the social media networks" have become a tool of recruitment, indoctrination, and training for potential lone actors.[33] Raphaeli even goes so as far to suggest that social media has become terrorist organizations' "most potent weapon."[33] Again, such robust networking debunks the commonly perceived notion that lone-actor terrorists are socially isolated. Even if one's connections are only virtual, many lone-actor terrorists are able to find niches online in which they are actively engaged and from which they receive consistent validation. For example, the two brothers who committed the Boston Marathon bombing were highly celebrated in a specially issued edition of al-Qaeda's Inspire magazine that "contained pages of glory and praises of the brothers" as martyrs.[33]

Unhealthy Social Interactions and Leakage

However, the social connections obtained through social media for lone-actor terrorists are often one-sided, lacking in the bidirectional exchanges of ideas that create a healthy relationship. Thus, there are often "leaks" that are evidence of such one-sidedness in virtual connections. One key finding of the CLAT study was that "lone-actor terrorists have often announced their intent to commit a terrorist act," although there were differences in intended audiences.[34] Gill et al. found it striking that in 82.4% of the cases they studied, others were cognizant of "the individual's grievances that spurred the terrorist plot."[31] Seventy-three percent of lone-actor terrorists had "offered oral or written justification for their actions."[30] Religiously inspired terrorists often publicize their ideologies and plans of violence before execution, and 45% of religiously inspired lone-actor terrorists were noted to disclose their plans to "to friends or families."[34] However, only 18% of right-wing–inspired lone actors had leakage to friends or families; instead 41% published their violent acts on social media after their attack.[34] Interestingly, lone-actor terrorists with single-issue grievances often justify their violent offense by appropriating popular grievances or political topics at the time. Such appropriation demonstrates that certain lone-actor terrorists commit violent acts on impulse alone, without any political or religious agenda. Furthermore, this lack of agenda and seeking out an "excuse" after the violence underscores the inherent vulnerability of potential lone-actor offenders to external stressors.

Many lone-actor terrorists are given positive validations through social media platforms. Internet-facilitated radicalization into extreme religious ideologies has been observed, and Flynn asserted that "technology and social media have fueled the rise of these lone actors."[33] The 2014 study by Gill et al. that studied 119 lone-actor terrorists showed that 35% "interacted virtually with a wider network of political activities," and 46.2% used virtual sources to "learn aspects of their attack method."[31] The rate of success based on online training is low, with the CLAT study noting only one case that caused a direct fatality; however, with possible advent of higher quality training manuals online, the potential for serious damage is worrisome.[30] Also, online newsletters and pamphlets that praise lone-actor terrorists as "heroes" or "martyrs," as seen with the Boston Marathon bombing culprits, continue to give positive reinforcement to those who are vulnerable and susceptible to instant gratification and adoration.[33] As mentioned before, the *Inspire* magazine issued by the Yemen branch of the al-Qaeda organization as another example of virtual connection "has led a campaign recommending solo terrorism and providing operational advice."[27]

CONCLUSION

In conclusion, rare events with disparate motives are something we cannot predict. We attempted to outline a lone-actor terrorist archetype, but, due to the low number of events, such analysis provides no clear way of identifying such individuals. However, we have proposed consideration of developmental inheritance, attachment patterns, character, exposures, and experiences that may influence those prone to violence. Being able to identify such patterns, characteristics, and experiences may enable the identification of such individuals as a means to intervene and prevent development of future lone-actor terrorists. There is much for us to learn about these rare events and the tipping points that preceded them. To decrease terrorism, we not only need to identify the individuals most likely to travel that pathway, but ultimately to modify wider society—from families to global communities—to favor nonviolent responses to the experience of ostracism and feeling disenfranchised.

NOTES AND REFERENCES

1. Burke J. Islamist terror has evolved toward lone actors—and it's brutally effective. *The Guardian*, 15 Jun 2016. https://www.theguardian.com/us-news/2016/jun/15/islam-jihad-terrorism-orlando-shooting-paris-attack
2. Ellis C, Pantucci P, de Roy van Zuijdewijn J, et al. Countering lone-actor terrorism series no. 11. Lone Actor Terrorism Final Report. 2016. https://static.rusi.org/201604_clat_final_report.pdf
3. Gill P, Horgan J, Deckert P. Bombing alone: Tracing the motivations and antecedent behaviors of lone-actor terrorists. *J Forensic Sci.* 2014;59(2):425–435.
4. Hamm M, Spaaij R. *Lone Wolf Terrorism in America: Using Knowledge of Radicalization Pathways to Forge Prevention Strategies*. Washington, DC: US Department of Justice; 2015.
5. Liem M, van Buuren J, de Roy van Zuijdewijn J, Schönberger H, Bakker E. European lone-actor terrorists versus "common" homicide offenders: An empirical analysis. *Homicide Stud.* 2018;22(1):45–69. doi:10.1177/1088767917736797.
6. National Research Council (US) and Institute of Medicine (US) Committee on Integrating the Science of Early Childhood Development; Shonkoff JP, Phillips DA, editors. From Neurons to Neighborhoods: The Science of Early Childhood Development. Washington (DC): National Academies Press (US); 2000. Available from: https://www.ncbi.nlm.nih.gov/books/NBK225557/doi:10.17226/9824
7. Binder E. The effects of early life stress on the epigenome: From the womb to adulthood and even before. *Provençal NExp Neurol.* 2015(268):10–20. doi:10.1016/j.expneurol.2014.09.001. Epub 9 Sep 2014.

8. Costa D, Yetter N, DeSomer H. Intergenerational transmission of paternal trauma among US Civil War ex-POWs. *Proc Natl Acad Sci.* 2018;115(44): 11215–11220. doi:10.1073/pnas.1803630115.

9. McDermott R, Tingley D, Cowden J, Frazzetto G, Johnson DD. Monoamine oxidase A gene (MAOA) predicts behavioral aggression following provocation. *Proc Natl Acad Sci U S A.* 2009 Feb 17;106(7):2118–2123. doi:10.1073/pnas.0808376106. Epub 2009 Jan 23. PMID: 19168625; PMCID: PMC2650118.

10. Raine A. A neurodevelopmental perspective on male violence. *Infant Ment Health J.* 2018;40(1):84–97; doi:10.1002/imhj.21761.

11. Timonen M, Miettunen J, Hakko H, et al. The association of preceding traumatic brain injury with mental disorders, alcoholism and criminality: The Northern Finland 1966 birth cohort study. *Psychiat Res.* 2002;113(3):217–226.

12. Arain M, Haque M, Johal L, et al. Maturation of the adolescent brain. *Neuropsychiatr Dis Treat.* 2013;9:449–461. doi:10.2147/NDT.S39776.

13. Sanchez R. Unsealed FBI docs paint disturbing portrait of Sandy Hook Shooter Adam Lanza. CNN, 25 Oct 2017. https://www.cnn.com/2017/10/24/us/sandy-hook-adam-lanza-unsealed-docs/index.html

14. Freeman H. What do many lone attackers have in common? Domestic violence. *The Guardian,* 28 Mar 2017. https://www.theguardian.com/commentisfree/2017/mar/28/lone-attackers-domestic-violence-khalid-masood-westminster-attacks-terrorism

15. Brennan P, Mednick S, Raine A. Biosocial interactions and violence: A focus on perinatal factors. In Raine A, Brennan P, Farrington D, Mednick S, eds. *NATO ASI series: Series A: Life Sciences, Vol. 292. Biosocial Bases of Violence.* New York: Plenum Press; 1997:163–174. doi:org/10.1007/978-1-4757-4648-8_10.

16. Illicit drug use. National Center for Health Statistics, Centers for Disease Control and Prevention, 3 May 2017. https://www.cdc.gov/nchs/fastats/drug-use-illegal.htm

17. Violence against women. World Health Organization, 29 Nov 2017. https://www.who.int/newsroom/fact-sheets/detail/violence-against-women

18. Turkheimer E, Pettersson E, Horn E. A phenotypic null hypothesis for the genetics of personality. *Annu Rev Psychol.* 2014;65:515–540.

19. Hazan C, Shaver P. Romantic love conceptualized as an attachment process. *J Pers and Soc Psychol.* 1987;52(3):511–524. doi:org/10.1037/0022-3514.52.3.511.

20. Inside McVeigh's mind. BBC News America, 11 May 2001. http://news.bbc.co.uk/2/hi/americas/1382540.stm

21. Profile: Timothy McVeigh. BBC News America, 11 May 2001. http://news.bbc.co.uk/2/hi/americas/1321244.stm

22. Meloy JR, Yakeley J. The violent true believer as a "lone wolf": Psychoanalytic perspectives on terrorism. *Behav Sci Law.* 2014;32:347–365. doi:10.1002/bsl.2109.

23. American Psychiatric Association. *Diagnostic and Statistical Manual of Mental Disorders.* 5th ed. Washington, DC: American Psychiatric Association; 2013. DSM-V. doi-org.db29.linccweb.org/10.1176/ appi.books.9780890425596. dsm02

24. De Roy van Zuijdewijn J, Bakker E. Analysing personal characteristics of lone-actor terrorists: Research findings and recommendations. *Perspect Terror.* 2016;10(2):42–49.

25. De Vogel V, Stam J, Bouman Y H, Ter Horst P, Lancel M. Violent women: A multicentre study into gender differences in forensic psychiatric patients. *J Forens Psychiatry Psychol.* 2016;27(2):145–168.

26. O'Toole M. *The School Shooter: A Threat Assessment Perspective.* Darby, PA: DIANE Publishing; 2009.

27. Nesser P. Research note: Single actor terrorism: Scope, characteristics and explanations. *Perspect Terror.* 2012;6(6):61–73.

28. Gill P, Corner E, Conway M, Thornton A, Bloom M, Horgan J. Terrorist use of the Internet by the numbers: Quantifying behaviors, patterns, and processes. *Criminol Public Policy.* 2017;16(1):99–117.

29. Spaaij R. *Understanding Lone Wolf Terrorism: Global Patterns, Motivations and Prevention.* Berlin: Springer Science & Business Media; 2011.

30. Ellis C, Pantucci R, de Roy van Zuijdewijn J, et al. Lone-actor terrorism: Analysis paper. Countering Lone-Actor Terrorism Series. No 4. London: Royal United Services Institute for Defense and Security Studies; February 2016.

31. Gill P, Horgan J, Deckert P. Bombing alone: Tracing the motivations and antecedent behaviors of lone-actor terrorists. *J Forensic Sci.* 2014;59(2):425–435.

32. de Roy van Zuijdewijn J, Bakker E. Policy Paper 1: Personal characteristics of lone-actor terrorists. Countering Lone-Actor Terrorism Series, No 5. The Hague: International Center for Counter Terrorism; 2016.

33. Fredholm M. ed. *Understanding Lone Actor Terrorism: Past Experience, Future Outlook, and Response Strategies.* New York: Routledge; 2016.

34. Ellis C, Pantucci R. Lone-actor terrorism: Policy Paper 4: "Leakage" and interaction with authorities. Countering Lone-Actor Terrorism Series, No. 8. Royal United Services Institute for Defence and Security Studies, February 2016.

6

The Role of Psychometrics in Investigating Lone-Actor Terrorism

NANCY P. MOCZYNSKI, ALLEN R. SCHILLER,
THEODORA NAJLA FARAH, AND ERIC Y. DROGIN

INTRODUCTION

The FBI defines terrorism as "the unlawful use of force and violence against persons or property to intimidate or coerce a government, the civilian population, or any segment thereof, in further-ance of political or social objectives."[1] Lone-actor terrorism—conducted by an individual with-out direct supervision—is by no means a novel development,[2] and it occurs with increasing fre-quency.[3] At present, however, systematic exami-nations of incidents and individuals are limited in both number and scope, such that precise dynam-ics have proved difficult to analyze in an aggregate fashion.

Theoretical perspectives on terrorist action have proved inconsistent over the course of the past several decades, with primary emphases that eventually shifted from individual characteris-tics to contextual variables. During the 1970s, for example, social scientists focused on identifying the components of the so-called terrorist per-sonality—a construct that has subsequently been refuted.[4] Terrorists were initially viewed as ratio-nal actors, but later as mentally unstable, emo-tionally vulnerable, and ideologically malleable. By the 1990s and early 2000s, explanatory models increasingly relied on group dynamics and reli-gious or political ideology.[5,6]

The lone-actor terrorist appears to defy many conclusions that were based on research on group-affiliated terrorism. In particular, more recent studies tend to indicate that mental ill-ness and other personal frailties are distinctly more common among lone-actor terrorists than among their peers who are provided the supervi-sion and reinforcement of a group.[7,8] A mere diag-nosis of mental illness, however, neither predicts

nor explains terrorist activity, particularly since most individuals with psychiatric disorders do not engage in violent behavior. For this reason, certain *symptoms* of mental illness become a sig-nificantly more important focus of contemporary research than diagnosis alone. Although no sin-gle, isolated psychological phenomenon "causes" terrorism, a host of intrapsychic factors appear to interact in complex and dynamic ways along the path to such activities.[9]

A greater understanding of the psychological attributes of lone-actor terrorists contributes to the ultimate goal of obviating physical and emo-tional harm and warding off broader threats to national security. In this chapter, we define and describe the science of psychometrics; enumerate and describe key instruments that this approach employs; identify the strengths, deficits, and behavioral inclinations that such instruments purport to measure; and specify how all of this complements efforts to prevent incidents of lone-actor terrorism. Such efforts represent a shared undertaking that calls for enhanced cooperation between professionals in security, law enforce-ment, and mental health.

PSYCHOMETRICS AND PSYCHOLOGICAL ASSESSMENT DEFINED

As an adjective, "psychometric" is a combina-tion of the word elements "psycho" (pertaining to the mind, spirit, or unconscious),[10] and "met-ric" (denoting the application of a standard of measurement).[11] The science of "psychometrics," therefore, brings statistically informed rigor to the investigation of psychological principles and ideas and provides the "mathematical underpinnings"[12] for the process of "psychological assessment," in which testing instruments, diagnostic clinical interviewing, and behavioral observations are employed to explore any of a range of factors that can include "intelligence, special abilities and disabilities, manual skill, vocational aptitudes, interests, and personality characteristics."[13] The most detailed and useful understanding of an individual results from combining the results of testing, interviewing, and observations with a thorough review of medical, psychological, and social histories gleaned from objective, external sources.[14]

ASSESSING RELEVANT DIAGNOSES AND CONDITIONS

It does not appear—at least to date—that psychological assessment has been particularly well-utilized in the investigation of lone-actor terrorism. Whether we understand this rarified form of violence as the end product of a developmental pathway[15] or as a changing and varied interaction between environmental and personal variables,[8] an increased understanding of this relatively unique population would surely contribute to more effective methods of detection, prevention, and amelioration. Following is a review of various diagnostic entities and other conditions worthy of investigation in this context.

Depressive Disorders

Depressive disorders have as their most salient common feature "the presence of sad, empty, or irritable mood, accompanied by somatic and cognitive changes that significantly affect the individual's capacity to function."[16] Recently conducted research has suggested that major depressive disorder, for example, may be a precipitating factor in an individual's vulnerability to terrorism-oriented radicalization.[17]

One would naturally inquire, in the course of a diagnostic clinical interview, into a number of potential depressive symptoms, including at a rather basic level how "depressed" an examinee currently feels. Although such data can be useful within the confines of treatment, they do little to afford objective comparison regarding the degree of distress commonly experienced by other individuals, by other groups of individuals, and—of critical relevance to forensically oriented evaluations—individuals being assessed by other evaluators.

One more objective approach could involve use of a research-validated, diagnosis-specific scale, such as the Beck Depression Inventory (in its current version, the BDI-2),[18] that addresses emotional and physical experiences typically associated with depressed mood. Examinees are asked, concerning each of 21 separate symptoms, to choose among four different statements that are arrayed in ascending order of personal distress, that statement representing the best approximation of how test-takers have been feeling during the course of the preceding 2 weeks. This measure and others like it are useful to the extent that they are both reliable (e.g., when repeated administrations result in similar responses, confirming consistency over time) and valid (e.g., when the test is proved to measure what it is intended to measure and not some other unintended or misidentified phenomenon).

Another similar but more expansive approach could involve the administration of a measure that addresses a much broader array of diagnostic entities—for example, the Minnesota Multiphasic Personality Inventory (in its current version, the MMPI-2, soon to become the MMPI-3)[19]—that was developed by refining test items with a large representative group (the "normative sample"). This enables evaluators to determine how individuals with varying diagnoses endorse the symptoms of a particular, targeted condition. This may be particularly helpful when the symptoms are not obvious or when the examinee has already denied the presence of such symptoms, perhaps in the context of a previously conducted diagnostic clinical interview. Here, also, the evaluator is more likely to uncover the presence of additional conditions that may not previously have been considered.

Intelligence

Intelligence may be conceptualized as the capacity to learn, understand, think, reason, and apply knowledge, as opposed to engaging a task automatically or merely by instinct.[20,21] David Wechsler, who developed the most widely used measure of intelligence—described in greater detail later—famously characterized what intelligence tests measure as "the capacity of an individual to understand the world about him and his resourcefulness to cope with its challenges."[22] The term "intelligence" itself, whether used colloquially or in a clinical context, reflects a composite of several often disparate factors. These factors can range from highly specific acquired knowledge (e.g., historical facts, technical definitions of words), to novel problem-solving (e.g., pattern recognition), to degrees of attention and concentration, to understanding social concepts, inference, and norms. "Intelligence," as a unified construct, can be regarded as the culmination—or at least the intersection—of each of these factors.

The concept of intelligence appears directly relevant to the psychological assessment of lone-actor terrorists. Research studies have asserted, for example, that lone actors may have higher intelligence than the average individual.[3] Notably, Ted Kaczynski, the so-called Unabomber,[23] had skipped two grades in school (6th and 11th) and matriculated at Harvard University at the age of 16. He claimed, in a psychiatric evaluation conducted during criminal proceedings, that his parents told him he was a genius and that he possessed a very high Full Scale Intelligence Quotient (IQ), perhaps in the range of 160 to 170 (an IQ of 100 is thought to represent the general population mean). Prior assessment records were unavailable at the time of Kaczynski's court-ordered evaluation, but updated testing yielded a Verbal IQ of 138, a performance IQ of 124, and a Full Scale IQ of 136—resting in the very superior range and higher than that of approximately 98% of the general population.[24]

In Kaczynski's case, his relatively high intelligence and abrupt, perhaps premature academic advancement may have contributed to the development of his lone-actor terrorist activities in that he had been emotionally unprepared and vulnerable when starting college and when he began to formulate and share his anti-technology formulations. This instance reflects a growing understanding on the part of researchers and clinicians that extremes of intelligence—either very high or very low—can foster a vulnerability to social pressure and a broader inability to function effectively with other individuals. Along these lines, Bellanti and Bierman[25] reviewed several studies that described how children who are identified as learning disabled, developmentally delayed, or otherwise low-achieving are more often subject to rejection by peers and that these poor social relationships, in turn, are predictive of difficulties later in life, including antisocial behavior. Although in general it is low intelligence that has been associated with a greater risk of mental illness[26] and social maladjustment,[27] Kaczynski's case illustrates how similar problems can develop at the opposite end of the cognitive spectrum.

The Wechsler Adult Intelligence Scale (in its current version, the WAIS-IV) is the most commonly utilized comprehensive test of intelligence. Its various IQ scores are normally distributed, with an average of 100 and a standard deviation of 15. Most scores cluster in the middle range, with 68% falling within the average range (i.e., 85–115), such that fewer individuals score at the extreme ends of the distribution.[28] The WAIS-IV is divided into four indexes, each made up of two to three subtests that measure different cognitive functions covering the domains of verbal understanding (verbal abstract reasoning, vocabulary, stored basic academic information), perception reasoning (visuo-spatial analysis and construction, visual integration/mental manipulation, and abstract visual reasoning), processing speed, and working memory (consciously retaining information while operating on it).

Personality Disorders

Personality disorders "can be described as the manifestation of extreme personality traits that interfere with everyday life and contribute to significant suffering, functional limitations, or both."[29] These disorders are characterized by deficient interactive styles, substandard coping strategies or resources, and excessively utilized defense mechanisms. It is not difficult to see how these conditions can be relevant to an understanding of lone-actor terrorism.

Narcissistic personality disorder, for example, is characterized by exaggerated self-evaluation that is nonetheless accompanied by an underlying fragility in one's sense of self.[16] This imbalance can lead to heightened sensitivity to perceived slights, with a marked reactivity that can be expressed verbally or otherwise. Anders Breivik, the perpetrator of a terrorist attack in Norway in 2011 that claimed 77 lives, was apparently described as narcissistic by one of the forensic teams to have evaluated him.[30] Breivik was seen by forensic psychiatrists during his trial, but it is unclear, on the basis of an open-source literature review, whether he submitted to formalized psychological testing.

Elliott Rodger, who perpetrated a drive-by shooting in California in 2014, killing six persons by shooting and collision, had been described as having narcissistic personality features. Based on a 137-page "manifesto" he uploaded to the internet,[31] a video he posted of himself just prior to the attack,[32] and an interview later granted by his father,[33] Rodger expressed his personal attributes in a notably grandiose fashion—describing himself in one instance, for example, as "gorgeous."

There are a number of psychological assessment measures currently employed to discern the presence of personality disorders. The MMPI-2 and the Personality Assessment Inventory (PAI)[34] are two of the most widely accepted and utilized examples. These measures use broad arrays of statements that range from directly reportable symptoms to more abstract views and positions. The Neuroticism-Extraversion-Openness (NEO) Inventory is another tool used to screen for personality disorders within the context of a five-factor theoretical model that also includes conscientiousness and agreeableness.[35] The PAI and NEO were both utilized in the case in the case of the Washington, DC, highway sniper Lee Boyd Malvo,[36] although it remains unclear what specific conclusions may have been reached based on results from these instruments.

Psychosis

Psychosis is ascribed when there exists evidence of hallucinations ("perceptions occurring in the absence of corresponding external or somatic stimuli"), delusions ("fixed false beliefs"), or both.[37] The broadly defined notion of psychosis is characterized by a disconnection from reality, disorganization of thought, or breakdown in logical inference. Auditory hallucinations in particular are associated with psychotic disorders, most notably those on the schizophrenia spectrum. The word element "schizo" derives from Latin meaning "division" or "split,"[10] incorporating the idea of the "splitting" of reality for the person with schizophrenia. Such hallucinations may take the form of "hearing voices" that exist solely within the examinee's mind but are misattributed to some external source. It will come as no surprise to learn that such symptoms can influence an individual's drift toward lone-actor terrorism.

Tamerlan Tsarnaev, who along with his brother Dzhokhar was responsible for the Boston Marathon bombing in 2013,[38] may have had a psychotic disorder, as suggested by his having reportedly mentioned to several people that he had begun hearing voices, that there were two people living in his head, and that he believed he was a victim of mind control.[39] These may have been valid symptoms of psychosis[40] and, as such, perhaps treatable. It is conceivable that pre-incident administration of psychological assessment instruments such as the MMPI and PAI could have provided further information regarding the presence of psychosis or at least have identified a level of distress and coping deficiency that might have led to the initiation of targeted clinical services.

Extreme Overvalued Beliefs

Extreme overvalued beliefs are among those that tend to become dominant over time and more resistant to change. Although objectively excessive,

these ideas stand in contrast to delusions and other indicia of psychosis in that they are shared by others in the person's cultural, religious, or other subgroup.[41] An individual can develop an emotional commitment to such beliefs and carry out violence in their service. Recent research has suggested that some lone-actor terrorists have inaccurately been characterized as psychotic when in fact it was extreme overvalued beliefs that motivated their illicit activities.[42] As of yet, there are no standardized psychometric tools specifically for evaluating such beliefs, though existing instruments such as the MMPI and PAI can provide useful information by querying such component elements as grandiosity, scrupulosity, and delusions.

Cognitive Disorders

Neuropsychological impairment may involve such cognitive domains as attention, executive function (higher order cognitive control), language (e.g., reading, understanding and producing words, reasoning with words), visuospatial ability (e.g., relationships in two and three dimensional space), motor and processing speed, memory (e.g., memory for newly learned information), and aspects of social emotional intelligence (e.g., recognizing facial emotion, perspective taking). Deficits in these domains (i.e., cognitive disorders) may leave an individual more susceptible to undue influence—including potential lone-actor terrorists who are being subjected to well-crafted, repetitive attempts at radicalization.

Assessment of executive function is particularly pertinent to an understanding of behavioral anomalies because it pertains directly to motor output (behavior) in ways that are not always obvious. While deficits in memory are often recognizable to the casual observer—for instance, when a person is incapable of retrieving information just recently presented—impaired problem-solving and lack of cognitive control may not be as readily obvious. Executive function spans a wide range of abilities that involve control of attention and integration of sensory input in order to serve the cognitive control of motor output (i.e., behavior). Executive abilities include sequencing, "multitasking" (shifting attention quickly between tasks), identifying and utilizing metacognitive strategies in learning and performance (e.g., organization of information to be learned), recognition of mistakes, response inhibition, and maintaining or switching cognitive sets. Executive systems also contribute to insight and self-awareness, as well as to emotional and affective regulation and modulation.

Instruments utilized for neuropsychological assessment measure cognitive functioning through engagement in tasks with varying cognitive demands. Inhibitory control, for example, can be measured by the number of impulsive errors made while engaged in different types of cognitive tasks (e.g., responding too quickly to a stimulus resulting in a false-positive error). Memory tasks typically involve the presentation of information to be learned (such as a story, list, or visual design) and require subsequent recall of the same information over varied time frames. Scores from cognitive testing are then compared to data collected from normal samples of individuals, generally stratified by variables such as age or level of education, or from those individuals with specified, relevant pathologies. By comparison of these scores and with knowledge of their base rates (normal frequency of occurrence), inferences can be drawn about the presence of pathology or other difficulties.

Neuropsychological assessment can be useful in identifying many areas of relative weakness and impairment that can reflect a variety of problems, including learning disorders (e.g., a reading disability), other neurodevelopmental disorders (e.g., attention deficit hyperactivity disorder), acquired impairment from trauma (e.g., brain injury), and neurodegenerative disorders (e.g., Alzheimer's disease). During the trial of Lee Boyd Malvo, neuropsychological assessment revealed that he had normal overall intelligence but that he also possessed a more difficult to discern impairment in attention and processing speed.[36] It is not known whether executive system weakness is a common factor in lone-actor terrorism; however, it is conceivable that problems with impulsivity, poor self-monitoring, and difficulty delaying gratification could contribute, for example, to rejection from a terrorist group and to difficulty sustaining employment—problems that have tended to surface repeatedly in detailed analyses of lone-actor terrorists.[8]

There exists some overlap between the measures employed in personality assessment and in neuropsychological assessment but with a predictable difference in focus and emphasis. While personality assessment emphasizes mood, personality, coping mechanisms, psychosis, and other psychological constructs (including psychological and emotional factors and often with only a cursory view of cognitive ability), neuropsychological assessment, conversely, takes a more cursory look at psychological and emotional factors, focusing primarily instead on cognitive functioning.

Deficits in Social Cognition

The notion of social cognition incorporates several constructs that relate to social competence as opposed to more traditional, achievement-oriented notions of intelligence. *Emotional intelligence* has been described as the ability to identify and monitor feelings and emotions (one's own and those of others), discriminate among those feelings and emotions, and use this information to guide one's own thinking and actions,[43] and it rests on abilities related to reasoning and problem-solving in the emotional domain.[44] Social intelligence includes the understanding of social norms with respect to how one (and others) should behave.[45] Theory of mind (TOM) can be conceptualized as the ability to model and reason about the intentions of others[46] and to use this information in the prediction and interpretation of behavior.[47] Overall, deficits in social cognition can also present as a vulnerability that may elevate risk for violent action; in addition, exposure to violence can in turn erode social cognition.[48,49]

Many aspects of social emotional behavior can be assessed in the context of a clinical interview accompanied by behavioral observations, such as give-and-take in the course of conversation, affective responsiveness, and eye contact. Psychometric tools used to augment these evaluations include rating scales like the Asperger Syndrome Diagnostic Scale (ASDS),[50] measures of emotion recognition (such as through auditory and visual modalities) and facial learning like the Advanced Clinical Solutions: Social Cognition (ACS:SC),[51] measures of TOM like the Reading the Mind in the Eyes Test[52] and the Edinburgh Social Cognition Test (ESCoT),[53] and measures of empathy like the Empathy Quotient (EQ).[54]

Social cognition has been correlated with academic achievement, successful workplace performance, social functioning, and overall well-being.[55] Deficits in social-emotional processing are key features of mental disorders such as autism spectrum disorder (ASD), with deficits that can result in interpersonal difficulties, failures in pair-bonding, and difficulties affiliating with groups.[16] Although the vast majority of autistic individuals do not engage in violent behavior, ASD has been identified as more prevalent among lone-actor terrorists than among the general population.[56]

Elliot Rodger was described by his father as having been very shy with very few friends,[33] and he had described himself as having difficulty in interpersonal relationships, particularly with women,[31] raising questions regarding deficits in social intelligence. His father opined publicly that Rodger might have had Asperger's disorder (now subsumed diagnostically as part of ASD)[16] and depicted him as prone to unusual sensory sensitivities and compulsive behaviors. Rodger indicated that he saw a violent act as a "final solution" to the perceived "injustice" he had encountered, which he blamed on women. To this end, he targeted and killed women in a sorority. According to his writings, he had planned the attack for 3 years. His mother, concerned, had reportedly wanted him to undergo a mental health evaluation and had requested that the police visit his residence.[57]

Adam Lanza, the Sandy Hook, Connecticut, Elementary School shooter, was described as having Asperger's disorder in a subsequent state's attorney's report of that incident.[58] Anders Breivik was depicted as having experienced difficulty dating and as having been rejected by peers in other contexts as well.[59,60] Whether or not any of these individuals met formal diagnostic criteria for ASD, an assessment-driven understanding of their interpersonal difficulties might have been helpful in recognizing their risk for committing violent acts.

Deficits in the ability to interact with one's social environment can increase the potential for eventual acts of interpersonal violence. Personal vulnerability has been identified as one of four key elements of the radicalization process with respect to political terrorism.[61] Another individual factor that has been associated with political violence is the experience of humiliation, which can be potentiated by many of the narcissistic attributes described in detail earlier.[62]

By extension, such factors can be applied directly to our understanding of lone-actor terrorism. These factors, interacting with several of what are described as "distal characteristics" associated with terrorist action—for example, deficits in attention and in executive system functioning, such as slowed processing—can make it difficult for persons to sustain gainful employment, thereby contributing to an overall thwarting of occupational goals.[63] Deficits in frontal executive systems, such as those occasioned by head trauma, can result in deficits in the ability to refrain from reacting to a given stressful or otherwise provocative situation. This can predispose one to ill-considered remarks, to acting without fully thinking through the consequences, and, ultimately, to impulsive violence.

DECEPTION AND LACK OF EFFORT

Under normal circumstances, deception is not invariably problematic and may indeed be virtually nonconsequential. Consider, for example, the offhanded proffer of a less-than-heartfelt compliment in order to finesse an awkward social situation. More significant deception, however, such as the sort that might enable a lone-actor terrorist to evade detection, may have dire consequences.

Feigned psychiatric disorders can be particularly prevalent in legal settings, where a desire to obtain money or evade incarceration can provide exceptionally powerful motivation. *Malingering*, one form of feigning, involves the intentional production of false or grossly exaggerated physical or psychological problems, motivated by external factors.[16] Participants in legal proceedings—including jurors and judges—may be reluctant to consider cognitive or other psychological deficits as "real" or "significant," especially when these factors are viewed as both difficult to quantify and susceptible to malingering. Overall, there may exist the perception that defendants can "act crazy" in order to evade responsibility for a criminal act. There is, however, a vast literature supporting the view that deception involving feigned mental and cognitive disorders can be detected with good reliability.[64]

Certain patterns of responding have been associated with deception, and their analysis can be instructive in understanding this phenomenon. Attention to response styles, such as endorsement of symptoms that are extremely rare for a given pathology or extremely rare in certain combinations, can help to clarify when consequential deception is present. While a nonstandardized interview alone has limited accuracy in the detection of efforts to deceive,[65,66] the inclusion of structured interviews and psychometric instruments greatly improves the capacity to detect deficient effort and deception. This approach is even more likely to be effective when supplemented by a review of prior treatment documentation and other collateral sources of information.[67]

Structured interview protocols commonly employed for this purpose include the Structured Interview of Reported Symptoms (in its current version, the SIRS-2)[68] or the Schedule of Affective Disorders and Schizophrenia (SADS).[69] Comprehensive personality assessment inventories such as the MMPI-2 or the PAI have built-in scales that are sensitive to such clinical phenomena as exaggeration, overendorsement, and malingering, on the one hand, and defensiveness, on the other hand.

In a similar vein, performance validity measures indicate whether a subject is giving good effort to perform well cognitively. Such measures tend to have high face validity in that they seem like a measure of cognitive function but are in actuality strong indicators of how hard the subject is trying. With the inclusion of such measures, there can be greater confidence that overall test findings are an accurate reflection of the examinee's true abilities.

WHAT WE KNOW SO FAR

The present store of publicly accessible psychometric data is insufficient for the identification of a robust, generalizable assessment profile for the lone-actor terrorist. Most information regarding psychological and psychosocial aspects of this population is drawn primarily from open source materials and typically does not include objective, statistically analyzable test scores. A literature review recently conducted by the current authors revealed a limited few instances in which reference to psychological assessment had been made at all. In those cases, neither evaluative reports nor test data were available for review, even when trial-related documentation was otherwise retrievable. This is perhaps not surprising, inasmuch as results from testing administered in the course of legal proceedings are often sealed by court order.

What knowledge we do possess suggests, however, that there are at least some psychological deficits, challenges, and vulnerabilities that have repeatedly surfaced in the shallow subject pool of this population.[8] Narcissistic traits and symptoms,[70] as well as reduced social competency,[71,72] have been ascribed to lone-actor terrorists on multiple occasions. Psychosis has been indicated in some cases as well.[73] Cognitive and/or intellectual deficits seem to have been identified less frequently, though they may be present in some instances.[36] Constructs such as impulsivity, inflexibility, and difficulty controlling anger have been identified in lone-actor terrorists,[9] suggesting executive system deficits, although these were characteristics inferred from open-source accounts and have not been measured directly.

HOW TO LEARN MORE

To move forward in our ability to predict those individual vulnerabilities that contribute to risk for lone-actor terrorism, we must undertake to study known and potential perpetrators as thoroughly as possible. This will be greatly potentiated when law enforcement and correctional systems see fit to lowering barriers to conducting evaluations of individuals who have been charged with acts of lone-actor terrorism. Furthermore, national security entities should consider providing funding for research on such individuals, which should include the development of a standardized—albeit flexible—assessment battery and a broadly accessible database of psychometric findings. Individuals who have been thwarted from carrying out violent attacks will also serve as important subjects of study, with the clearly perceivable benefit of providing vital mechanisms for identifying such persons by law enforcement.

Expanding opportunities for research and study of convicted perpetrators should be encouraged by the provision of grant-based academic resources to support this work. When the necessary information is available, a confounding factor of bias may have an effect on interpretation of the data,[74,75] particularly for measures that are more subjective or open to interpretation (e.g., with lower reliability). Considering this potential for bias, reports describing data alone are insufficient, and raw data need to be reviewed directly by a trained clinician with no ties to a case or its outcome. Improving access to psychological test data procured during the course of legal proceedings and analyzed with due sensitivity to the protection of civil liberties, may be challenging but still possible. To circumvent related problems, obtaining data outside of a highly adversarial legal proceeding would be ideal, though the collection of such psychometric data on the relatively rare lone-actor terrorist currently presents daunting practical hurdles.

WHEN TO EVALUATE

With the ultimate goal of prevention, greater vigilance concerning risk factors for violent actions will more readily prompt mental health professionals to consider comprehensive evaluation, including psychometrics. Increased awareness regarding signs of threat should be encouraged. Evidence for the presence—among other factors—of significant grievances, related all-or-none thinking, grandiose or extreme beliefs, violent ideation, a history of humiliation, thwarting of occupational goals, disillusionment with the existing social order, and resentment should immediately raise concerns. Comprehensive assessment in the context of such risk factors should be encouraged, and aggressive intervention for mental health and social setbacks and deficiencies should be funded and implemented where possible.

When there exists a predictable reluctance to participate in mental health evaluation and treatment, balancing the rights of the individual on the one hand against the rights of society for safety and security on the other will never be a simple matter. Both law enforcement and mental health professionals nonetheless need to be vigilant with respect to warning signs and to follow through concerning opportunities for evaluation when this is legally and ethically feasible.

EVALUATION PROCESSES AND GOALS

What would we want to derive from the psychological assessment of a lone-actor terrorist? Neuropsychological and psychological assessment has the potential for identifying important personal vulnerabilities. Childhood weaknesses in learning and cognition, for example, are frequently associated with school failure and are not always identified at that time. Such academically related problems—particularly when they remain inadequately addressed during primary school years—can ultimately contribute to significant self-esteem problems in later years for adolescents and adults.[76,77] Persistent learning disabilities, such as in reading or mathematics, can be discovered in adults with the use of broad as well as subject-specific academic achievement measures. Poor impulse control and incapacity to delay gratification can lead to actions that are performed without adequate consideration for consequences, so scanning for these issues should be included in evaluations for this population. Impaired problem-solving, limited planning capacity, and lack of insight can similarly have a negative impact on social relationships and on the ability to sustain gainful and meaningful employment.

Psychometric tools are available to measure and quantify planning, concept formation, and cognitive flexibility in addition to other executive skills. Serious attention deficits contribute to similar social challenges, and, for this reason, measures of focused attention, sustained attention, and processing speed should be included. Social intelligence factors, including perspective taking, TOM, and recognition of affective/emotion information—as from gestures, facial expressions, and prosody—may contribute to social isolation-based ineptitude. Measures of social intelligence and social cognition should also be included in a comprehensive evaluation. Assessment of overall intellectual capacity, with particular attention to domains of associated deficits at the subtest level, may further identify personal cognitive vulnerabilities.

Psychological evaluations that incorporate the assessment of mood, distress levels, personality, reality testing, and coping resources may reveal further personal challenges. Affective states such as depression and anxiety are risk factors and should be assessed with careful attention to motivation, defensiveness, or exaggeration. A measurement such as the MMPI-2 or PAI may uncover and quantify abnormal personality features, including narcissism and emotional instability. Evaluation for psychosis, especially paranoid thinking, can be enhances by these and similar measures, which may additionally be helpful in identifying the presence and severity of extreme overvalued beliefs.

Cognitive factors—such as attention, executive system function, learning, memory, and the ability to use and understand language and visuospatial information—are critically important bases for understanding individuals and their manner of functioning in the world at large. Psychological assessment utilizing psychometric tools can aid in the specification of such relevant conditions such as learning disabilities, attention deficit hyperactivity disorder, head trauma, dementia, schizophrenia, depression, and ASD. When conducting evaluations in the context of lone-actor terrorism, focusing on a predetermined list of diagnostic entities may be less important than identifying relevant personal vulnerabilities as one seeks to predict and understand susceptibility to radicalization and the subsequent potential for violent action.

CONCLUSION

Why do some individuals engage in terrorist actions on their own? While there is not currently a comprehensive answer to this question, much has been learned, and research-based efforts are ongoing. It has become evident that psychological factors are relevant and significant contributors to vulnerability concerning lone-actor terrorism. Efforts to understand these factors and their dynamic interactions within an individual—and with external circumstances and the environment—have improved our knowledge of this phenomenon. The inclusion of psychometric approaches has the potential to refine this knowledge and facilitate the identification of lone-actor terrorists.

NOTES AND REFERENCES

1. 28 C.F.R. § 0.85 (1969).
2. Pantucci R, Ellis C, Chaplais L. *Lone-Actor Terrorism: Literature Review*, Dec 2015. https://www.chathamhouse.org/sites/default/files/publications/research/20160105LoneActorTerrorismLiteratureReviewRUSI.pdf
3. Spaaij R. *Understanding Lone Wolf Terrorism: Global Patterns, Motivations and Prevention.* New York: Springer; 2012.
4. Borum R. *Psychology of Terrorism.* Tampa: University of South Florida; 2004.
5. Moghadam F. The staircase to terrorism: A psychological exploration. *Am Psychol.* 2012; 60(2):161–169.
6. Crenshaw M. The causes of terrorism. In Kegley CW, ed. *The New Global Terrorism: Characteristics, Cosmos, Controls.* Upper Saddle River, NJ: Prentice Hall; 2003:92–105.
7. Corner E, Gill P. A false dichotomy? Lone actor terrorism and mental illness. *Law Hum Behav.* 2015;39(1):23–24.
8. Gill P. *Lone-Actor Terrorists: A Behavioural Analysis.* New York: Routledge; 2015.
9. Corner E, Bouhana N, Gill P. The multifinality of vulnerability indicators in lone actor terrorism. *Psychol Crime Law* 2019;25(2):111–132.
10. Online Etymology Dictionary. Schizo-. 10/25/17 https://www.etymonline.com/word/schizo-
11. Merriam-Webster. Metric. 12/12/21 https://www.merriam-webster.com/dictionary/metric
12. Viloratou S, Pickles A. A note on contemporary psychometrics. *J Ment Health.* 2017;26(6):486–488.
13. Campbell R. *Campbell's Psychiatric Dictionary.* 9th ed. New York: Oxford; 2009.
14. Hopwood C, Bornstein R. *Multimethod Clinical Assessment.* New York: Guilford; 2014.
15. Calhoun F, Weston S. *Threat Assessment and Management Strategies: Identifying the Howlers and the Hunters.* Boca Raton, FL: Taylor & Francis; 2009.
16. American Psychiatric Association. *Diagnostic and Statistical Manual of Mental Disorders.* 5th ed. Arlington, VA: Author; 2013.
17. Bhui K, Otis M, Silva M, Halvorsrud K, Freestone M, Jones E. Extremism and common mental illness: Cross-sectional community survey of white British and Pakistani men and women living in England. *British J Psychiatry.* 2020;217(4):547–554.
18. Beck A, Steer R, Brown G. *Beck Depression Inventory-II Manual.* San Antonio, TX: Psychological Corporation; 1996.
19. Butcher J, Graham J, Tellegen A, Kaemmer B. *Manual for the Restandardized Minnesota Multiphasic Personality Inventory: MMPI-2.* Minneapolis, MN: University of Minnesota Press; 1989.
20. Lexico. Intelligence. 2021. https://www.lexico.com/definition/intelligence
21. Merriam-Webster. Intelligence. 6 Dec 2021 https://www.merriam-webster.com/dictionary/intelligence
22. Wechsler D. Intelligence defined and undefined: A relativistic appraisal. *Am Psychol.* 1975;30(2):135–139.
23. Norman M. The Unabomber strikes again: An investigation into whether the Victim and Witness Protection Act of 1982 violates the First Amendment or conflicts with the Copyright Act of 1976. *So Cal Law Rev.* 2008;81:1281–1340.
24. Johnson S. Psychological evaluation of Theodore Kaczynski. 1/16/98 https://paulcooijmans.com/psychology/unabombreport.html
25. Bellanti CJ, Bierman KL, Conduct Problems Prevention Research Group. Disentangling the impact of low cognitive ability and inattention on social behavior and peer relationships. *J Clin Child Psychol.* 2000;29(1):66–75.
26. Gale C, Hatch S, Batty G, et al. Intelligence in childhood and risk of psychological distress in adulthood: The 1958 National Child Development Survey and the 1970 British Cohort Study. *Intell.* 2009;37(6):592–599.
27. Grossberg I, Cornell D. Relationship between personality adjustment and high intelligence: Terman versus Hollingworth. *Except Children.* 1988;55(3):266–272.
28. Groth-Marnat G. *Handbook of Psychological Assessment.* 4th ed. Hoboken, NJ: Wiley; 2003.
29. Ekselius L. Personality disorder: A disease in disguise. *Ups J Med Sci.* 2018;123(4):194–204.
30. Orange R. Anders Behring Breivik "should be declared insane." *The Telegraph*, 21 Jun 2012. https://www.telegraph.co.uk/news/worldnews/europe/norway/9347018/Anders-Behring-Breivik-should-be-declared-insane.html
31. Rodger E. The Manifesto of Elliott Rodger. *New York Times*, 25 May 2014. https://www.nytimes.com/interactive/2014/05/25/us/shooting-document.html
32. Rodger E. Retribution. *New York Times*, 24 May 2014. https://www.nytimes.com/video/us/100000002900707/youtube-video-retribution.html
33. Springer A. The agony of Peter Rodger, a dad whose son became a mass killer. *ABC News*, 27 Jun 2014. https://abcnews.go.com/US/agony-peter-rodger-dad-son-mass-killer/story?id=24317702
34. Morey L. *Personality Assessment Inventory Professional Manual.* Lutz, FL: Psychological Assessment Resources; 2007.
35. Costa P, McCrae R. *Revised NEO Personality Inventory (NEO-PI-R) and NEO Five-Factor Inventory (NEO-FFI) Professional Manual.* Odessa, FL: Psychological Assessment Resources; 1992.
36. Albarus C, Mack J. *The Making of Lee Boyd Malvo: The D.C. Sniper.* New York: Columbia University Press; 2012.

37. Arciniegas D. Psychosis. *Continuum*. 2015; 21(3)715–736.

38. Winter T. Russia warned U.S. about Tsarnaev, but spelling issue let him escape. *NBC News*, 25 Mar 2014. https://www.nbcnews.com/storyline/boston-bombing-anniversary/russia-warned-u-s-about-tsarnaev-spelling-issue-let-him-n60836

39. Daily Mail Reporter. Was Tamerlan Tsarnaev schizophrenic? Boston bomber told friends and family he "had two people living in his head" was the victim of mind control. control. *Daily Mail.com*, 16 Dec 2013 https://www.dailymail.co.uk/news/article-2524891/Was-Boston-bomber-Tamerlan-Tsarnaev-schizophrenic.html

40. Cotti P, Meloy R. The Tamerlan Tsarvaev case: The nexus of psychopathology and ideology in a lone actor terrorist. *J Threat Assess and Manag*. 2019;6(3-4):135–158.

41. Rahman T, Meloy R, Bauer R. Extreme overvalued belief and the legacy of Carl Wernicke. *J Am Acad Psychiatry Law* 2019;47(2):180–187.

42. Rahman T, Hartz S, Xiong W, et al. Extreme overvalued beliefs. *J Am Acad Psychiatry Law* 2020;48(3)(in press). doi:10.29158/JAAPL.200001-20.

43. Salovey P, Mayer J. Emotional intelligence. *Imagin Cogn Pers*. 1990;9(3):185–211.

44. Mayer J, Roberts R, Barsade S. Human abilities: Emotional intelligence. *Annu Rev Psychol*. 2008;59:507–536.

45. Baez S, Rattazzi A, Gonzalez-Gadea ML, et al. Integrating intention and context: Assessing social cognition in adults with Asperger Syndrome. *Front Hum Neurosci*. 2012;6(1):1–21.

46. Baron-Cohen S, Ring HA, Wheelwright S, et al. Social intelligence in the normal and autistic brain: An fMRI study. *Eur J Neurosci*. 1999;11(6):1891–1898.

47. Premack D, Woodruff G. Does the chimpanzee have a theory of mind? *Behav Brain Sci*. 1978;1(4):515–526.

48. Guerra N, Huesmann L, Spindler A. Community violence exposure, social cognition, and aggression among urban elementary school children. *Child Dev*. 2003;74(5):1561–1576.

49. Heleniak C, McLaughlin K. Social-cognitive mechanisms in the cycle of violence: Cognitive and affective theory of mind, and externalizing psychopathology in children and adolescents. *Dev Psychopathol*. 2019;32(2):735–750.

50. Myles B, Jone-Bock S, Simpson R. *Asperger Syndrome Diagnostic Scale Manual*. North Tonawanda, NY: MHS; 2001.

51. Wechsler D. *Advanced Clinical Solutions for WAIS-IV and WMS-IV*. San Antonio, TX: Psychological Corporation; 2009.

52. Baron-Cohen S, Wheelwright S, Hill J, et al. The "Reading the Mind in the Eyes" test revised version: A study with normal adults, and adults with Asperger syndrome or high-functioning autism. *J Child Psychol Psychiatry* 2001;42(2):241–251.

53. Asaad Baksh R, Abrahams S, Bertlich M, et al. Social cognition in adults with autism spectrum disorders: Validation of the Edinburgh Social Cognition Test (ESCoT) [Published ahead of print Mar 19, 2020]. *Clin Neuropsychol*. doi:10.1080/13854046.2020.1737236.

54. Baron-Cohen S, Wheelwright S. The empathy quotient: An investigation of adults with Asperger syndrome or high functioning autism, and normal sex differences. *J Autism Dev Disord*. 2004;34(2):163–175.

55. Brackett MA, Rivers SE, Salovey P. Emotional intelligence: Implications for personal, social, academic, and workplace success. *Soc Personal Psychol Compass* 2011;5(1):88–103.

56. Corner E, Gill P, Mason O. Mental health disorders and the terrorist: A research note probing selection effects and disorder prevalence. *Stud Confl Terrorism* 2015;39(6):560–568.

57. Blood MR. Why didn't anyone stop Elliot Rodger? Associated Press, 28 May 2014. https://www.emsworld.com/news/11488222/why-didnt-anyone-stop-elliot-rodger

58. Sedensky S. Report of the State's Attorney for the Judicial District of Danbury on the shootings at Sandy Hook Elementary School and 36 Yogananda St, Newtown, Connecticut on Dec 14, 2012. *New York Times*, 25 Nov 2013. https://archive.nytimes.com/www.nytimes.com/interactive/2013/11/26/nyregion/26newtown-report.html?ref=nyregion

59. Liddle R. A father's tale: Rod Liddle meets Jens Breivik. *The Times*, 25 Jan 2015. https://www.thetimes.co.uk/article/a-fathers-tale-rod-liddle-meets-jens-breivik-s5vfqfh7l2t

60. Pidd H. Anders Behring Breivik spent years training and plotting for massacre. *The Guardian*. 24 Aug 2012. http://www.guardian.co.uk/world/2012/aug/24/anders-behring-breivik-profile-oslo

61. Speckhard A. Contextual and motivational factors in the pathways to radicalization: Why location matters. In Festermacher L, Kuznar L, Rieger T, et al., eds. *Protecting the Homeland from International and Domestic Terrorism Threats: Current Multi-Disciplinary Perspectives on Root Causes, the Role of Ideology, and Programs for Counter-Radicalization and Disengagement*. https://www.researchgate.net/publication/271195304_Contextual_and_Motivational_Factors_in_the_Pathways_to_Radicalization_Why_Location_Matters

62. Lemieux A. Psychological factors, individual factors, and triggers. In Festermacher L, Kuznar L, Rieger T, et al., eds. *Protecting the Homeland from International and Domestic Terrorism Threats: Current Multi-Disciplinary*

Perspectives on Root Causes, the Role of Ideology, and Programs for Counter-Radicalization and Disengagement. Jan 2010. https://start.umd.edu/sites/default/files/files/publications/U_Counter_Terrorism_White_Paper_Final_January_2010.pdf

63. Meloy J. The operational development and empirical testing of the Terrorist Radicalization Assessment Protocol (Trapp 18). *J Pers Assess.* 2018;100(5):483–492.

64. Rogers R. Detection of strategies for malingering and defensiveness. In Rogers R, Bender S, eds. *Clinical Assessment of Malingering and Deception.* 4th ed. New York: Guilford; 2018:18–41.

65. Rogers R, Bender S. Evaluation of malingering and deception. In Goldstein A, Weiner IB, eds. *Handbook of Psychology.* Vol. 11. Hoboken, NJ: Wiley; 2013:109–129.

66. Ekman P, O'Sullivan M. Who can catch a liar? *Am Psychol.* 1991;46(9):913–920.

67. Pirelli G, Otto R, Estoup A. Using internet and social media data as collateral sources of information in forensic evaluations. *Prof Psychol Res Pr.* 2016;47(1):12–17.

68. Rogers R, Sewell K, Gillard N. *Structured Interview of Report Symptoms, 2nd Edition: Professional Manual.* Lutz, FL: Psychological Assessment Resources; 2010.

69. Spitzer R, Endicott J. *Schedule for Affective Disorder and Schizophrenia.* 3rd ed. New York: Biometrics Research; 1978.

70. Bondu R, Scheithauer H. Narcissistic symptoms in German school shooters. *Int J Offender Ther Comp Criminol.* 2014;59(14):1520–1535.

71. Erlandsson A, Meloy J. The Swedish school attack in Trollhättan [Published ahead of print Apr 23, 2018]. *J Forensic Sci.* doi:10.1111/1556-4029.13800.

72. Gruenwald J, Chermak S, Freilick J. Distinguishing "loner" attacks from other domestic extremist violence: A comparison of far-right homicide incident and offender characteristics. *Criminol Public Policy* 2013;12(1):65–91.

73. Corner E, Gill P. The nascent empirical literature on psychopathology and terrorism. *World Psychiatry* 2018;17(2):147–148.

74. Murrie D, Boccaccini M, Guarnera L, et al. Are forensic experts biased by the side that retained them? *Psychol Sci.* 2013;24(10):1889–1897.

75. Murrie D, Boccaccini M, Johnson J, et al. Does interrater (dis)agreement on psychopathy checklist scores in sexually violent predator trials suggest partisan allegiance in forensic evaluations? *Law Hum Behav.* 2008;32(4):353–363.

76. Booth M, Gerard J. Self-esteem and academic achievement: A comparative study of adolescent students in England and the United States. *Compare.* 2011;41(5):629–648.

77. Heyman W. The self-perception of a learning disability and its relationship to academic self-concept and self-esteem. *J Learn Disabil.* 1990;23(8):472–475.

7

Understanding Lone-Actor Violence Through Linguistic Analysis

ISABELLE W. J. VAN DER VEGT, BENNETT KLEINBERG, AND PAUL GILL

INTRODUCTION

This chapter focuses on the language of lone-actors and synthesizes the efforts that have been made, as well as the tasks that lie ahead in order to best understand lone-actor violence through linguistic data. This is an important area of research because lone-actor terrorists—as all types of extremist populations are increasingly doing—use the internet to consume and spread their ideas.[1] Thus, this chapter focuses on their written communications, including manifestos, pre-attack threats, and online activity including extremist forum postings. Since the literature specifically examining lone-actor terrorist language is relatively scarce, we also draw on relevant studies on radicalized individuals and group-based terrorists as well as communications related to analogous forms of grievance-fueled targeted violence.[2,3] This enables us to make suggestions about how the study of lone-actor terrorist language may benefit from these related lines of research. The increased importance of detecting and countering the narratives of potentially violent individuals online further necessitates focusing on automated approaches to linguistic analysis. The chapter first explains why linguistic approaches to mitigating lone-actor terrorism are worthwhile. Then we examine studies on automated linguistic assessment of lone-actor terrorist language and other radicalized and aggrieved populations. We discuss word count- and weight-based approaches to linguistically examining warnings signs of violence, including measures of psychological and social processes. Finally, we identify gaps in the literature and make suggestions for the furtherance of the field of automated linguistic analysis of lone-actor terrorist language.

WHY STUDY LONE-ACTOR LANGUAGE?

In a study of 119 individuals convicted for lone-actor terrorism in the United States and Europe since 1990, Gill, Horgan, and Deckert (2014) found that, in the majority of cases, somebody knew something about the perpetrator's grievance and/or intent to commit violence.[4] In 82.4% of the incidents, other people were aware of the perpetrator's grievance, and in 79% of the cases, others were aware of their commitment to an extremist ideology.[4] In the same study, it was found that, in 63.9% of lone-actor terrorism activity, the perpetrator verbally told others of their plans, and 58.8% produced some form of public statement about their beliefs prior to their plot.[4] These communications happened both on- and offline. In another study, Gill et al. (2017) analyzed internet usage by convicted UK terrorists and found that some discussed target selection online, including whether to target civilians, civil servants, or the police.[5]

Online communications pose several problems and opportunities for security practitioners. Imagine the following scenario: an unknown individual threatens to bomb an event where a well-known politician will be speaking. The messages arrive via the politician's Facebook page. Having access to the threatener may offer the most insight into their intentions and motivation. However, the person behind the Facebook account appears to be untraceable, so security officials have not been able to gain access to the subject. If they had, the subject may have denied involvement or cooperation, they may not have been able to cooperate appropriately (e.g., due to significant mental illness), the individual may have concealed or downplayed their intentions, or the risk of violence may have increased if officials engaged with the subject.[6,7] In this case, it is necessary to resort to other sources of information, such as the subject's use of language in the threatening messages and other social media posts. Indeed, linguistic data may sometimes be the only evidence available. On such occasions, security practitioners may gain insight into the subject's pathway to violence by analyzing the texts produced by the individual. (Please note that we use "text" and "language sample" interchangeably, referring to any type of linguistic data produced by an individual [e.g., forum postings, letters, instant messages]). In other cases where security professionals do have access to the individual in question, linguistic information may provide additional insights or serve as important supplementary evidence, for example in police investigations.

Psychological and computational research increasingly examines language use to gain insight into psychological processes. Applications of linguistic analysis include detecting deception,[8,9] measuring emotion, and gauging social relationships,[10] as well as predicting traits such as age[11] and gender.[12] The relative success of linguistic analysis within the field of psychology suggests that a similar approach is worthwhile within the specific domain of studying lone-actor terrorism.

The internet drastically simplified sharing extremist ideas with like-minded individuals, as well as the process of transmitting threats. The scale on which this problem occurs is large, illustrated by the record number of female MPs in the UK standing down before the December 2019 elections, citing constant abuse and threats.[13] In the earlier example of online threats made to the politician, the target may receive hundreds of messages a day, all of which require time and effort to review. Moreover, many of these messages may contain some worrying element or an (in)direct threat, but it may be unclear which of these needs to be taken seriously. In other instances, manually processing lengthy terrorist manifestos, repeated threat letters, extensive social media profiles, or multitudes of forum postings demands resources that could be spent elsewhere. An automated approach to linguistic threat assessment, in which computer software processes texts, offers a potential solution. First, automated procedures process large amounts of data in a short amount of time. Second, computer software can identify patterns in data that might be indistinguishable to the human eye. Third, automatic procedures can be combined with human judgment, so that an algorithm serves as an initial filter, removing low-risk, irrelevant texts and thus reducing the workload for an expert threat manager who makes a final decision about whether an individual warrants attention. Such a filter system would, however, need to be based on indicators that are independent of each other (i.e., the measures must be uncorrelated), so as to not propagate false positive and false negative rates.[14] Indeed, an automated procedure may aid in situations like the aforementioned threat to the politician, by contributing to the detection of potential high-risk messages, or assist in the decision-making process of having law enforcement follow up on a threat. The research discussed below encapsulates the emerging field of automatic linguistic threat assessment and how it relates to violent lone-actor terrorism. In addition, we describe linguistic research on aggrieved, radicalized, and extremist populations more generally, in order to draw lessons for the understanding of lone-actor violence through linguistic analysis.

AUTOMATED LINGUISTIC ANALYSIS OF LONE-ACTOR, AGGRIEVED, RADICALIZED, AND EXTREMIST POPULATIONS

Approaches to automatically analyzing texts vary in terms of the type of linguistic information that is exploited. To clarify this, we categorized the studies by the way in which texts were represented quantitatively. First, we synthesized research that seeks frequencies of words that are considered markers of different psychological and social processes (e.g., word count-based approach). Second, we summarized studies in which words in a text are assigned a score representing a specific psychological concept, such as sentiment, affect, or abusiveness (i.e., weight-based approach). Both sections describe research in which these methods have been applied to studying language samples from lone-actor terrorists and analogous groups. All linguistic research described focuses on English language samples unless otherwise specified.

WORD COUNT-BASED APPROACHES TO LINGUISTIC ANALYSIS

Linguistic inquiry and word count (LIWC) software is a commonly used resource in psycholinguistic research to study a large range of psychological and social constructs through counting word occurrences.[15] The assumption behind LIWC software is that specific words in a text reflect the author's emotions and cognitive processes.[10] The LIWC software processes each word in a piece of text and determines whether the same word appears in a dictionary consisting of almost 6,400 words.[15] The words in the dictionary are organized into grammatical categories (e.g., pronouns, articles), psychological concepts and processes (e.g., power, positive emotion), and content categories (e.g., family, money). The output of running a text through LIWC software consists of frequencies and proportions for each word category, thereby providing an indication of the presence of certain constructs and processes in a text.

Baele (2017) examined pieces of text written by lone-actor terrorists, measuring various psycho-social variables using LIWC software.[16] The aim of the study was twofold. First, the study assessed whether texts written by lone-actor terrorists were characterized by higher levels of anger and negative emotion than texts written by nonviolent individuals. Baele (2017) notes that this question stems from claims that violence is typically linked to anger, especially in the case of political violence.[16] The second line of inquiry concerns the way in which lone-actor terrorists cognitively function. Some theories suggest that lone-actor terrorists think and process information in a rigid and inflexible way. The theory that cognitive and ideational inflexibility is associated with extremism and violence has been widely considered in the field of terrorism research.[17,18] It has been argued that terrorists are limited to black-and-white thinking and oversimplified "us versus them" reasoning.[15] Baele (2017) examined the anger and cognitive inflexibility hypotheses by testing lone-actor terrorist writings for LIWC categories related to emotion and cognitive processes.[16] The scores for the lone-actor texts were compared to scores for texts written by non-violent activists (e.g., Martin Luther King, Nelson Mandela) as well as samples of standard control writings and emotional writings ("baseline" texts provided by LIWC developers expressing low and high emotionality, respectively).[16] Lone-actor texts contained higher proportions of negative emotion words (resentment and anger) than did the non-violent activist texts, standard control texts, and emotional texts. Furthermore, the lone-actor texts showed high cognitive sophistication and low cognitive inflexibility based on the proportions of LIWC categories for "cognitive processes," "causality," "certainty," "tentative," words

with more than six letters, and a separate measure of cognitively complex language.[19] In short, Baele (2017) argued that the psycho-social characteristics of lone-actor terrorist texts support the idea that perpetrators exhibit high levels of anger but are characterized by high cognitive complexity rather than inflexibility.[16]

In a similar vein, Kaati, Shrestha, and Cohen (2016) compared writings from 10 lone-actors to 714,000 "control" texts retrieved from personal blogs (on Blogs.com and LiveJournal.com).[20] Using LIWC software, the aim was to identify the drives and emotions preceding an attack. The results showed that lone-actor texts contain significantly higher levels of negative emotion as well as significantly lower levels of positive emotion and friendship-related words than the control texts. Texts written by lone-actors also scored higher in terms of power-related language as well as anger when compared to the control writings. Lone-actor texts showed higher proportions of the LIWC category "certainty" than did the control writings, which was used to measure the extent of cognitive flexibility in the texts. The category denoting "big" words longer than six letters was used to measure psychological distancing from a violent act and was found to a higher extent in the lone-actor group. Last, lone-actor texts contained more third-person pronouns than the control texts, which was considered a response to outgroup threat and "us versus them" thinking.[20]

In a similar investigation, Kaati, Shrestha, and Sardella (2016) examined 10 lone-actor terrorist manifestos for psychological warning signs of targeted violence.[21] The manifestos were compared to texts written by non-violent activists, texts from personal blogs, forum postings on a white supremacy forum, and personal interest forum postings in order to discern the linguistic characteristics of texts written by violent lone offenders. Psychological constructs were extracted through LIWC. Certain LIWC categories were particularly important for distinguishing between offender and non-offender texts. These included linguistic variables (i.e., pronouns, articles, and prepositions) as well as certain psychological processes, such as negative emotion (e.g., "hate," "kill"), perceptual processes (e.g., "see," "heard," "feel"), differentiation (e.g., "but," "without"), affective processes (e.g., "laugh," "sad"), and biological processes (e.g., "eat," "blood").

A synthesis of both works by Kaati et al. (2016a, 2016b) forms the basis of a proposed tool for risk assessment in written communication entitled the Profile Risk Assessment Tool (PRAT).[22] The tool measures the presence of certain psychological variables in a text; this comprises the "profile" of a text, which is then compared to a sample of profiles of known risk texts. The comparison sample consists of texts extracted from radical Islamic forums, right-wing extremist forums, texts written by school shooters, and lone-actor terrorist manifestos and communications. A normative comparison sample is also provided in the form of personal blog posts. The PRAT computes the similarity between a text of interest and the texts in the comparative samples, providing intraclass correlations between the text and aforementioned datasets. The average similarities are computed with a dictionary-based approach, measuring concepts including social processes, leakage, and fixation behavior. For instance, radicalized individuals may exhibit an "inflated self" in texts, demonstrated by frequent use of the pronoun "I," as well as a tendency to frequently use "we," signifying boundaries between groups.[22] PRAT measures warning behaviors by assessing references to killing, power, weapons, and military terms, as well as mentions of well-known previous lone offenders and school shooters. PRAT additionally measures a fixation on topics related to Judaism, migration, Islamization, Islamic State terminology, and "involuntary celibate" terminology.[22] The developers of the PRAT also describe constructing a personality profile for the text authors based on previous research that stressed the importance of personality factors to political extremism as well as behavior in general.[23] The researchers also mention that the PRAT assesses the "Big Five" personality factors through language, resulting in scores for neuroticism, extraversion, openness to experience, agreeableness, and conscientiousness. The PRAT tool is also used to measure sentiment in texts; this weight-based method is described later.

In an exploration of an "incel" (i.e., "involuntary celibate") forum, Jaki et al. (2019) conducted several linguistic analyses to assess whether the forum fostered radicalization.[24] The incel community generally consists of "men united by their inability to convince women to have sex with them."[25] Like-minded individuals gather in online forums to discuss the perceived injustice of women not being attracted to them, among other frustrations. Some acts of lone-actor violence have been committed by individuals with similar ideas (e.g., Elliot Rodger in 2014, Isla Vista, California).[26] Comparing 50,000 messages from an incel forum to 50,000 "neutral" control texts extracted from Wikipedia articles and random

English tweets via LIWC software, the researchers found that incel messages contained more swear words, personal pronouns, modal adverbs, and negative adjectives but fewer positive adjectives than the control texts.[24] The incel texts also expressed more negative emotion (anger and uncertainty categories) and social inhibition (avoidance and anxiety categories). In terms of topics, the incel texts discussed relationships and sexuality to a larger extent than the control texts, but family, work, hobbies, goals, and beliefs to a lesser extent.[24]

Figea, Kaati, and Scrivens (2016) measured affect on a white supremacy forum, focusing on racism, aggression, and worries.[27] In the study, three independent human annotators scored 300 posts from the forum on a scale from 0 to 7 for racism, aggression, and worries. Thereafter, several different linguistic variables were extracted from the dataset: all 73 LIWC categories, the number of misspellings, the number of words, part-of-speech tags, and words from three "expert knowledge dictionaries relating to worries, racism and aggression," as well as the 100 most frequent words in posts with a high affect (i.e., level 6–7 for racism, aggression, or worries) and the 100 most frequent words that differed between high and low affect posts. Important linguistic characteristics for recognizing racism were LIWC categories for religion (e.g., Muslim, church), seeing (e.g., view, saw), and third-person pronouns (e.g., they, them). The LIWC categories for anger (e.g., hate, kill) and an expert dictionary category for aggression were important for recognizing both worries and aggression.

In addition to the LIWC approach to quantitative text analysis, other methods also measure the presence of key words. For instance, in a case study of the Fort Hood shooter's correspondence, Zahedzadeh (2017) made use of the keyword in context (KWIC) method to identify thought patterns and individual trajectories toward terrorism.[28] More specifically, KWIC extracts frequent words in a text and identifies the context (i.e., a fixed number of words) preceding and following the keyword. The initial set of texts consisted of a speech and slides presented by the perpetrator as part of his training as a military psychiatrist. The speech focused on Islam, Muslims in US military, and jihad. The most frequent terms in this presentation were "god," "submission," and "heartedly." The second set of texts comprised e-mails exchanged between the perpetrator and Anwar al-Awlaki, a preacher and imam strongly involved with al-Qaeda in the Arabian Peninsula

(AQAP). Studying the context surrounding the most common term "God" in the e-mails, it was argued that the perpetrator implied "full loyalty to God is fundamental" and that use of force to establish an Islamic state would be condoned.[28] Specifically examining the occurrence of word pairs in one of the last emails sent by the perpetrator, "suicide" and "permissible" occurred most frequently together.[28] Zahedzadeh (2017) argues that the text analysis reveals that the subject of study had attempted to justify the violent attack that followed.

Neuman et al. (2015) used a different approach to measure the presence of personality and other mental health disorders in language samples from school shooters and non-offender males of a similar age.[29] This method—called *vector space model of semantics*—assumes that the meaning of a word can be determined based on the words that co-occur with it. Thus, a word's meaning can be represented as a vector in high-dimensional space, with each dimension representing a co-occurring word.[29] For example, the word "depressed" may co-occur with the words "anxious," "angry," "suicidal," and "sad." Importantly, a single text can similarly be represented as a vector. The level of a specific (group of) word(s) in the text is then calculated by measuring the distance between the vector of the word and the vector of the text (i.e., the closer a vector of a text is to a vector of interest, the more similar it is to it).

When the school shooter texts were compared to the non-offender male blogger texts, school shooters' texts had smaller distances to the following vectors: "revengeful," "humiliated," and those associated with narcissistic personality disorder (e.g., "arrogant," "egocentric"). From there, Neuman et al. (2015) used different statistical models to predict whether certain texts originated from a school shooter, producing a ranking of texts that need to be screened in order to identify all school shooters. Of particular interest to law enforcement and mental health practitioners, the authors argue that this ranking and prioritization method can identify "red flag language" while only searching through a small amount of the corpus.[29]

WEIGHT-BASED APPROACHES TO LINGUISTIC ANALYSIS

Similar to word count-based approaches, weight-based approaches typically rely on a dictionary. However, words in these dictionaries are additionally assigned a weight that signifies the intensity of a particular concept (e.g., a score for sentiment or abusiveness). A dictionary-based sentiment analysis is perhaps one of the most widely known weight-based approaches. This method specifically serves to measure the polarity of a text, also known as the extent to which a text signifies positive or negative emotion. For this purpose, sentiment dictionaries are used in which a large number of words' polarity scores (e.g., ranging from −1 for highly negative words to +1 for highly positive words) are represented. When a sentiment analysis is conducted on a text, the words that also appear in the sentiment dictionary are extracted and assigned the according weight. After correcting for text length, an average sentiment score is typically reported for a piece of text. In contrast, a LIWC approach to measuring positive and negative emotion measures the proportion of words that are considered to refer to the former or the latter. As such, a sentiment analysis is usually more comprehensive in that it considers the polarity of a wider range of words and also provides an average polarity score instead of a proportion score. Affect analysis extends basic sentiment analysis by considering a wider range of emotions, such as anger, surprise, sadness, and joy. Again, emotions are measured with a dictionary approach, where words are scored for the extent to which they represent a specific emotion. For example, the PRAT tool employs both sentiment and affect analysis, measuring positive sentiment, negative sentiment, and anger, arguing that emotions are an important predictor of violent extremism.[22] Further studies discussed later similarly apply sentiment and affect analyses to extremist, radical, grievance-fueled, and lone-actor texts.

Scrivens, Davies, and Frank (2018) used sentiment analysis to identify radical users of four Islamic web forums (*Gawaher*, Islamic Awakening, Islamic Network, and Turn to Islam).[30] An average sentiment score (per posting) was computed for approximately 1 million postings. Then, in order to identify radical forum users, the authors considered four components: (1) the average sentiment score across all posts from a single author, (2) the volume of negative posts (i.e., the number of posts with a negative polarity value as well as the number of negative posts in proportion to all posts), (3) severity of negative posts (i.e., the number of very negative posts with a standardized count score above 3 as well as the number of very negative posts in proportion to all posts), and (4) the duration of negative posts (i.e., the time difference [date] between the first and last negative post). All components result in a score between 1 and 10. When summed, the components result in a "radical score" between 1 and 40. Based on the radical score for 26,171 users across all four forums, it was found that the most radical users were concentrated within two forums (i.e., Islamic Awakening and *Gawaher*), with the most radical poster achieving a score of 39.03 out of 40.[30] The authors emphasize that no single profile or behavior pattern was found that describes a radical author. Instead, the results illustrate the importance of considering multiple factors when analyzing online radical behavior.

Some research applied affect analyses to extremist and violence-related texts. For example, Abbasi and Chen (2007) measured the intensity of hate and violence on American and Middle Eastern dark web forums.[31] A custom affect lexicon was developed containing words and phrases from the forums related to violence and hate, each manually scored for intensity (on a scale from 1 to 20). Messages from 16 US white supremacist and Middle Eastern extremist group forums were compared against the hate and violence lexicons. Results indicated that Middle Eastern forums scored significantly higher than American forums in terms of violent affect. Forums from both regions did not differ in terms of hate intensity. In addition, a correlation between hate and violence was found across messages and forums from the Middle East.

In a similar vein, Chen (2008) proposed an automated method for analyzing affect within two jihadist dark web forums.[32] Up to 909,039 messages were collected from the forums, of which 500 were utilized to manually construct a custom lexicon for violence, anger, hate, and racism affects. One of the forums, known to be more radical, was indeed found to contain higher levels of violence, anger, hate, and racism than the other.[32] A simple sentiment analysis was also conducted, indicating that the entire radical forum could be classified as having a negative sentiment polarity, while the moderate forum was found to be neutral in terms of sentiment polarity.

In addition to sentiment and affect, abusive language is also frequently measured with a weight-based approach. For instance, the website Hatebase records hate-speech terms and an associated rating for offensiveness as well as their sightings across the world.[33] The website categorizes hate speech terms into nationality, ethnicity, religion, gender, sexual discrimination, disability, and class. The repository has frequently been

employed in computational approaches to detect hate speech, for example on social media[34] and the white supremacist forum Stormfront.[35,36] De Gibert et al. (2018) extracted sentences from the Stormfront forum and manually annotated them for containing hate speech or not (defined as "a deliberate attack directed at a specific group motivated by aspects of the group's identity").[35] Thereafter, the authors calculated a hate score for individual words by means of the correlation between the word and the category of hate sentences as well as the category of no-hate sentences. For this particular dataset of Stormfront posts, words with the highest hate score include "ape," "scum," and "savages."[35]

Wiegand et al. (2018) developed another more domain-independent lexicon by annotating words with a negative polarity for their abusiveness.[37] Five annotators judged a sample of 500 nouns, adjectives, and verbs with a negative polarity for abusiveness (yes/no). Words were only considered abusive if four out of five annotators agreed. In addition to this base lexicon, other linguistic features were also considered for later detection of abusive language. Wiegand et al. (2018) also determined a finer-grained measure of intensity by extracting the words from online reviews (including abusive "reviews" of persons) and computing the weighted mean of the star ratings in which the word occurred.[37] The underlying assumption is that 1-star review of persons (e.g., celebrities, politicians) are abusive comments. Among other things, further linguistic features included affect categories, sentiment views (the perspective of the opinion holder of a polar expression[38]), semantic associations, and word embeddings. The authors then applied the initial lexicon extended by the linguistic features to detect abusive posts in several different datasets (Twitter, Wikipedia comments). It was found that the lexicon, supplemented by aforementioned features, performed better at detecting abusive online posts than other lexicons considered, such as the Hatebase lexicon.

CURRENT LIMITATIONS TO THE STUDY OF LONE-ACTOR LANGUAGE

It is important to note that the current approach to the automatic linguistic analysis of lone-actor terrorist texts still has many limitations. Some of the most important, discussed in this section, include (1) a lack of empirical evidence and replications, (2) lack of adequate datasets, (3) lack of adequate dictionaries and transparent construction procedures, (4) lack of context-sensitive measures, and (5) lack of dynamic measures.

Lack of Empirical Evidence

Many of the studies discussed thus far are based on theories about the psychological characteristics of lone-actor terrorists and other potentially violent individuals and have set out to quantitatively measure these concepts through language. In some cases, this means that theoretical claims determined what linguistic features were measured. This includes assumptions about the thinking style and emotions of terrorists,[16,20] mental health disorders believed to be associated with terrorism,[29] and personality traits attributed to violent individuals.[22] This procedure may be problematic for three reasons. First, although many of these assumptions about the characteristics of violent lone-actors make intuitive sense, it is important to also find empirical support for them. In cases where such evidence is lacking, the theory in question should not warrant linguistic study. In a field where the implications of false negatives and false positives are far-reaching, attempts at linguistic detection should be supported by extensive evidence confirming that a psychological construct one intends to measure is indeed of importance. This does not only include empirical inquiries into the postulated traits of violent individuals, but also consistently replicated effects.

Second, previous research has shown that no single profile for a lone-actor terrorist exists.[4] Although mental health disorders may often be present in lone perpetrators of violence,[39] linguistic measures of such disorders should not be used as a single detection measure. Just as every lone-actor terrorist will have a unique combination of traits, so will their language consist of a unique combination of features.

Third, for specific characteristics that are found to be more prevalent among violent terrorists, it still remains to be seen whether the concepts can indeed be measured through language. Again, this matter requires empirical study, specifically into whether different levels of the trait also manifest in language. Such an enquiry may, for example, take the shape of an experiment where individuals are tested on a particular trait (e.g., narcissism, anxiety) and then are instructed to write a piece of text. If differences in language use reflect differences in the trait among the text authors, this finding would support the idea that the trait in question is worthy of linguistic study and potential practical applications.

Lack of Adequate Datasets

While the amount of texts produced by lone-actor, radical, and extremist individuals (e.g., through social media) will likely continue to increase, the seriousness of threats or (linguistic) signals of impending violence will often not become apparent until after a violent act has taken place. The problem of detecting texts authored by potentially violent individuals has been compared to "searching for a needle in a haystack,"[40] referring to the small number of relevant texts dispersed among all text available online. Small sample sizes characterize many studies on lone-actor terrorist, radical, or extremist-authored texts. As a result, a large part of automated analyses of lone-actor language compares their writing to an often larger sample of "control" writings. The control group has comprised personal blog entries,[20-22] unrelated texts written by individuals matched for gender and age,[29] and standard "baseline" texts or emotional texts provided by the developers of LIWC[16] or Wikipedia articles.[24] This approach has often resulted in statistically significant differences between the violent lone-actor and non-violent control group on various linguistic markers. Indeed, lone-actor texts seem to have largely been compared to texts that are completely unrelated in nature and often concern entirely different topics, thus raising concerns about the validity of the tests that are performed. In other words, the question arises whether the distinguishing characteristics of lone-actor texts are measured or merely the difference between lone-actor and innocent texts in terms of topic(s).

Furthermore, the approach in question fails to address a matter that may be of most interest to security professionals and threat managers. Perhaps the most interesting (but highly difficult) task for the current field is to understand what distinguishes the language use of individuals who are serious about committing violence out of a larger group in which all texts discuss concepts of violence and extremist ideals. Approaches where violent texts are compared to, for example, Wikipedia articles fail to address this issue since these control texts concern highly different matters than violence and extremism and often lack any emotional valence in the first place.

Noteworthy attempts at addressing this issue have been made, for example by Kaati, Shrestha, and Sardella (2016) and Baele (2017), who additionally compared terrorist writings to texts written by non-violent extremists or so-called peaceful radicals.[16,21] However, these peaceful texts likely lack references to violence and extremist ideology. One of the few instances in which this problem has been addressed is the comparison between lone-actor terrorist manifestos to posts on the right-wing extremist forum Stormfront,[21] on which the users may be considered similar in terms of extremism to the lone-actor sample. However, this comparison remains problematic, seeing that it is impossible to rightfully assume none of the (anonymous) forum posters has engaged in violence based on their beliefs. Another noteworthy example is the comparison between tweets by supporters of the Islamic State in Iraq and al-Sham (ISIS) and those by non-ISIS supporters, where both groups discuss similar concepts.[41] This is an important endeavor, seeing that the detection of radical language is faced with the problem that texts written by non-radical individuals may commonly include radicalization terminology (e.g., journalists reporting on radicalization), thus engendering false positives. This issue was addressed by examining semantic contexts surrounding common radicalization terms, thus allowing for better discrimination between radical content and non-radical content containing radical terminology.[42]

In short, perhaps the most challenging task for the field of linguistic threat assessment is acquiring datasets that allow for valid linguistic comparisons between violent and non-violent populations. In doing so, it is especially important to consider control groups whose content may be similar to that of the experimental group so that detection systems can be fine-tuned through discovering true discriminatory linguistic variables rather than differences in topic alone. Moreover, it is now clearly possible to discriminate between texts written by violent persons and a sample of neutral texts written by non-violent persons, but the challenge ahead is to accurately and reliably discriminate between a violent text authored by a violent individual and a text discussing violence authored by an individual who does not intend to commit such violence.

Lack of Adequate Dictionaries and Transparent Development

The majority of studies discussed thus far relied on a dictionary-based approach. This includes investigations that made use of word-count approaches such as LIWC,[16,20,21] as well as any dictionary-based sentiment analyses.[30] An important limitation of a dictionary approach to automated linguistic analysis is the constrained nature of any given dictionary because of the difficulties associated with creating a fully comprehensive

dictionary, thus creating the risk that markers of certain concepts are missed. Furthermore, the meaning of certain words in a dictionary can be highly context-dependent.[22,32] Some words may be incorrectly considered simply because they appear in a dictionary. For example, the word "ape" can be used as a racist slur when directed at people but may also occur in an innocent context where the animal is described. Furthermore, some words may not be picked up due to misspellings or spelling variations, especially if one studies noisy online text data. Although solutions to this problem exist, such as automatic spelling correction or substitution based on a dictionary of word variations,[43,44] this problem may not be adequately circumvented in all cases.

Perhaps most importantly, existing dictionaries may not capture the relevant concepts that are needed to detect and counter extreme messages. Researchers in this domain may be interested in assessing concepts such as grievance, aggression, or hate, which for example do not appear in LIWC. Although commonly used for this purpose, the LIWC dictionary has indeed not been specifically developed for the study of lone-actor terrorist language or the purpose of threat assessment. The study of lone-actor terrorist language is thus far lacking a dictionary tailored to measure linguistic concepts that are of specific interest to threat assessment and security professionals. Furthermore, even though some custom dictionaries can be used to extract terms used by right-wing extremists or radicalized Muslims,[27,31] the specific jargon likely to feature in these dictionaries precludes the possibility of applying the dictionary to communications resulting from other types of grievances. In short, the field of linguistic threat assessment may greatly benefit from a dictionary that is specifically developed for this purpose and that can be utilized across the full domain of grievance-fueled communications.

A further matter to consider is that dictionaries are often constructed by humans. The LIWC documentation notes that categories and word instances were constructed through brainstorm sessions and crowd-sourced initiatives on discovering word associations.[15] Such a procedure is highly sensitive to human biases that may influence what words are included in the word categories and dictionary. Likewise, parts of the dictionary critical to the PRAT tool were developed through consultations with domain experts on the topic of risk.[22] The themes that experts were consulted on were then supplemented with distributional semantic models and consequently manually verified by experts again. Furthermore, other investigations[27,31] also report relying on expert annotations to construct custom dictionaries for concepts such as violence and aggression.

While consultation with domain experts likely promotes the validity and applicability of a tool, the exact procedure of this consultation remains opaque. That is, characteristics of the experts are not described and therefore the reader cannot verify the quality of the judgments given by the experts in question. In addition, little information is given as to how and why certain words and concepts were selected by the experts for inclusion in the dictionary. It is highly likely that various custom dictionaries that may have been intended to measure the same construct vary in terms of validity and scope because the procedure of developing the dictionaries varies across research groups. Unfortunately, the exact procedures of development for the dictionaries are sparsely documented and the contents of dictionaries are rarely made publicly available. While expert consultation and brainstorm sessions are arguably a good starting point, researchers intending to build their own dictionary should foster transparency about the procedure in which it is constructed. Questions that arise are (1) who are the experts consulted? (2) What are they consulted on? (3) To what extent do they have experience with the construct that needs to be measured through the dictionary? (4) What are the constructs they suggested? And (5) Which concepts were eventually chosen for inclusion in the dictionary? If researchers are open about procedures and materials, then the wider research community and security professionals can make a fair judgment about those instances in which the dictionary may or may not be useful and to what extent it is comprehensive in its measurements, as well as make inferences about any potential biases that may have resulted from the annotator or expert sample.

Lack of Context-Sensitive Measures

As raised in our discussions of dictionaries and datasets, the present approach to understanding and detecting radical and violent language is faced with the issue of context-dependent meanings. This manifests in the difficulties associated with detecting radical users based on jihad-related terms because this procedure may also falsely identify users who use the same terms to condemn the ideology, report news related to the topic, or offer counter-narratives.[41] Therefore, efforts should be made to develop

context-sensitive measures for linguistic threat assessment. A good example of this was described in the vector space model approach to identifying school shooters, which relies on co-occurrences of words rather than static individual instances in a dictionary.[29] This context-sensitive approach, also known as *word embeddings*, has gained considerable traction in the wider field of computational linguistics, where it is frequently used to detect hate speech,[45,46] sometimes outperforming approaches that rely on word frequencies alone.[43] An alternative approach to considering context is extracting the segments surrounding words of interest, which is done in a KWIC analysis.[28] The contexts may then be qualitatively or quantitatively (e.g., through sentiment) studied in order to promote an understanding of word occurrences and their contexts.

Lack of Dynamic Measures

Across the different approaches to linguistic analysis, including those considering psycho-social features, sentiment, and affect, a dominant characteristic is to report the aforementioned features in a static manner. That is, a single score is computed for a concept (e.g., the proportion of words related to power or an average score for sadness). This procedure is especially pervasive in the case of sentiment analysis. For example, in Scrivens et al. (2018), a cumulative "radical score" was calculated based on average sentiment across forum postings as well as the volume, severity, and duration of negative posts.[30] In another case, a single average sentiment score was calculated across all posts of two entire forums.[32] In short, it appears to be common procedure to compute averages for sentiment to represent the polarity of a single text or average polarity across multiple texts.

A downside to this approach is that shifts in sentiment may be obscured when a text is represented by a single score. If a text author is highly negative in one section of text but highly positive in another, the polar scores may average each other out, resulting in a neutral sentiment score for the text.[47,48] In such cases, the resulting single static score is not informative, especially when the purpose is to detect highly negative language use within or across texts or pathways toward negative language use across texts. Indeed, within the context of mitigating extremist violence, it may be of particular interest to detect a highly aggressive forum posting, model trajectories toward more radical language, examine fluctuations of positive and negative language use and the topics that give rise to these sentiments, or study the effects of external events—like a lone-actor terrorist attack—on sentiment trajectories over time.[49] Alternatively, researchers may be interested in detecting bursts of positive sentiment prior to a violent attack if an individual is perhaps excitedly anticipating the impending act of violence. It has been suggested that sentiment deterioration or escalation may be useful linguistic signals of threat,[50] a process that can only be linguistically measured if language use over time is considered.

Language use will need to be modeled dynamically, and efforts should be made to move away from single static scores. Instead, a text or sequence of texts can be represented in terms of linguistic trajectories. That is, concepts such as sentiment and abusive language, but also specific topics, such as religion and family, can be gauged at several points within and across texts. Consequently, texts can be represented as a function of the concept or topic in question, showcasing shifts at a more granular level. This approach has been implemented in research on lone-actor terrorist manifestos,[49] where shifts of positive and negative language use are modeled throughout texts. The same approach has also been applied to right-wing extremist forum posts, albeit across multiple posts in chronological order.[51] In this case, the dynamic approach to modeling sentiment and abusive language makes visible transitions to more extreme language over time. Furthermore, a similar approach (measuring average sentiment of specific keywords at multiple time points) has been applied to measure shifts in sentiment toward specific concepts and the influence of external events on this trajectory.[52]

CURRENT PRACTICES AND OUTLOOK
At present, the approaches discussed in this chapter, as well as their respective limitations, describe an emerging field of research. Some researchers have set out to implement these efforts into usable tools such as the PRAT.[22] At the same time, related methods are applied within tech companies that similarly work to tackle terrorist and extremist content on their (social media) platforms.[53] In contrast, these methods will not (yet) be available to general forensic practice or small-scale law enforcement. This is partly due to the closed nature of systems developed in-house by tech companies as well as the limited availability of academic research on the topic of terrorist language use and the very few cases where research has been translated into practical tools. Once automatic linguistic threat assessment tools

become available on a wider scale (e.g., in police departments), it remains important to retain human expertise in the decision-making process due to the danger associated with false positives and negatives produced by automatic systems. Furthermore, it is of great importance for automated linguistic threat assessment tools to be constantly evaluated and adapted as the nature of terrorist language and online behavior evolves simultaneously. Again, this is an important point to consider for small-scale threat assessment firms or law enforcement agencies that may not have the capacity or resources to monitor ongoing changes, both in terms of online behavior and technological developments. Therefore, any party offering an automated threat assessment tool should assume responsibility for constantly adapting its product to meet the demands brought about by the constantly evolving nature of violent threats.

CONCLUSION
The automatic linguistic analysis of lone-actor, radical, extremist, and grievance-fueled texts is receiving increasing attention because of the increasing presence of these populations in the online sphere. As such, it has become even more important to understand, detect, and counter these messages. The body of research reviewed in this chapter has highlighted the various ways in which psychological, social, and emotional characteristics of lone-actor terrorist and other (potentially) violent individuals have been measured through language.

Considerable strides have been made at discovering linguistic features that are of interest when studying these populations. At the same time, a number of limitations to the study of lone-actor language remain to be addressed. First, linguistic inquiries should be based on empirically evaluated claims regarding the psychological characteristics of lone-actors and other violent individuals. Furthermore, better control sample texts will need to be obtained and implemented to effectively understand warning signs of violence. An ideal study would compare a sample of threatening or extreme texts for which it is known that the authors did not turn to violence (i.e., the threats were a bluff) to a sample of similarly threatening or extreme texts for which it is known that the authors did engage in violence. While this may be a highly challenging endeavor, collaboration between threat assessment professionals who may possess such data and researchers familiar with linguistic analysis may address this important limitation and thereby significantly advance the field of linguistic threat assessment.

Collaboration between threat assessment professionals and academics is also essential for the development of effective dictionaries that measure concepts of specific interest to the study of lone-actor language. When embarking on such ventures, it is important to foster openness about the procedures used to construct and contents of the dictionaries so that their quality can be judged in the wider academic and security community if these works are to stand the test of time. We have also stated the importance of implementing and further developing context-sensitive measures in order to appropriately measure linguistic constructs of interest and further reduce false positives. In applying word count- or score-based dictionaries, we have emphasized that dynamic measures should be utilized to adequately represent trajectories of a concept, instead of static single scores. In a field where understanding pathways to radicalization or violence are of extreme importance, modeling linguistic trajectories will likely prove useful.

This chapter illustrates that an automated linguistic approach to understanding lone-actor terrorists not only provides highly interesting insights, but it has also demonstrated that this approach may contribute to ongoing efforts at detecting and countering terrorist and extremist narratives. In short, the main facets of the measures needed for this field to develop into its full potential are the concepts of openness and collaboration. Together, security professionals and researchers can deepen our understanding of this pressing problem and ultimately improve our ability to counter it.

NOTES AND REFERENCES

1. Gill P, Corner E. Lone actor terrorist use of the Internet and behavioural correlates. *Terrorism Online: Politics, Law and Technology*, Lee Jarvis, Stuart MacDonald, Thomas M. Chen (London, UK, Routledge) 2015:34–53.
2. Corner E, Gill P, Schouten R, Farnham F, Corner E, Gill P, et al. Mental Disorders, Personality Traits, and Grievance-Fueled Targeted Violence: The Evidence Base and Implications for Research and Practice. Journal of Personality Disorders, 2018;3891. https://www.tandfonline.com/doi/abs/10.1080/00223891.2018.1475392
3. Silver J, Horgan J, Gill P. Shared Struggles? Cumulative Strain Theory and Public Mass Murderers from 1990 to 2014. Homicide Studies. 2018;23(1):64–84 2018; https://journals.sagepub.com/doi/abs/10.1177/1088767918802881
4. Gill P, Horgan J, Deckert P. Bombing alone: Tracing the motivations and antecedent behaviors of lone-actor terrorists. J Forensic Sci. 2014;59(2):425–435.
5. Gill P, Corner E, Bloom M, Horgan J. Terrorist use of the internet by the numbers; Quantifying Behaviors, Patterns, and Processes. Criminol Public Policy Rev. 2017;16(1):99–117. https://doi.org/10.1111/1745-9133.12249
6. Geurts R, Granhag PA, Ask K, Vrij A. Taking threats to the lab: Introducing an experimental paradigm for studying verbal threats. J Threat Assess Manage. 2016;3(1):53–64.
7. Meloy JR, Hart S, Hoffmann J. *International Handbook of Threat Assessment.* New York: Oxford University Press; 2014.
8. Bond GD, Holman RD, Eggert JL, Speller LF, Garcia ON, Mejia SC, et al. "Lyin' Ted," "Crooked Hillary," and "Deceptive Donald": Language of lies in the 2016 US Presidential Debates.Applied Cognitive Psychology. 2017;31(6):668–677. https://onlinelibrary.wiley.com/doi/10.1002/acp.3376
9. Newman ML, Pennebaker JW, Berry DS, Richards JM. Lying words: Predicting deception from linguistic styles. Personality Soc Psychol Bull. 2003 May 2;29(5):665–675.
10. Tausczik YR, Pennebaker JW. The psychological meaning of words: LIWC and Computerized text analysis methods. J Lang Soc Psychol. 2010;29(1):24–54.
11. Nguyen D, Gravel R, Trieschnigg D, Meder T. "How old do you think I am?": A study of language and age in Twitter. Proceedings of ICWSM. 2013;439–448.
12. Burger JD, Henderson J, Kim G, Zarrella G. Discriminating gender on Twitter. Emnlp. 2011;1301–1319.
13. Perraudin F, Murphy S. Alarm over number of female MPs stepping down after abuse. *The Guardian*, 31 Oct 2019 [cited 2019 Nov 8]. https://www.theguardian.com/politics/2019/oct/31/alarm-over-number-female-mps-stepping-down-after-abuse
14. Kleinberg B, Arntz A, Verschuere B. Detecting deceptive intentions: Possibilities for large-scale applications. In Docan-Morgan T, ed. *The Handbook of Deceptive Communication.* New York: Palgrave; 2019:403–417, https://doi.org/10.1007/978-3-319-96334-1
15. Pennebaker JW, Boyd RL, Jordan K, Blackburn K. *The Development and Psychometric Properties of LIWC2015.* Austin: University of Texas at Austin; 2015.
16. Baele SJ. Lone-actor terrorists' emotions and cognition: An evaluation beyond stereotypes. Political Psychology. 2017;38(3):449–468.
17. Loza W. The psychology of extremism and terrorism: A Middle-Eastern perspective. Aggression Violent Behav. 2007;12(2):141–155.

18. Schwartz SJ, Dunkel CS, Waterman AS. Terrorism: An identity theory perspective. Studies Conflict Terrorism. 2009;32(6):537–559.

19. Pennebaker JW, Chung CK, Frazee J, Lavergne GM, Beaver DI. When small words foretell academic success: The case of college admissions essays. Gong Q, ed. PLoS ONE. 2014 Dec 31;9(12):e115844.

20. Kaati L, Shrestha A, Cohen K. Linguistic analysis of lone offenders manifestos. In *IEEE International Conference on Cybercrime and Computer Forensic (ICCCF)*. 2016:1–8.

21. Kaati L, Shrestha A, Sardella T. Identifying warning behaviors of violent lone offenders in written communication. In *2016 IEEE 16th International Conference on Data Mining Workshops*. 2016:1053–1060.

22. Akrami N, Shrestha A, Berggren M, Kaati L, Obaidi M, Cohen K. Assessment of risk in written communication: Introducing the Profile Risk Assessment Tool (PRAT). Paper presented at the 2nd European Counter-Terrorism Centre (ECTC) Advisory Group conference, 17–18 April 2018, at Europol Headquarters, The Hague. https://www.europol.europa.eu/publications-events/publications/assessment-of-risk-in-written-communication, 2–24.

23. Thomsen L, Obaidi M, Sheehy-Skeffington J, Kteily N, Sidanius J. Individual differences in relational motives interact with the political context to produce terrorism and terrorism-support. Behav Brain Sci. 2014 Aug 27;37(04):377–378.

24. Jaki S, Smedt T De, Gwó M, Panchal R, Rossa A, Pauw G De. Online hatred of women in the incels. me Forum: Linguistic Analysis and Automatic Detection. Journal of Language Aggression and Conflict. 2019;7(2):1–30.

25. Beauchamp Z. Incel, the ideology behind the Toronto attack, explained. Vox, 2018 [cited 2018 Nov 29]. https://www.vox.com/world/2018/4/25/17277496/incel-toronto-attack-alek-minassian

26. BBC News. How rampage killer became misogynist "hero." BBC News, 26 Apr 2018 [cited 2019 Oct 13]. https://www.bbc.com/news/world-us-canada-43892189

27. Figea L, Kaati L, Scrivens R. Measuring online affects in a white supremacy forum. In *IEEE International Conference on Intelligence and Security Informatics: Cybersecurity and Big Data, ISI 2016*. 2016:85–90.

28. Zahedzadeh G. Overt attacks and covert thoughts. *Aggression Violent Behav*. 2017;36(Oct 2016):1–8.

29. Neuman Y, Assaf D, Cohen Y, Knoll JL. Profiling school shooters: Automatic text-based analysis. Front Psychiatry. 2015;6(86).

30. Scrivens R, Davies G, Frank R. Searching for signs of extremism on the web: An introduction to sentiment-based identification of radical authors. Behav Sci Terrorism Political Aggress. 2018;10(1):39–59.

31. Abbasi A, Chen H. Affect intensity analysis of dark web forums. In *2007 IEEE Intelligence and Security Informatics*. 2007:282–288.

32. Chen H. Sentiment and affect analysis of Dark Web forums: Measuring radicalization on the internet. *IEEE International Conference on Intelligence and Security Informatics, 2008, IEEE ISI 2008*. 2008:104–109.

33. Hatebase. https://hatebase.org

34. Mondal M, Silva LA, Benevenuto F. A measurement study of hate speech in social media. *Proceedings of the 28th ACM Conference on Hypertext and Social Media*. 2017:85–94, https://dl.acm.org/doi/proceedings/10.1145/3078714

35. de Gibert O, Perez N, García-Pablos A, Cuadros M. Hate speech dataset from a white supremacy forum. In Proceedings of the 2nd Workshop on Abusive Language Online (ALW2), 2018.

36. Sahlgren M, Isbister T, Olsson F. Learning representations for detecting abusive language. 2018:11–20. https://aclanthology.org/W18-5102/

37. Wiegand M, Ruppenhofer J, Schmidt A, Greenberg C. Inducing a lexicon of abusive words: A feature-based approach. In *Proceedings of the 2018 Conference of the North American Chapter of the Association for Computational Linguistics: Human Language Technologies*. 2018:1046–1056. https://aclanthology.org/volumes/N18-1/

38. Wiegand M, Schulder M, Ruppenhofer J. Separating actor-view from speaker-view opinion expressions using linguistic features. In *Proceedings of NAACL-HLT*. 2016:778–788. https://aclanthology.org/N16-1092

39. Corner E, Gill P. A false dichotomy? Mental illness and lone-actor terrorism. Law Hum Behav. 2015 Feb;39(1):23–34.

40. Cohen K, Johansson F, Kaati L, Mork JC. Detecting linguistic markers for radical violence in social media. Terrorism Political Violence. 2014;26(1):246–256.

41. Fernandez M, Alani H. Contextual semantics for radicalisation detection on Twitter. Semantic Web for Social Good Workshop (SW4SG) at International Semantic Web Conference 2018, 9 Oct 2018, CEUR. https://sw4sg.github.io/ISWC2018/

42. Fernandez M, Asif M, Alani H. Understanding the roots of radicalisation on Twitter. WebSci '18: Proceedings of the 10th ACM Conference on Web Science. https://doi.org/10.1145/3201064.3201082, 2018; 1–10.

43. Han B, Baldwin T. Lexical normalisation of short text messages: Makn sens a #twitter. In *Proceedings of the 49th Annual Meeting of the Association for Computational Linguistics: Human Language Technologies - Volume 1*. Stroudsburg, PA, Association for Computational Linguistics; 2007:368–378.

44. Clark E, Araki K. Text normalization in social media: Progress, problems and applications for a pre-processing system of casual English. Procedia Soc Behav Sci. 2011 Jan 1;27:2–11.

45. Djuric N, Zhou J, Morris R, Grbovic M, Radosavljevic V, Bhamidipati N. Hate speech detection with comment embeddings. In *Proceedings of the 24th International Conference on World Wide Web - WWW '15 Companion*. New York: ACM Press; 2015:29–30.

46. Nobata C, Tetreault J, Thomas A, Mehdad Y, Chang Y. Abusive language detection in online user content. In *Proceedings of the 25th International Conference on World Wide Web - WWW '16*. New York: ACM Press; 2016:145–153.

47. Jockers M. Revealing sentiment and plot arcs with the syuzhet package. 2015. https://www.matthewjockers.net/2015/02/02/syuzhet/

48. Kleinberg B, Mozes M, van der Vegt I. Identifying the sentiment styles of YouTube's vloggers. In *Proceedings of the 2018 Conference on Empirical Methods of Natural Language Processing*. 2018.

49. van der Vegt I, Kleinberg B, Gill P (forthcoming). Understanding sentiment trajectories in lone-actor terrorist manifestos.

50. Spitzberg BH, Gawron JM. Toward online linguistic surveillance of threatening messages. J Digital Forensics Security Law. 2016;11(3):43–78.

51. van der Vegt, I., Kleinberg, B., & Gill, P. Understanding sentiment trajectories in lone-actor terrorist manifestos [Conference presentation]. Society for Terrorism Research Conference, Liverpool John Moores University, Liverpool, UK; 2018, September 6–7.

52. van der Vegt I, Mozes M, Kleinberg B, Gill P. Online influence, offline violence: Linguistic responses to the 'Unite the Right' rally. April 2020, https://arxiv.org/abs/1908.11599

53. van der Vegt I, Gill P, Macdonald S, Kleinberg B. Shedding light on terrorist and extremist content removal. Global Research Network on Terrorism and Technology, 2019. https://rusi.org/publication/other-publications/shedding-light-terrorist-and-extremist-content-removal

8

Propaganda and Lone-Actor Terrorism

ERIC Y. DROGIN

INTRODUCTION

Propaganda and lone-actor terrorism enjoy a distinctly symbiotic relationship. Scholarly essays offer differing perspectives on the extent to which lone-actor terrorists are truly "alone" in their endeavors: for example, American sociologist David Hoffman has utilized techniques of social network analysis to challenge the notion that such persons ultimately "radicalize, operate, plan, and execute plots . . . with little connection to formal or more organized terrorist groups and networks."[1] To the extent that the lone-actor terrorist's activities are not solely the product of a self-conceived, self-driven scheme, they are influenced by exposure to a campaign of attraction, indoctrination, and operationalization that is a hallmark of the most effective politically oriented propaganda. Inversely, propagandists gleefully rely—in addition to scapegoating, repetition, and hyperbole—on the alleged heroism and the flamboyant, outsize martyrdom so starkly typified by the exploits of the lone-actor terrorist.

Much of this volume is devoted to an understanding of the experiential and psychological underpinnings of lone-actor terrorism, including childhood adversity, socioeconomic marginalization, sociopathy, sadism, and dependent as well as histrionic personality characteristics. This chapter's distinct focus is on propaganda as a historical and modern phenomenon, distinguishing it from other means of persuasion—both benign and sinister—and describing the different forms it takes as a weapon of opinion formation in the political arena. Emerging from these analyses will be an accounting of how propaganda and lone-actor terrorism are ultimately inseparable, as each requires the existence of the other to flourish to its fullest potential.

PROPAGANDA GENERALLY DEFINED

At the end of the nineteenth century, in his classic treatise on *The Crowd: A Study of the Popular Mind*, French psychologist Gustave Le Bon wrote that "[t]he masses have never thirsted after truth . . . [w]hoever can supply them with illusions is easily their master."[2] In keeping with this foundational notion, Austrian-American public relations pioneer Edward Bernays characterized propaganda almost 30 years later as "a mechanism which controls the public mind" and that is "manipulated by the special pleader who seeks to create public acceptance for a particular idea."[3] It was around the same time that American political commentator Walter Lippman defined this practice as "the effort to alter the picture to which men respond" as a means "to substitute one social pattern for another" and concluded—with eloquent simplicity—that what propaganda ultimately constitutes is "the manufacture of consent."[4]

American psychology professors Anthony Praktanis and Elliot Aronson have pinpointed the far more distant origins of the term "propaganda" itself.

> Its first documented use occurred in 1622, when Pope Gregory XV established the Sacra Congregatio de Propaganda Fide. . . . Pope Gregory established the papal propaganda office as a means of coordinating efforts to bring men and women to the "voluntary" acceptance of church doctrines. The word *propaganda* thus took on a negative connotation in Protestant countries but a positive one (similar to that of *education* or *preaching*) in Catholic areas.[5]

From a modern clinical perspective, *Campbell's Psychiatric Dictionary* defines "propaganda" as "[a]ny organized effort to spread a belief, doctrine, value system," noting that this concept is "of particular interest to psychiatry because of the possibility of controlling behavior with nonphysical means."[6] *Black's Law Dictionary* weighs in with the currently authoritative legal definition, which addresses this phenomenon in terms of "[t]he systematic dissemination of doctrine, rumor, or selected information to promote or injure a particular doctrine, view, or cause."[7]

PROPAGANDA DISTINGUISHED FROM OTHER MEANS OF PERSUASION

Apart from statements of simple, unadorned facts, feelings, or opinions, with no investment in what may occur as a result, all attempts at communication contain a palpable element of persuasion.[8] This includes any and all exhortations to think or act in a particular fashion, ultimately in service of what French philosopher Jacques Ellul characterized as attempts to "modify the structure of public opinion."[9] Posted notices on proper public comportment, invitations to seek one form of televised entertainment over another, and self-help texts on the virtues of exercise, relaxation, and a proper diet—all of these share a common goal, at differing levels of specificity and intensity, to control, cajole, coax, or convince. In general, none of these would properly be characterized as "propaganda," although the term is often applied rather freely in modern times to various forms of persuasion that a particular group or individual does not like or appreciate.[10]

Rhetoric

Rhetoric previously enjoyed centuries of recognition and positive regard as the legitimate, academically based art and study of oral persuasion, thus standing in contrast to propaganda's inherently sinister role as "an instrument of control and conformity by the dominant social power."[11] Although it "once formed the very core of the educational curriculum, where it was linked closely with logic and grammar,"[12] rhetoric as a skill-based communications discipline has fallen out of mainstream professional and pedagogical favor, largely due to its association with modern propaganda.[13] Rhetoric's relation to propaganda is best viewed as that of a technique to an application. Although the contemporary research literature contains ample references to "positive" as opposed to "negative" rhetoric,[14] these

designations are used to distinguish between self-supportive as opposed to externally derogative observations, but all within the same allegedly manipulative context.

Religion

Perhaps the most long-standing, concerted efforts at persuasion involve fostering adoption of—and adherence to—any of a variety of religious beliefs. In addition to messages conveyed during in-person worship services, nearly every major faith system can refer its constituents to one or more sacred texts.[15] Although the notion of the "state religion" is firmly entrenched and actively persists to the present day,[16] the texts in question are not easily revised and subverted to the whims of a current ruling party. Effective propaganda must be nimble and readily modifiable to reflect contemporary shifts in political circumstance. One could argue that Bible, the Torah, and the Quran, for example, are decidedly not.

The relationship between lone-actor terrorism and religion is well-documented,[17] and, similarly, it would be transparently absurd to assert that propaganda does not draw on religious themes. Even the Soviet Communists, for whom a frontal assault on all trappings of organized religion was a political staple during the 1920s and 1930s, found themselves compelled during World War II to incorporate classic Christian themes into propaganda posters aimed at generating support among persons born during the Tsarist era.[18] This was a far cry, however, from any attempt on the part of political or religious authorities—if only because no organized vestiges of the Church remained at that juncture—to attempt the reinstitution of Christian ceremony or principles in the Soviet Union via propaganda. As discussed later, however, churches themselves were to make considerable use of propaganda during various periods throughout history.

Political Campaigning

In the United States, political campaigning is as old as our democratic system itself and has seemingly never been without an edge of personalized nastiness. In 1852, for example, Presidential candidate Franklin Pierce, having been tagged with the nickname "Fainting Frank" as a result of a horse-riding accident during the Mexican-American War, had to combat allegations of cowardice that were woven into his opponent's national campaign.[19] A quarter of a century earlier, Andrew Jackson's bid for the presidency had been dogged by accusations that he was not only power-hungry and deranged, but also that he was neglectful of standard religious observances.[20] In the present day, of course, examples of personal taunting in presidential races have reached unprecedented levels.[21]

Political campaigning, although it clearly possesses—and from time to time directly emphasizes—propagandistic elements, functions so that such components remain as distinct as possible from the traditional, recognized context of the electoral process. Elections occur within a prescribed external structure, allowing for a give-and-take between participants, and, by their very existence, they do not anticipate the prospect of a single-party state dictating the tone and content of messaging at the national level. Overall, propaganda can be employed during a political campaign, but the campaign itself has a sanctioned, periodically recurring goal that at least in theory can be reached either with or without resorting to accusation, belittlement, and systematic misrepresentation.

Advertising
Of any of the other forms of persuasion, advertising could most be readily seen as equivalent to propaganda. The readiest distinction can be drawn on the basis of the acknowledged medium of exchange. Modern propaganda is first and foremost about politics, while advertising has to do with sales, if necessary via the overt promotion of what American linguist Noam Chomsky termed "fashionable consumption."[22] Finance is, of course, by no means a domain that exempts itself by definition from moral concerns, but it is if nothing else a transparent means to an end: the goal is to meet a payroll, reduce inventory, and otherwise maximize profits. Both activities draw on social science lore to stimulate an identification of need in their target audiences—to the extent that such stimulation is truly necessary. Advertising is complexly and exhaustively regulated,[23] and business in the twenty-first century is almost unthinkable without it. Propaganda, however, answers to no controlling authority but that of the entity that spawns it.

PROPAGANDA: HISTORICAL ORIGINS AND DEVELOPMENT
The documented history of propaganda extends back many centuries. According to American communications scholars Garth S. Jowett and Victoria O'Donnell, the possession of only primitive tools for influencing a targeted demographic

has never been a decisive impediment to the assertion of political dominance.

> [W]hile the ancient Egyptians developed no method of printing or other techniques of mass dissemination of their messages, nevertheless for nearly three millennia they exerted a tight psychological control over a large and geographically spread population. The rulers of Egypt demonstrated their understanding of the techniques of propaganda by using a sophisticated palette of intimidating images, particularly depicting the savage treatment of enemies, as well as a highly controlled set of widely recognized symbols to communicate and consolidate their power.[24]

Similar stirrings of the propagandist's craft were detectable not long afterward, thousands of miles away.

> Mayan texts and monuments often manipulated historic dates, life spans of rulers, astronomical cycles, and real events to place a current ruler in a favorable light—for example, alignment of the birth date of a current leader with the birth date of a stronger leader of the past to suggest the old leader's reincarnation, or depicting slain enemies and captives in an exaggerated way to make a leader appear strong and to strike fear into the masses. Given that only leaders and their priests could decipher hieroglyphic images and symbols, the nature of persuasion . . . was unidirectional—from the ruler to the masses.[5]

Indian Philosopher Kautilya (ca. 350–275 BCE) authored the *Arthashatra*, a guide to the use of propaganda that was arguably centuries ahead of its time. Subsequently recognized—particularly in contrast to later texts on mass communication themes—as an example of "brutal realism,"[25] this influential volume focused in particular on the consolidation of authoritarian power.

> Thus the King is canonized from being a mere ruler to that of an agent of God on earth. This makes the subjects more content and they would believe that their King is the best person to rule them and that they would lead peaceful and prosperous lives hereafter. The core is now shifted from fear to God. Since God is the considered supreme, the King's feigned allegiance with God has now made him more powerful than any other ruler.

Thus he easily begins to control them through their mind and not physical body.[26]

Propaganda in the Middle Ages was the almost exclusive province of the established Church. This circumstance establishes definitively that a power structure that eventually neutralizes any identifiable opposition still has no less need for affirmative mechanisms of social control. In this instance, of course, there was also a need to galvanize the home population for the participation in a rolling series of Holy Wars,[27] as well as to bolster religious adherence more generally.

> The Christian church . . . spent the eight centuries preceding the First Crusade proselytizing and Christianizing Europe, often in the face of extreme pagan opposition. In the process, ecclesiastical missionaries gradually honed their propagandistic tools to the point at which their message could be couched in a universally intelligible and acceptable terminology. They created a pan-European community of concepts whose spirit was clearly manifested in the mass response to the Crusade's call.[28]

The above-noted works of Pope Gregory XV in his establishment of the Sacra Congregatio de Propaganda Fide[5] constituted the classic example of Renaissance-era efforts in promoting and entrenching the role of Church at all levels of contemporary society. The late British communications expert Philip M. Taylor, observing that "propaganda appears most effective when it preaches to the already converted," cited the Congregatio de Propaganda Fide as the inspiration for "a new generation of Catholic propagandists who were given a remarkable amount of discretion concerning the methods to be employed in the field" and claimed that "this often involved secrecy, whether of production or distribution of material, and these characteristics have left a cloud of suspicion over the word 'propaganda' ever since, especially in north European Protestant countries."[29] This is not, of course, the sole perspective on such matters—particularly as they continued to persist into the modern era.

> If just and reasonable pride may be permitted in the work of carrying the message of the Gospel to the children of men, the Congregation may indeed be proud of its success in the United States. . . . [T]o no other department of the Curia do we owe so much

in the phenomenal progress of the faith in the United States as to Propaganda. And yet, one would search fruitlessly in American Catholic literature during the past century for any adequate appreciation of Propaganda's services.[30]

The flourishing of mass media in the nineteenth century—including, in particular, the popular press—allowed for broader and quicker dissemination of propaganda. In Great Britain, to cite one example, the Indian Rebellion of 1857 was a conflict in which

> Both sides committed atrocities, but the propaganda in the English homeland elicited a violent outcry against the Sepoys. . . . Some of the primary vessels for stirring up these sentiments were political cartoons. The cartoons relating to the rebellion emphasized racial differences and styed Britain as the keeper of peace and justice in India. Portrayal of the rebellion in the media successfully instilled fear of the Indians in the minds of the British people.[31]

In the United States, the American Civil War witnessed a country embroiled in a social as well as military struggle that was destined to highlight the most aggressive conveyance of bitter, longstanding grievances. American historian George Winston Smith, characterizing propaganda "as an inevitable component of war," described how "[a]ccording to the propaganda ritual of 1861, the pro-slavery South hated Northern ideals, hated the Northern way of life, her free schools, her economic power, and her enterprising spirit."[32] The Southern perspective, in turn, was popularized with particular attention to how it might play overseas, given the Confederacy's cherished hope that Europe might somehow be enticed to intervene in the struggle—perhaps militarily, but at least economically—on its behalf.[33] In 1861, the South dispatched an agent by the name of Henry Hotze to London in order to "sell the public on the ability of the Southern States" to prevail, with an understanding that "[h]e would focus on England, the leading industrial power, but his propaganda would carry to the continent through the British press and his own public tours."[34]

World War I coincided with the dawn of air power as a burgeoning factor in the unprecedentedly vast distribution of leaflet propaganda,[35] which could be delivered in this fashion independently as well as in concert with nascent attempts at strategic bombing.[36] Also at this time, drawing momentum from the astonishing pace of development in modern graphic design,[37] poster propaganda—also capable of being conveyed in leaflet form—evolved from simple themes of national pride and community to complex and increasingly savage depictions of the enemy as an entity wholly despicable.[38] As noted by British propaganda expert Charles Roetter,

[h]aving sought to pin war-guilt and all the moral condemnation this entails on the enemy, the next step is virtually inescapable: to make the enemy appear inhuman, degraded, foul, incapable of any humane or decent instinct. Until the faith of one side or the other in ultimate victory begins to crack, efforts to place responsibility for the outbreak of war on the other side is bound to be followed by propaganda about the atrocious way the other side is behaving.[39]

Film and radio propaganda flourished during World War II, in step with technological advances that no longer required messages to be transmitted in three-dimensional formats. National Socialist Germany's totalitarian regime proved particularly adept at corralling the power of the state to exert control over all forms of filmed news and entertainment, such that the output of an entire industry was subjected to review by a single government entity—and typically on an individual basis—by that entity's primary architect and overseer, Minister of Propaganda Joseph Goebbels.[40] The anti-Semitic diatribe *Jew Suss* (1940) was profoundly influential in potentiating a pattern of rationalization and acceptance that culminated in the Holocaust.[41,42] During that period when Germany could brag without contradiction of an uninterrupted series of military victories, *Victory in the West* (1940)[43] was a particularly effective cinematic calling card.

Triumph of the Will (1935) had presented Germany, teetering on the edge of war, as an inexorable political and military force.[44] Its director, Leni Riefenstahl, was also responsible for *Olympia* (1938), which touted both German athletic prowess and the architectural grandeur of a newly revitalized Berlin—adroitly accommodating the multiple victories of African American athlete Jesse Owens.[45] Riefenstahl's gift for potent iconography and a nimble ability to intercut scenes and juxtapose images exerted a powerful influence on subsequent propaganda films of decades to come, decisively bringing this use of the medium into its own.[46] Among other innovations, critics

recognize Riefenstahl's work as a clear antecedent to the modern use of "deepfakes,"[47] which are technologically fabricated but almost undetectable realistic video manipulations that have increasingly been employed as tools for spreading politically oriented disinformation.[48]

The advent of full-scale radio propaganda during World War II provided virtually unrestricted access by anyone within receiving range—except, as was to occur with increasing frequency, when transmission signals were impeded via the application of an electronically generated blocking technique known as "jamming."[49] No nationally sponsored disinformation campaign even approached in scope and effectiveness the radio-borne escapades conducted by the Political Intelligence Department of British Foreign Office, as directed by German-born Sefton Delmer.[50] What Delmer pioneered was a form of "black propaganda," a means of persuasion defined by the Central Intelligence Agency (CIA) as "misinformation that identifies itself with one side of a conflict, but is truly produced by another opposing side."[51] Delmer's broadcast programs contained the direst anti-German propaganda but were disguised as consisting of transmissions that emanated from within Germany itself or within its occupied territories.[52] For example, the station "Gustav Siegfried Eins" starred a character known as "Der Chef" ("The Chief"), purported for fictional purposes to be a disgruntled, disillusioned German military veteran,[53] appalled at goings-on in the upper hierarchy of the Nazi Party. Delmer once recalled that

[w]hat pleases me most was when I found a story we had invented being retailed as fact by the Germans without any mention of Gustav Siegfried Eins at the source. Great was my delight, for instance, when in the P.O.W. monitoring reports I found a freshly captured German Luftwaffe officer telling the story about Nazi boss Robert Ley and the "Diplomat Rations" which "Der Chef" had invented and broadcast only three weeks before. . . . Gustav Siegfried Eins made out that the Party big shots had all got themselves fixed up with "Diplomat Rations" as a way of evading the rationing laws to which the common man was subject.[54]

As battles for geopolitical supremacy evolved for the most part beyond traditional, set-piece armed conflict such as declared wars, nationally sponsored propaganda operations strove for the sort of international listenership composition and ostensible credibility epitomized by the British Broadcasting Corporation (BBC) during World War II. The BBC's willingness to disclose both good news as well as bad established its reputation for veracity but it has been a hard standard for other liberal western powers to duplicate. In the United States, the closest analogy is probably Voice of America (VOA).[56] By contrast, for example, propaganda efforts on the part of Chinese Communism tended instead to look inward,[57] constituting a tacit admission that the message they reflected was not focused on international audiences and would in any event be viewed with as much incomprehension as suspicion.

What all efforts at propaganda have held in common—certainly from their almost prehistoric origins through the all-consuming global conflicts of the twentieth century—is an attempt to sway as many persons as possible toward a unified perspective on such notions as the true path to religious salvation, the best candidate for political office, the most desirable commercial products, and the utter perfidy of a nation's internal and external enemies. From the pulpit to the printing press, and then from airdrops to the airwaves, propaganda's pervasiveness has been limited only by the reach and accessibility of the technology employed to diffuse it.

The same can be said of the damage caused by those individuals who have been attracted, inflamed, and set on a path of destruction by finely tuned and precisely targeted persuasion. The ability of the lone-actor terrorist to harm and horrify has never been greater, abetted—and glorified—by an internet that extends to nearly every location on Earth. What circumstances and processes inform and potentiate the symbiotic relationship between propaganda and lone-actor terrorism?

LOW-HANGING FRUIT: RECRUITMENT OF THE LONE-ACTOR TERRORIST

Paul Gill and colleagues conducted an exhaustive review of the behavioral characteristics of 119 lone-actor terrorists. That review identified a number of factors common to—or overrepresented among—this population, some of which point to a distinct susceptibility to propagandistic overtures:

- Prior criminal convictions,
- A history of diagnosable mental illness,
- Religious radicalization and/or recent religious conversion,

- Unemployment and/or underemployment, and
- A subjective experience of having been victimized.[58]

These findings are consistent with other contemporary research sources. Jails and prisons are frequently identified as problematic sites for the dissemination of propaganda.[59,60] Mental status is known to be a relevant factor in susceptibility to disinformation.[61] Religious radicalization is recognized as an ongoing phenomenon with an established precursor role regarding lone-actor terrorism.[62] The role of economic hardship in vulnerability to influence has long been recognized by social scientists.[63,64] Exploitation of personal grievances in laying the groundwork for responsiveness to inflammatory propaganda is a frequently employed technique.[65]

It is not necessary for potential lone-actor terrorists to be radicalized by propaganda to the extent of outright, predictably inevitable martyrdom. Along these lines, "both ISIS and Al-Qaeda have encouraged readers of their propaganda to conduct lone-actor terrorist plots for the simple reasons that they cause casualties and cannot be easily detected."[66] This having been acknowledged, there also exists in some cases a "cult of martyrdom" characterized by lone assailants who sacrifice their own lives and "justify their act of violence primarily in terms of their own victimhood."[67]

Researchers unsurprisingly surmise that the internet plays a critical role in present-day lone-actor terrorism. This medium "is considered by some to be a driver of the threat, by others as an accelerator, and by some commentators as a surrogate community—a social environment in which lone actors feel they belong."[68] Overall, as noted by German conflict and violence authority Nils Böckler and colleagues,

> The Internet plays a central role in the triumphal possession of the "lone-wolf" tactic. It is an instrument for disseminating propaganda and a social context for radicalization. Individuals dealing with personal and/or collective grievances, seeking a cause or preparing for an attack, find broad support and instructions in numerous jihadist forums and online magazines such as Al Qaida's *Inspire* or the Islamic State's *Dabique*.[69]

While internet-based instigation may take on the complex, often longer term role of deliberately inspiring resentment and then shaping desired behaviors, much of what the internet involves is of a repetitive rather than original, creative nature.[70] Stepwise programming will not be required if broader propaganda broadsides capture the disaffected target's imagination. So-called copycat perpetrators can foster terroristic acts—deliberately or unintentionally—via online or more traditional media.[71]

RECYCLING HATE: EXPLOITING THE ACTIONS OF THE LONE-ACTOR TERRORIST

Recent history abounds with examples of how entities that inspire terror feed on specific incidents of violence they have incurred, thus ensuring that they can ensnare subsequent waves of violent adherents. Paul Gill has identified—among others—a number of such examples, including "a video titled 'A Call to Arms' that encouraged people to 'undertake lone-wolf operations in the West' and praised the actions of Nidal Malik Hassan (the Fort Hood shooter)," an issue of the al-Qaeda magazine *Inspire* featuring "Umar Farouk Abdulmutallab who attempted to bomb a civilian aircraft while on board in December 2009," as well as "public mass shooting attacks like those of lone actors Nidal Malik Hassan and Abdul Hakim Mujahid Muhammad and IEDs [improvised explosive devices] constructed from pressure cookers (like those used in Boston in 2013)."[72]

It is not necessary, of course, for propagandists—and the organizations they represent or champion—to restrict their focus to those incidents to which they can properly substantiate—or even prove to themselves—some sort of direct or more attenuated involvement. The European Counter-Terrorism Center at Europol describes a "flawed claim for the Las Vegas shooting" in 2017, as well as another such claim concerning a 2018 incident in which "a man crashed his car into shop fronts in a Melbourne street, exited and started stabbing passers-by, killing one person."[73] In some cases, those making these assertions may not even know themselves if the acts in question are examples of lone-actor terrorism or instead the work of what may be designated "common" homicide offenders.[74]

COUNTERING THE SYMBIO-SIS OF PROPAGANDA AND LONE-ACTOR TERRORISM

While it is intriguing and informative to identify the relationship between agitation and action—and to describe the dynamics that lay the groundwork for its inception and development—it is incumbent upon those who seek more than mere insight to consider how the problem might be prevented or at least curtailed. Armed with an enhanced understanding of relevant factors, how can authorities address the symbiosis of propaganda and lone-actor terrorism, using the input of social scientists and other consultants?

- *Remove the basis for the problem.* This remedy, if capable of being applied, would probably do more than anything else to eradicate the context for propaganda and the receptivity of its intended targets. Withdrawal of occupying forces, recalibration of economic relationships with aggrieved nations, overt expressions of respect for religious observance and social custom, and material support for scientific endeavors[75] are examples of such actions. Noting the existence of these options does not constitute advocacy for a sea change in international relations; rather, it constitutes merely the identification of one arguably logical and potentially effective solution, in full recognition that this would run very much counter to the conventional wisdom of contemporary politics and present-day perspectives on military and security interests.

- *Remove the means for potentiating the problem.* Historically, when propaganda was primarily preached from the pulpit, printed on presses, or broadcast with the use of radio and television transmitters, those seeking to staunch its flow could mount an attack on such activities at their physical source. In modern times, however, propaganda is often generated on the fly, via the medium of the internet, requiring little more than a laptop-enabled camera and some form of online hookup.[76] Such military remedies can also constitute a political liability, compelling political authorities to scramble for a means to describe the necessity for such operations and to apologize for what would likely be characterized—even if in vain—as unavoidable collateral damage.[77]

- *Impose internet censorship.* China, for example, has chosen to approach the problem in this fashion, with what at least one study has suggested may be a fair degree of internal approval and support.[78] Countries lacking centralized control over the internet and other consumer habits of their citizens may find this solution far less feasible, not mention far less politically acceptable both at home and abroad. There may, in fact, be local laws that obviate such approaches from the outset.[79] In addition, just as physical sources of externally generated messaging are difficult to track down for purposes of destruction, the act of tracking and blocking electronic sources can prove equally challenging as domain names change, messages are reposted, and content is retweeted.[80]

- *Employ "black propaganda."* This phenomenon, as referenced earlier, emanates from an "undisclosed source"[81]—or at least one whose *true* source is not revealed, inasmuch as it purports to be the product of another author or movement. This would ultimately involve, within the context of propaganda and lone-actor terrorism, a scheme by which clumsily conveyed and off-putting views and exhortations are attributed to the very organization seeking to sponsor violent and disruptive acts. The potential lone-actor terrorist would be encouraged by this device to question and ultimately reject the goals of potential agitators by seeing these goals conveyed in a fashion that is either overstated or deliberately inaccurate. If carried out properly in terms of tone, distribution, and camouflaged origins, this scheme could diminish the effects of—or perhaps prevent outright—radicalization of the target audience.
- *Employ "white propaganda."* As defined by American communications experts Garth Jowett and Victoria O'Donnell, this brand of information involves statements "neither deceitful nor false" for which "the source was known."[82] White propaganda can be utilized proactively to propound a worldview that the sponsoring entity is proud to endorse and serves the purpose of furthering acknowledged interests in a fashion calculated to appeal to an extended audience. It also has a reactive function, in that it can be employed in the form of a response to allegations that stand a decent chance of being disproved on the basis of objective facts. Such tactics can play a valuable role in "winning the support or neutrality of other nations"[83] and can, at very least provide, a credible, alternative source of input for potential lone-actor terrorists on the verge of becoming radicalized.
- *Ignore the problem.* This approach is not as passive or indifferent as it might seem. It is a long-standing tenet of counter-propagandistic efforts that the reach of an adversary's

damaging rumor or other inaccurate assertion is only potentiated by drawing attention to it in the wrong fashion. Such second-hand distribution has in modern times become easier than ever due to relaxed restrictions in the wake of overt recognition that this is "protected by the Bill of Rights and public's right to know."[84] Avoiding drawing attention to propaganda is not tantamount to "a tendency to assume that propaganda no longer exists,"[85] but rather a recognition that one scarcely suppresses negative information by granting it a broader audience.

CONCLUSION

The phenomena of propaganda and lone-actor terrorism are inextricably intertwined. Radicalization is necessary for spreading fear-inducing violence. Martyrs and other heroes are a necessary narrative focus for the delineation of grievances—real or imagined, but always inflated—that inspire each new generation of homicidal converts.

Social scientists require an understanding of propaganda as a tool of persuasion and an understanding of lone-actor terrorism as a unique form of threat. There are numerous ways in which the symbiosis of recruitment and compliance can be addressed proactively, depending on the confluence of shared purpose, will, and resources.

NOTES AND REFERENCES

1. Hoffman D. How "alone" are lone-actors? Exploring the ideological, signaling, and support networks of lone-actor terrorists. *Stud Conflict Terrorism*, 2 Oct 2018. https://www. tandfonline. com/doi/abs/10.1080/1057610X.2018.1493833?journalCode = uter20
2. Le Bon G. *The Crowd: A Study of the Popular Mind.* 2nd ed. London: T. Fisher Unwin; 1896:67.
3. Bernays E. *Propaganda.* New York: IG Publishing; 1928:45.
4. Lippman W. *Public Opinion.* New York: Simon & Schuster; 1922:16, 158.
5. Pratkanis A, Aronson E. *Age of Propaganda: The Everyday Use and Abuse of Persuasion.* Rev. ed. New York: Henry Holt & Co.; 2001:11–12.
6. Campbell R. *Campbell's Psychiatric Dictionary.* 9th ed. New York: Oxford University Press; 2009:789.
7. Gardner B, ed. *Black's Law Dictionary.* 11th ed. 2019. https://lawschool.westlaw.com
8. Bernays E. *Crystallizing Public Opinion.* New York: IG Publishing; 1923.
9. Ellul J. *Propaganda: The Formation of Men's Attitudes.* New York: Alfred A. Knopf; 1965:203.

10. Walton D. What is propaganda, and what exactly is wrong with it? *Public Aff Q.* 1997;11(4):383–413.

11. Fitzmaurice K. Propaganda. *Brock Educ J.* 2018; 27(2):63–67:64.

12. Sloane T, ed. *Encyclopedia of Rhetoric.* New York: Oxford University Press; 2001:xi.

13. McCerrick R. Critical rhetoric and propaganda studies. *Annals Int'l Communic Assoc.* 1991;14(1):249–255.

14. Chavez L, Campos B, Corona K, Sanchez D, Ruiz C. Words hurt: Political rhetoric, emotions/affect, and psychological well-being among Mexican-origin youth. *Soc Sci Med.* 2019;228:240–251.

15. Wilson A, ed. *World Scripture: A Comparative Anthology of Sacred Texts.* St. Paul, MN: Paragon House; 1998.

16. Fox J. *A World Survey of Religion and the State.* Cambridge: Cambridge University Press; 2008.

17. Capel M, Sahliyeh E. Suicide terrorism: Is religion the critical factor? *Secur J.* 2007;29(4):267–283.

18. Rhodes A. *Propaganda: The Art of Persuasion: World War II.* Broomall, PA: Chelsea House Publishers; 1976.

19. McCullough N. *The Essential Book of Presidential Trivia.* New York: Random House; 2007.

20. Cummins J. *Anything for a Vote: Dirty Tricks, Cheap Shots, and Oct Surprises in U.S. Presidential Campaigns.* Philadelphia, PA: Quirk Books; 2007.

21. Korostelina K. *Trump Effect.* New York: Routledge; 2017.

22. Barsamian D, Chomsky N. *Propaganda and the Public Mind: Conversations with Noam Chomsky.* Cambridge, MA: South End Press; 2001:151.

23. Irving L, ed. *Ad-Infinitum: Legal Checklists for the Advertising Industry.* Manhattan Beach, CA: Manhattan Advertising & Media Law; 2015.

24. Jowett G, O'Donnell V. *Propaganda and Persuasion.* 7th ed. Thousand Oaks, CA: Sage; 2019:49.

25. Boesche R. Moderate Machiavelli? Contrasting the prince with the Arthashastra of Kautilya. *Crit Horiz.* 2015;3(2):253–276:253.

26. Aravind G, Dwivedi L. Kautilya's The Arthashastra. *Mediterranean J Soc Sci.* 2015;6(6):678–683:680.

27. Maier T. *Crusade Propaganda and Ideology.* Cambridge: Cambridge University Press; 2000.

28. Cohen E. The propaganda of saints in the middle ages. *J Commun.* 2006;31(4):16–26:16.

29. Taylor P. *Munitions of the Mind: A History of Propaganda from the Ancient World to the Present Day.* 3rd ed. Manchester, UK: Manchester University Press; 2003:8, 111.

30. Guilday P. The sacred Congregation de Propaganda Fide (1622–1922). *Cathol Hist Rev.* 1921;6(4):478–494, at 482.

31. Summers C. The Indian rebellion of 1857. *Tenor Times.* 2015;4(6):42–49, at 46.

32. Smith G. Union propaganda in the American Civil War. *Soc Stud.* 1944;35(1):26–32, at 26.

33. Tilley N. England and the Confederacy. *Am Hist Rev.* 1938;44(1);56–60.

34. Oates S. Henry Hotze: Confederate agent abroad. *History.* 1965;27(2):131–154:131.

35. Taylor P. *British Propaganda in the Twentieth Century: Selling Democracy.* Edinburgh, UK: Edinburgh University Press; 1999.

36. Lamberton W. *Reconnaissance and Bomber Aircraft of the 1914-1918 War.* Fallbrook, CA: Aero Publishers; 1962.

37. Poulin R. *Graphic Design and Architecture, A 20th Century History: A Guide to Type, Image, Symbol and Visual Storytelling in the Modern World.* Beverly, MA: Rockport Publishers; 2012.

38. Bownes D, Fleming R. *Posters of the First World War.* London: Bloomsbury Publishing; 2014.

39. Roetter C. The Art of Psychological Warfare: 1914-1945. New York: Stein & Day; 1974:43.

40. Winkler A. *The Politics of Propaganda: The Office of War Information 1942-1945.* New Haven, CT: Yale University Press; 1978.

41. Sheffi N. Jews, Germans and the representation of Jud Süss in literature and film. *Jewish Cult Hist.* 2003;6(2):25–42.

42. Levin H. Anti-semitism in German "volk" culture by propaganda through the pen and screen. *Earlham Hist J.* 2014;7(1):34–63.

43. Herzstein R. *The War That Hitler Won: The Most Infamous Propaganda Campaign in History.* New York: G. P. Putnam; 1978.

44. Barsam R. Filmguide to Triumph of the Will. Bloomington: Indiana University Press; 1975.

45. Milford M. The "reel" Jesse Owens: Visual rhetoric and the Berlin Olympics. *Sport Hist.* 2018;38(1): 96–117.

46. Włodarczyk A. *Olympia* by Leni Riefenstahl: Propaganda, document, or art? *Stud Sport Humanit.* 2016;19:37–41.

47. Coggin W. "Deepfake" viral videos have worrying propaganda potential. *The Post and Courier,* 1 Apr 2019. https://www.postandcourier.com/opinion/commentary/deepfake-viral-videos-have-worrying-propaganda-potential/article_981edc88-54a9-11e9-9630-8b6c80922187.html

48. Dobber T, Metoui N, Trilling D, Helberger N, de Vreese C Do (microtargeted) deepfakes have real effects on political attitudes? *Int'l J Press/Polit.* 2020;26(1):69–91. https://journals.sagepub.com/doi/ full/10.1177/1940161220944364

49. Wood, J. *History of International Broadcasting.* London: P. Peregrinus; 1992.

50. Rankin R. *A Genius for Deception: How Cunning Help the British Win Two World Wars.* Oxford: Oxford University Press; 2011.

51. Central Intelligence Agency. The Office of Strategic Services: Morale Operations Branch. News and Information, 29 Jul 2010. https:// www.cia.gov/

news-information/featured-story-archive/2010-featured-story-archive/oss-morale-operation

52. Argemi M, Fine G. Faked news: The politics of rumour in British World War II propaganda. *J War Cult Stud*. 2019;12(2):176–193.

53. Wortman M. The fake British radio show that helped defeat the Nazis. Smithsonian.Com, 8 Feb 2017. https://www.smithsonianmag.com/history/fake-british-radio-show-helped-defeat-nazis-180962320

54. Delmer S. *Black Boomerang*. London: Secker & Warburg; 1962:73–74.

55. Tandoc EC, Lim ZW, Ling R. Defining "fake news": A typology of scholarly definitions. *Digit Journal*. 2018;6:137–153.

56. Rawnsley GD. *Radio Diplomacy and Propaganda: The BBC and VOA in International Politics, 1956-1964*. New York: St. Martin's Press; 1996.

57. Brady A. *Marketing Dictatorship: Propaganda and Thought Work in Contemporary China*. Plymouth, UK: Rowman & Littlefield; 2008.

58. Gill P, Horgan J, Deckert P. Bombing alone: Tracing the motivations and antecedent behaviors of lone-actor terrorists. *J Forensic Sci*. 2014;59(2):425–435.

59. Office of Public Affairs, Department of Justice. Bronx man sentenced in Manhattan federal court to 22 years in prison for attempting to provide material support to ISIS. *Justice News*, 6 Dec 2019. https://www.justice.gov/opa/pr/bronx-man-sentenced-manhattan-federal-court-22-years-prison-attempting-provide-material

60. Dearden L. Man jailed for stabbing own mother shared "horrific" Isis propaganda with inmates. *Independent*, 21 Jun 2019. https://www.independent.co.uk/news/uk/crime/isis-propaganda-prison-jail-young-offenders-gul-phone-a8969821.html

61. Hambrick D, Marquardt M. Cognitive ability and vulnerability to fake news. *Scientific American*, 6 Feb 2018. https://www.scientificamerican.com/article/cognitive-ability-and-vulnerability-to-fake-news

62. Prats M, Raymond S, Gasman I. Religious radicalization and lone-actor terrorism: A matter for psychiatry? *J Forensic Sci*. 2019;64(2):1253–1258.

63. Eisenberg P, Lazarsfeld P. The psychological effects of unemployment. *Psych Bull*. 1938;35(6):358–390.

64. Liem R, Liem J. Psychological effects of unemployment on workers and their families. *J Soc Issues*. 1988;44(4):87–105.

65. Awan I. Cyber-extremism: Isis and the power of social media. *Society*. 2017;54(2):138–149.

66. Palombi S, Gomis B. *Lone-Actor Terrorism, Policy Paper 2: Attack Methodology and Logistics*, Feb 2016. https://www.isdglobal.org/wp-content/uploads/2016/03/CLAT_Policy-Paper-Chatham-House.pdf

67. Böckler N, Leuschner V, Roth V, Zick A, Scheithauer H. Blurred boundaries of lone-actor targeted violence: Similarities in the genesis and performance of terrorist attacks and school shootings. *Viol Gender*. 2018;5(2):70–80:74.

68. Pantucci R, Ellis C, Chaplais L. Lone-actor terrorism: Literature review. Dec 2015. https://www.chathamhouse.org/sites/default/files/publications/research/20160105LoneActorTerrorismLiteratureReviewRUSI.pdf

69. Böckler N, Hoffman J, Zick A. The Frankfurt airport attack: A case study on the radicalization of a lone-actor terrorist. *J Threat Assess Manage*. 2015;2(3-4):153–163:154.

70. Carr N. *The Shallows: What the Internet Is Doing to Our Brains*. New York: Norton; 2010.

71. Parker D, Pearce J, Lindekilde L, Rogers M. Press coverage of lone-actor terrorism in the UK and Denmark: Shaping the reactions of the public, affected communities, and copycat attackers. *Crit Stud Terrorism*. 2019;12(1):110–131.

72. Gill P. *Lone-Actor Terrorists: A Behavioural Analysis*. London: Routledge; 2015:8–9.

73. Staff Member. Caliphate soldiers and lone actors: What to make of IS claims for attacks in the West 2016-2018. International Center for Counter-Terrorism—the Hague, Apr 2019. https://www.europol.europa.eu/sites/default/files/documents/icct-caliphate-soldiers-and-lone-actors-may2019.pdf

74. Liem M, van Buuren J, van Zuijdewijn J, Schönberger H, Bakker E. European lone actor terrorists versus "common" homicide offenders: An empirical analysis. *Homicide Stud*. 2018;22(1):45–69.

75. Verma I. Illiteracy, ignorance, intolerance = terrorism. *Molecular Ther*. 2003;8(1):1.

76. United Nations Office on Drugs and Crime. The use of the internet for terrorist purposes. Sep 2012. https://www.unodc.org/documents/frontpage/Use_of_Internet_for_Terrorist_Purposes.pdf

77. Norton-Taylor R. Serb TV station was legitimate target, Blair says. *The Guardian*, 23 Apr 1999. https://www.theguardian.com/world/1999/apr/24/balkans3

78. Guo S, Feng G. Understanding support for Internet censorship in China: An elaboration of the theory of reasoned action. *J Chin Polit Sci*. 2012;17:33–52.

79. Brown I. The Global Online Freedom Act. *Georget J Int'l Aff*. 2013;14(1):153–160.

80. Ferrara E. Contagion dynamics of extremist propaganda in social networks. *Info Sci*. 2017;418-419(12):1–12.

81. Brunello A. A moral compass and modern propaganda? Charting ethical and political discourse. *Rev Hist Polit Sci*. 2014;2(2):169–197:175.

82. Jowett G, O'Donnell V. *Propaganda and Persuasion*. 7th ed. Thousand Oaks, CA: Sage; 2018:2.

83. Ingram H. A brief history of propaganda during conflict: Lessons for counter-terrorism strategic communications. International Center for Counter-Terrorism, Jun 2016. https://icct.nl/wp-content/uploads/2016/06/ICCT-Haroro-Ingram-Brief-History-Propaganda-Jun-2016-3.pdf

84. Armstrong M. Censoring the Voice of America. *Foreign Policy*, 6 Aug 2009. https:// foreignpolicy.com/2009/08/06/censoring-the-voice-of-america

85. Koppang H. Social influence by manipulation: A definition and case of propaganda. *Middle East Crit.* 2009;18(2):117–143:117.

9

Lone-Actor Mass Casualty Events and Linkages to Organized Violent Salafist-Jihadist–Inspired Terror Groups

*ANDREA J. DEW AND DANIEL STARR**

INTRODUCTION

This chapter examines the current trends in lone actor mass casualty (LAMC) attacks carried out by individuals inspired by organized violent Salafist-jihadi terror groups such as al-Qaeda and the Islamic State in Iraq and al-Sham (ISIS). The examples are drawn from the University of Maryland's START Database from 2001 onward and include only attacks that have a qualitative description in the database that includes possible Salafist jihadi terror links.

To better understand the range of linkages between attackers and organized groups, the chapter discusses qualitative background on a range of attacks. In some cases, this included close linkages: the attacker was closely linked to an organized group through direct recruitment, attending a training camp, and receiving specialized technical knowledge. In other cases, interacting on social media websites, watching propaganda videos, and reading or listening to recorded messages were sufficient for the attacker to be drawn to the messaging of the group and motivated to carry out an attack. In other cases, although there is evidence that the attacker watched online videos and may have left their own recorded message, the linkages to an organized group are much more tenuous.

The chapter begins with a vignette from 2016, which contains many of the elements of current violent Salafist jihadi attacks and which also has many unanswered questions about why the attacker carried out the attack. Next, the chapter

discusses the database and methodology of the chapter. The focus of the discussion is on violent Salafist jihadist-linked cases because the number of cases and the complexity of linkages and inspirations has rapidly evolved since 2014 and the emergence of the ISIS. These elements include an attacker who lives or has close connections to the geographic location of the attack, whose connections to an organized group are difficult to establish, and who are prepared to resist law enforcement or by-stander attempts to disarm or arrest them.

Next the chapter considers the trends for these kinds of LAMC events between 2001 and 2014 and after 2014. The role of key individuals, including Anwar al-Awlaki, in inciting and inspiring more domestic attacks is discussed. In addition, the social media strategies of ISIS and how attackers interacted with its media products are discussed.

The chapter concludes by emphasizing trends over time in order to consider the law enforcement, social, medical, and legal challenges that these trends may create. The conclusion suggests paths for future research to consider especially given the renewed US focus on domestic extremist including nationalist terror groups and right-wing terror groups.

VIGNETTE: LOOSE ASSOCIATION WITH MANY UNANSWERED QUESTIONS

Just after 11 PM on July 14, 2016 in Nice, France, as the throngs of locals and tourists prepared to

---

* The opinions in this chapter are those of the chapter authors and not that of the US Navy, US Naval War College, the Dept. of Defense, or the US State Department.

celebrate Bastille Day, a 31-year-old man drove a 19-tonne white truck onto the *Promenade des Anglais*. The pedestrian zone overlooks the Mediterranean Sea and was filled with families enjoying the late summer evening. For 2 kilometers, the attacker ploughed through the crowds leaving 84 people, including 10 children and teenagers, dead in his wake. His bloody rampage was only stopped after a by-stander leaped in front of the truck, causing the attacker to open fire and Nice police were able to shoot and kill him in the truck cab. The man was identified based on cards in his wallet and was accompanied in the cab by two automatic weapons and more ammunition.[1]

The attack capped off a grim 18 months for France. In January 2015, 17 people were killed by a group of gunmen at the *Charlie Hebdo* offices in Paris. A Moroccan national's attack on a train between Amsterdam and Paris was foiled by passengers in August 2015. In addition, in November 2015, a group attack on the Bataclan nightclub and nearby restaurants killed 130 people.[2] Individuals were also accused of carrying out politically motivated violence elsewhere in France, including beheadings, knife attacks, and at least one attempt to ram security forces with a truck.

The Bastille Day attack, however, was a watershed event: the attacker planned his attack beforehand—he rented the truck and deliberately moved barriers to maneuver the truck onto the promenade. In addition, there was no personal link to any of the victims, and he was not directly tied to an organized terror group. On Bastille Day 2016, the scale of this post-bin-Laden, LAMC terrorism attack shocked France.

As France reeled from the Bastille Day attack news, the questions started immediately from politicians, the public, the press, and the French prosecutor's office: Who was the attacker, and why did he carry out this heinous attack in Nice? Was he recruited? Religious? Self-motivated? And could his personal journey from small-time violence thug to mass murder have been prevented or disrupted?

The answers—that he was born in Tunisia, estranged from his family and two young children, unknown at the local mosques but definitely known for liking women and gambling—brought more questions. He did not fit a profile of a devout and isolated zealot. He did not leave behind a manifesto or recorded message justifying his actions. He may, or may not, have had direct contact with known violent political Salafists in Nice. He may also have been part of the new wave of LAMC terrorists that seem to fit into four overlapping criteria: first, they aim themselves, with deadly intent, at the societies in which they live; second, their connections to organized terror groups range from immediate direct contact to more distant inspired by media; third, the extent of their connections to hubs of other jihadists can also vary greatly, from part of a loose network to unconnected; and, fourth, their path from inspiration to violent action leaves many questions behind them, which compounds the complexity law enforcement and medical policy challenges.

METHODOLOGY: A QUALITATIVE APPROACH

The chapter uses a framework of message, messenger, and media to examine the evolution of the phenomena of individuals who have loose connections to violent political Salafists and who carry out LAMC attacks.[3] This section gives a brief overview of the University of Maryland's Global Terrorism Database (GTD) on political terrorism attacks, which provides qualitative descriptions of the lone-actor events used in this chapter. Cases were drawn from North Atlantic Treaty Organization (NATO) states plus European Union (EU) countries using English language sources.[4]

Our qualitative analysis was based on cases drawn from the National Consortium of Terrorism and the Study of Terrorism Project in their Global Terrorism Database (GTD), which is housed at the University of Maryland.[5] In addition, the US cases were supplemented by cases from the Terrorism and Extremist Violence in the United States (TEVUS) portal, which allows for searches of court cases for attacks in the United States.[6] These were cross-referenced with a broader study that focused on all jihadi-inspired terror attacks by groups or individuals from 2014 to 2017 in NATO plus EU countries by scholars at the Program on Extremism at the George Washington University and International Centre for Counter-Terrorism (ICCT) in The Hague.[7]

Qualitative Focus on Organized Group Linkages

Other scholars, such as Paul Gill, have examined the broader lone-actor terrorism phenomena in detail.[8] Scholars such as Thomas Hegghammer and Lorenzo Vidino et al. have also examined the ISIS linkages to lone-actor terrorism in Western countries early in the movement's evolution from 2014 to mid-2017.[9] For the purposes of this chapter, we broadened the time period—2001 to 2018—and included attackers who had some connections to al-Qaeda or al-Qaeda affiliated groups or to ISIS. Vidino et al. discuss the challenges of using "jihadi" as a description for these motivations; however, since the databases use this terminology and it is widely used in other English-language sources, it is used in this chapter to minimize mis-sorting examples.[10]

LAMC attacks listed as unaffiliated or "jihadi-inspired" rather than directly linked to organized Salafist terror groups were included. From the narratives, we searched for terms such as "pledged," "claimed," and "confirmed" to determine whether the attacker had pledged allegiance, whether a known group had claimed responsibly for the attack, and whether state authorities had confirmed these links based on publicly available sources. Not surprisingly, one of our early findings was that each case included widely varying terminologies for these connections and confidence in these determinations, which, as we note in the Conclusion, will make future quantitative analysis challenging. It is important to also note that terror attacks can have multiple intended audiences and public policy responses; thus, the narratives of the attacks were developed from English-language news sources or translations, which also helped to confirm the identities and linkages to organized terrorist groups as noted.

We hand-sorted using the database term of "unaffiliated" those individuals in the narrative section of the Global Terrorism Database and included them in this chapter if they fit the following criteria:

Lone actors: Individuals, not small groups, even though they may have contact, motivation, or training from a larger network.

Acts of terrorism: Using the definition used by the US Department of Defense of "The unlawful use of violence or threat of violence, often motivated by religious, political, or other ideological beliefs, to instill fear and coerce governments or societies in pursuit of goals that are usually political."[11]

Mass casualty events: The threshold for inclusion as a mass casualty event in this chapter is defined as four or more people seriously injured or killed, not including the attacker. This follows the approach set out by John G. Horgan et al., which is based on the FBI threshold for mass murder but is broadened by us to include survivors.[12]

Unaffiliated or jihadi-inspired: LAMC attacks listed as unaffiliated or "jihadi-inspired" were included to more closely examine how LAMC attacks relate to organized Salafist terror groups.

Inclusions/Exclusions: Per the editorial guidelines for this edited volume and to de-emphasize the glorification of individuals, the names of perpetrators are not included in the chapter. Cases are drawn from English-language sources and reporting of incidents, which includes attacks in non–English-speaking countries if media coverage is available. Geographic areas were limited to NATO plus EU countries. White supremacist and xenophobic-type motivations were excluded in order to focus on attacks related to organized Salafist groups, which allowed us to isolate trends related to these groups. Notes in the Conclusion on the next steps for further research suggest future comparisons between different motivations.

Time range: The time range for data is September 2001 to September 2018.[13] Since the focus of this chapter is on LAMC attacks inspired by and linked to al-Qaeda and groups that are following in its wake, this date range was selected to give a snapshot of LAMC attacks before al-Qaeda's attacks on 9/11, through the bin Laden years, and until ISIS was pushed out of Mosul in Iraq. The qualitative discussion focuses on 2014–2018, at the height of the ISIS cyber campaigns outside of Syria and Iraq.

Using these parameters, we found 48 cases in which the LAMC events were subjectively characterized as either "unaffiliated" but with narrative comments that linked the attacker to known jihadi terror groups or "jihadi-inspired," in NATO plus EU countries, in English-language sources, and either killed by security forces or convicted. Although this list may not be exhaustive, it provided a foundational range of actors, ages, geographic locations, and dates to examine variations in linkages. LAMC events that were more directly linked to al-Qaeda or ISIS were not included in this list. Foiled attempts that had the potential to become mass casualty events were not included in this list. As a result, the following cases were included

- al-Qaeda era: 2001–2011: Total (5): USA (4), Germany (1)
- Post bin Laden's death: 2012–2013: Total (2): France (2)
- ISIS era: 2014–2018: Total (41): USA (12), France (10), Germany (6), UK (4), Canada (2), Denmark (2), Sweden (2), Spain (2), Italy (1)

WITH DEADLY INTENT

This section contextualizes al-Qaeda's rise to prominence and the amplifying effect of the September 11, 2001 attacks on the United States on Osama bin Laden's ability to connect his message to an audience.

The attacks on the United States by al-Qaeda on 9/11 ushered in a new era of scholarship and political attention to terrorism. Some of the groundbreaking scholarly work focused on how al-Qaeda is organized, how it recruits, its ideological message, and the power of its messengers. In particular, the role of Osama Bin Laden as the leader of al-Qaeda was examined by a spectrum of researchers. In the realm of popular journalism, Fareed Zacharia's "The Politics of Rage: Why Do They Hate Us?" became an instant classic, while in the academic realm, work by scholars such as Bruce Hoffman drew on decades of studying terrorism to provide an analytical window into how al-Qaeda was formed, organized, and recruited, and its motivations.[14]

One of the most complex topics scholars and practitioners grappled with was the ideological underpinnings of the al-Qaeda movement and how it motivated people to join, fight for, and die for the al-Qaeda cause. Sometimes referred to as a *takfiri* group and later as *Salafists* in the scholarly literature, the al-Qaeda movement is underpinned by violent political Salafism ideas.[15] *Takfiri* means the practice of "excommunicating or declaring a Muslim an apostate, which is punishable by death."[16] The violent political Salafist-jihadist perspective has its roots in the Salafist movement that follows an ultra-conservative version of Sunni Islamic teachings that date back to the third generation of Islamic scholars after the death of the Prophet Mohammad in 632 AD. Simply put, Salafism refutes developments—secular, technological, and religious—since that point in time and requires its adherents to reject them and live within the rules and teachings of that distant point in time.[17]

The *violent* and *political* Salafist movements developed from the turn of the twentieth century and found their muse in the writing of jailed Egyptian author, Sayyid Qutb, whose visit to the United States in the late 1940s shaped his views of secular Western culture. He joined the Muslim Brotherhood in Egypt and, after their assassination attempt on Egypt's president, Gamal Nasser, was jailed in 1954. In jail and briefly out again until his execution in 1966, Qutb's writings have inspired three generations of violent political Salafists, including Ayman Zawahiri, the former second in command in al-Qaeda and the current leader of the group.[18]

Qutb's powerful ideas about who could be considered *takfir*—unrighteous—extended to entire Muslim governments and his emphasis on not co-existing with such systems are foundational to al-Qaeda's worldview. Coupled with an even more extreme view, *kefhir*—that it is a duty of the righteous to kill the unrighteous—*takfirism* is one of the most potent and controversial justifications used by al-Qaeda and its followers for their violent attacks.

These extreme twin pillars of belief, however, also created an unwieldy strategic dilemma for Osama bin Laden and Ayman Zawahiri in the early 1990s, after their departure from Afghanistan: Whom to target first, and how to craft the message around the attacks? Should al-Qaeda, which began with the logistical networks used to supply foreign fighters against the Russian Red Army in the 1980s in Afghanistan, first turn its attention to what they called "the near enemy"—the apostate regimes of the Muslim world? Or should they turn first to the United States as the sole remaining superpower with thousands of troops still stationed in Saudi Arabia after the Gulf War in 1992?

Shut out of Saudi Arabia due to his own behavior, Bin Laden's strategy was to focus first on the far enemy—the United States—with the 1998 US Embassy attacks in Kenya and Tanzania and with the 9/11 attacks on US soil.[19] Zawahiri, however, especially after Bin Laden's death in 2011 and again with his strategic reboot in 2014, used the fissures created by the original attacks to focus on building a base deep inside Muslim countries—the near enemy—in order to challenge and eventually overthrow those regimes.

Scholars such as Assaf Moghadam and Jessica Stern have examined the recruitment process and the potency of the idea of martyrdom in motivating individuals to carry out the attacks. In *The Globalization of Martyrdom*, Moghadam, for example, provides an early linking mechanism to understand why LAMC attacks that often end with the death of the attacker have such a potent draw, even while the leadership of organized groups fight among and between themselves. Moghadam overlays an additional phenomenon on these ideological foundations and strategic dilemmas; a viral idea about the role of the individual, their sacrifice, their duty, and their reward in these clashes of worldviews.[20] As Thomas Hegghammer and others have argued, this idea of suicide attacks as a form of martyrdom has picked up new resonance with ISIS groups focused toward Western countries since 2014.[21]

For context, two of the LAMC attacks from the database in the United States in this time period were anti-Israeli: an attack on the El Al Israeli Airlines ticket counter at LAX airport in 2002, in which the attacker was killed, and an attack against the headquarters of a Jewish organization accompanied by anti-Israeli messages in Seattle, Washington, in 2006. Neither attacker was directly linked to organized jihadi terrorist groups. However, the 2006 attack in Chapel Hill, North Carolina, in which the attacker used a car, had elements that became steadily more common: a LAMC attack in which the attacker was not directly or closely affiliated with a known group but who claimed his actions were inspired by their cause. In the Chapel Hill case, the attacker pleaded guilty to nine counts of attempted first-degree murder in August 2008.[22] He described his motivation as "revenge for Muslim deaths overseas" and was not clearly linked to any organized terrorist group.

A US Army Major's testimony in his Article 32 military court hearing after the attack in Ft. Hood, Texas, in 2009, in which he was convicted of first-degree murder charges, followed a similar pattern. According to the US Army's official final report, while on active duty, he killed 15 people and wounded 42 more during the Ft. Hood attack.[23] The attacker was not directly connected to an organized terrorist group, although, as discussed later, he had listened to messages by Anwar al-Awlaki, and he justified his actions as choosing sides: "There was adequate provocation—that these were deploying soldiers that were going to engage in an illegal war."[24]

The lack of strong connection to an organized jihadist group is of particular note in comparison to others in which the connection was clear: for example, the foiled attempt by the attacker dubbed the "Shoe Bomber" who admitted he was an al-Qaeda member during his guilty plea on charges of trying to blow up American Airlines flight 63 between Paris and Miami in December 2001.[25] Another foiled attempt was by a lone actor who tried to explode a bomb in an SUV in Times Square, New York City, in May 2010. This attacker was directly linked, trained, and funded by a jihadi terrorist organization. Indeed, the attacker had traveled to Pakistan and received training from the terrorist group, Tehrik-e-Taliban before returning to the United States to rent his SUV for the attack.[26] He pleaded guilty to 10 federal crimes surrounding the attempted attack.[27]

In summary, between the 9/11 attacks and the death of bin Laden in 2011, LAMC attacks in the NATO plus EU states were rare, but world events also amplified the potency of al-Qaeda's messages and the viral nature of the martyrdom idea: the US-led invasion of Iraq in 2003, Operation Iraqi Freedom, opened up a new fighting front in an easily accessible area. Iraq, with multiple routes of access and seething resentment of both Saddam Hussein's Ba'athist regime and US invasion forces, amplified the appeal of al-Qaeda's message while raising the profile of its ideology. There were very few lone-actor plots in our study parameters, but we saw both "inspirational" linkages *and* groomed and directly trained operatives of organized groups; the Ft. Hood attack shows one of the early linkages to an influential individual in inspiring attacks.[28]

DEBATE AROUND THEIR CONNECTIONS TO CENTRALLY ORGANIZED GROUPS

This section examines the early academic debates on the role of individuals in carrying out al-Qaeda's missions in lone-actor (or small group) violent attacks to analyze the recruitment and radicalization strategies followed by al-Qaeda after bin Laden's death in 2011.

As US-led operations against al-Qaeda, its franchises, and its affiliates seemed to broaden by the week in 2009, the question for scholars studying this phenomenon turned to what would become the future of al-Qaeda's recruitment and mobilization strategy? Despite setbacks due to the brutality used by al-Qaeda's first franchise in Iraq, run by the Jordanian Abu Musab al-Zarqawi, the potent combination of message, messengers, and media coverage at the global and regional levels helped to amplify al-Qaeda's reputation and draw fighters and martyrs to its cause. Analysts were divided about what this meant for the future of al-Qaeda's organization: some argued that al-Qaeda was done as a fighting organization, its message undermined, and that it would retreat into a much-diminished group. Other analysts argued that al-Qaeda's actions had created an inspirational focal point that would continue to inspire more attacks in countries distant from the fighting fronts.

Bruce Hoffman and Marc Sageman became embroiled in a debate about the future of al-Qaeda's operations, particularly in terms of the domestic terrorism phenomenon. Sageman, a forensic and clinical psychiatrist, argued in his book, *Leaderless Jihad*, that al-Qaeda's brand of ideology and appeal would generate a new generation of individuals and small groups willing to carry out suicide attacks in the name of al-Qaeda's goals.[29]

In contrast, Hoffman argued that the potency of al-Qaeda lay in its leadership, the strategic communications tied to its real-world attacks in the multiple new fronts in Iraq and Afghanistan, and the organization of the group that included a sophisticated cyber and information capability.[30]

An early focal point for these clashing perspectives were the suicide attacks on July 7 2005, directed against the London underground and buses, in which 52 people were killed. All the attackers died in the attacks.[31] At first it seemed that they had self-radicalized—seemingly under the noses of families and communities. However, Hoffman argued that, far from being self-radicalized, they were part of an earlier pattern of recruitment and had strong group ties: they had a strong connection to a senior al-Qaeda leader and had traveled overseas as part of their preparation for the attack.[32]

The debate between the two scholars over the future of al-Qaeda's source of appeal and power had real-world implications for military strategy and domestic security. If citizens were willing to stay home, self-radicalize without command and control contact from al-Qaeda, and carry out attacks in their home countries, what laws and powers would be required to predict and prevent those attacks? If the source of inspiration and coordination was the al-Qaeda core organization, could domestic security be improved by directing more resources to disrupting al-Qaeda's activities overseas?

After Bin Laden's death in 2011, moreover, there was a vigorous debate about what would happen to the LAMC terrorism attacks. The 2011 LAMC attack in Montauban and Toulouse, France, against off-duty soldiers and a Jewish school that left seven people dead, seemed to fit this new hybrid pattern of both inspired by an organized group, but also acting independently of its direction.[33] Another attacker, who was killed

by police after a standoff in Toulouse, appeared to be "part of the new generation of Islamic terrorists who act alone, abetted by jihadi Web sites and their own anger," said Jean-Louis Bruguière, a former French counterterrorism judge and expert on European terrorism."[34]

This became a new watershed in the evolution of violent Salafist groups. The counter-terrorism scholars and analysts tried to predict whether the resonance of al-Qaeda's messages would be disrupted by Bin Laden's death and the leadership transition to al-Zawahiri.[35] The emergence of new messengers of violent political Salafist movements, such as Anwar al-Awlaki and Abu Mohammed al Adnani, the spokesman for ISIS, moreover, used social media to capture the attention of a younger generation.[36]

THE CYBER CALIPHATE

This section examines the catalyzing effect of the message and media used by ISIS from 2014 onward.[37] This section also highlights the role of key messengers, especially Anwar al-Awlaki and Abu Mohammed al Adnani, in inspiring a new generation of lone-actor attacks during the height of ISIS operations in Syria and Iraq (2014–2018).[38]

Anwar al-Awlaki, a Yemini-American Sunni imam, seems to have played an outsize role as a messenger—an influencer—in bridging al-Qaeda's mission and ISIS's incitement to violence. Al-Awlaki's shift from preaching in a US mosque to exhorting true believers to use violence against the societies in which they live occurred after the attacks of September 11, 2001. Using digital media—first through a series of recorded sermons and then via a slick online publication in English called *Inspire* magazine—al-Awlaki had an outsized reach on a new generation of Sunni Muslims who had watched the US-led invasion of the Iraq in 2003 on media screens. In particular, al-Awlaki's American-accented English was credited with creating a relatable bridge between events in the Middle East and young Muslims in English-speaking countries such as the United States and the United Kingdom.[39]

Scott Shane, a *New York Times* reporter who earned the Lionel Gelber Prize for his extensive investigations into al-Awlaki, noted the connection between viewing al-Awlaki sermons and a slew of attacks. By 2016, the digital Counter Extremism Project had mapped al-Awlaki's connection to multiple violent attacks in the United States, including the Pulse nightclub in Orlando, Florida, June 12, 2016, which killed 49 people and injured 53 more. In addition, attackers who listened to al-Awlaki included the Fort Hood attacker in 2009 and the foiled so-called "under-wear bomber's" attack in 2009. One of the Boston Marathon bombers (2013) listened to al-Awlaki's sermons, as did the perpetrators the 2015 San Bernardino attacks, the lone actor involved in the New York/New Jersey bombings (2016), and the Ohio State University attacker (2016).[40] The brothers who carried out the *Charlie Hebdo* attack in Paris in January 2015, and the attacker who killed five people in a dual attack at a US Marine Recruiting base and US Navy office in Chattanooga, Tennessee in July 2015 also listened to al-Awlaki.[41]

Although al-Awlaki was killed in a US drone strike in Yemen in September 2011, his sermons and his digital magazine—*Inspire*—continue to influence a new generation of jihadists.[42] Indeed, ISIS incorporated al-Awlaki into their own social media operations by naming an English-speaking fighting brigade after him and editing his voice over ISIS recruitment videos.[43]

As ISIS expanded its territorial holdings in Syria and Iraq in 2014, it was also pursuing a cyber strategy that set it apart from al-Qaeda's cyber brigades.[44] By 2016, Western analysts had dubbed this effort a virtual or "Cyber Caliphate" in acknowledgment of how far-reaching and strategically important this effort was to ISIS recruitment, financing, and influence.[45] As we noted in a previous publication:[46] Charlie Winter and Jordan Bach-Lombardo's analysis of the ISIS propaganda machine shows how effective ISIS was at combining negative and positive themes to create a core narrative—of a successful model society—to a wide range of audiences around the world. Moreover, its central coordination office or "Base Foundation" set a core message, which was communicated by 48 dispersed media offices around the world, and actively cultivated unofficial spokespeople who help to connect ISIS messages to local audiences. Concurrent with ISIS's social media activities, a slew of individuals and small groups began carrying out violent attacks far from the fighting fronts in Iraq and Afghanistan. Vidino et al.'s report on the domestic threat to the Western countries included both lone-actor and small-group attacks from 2014 to 2017 and catalogued cases, deaths, and trends for all terror attacks (lone actor and group) in Western countries.[47] Their findings included:[48] In the three years following the Caliphate's proclamation, a total of 51 attacks were successfully carried out in North America and Europe by individuals motivated by jihadist ideology. These 51 attacks included in the

database took place in a relatively limited number of countries (8 out of 32). The country with the largest number of attacks was France (17), followed by the United States (16), Germany (6), the UK (4), Belgium (3), Canada (3), Denmark (1) and Sweden (1). Therefore, 32 attacks were executed in Europe (63%) and the remaining 19 in North America (37%).

Moreover, ISIS's ease with social media and chat applications allowed it to reach deep into the living rooms of potential recruits and influence them at home, particularly the messages from Abu Mohammed al Adnani, ISIS spokesman on its media network.[49] This combination of negative and positive messaging reached far beyond the fighting fronts in Syria and Iraq, especially ISIS spokesman al-Adnani's encouragement in 2016 to kill "disbelieving Americans or Europeans" and stay home in Western countries to do so.[50] This was amplified in early 2016 through shocking ISIS videos of the beheadings of prisoners, and its use of slick video productions amplified the reach of their message and enhanced their recruitment of Westerners to fight in Syria and Iraq.[51]

Vidino et al. also make note of the role of Abu Mohammed al Adnani, whose messages exhorted ISIS followers to attack unbelievers in their own communities however they could.[52]

> Do not ask for anyone's advice and do not seek anyone's verdict. Kill the disbeliever whether he is civilian or military, for they have the same ruling. Both of them are disbelievers. . . . If you are not able to find an IED or a bullet, then single out the disbelieving American, Frenchman, or any of their allies. Smash his head with a rock, or slaughter him with a knife, or run him over with your car, or throw him down from a high place, or choke him, or poison him.

The analysis also came with acknowledgment of a disturbing trend: of the 65 people involved in the attacks (in groups and as lone actors) 27 (42%) were connected to an organized terrorist group such as ISIS or al-Qaeda, although sometimes it was difficult to fully prove the connections.[53]

In our analysis of just LAMC events between 2014 and 2018, the linkages to organized terrorist groups covered an even wider spectrum of loose to strong connections, and those links were difficult to establish. Indeed, in many cases we examined, the attacker may not have left a manifesto or may have placed blame for their actions on the foreign policy of the state rather than framed their actions as in support of a particular group. They may have possessed paraphernalia for ISIS such as an ISIS flag, but they may also have had no apparent direct connections with the group; the flag may symbolize an aspiration or an inspiration, but not an affiliation.[54] They may have claimed to be acting for ISIS, and ISIS may have claimed their attack, but, in many cases, the linkages are unproved. Even more problematic for public policy and those crafting legal approaches to deter such attacks, while some lone actors had a history of violence, others had a history of misdemeanor offenses or no criminal record.

One example of a very complex nexus of influence and relationships is the January 2015 attack that killed five people and wounded three more at the Hyper Cache kosher supermarket in Paris. The lone attacker, who was killed by security forces, shared an external handler with a pair of attackers who were responsible for the simultaneously occurring *Charlie Hebdo* attacks. Indeed, although the Hyper Cache attacker carried out his attacks alone, directed via an email account, his handlers used him as part of a distraction from the *Charlie Hebdo* attacks. According to French investigators, the attacker was also directed to make a video to help amplify the effects of the attack. However, while the *Charlie Hebdo* attackers were linked to al-Qaeda in the Arabian Peninsula (AQAP), the Hyper Cache attacker was linked to ISIS (which had already declared itself to be a rival jihadist group.)[55]

In contrast, the April 2017 attack on Paris's Champs-Élysées Avenue, which killed one police officer and resulted in the death of the attacker, was shrouded in questions. ISIS claimed responsibility for the attack much more quickly than usual and named another individual as the attacker. The actual perpetrator was on France's list of radicalized individuals, had served 14 years in prison for attempted murder, and in 2016 had attempted to purchase firearms. A note linking his actions to ISIS was found near his body, but ISIS did not claim the attacker as one of their "soldiers of IS" as they have done in previous attacks, which again left behind questions: Was the attacker directly linked or simply inspired by ISIS social media campaigns? As discussed in the Conclusion, this also resulted in lingering questions about whether intervention through social programs would have helped divert his path to attempted mass violence or whether his anger against French police officers and sentiments about France's role in Syria were a combination that would have exploded regardless of ISIS propaganda.[56]

Moreover, these confusing sets of signals have not been limited to France. The spate of LAMC attacks in Germany in 2016 also showed similar traits: on July 18, in an attack on a commuter train near Würzberg, an assailant with a knife and axe injured five passengers. The 17-year-old attacker was killed by police. According to German investigators, he had recently arrived as an asylum seeker, watched ISIS videos, and left his own video in which he brandished a knife in his foster family's house before the attack. ISIS claimed his attack, but German security officials suggested that his actions were more those of a suicidal teenager and less of a hardened ISIS killer.[57] The confusion after this attack in Germany had policy, legal, and social implications. For example, how would clinicians and the police have approached his case if they had been able to intervene before the attack? Would clinical interventions have helped his suicidal ideation and disrupted the attraction to ISIS's messages? Why did the ISIS message or particular media products draw this suicidal teenager to them, and how can we disrupt the resonance of that messaging?

This also refocuses our attention on the role of social media in making ISIS videos available and the role of algorithms in suggesting the next video on a playlist, which allows viewers to dive deeper and deeper into extremist media. Nongovernmental organizations (NGOs) and states have all turned their attention to how to disrupt the glorification and amplification of LAMC events via traditional and social media. One example comes from the Counter Extremism Project (CEP), a not-for-profit organization that "combats extremism by pressuring financial and material support networks; countering the narrative of extremists and their online recruitment; and advocating for smart laws, policies, and regulations."[58] As part of their technology project, the CEP drew attention to the al-Awlaki videos and ISIS videos on You Tube, links on Facebook, and the use of Twitter by ISIS. CEP has lobbied for social media companies to fine-tune their search algorithms to make it more difficult to find al-Awlaki's speeches and not automatically play related videos that may draw the viewer deeper into the ISIS propaganda web. Although completely voluntary, CEP's Digital Disruption project may provide a pattern for social media companies to consider their responsibilities for promulgating extremist propaganda even as states begin to consider their own far-right and ultra-nationalist extremist challenges.

Two more attacks in Germany in July 2016, followed a different pattern. Both occurred in Bavaria: one on July 22 at a Munich shopping mall and one on July 24 at a music festival. Nine people were shot and killed in the Munich attack by an 18-year old man who appears to have planned the attack for at least a year after his visit to the scene of a previous mass shooting in Winnenden. German police found no connection to ISIS or political motivations for his attack.[59] In contrast, the music festival attacker, a 28-year old man, left behind a video post pledging allegiance to ISIS. In this case, the attacker was a Syrian asylum seeker who detonated a backpack filled with chemicals and sharp metal that wounded 15 people and killed him as well. He had no criminal record or history of mental health issues but was facing deportation from the EU after his refugee application and appeals had been unsuccessful.[60] These attacks and others in Germany provoked furious public policy debates about Germany's refugee policy and encouraged anti-refugee sentiments.[61]

Other authors in this edited volume have covered in detail two of the bloodiest American cases between 2014 and 2018: the 2015 San Bernardino attacks at the Inland Regional Center involving a pair of attackers who killed 16 people and injured at least 17, and the 2016 Pulse nightclub attack in Orlando, Florida that killed 50 people and wounded at least 50 more. In both cases, the attackers seem to have been inspired by but not directly controlled or trained by ISIS. In other LAMC attacks in the United States, moreover, the connections between ISIS and the attackers were claimed by the attackers but hard to establish. For example, the attack at the Ft. Lauderdale Airport in January 2017, in which four people were shot and killed and six more wounded[62]; the explosion at the Port Authority in New York City in December 2017, in which three people were injured;[63] and the explosion in a Chelsea neighborhood in New York City that injured 29 people in September 2016 were all carried out by individuals who claimed linkages to ISIS but for whom those linkages were not clearly established by authorities.[64]

Finally, one of the British cases involving explosives may best summarize these tangled webs of connections, inspirations, and the public policy challenges in preventing such attacks. The Parsons Green Underground attack injured 51 people and resulted in the conviction for attempted murder of the 19-year-old lone-actor attacker in March 2018.[65] The participation of the attacker, an asylum seeker from Iraq, in the

UK's Prevent strategy—a program of de-radicalization for at-risk individuals—was debated and challenged after the attack. Other authors in this edited volume return to the question of who should be included in the UK government's Prevent program, whether participation should continue to be voluntary, and its effectiveness in diverting and preventing violence.[66]

CONCLUSION

This concluding section considers the key challenges going forward as the international and local threat from violent political Salafist groups continues to evolve. The distance between active conflict zones, such as Afghanistan or Syria, and the place of the attacks in NATO plus EU countries has amplified the shock value of these attacks in many societies. Moreover, the connections can be in-person or via the cyber world, which makes tracing and confirming the degree of connections even more challenging for prevention, de-radicalization, and law enforcement efforts. In addition, understanding these trends may also have utility for further research into LAMC attacks linked to nationalist terror groups and right-wing terror groups.

This chapter draws from a framework developed to examine how leaders communicate ideas— message, messenger, media—to examine the why and how the next generation of violent political Salafists have been successful in inspiring the next wave of attacks by lone actors (and small groups) and the policy implications of these developments.

The four characteristics of these LAMC attacks reveal the following: first, they aim themselves, with deadly intent, at the societies in which they live; second, their connections to organized terror groups range from immediate direct contact to more distant inspired by media; third, the extent of their connections to hubs of other jihadists can also vary greatly, from part of a loose network to unconnected; and, fourth, their path from inspiration to violent action leaves many questions behind them, which compounds the complexity law enforcement and medical policy challenges.

As noted in the methodology section of this chapter, attacks with these characteristics present immediate challenges for future quantitative research. These include how to determine the degree of connection and code for confidence that these individuals are really connected to hubs, networks, or groups in the way they claim. What is the threshold for determining that connection: Is a video claiming connection sufficient? A manifesto? Or an off-hand remark to a co-worker? All of these have been thresholds for legal investigations into individuals suspected of radicalization, but they are difficult to establish before and after the fact. In addition, terrorist groups may seek to overclaim responsibility in order to amplify their reach, while lone actors may overclaim to amplify their own importance.

Moreover, the first, second, and third characteristics also create complex policy and law enforcement challenges. One example is the LAMC attack at the Manchester Arena after an Arianne Grande concert that killed 22 and injured more than 800 people in May 2017.[67] ISIS claimed responsibility for the attack.[68] The attacker, who was born in Manchester, traveled to Libya with his father as a teenager and subsequently returned to meet with ISIS networks in Libya—the group Katibat al-Battar al-Libi.[69] Analysts suggest that the al-Battar group became a magnet for French-speaking ISIS supporters, some of whom fought in Syria and Iraq, and helped operationalize martyrdom ideas for a new generation.[70] Indeed, the group was also connected to the squad of young men who were responsible for the 2015 Paris terror attacks that killed 130 people, wounded hundreds more, and targeted restaurants and bars, the Bataclan concert hall, and the soccer stadium, Stade de France.[71] The challenge for policy-makers is how to treat these kinds of encounters in which an individual is clearly linked to an organized terrorist group. As new hubs emerge, such as the al-Battar group, should new laws criminalize in-person contact with them? Should travel watch lists alert authorities to simple travel to a country—in this case Libya—from which a group is operating? What about cyber contact? How could these encounters be monitored, and what are the civil liberty repercussions?

And, fourth, the intersections among policy, law enforcement, and medical issues generated from this new generation of LAMC attackers are also complex. One of the attacks included in this study occurred in Milan, Italy (May 18, 2017). The attacker stabbed a police officer and two soldiers at a train station and injured three others.[72] He was sentenced to 7 years in prison for the attacks by a court in Italy.[73] However, the ruling mentioned consideration of his "diminished mental state," he shouted "I'm alone and abandoned" to security forces just before the attack, and his Facebook page had some ISIS videos posted to it.[74] The attack was included in the study to capture the range of individuals that ISIS social media has reached, but it raises the issue of how mental health issues are treated in relation to terror attacks and who is vulnerable to ISIS messaging.

This attacker's linkages to an organized violent Salafist group seem tenuous, whereas his erratic behavior had drawn notice in other venues. In this case, perhaps recognizing the appeal of violent ideologies and their trends on social media would be helpful to clinical and social work professionals working with vulnerable individuals.

The work of the CEP, as discussed earlier, provides a framework for considering how digital disruption by technology companies can make propaganda more difficult to find.[75] This case also suggests areas for further study considering how law enforcement agencies prosecute these kinds of attack. On the one hand, ISIS laid claim to the attack and benefitted from more publicity and notoriety in the aftermath. However, for the same reason that the names of attackers are not used in this chapter, more research is needed to examine whether separating out vulnerable individuals from true believers might also undercut the strategic communication value of such attacks.

Finally, to return to the opening vignette, the Nice Bastille Day attack in 2016 presents many of the most difficult dimensions of this phenomena: the attacker had no overt signs of radicalization, did not demonstrate overt connections to known organizations, and did not travel to an areas where a hub existed. One of the elements that was present in multiple attacks was a prior criminal history—in the case of the Bastille Day attacker, petty violence and crimes. Some might argue that this is a new indicator to track, but this raises legal questions about what kinds of interactions should raise red flags and what civil liberties are at risk in the process. Moreover, would any prior interventions reduce, disrupt, or prevent future recruitment or attacks, or are they political theater for domestic audiences, intended to reassure but inadequate to protect citizens?

In this chapter, we discussed the Paris 2015 attacks in which a lone actor was motivated by one set of ideas but linked through a handler to another more complex attack motivated by different ideas. This intersection between individuals and small groups motivated or manipulated by outside actors may add further complexity to the study of LAMC events. In March 2021, for example, FBI Director Wray called the attacks on the US Capitol in January an act of domestic terrorism.[76] In addition, the US Capitol attack drew together individuals, small groups linked by a web of common social media sites, and more tightly organized groups; thus, although this chapter and this volume focus on LAMC events, future research must consider the intersection of such actors and others in a single event. Further academic research is also necessary to determine whether similar trends have emerged—or are emerging—in attacks linked to other types of organized terror groups, such as nationalist, right-wing, or eco-terrorist groups.

NOTES AND REFERENCES

1. Yuhas A, Weaver M, Malkin B, Rawlinson K. Nice attack: Truck driver named as France mourns 84 killed in Bastille Day atrocity – as it happened. Guardian.com, 15 Jul 2016. https://www.theguardian.com/world/live/2016/jul/14/nice-bastille-day-france-attack-promenade-des-anglais-vehicle
2. Charlie Hebdo: 14 suspects on trial over Paris massacre. 2 Sep 2020. https://www.bbc.com/news/world-europe-53975350
3. Dew AJ, Genest MA, Paine SCM. *From Quills to Tweets* Washington, DC: Georgetown University Press; 2019. https://ebookcentral.proquest.com/lib/[SITE_ID]/detail.action?docID = 5965278
4. The National Consortium of Terrorism and the Study of Terrorism project, University of Maryland. https://www.start.umd.edu
5. Codebook for the START database. https://www.start.umd.edu/gtd/downloads/Codebook.pdf
6. https://tap.cast.uark.edu
7. Vidino L, Marone F, Entenmann E. *Fear Thy Neighbor.* Ledizioni, Milano—Italy; 2017. https://icct.nl/wp-content/uploads/2017/06/FearThyNeighbor-RadicalizationandJihadistAttacksintheWest.pdf
8. Gill P. *Lone-Actor Terrorists.* London: Routledge; 2015. http://bvbr.bib-bvb.de:8991/F?func=service&doc_library=BVB01&local_base=BVB01&doc_number=027860410&sequence=000003&line_number=0001&func_code=DB_RECORDS&service_type=MEDIA.
9. Hegghammer T, Nesser P. Assessing the Islamic State's commitment to attacking the West. *Perspect Terrorism.* 2015;9(4):9. http://www.terrorismanalysts.com/pt/index.php/pot/article/view/440. See also Vidino, Marone, Entenmann *Fear Thy Neighbor.*
10. See Vidino, Marone, Entenmann *Fear Thy Neighbor*, chapter 2.
11. US Department of Defense. Joint Publication 3-07.2 Antiterrorism. 2010. http://navybmr.com/study%20material/JOINT%20PUBLICATION%203-07.2%20(2014),%20ANTITERRORISM.pdf
12. Horgan J, et al. Final report: Across the universe? A comparative analysis of violent behavior and radicalization across three offender types with implications for criminal justice training and education. 2016. https://www.ncjrs.gov/pdffiles1/nij/grants/249937.pdf
13. National Consortium for the Study of Terrorism and Responses to Terrorism (START), University of Maryland. The Global Terrorism Database (GTD). 2019. Retrieved from https://www.start.umd.edu/gtd
14. Zakaria F. The politics of rage: Why do they hate us? *Newsweek,* 15 Oct 2001:22; Hoffman B. The changing face of al Qaeda and the global war on terrorism. *Stud Conflict Terrorism.* 2004;27(6):549–560. https://doi:org/10.1080/10576100490519813
15. Ryan MWS. *Decoding al-Qaeda's Strategy.* Columbia Studies in Terrorism and Irregular Warfare. New York: Columbia University Press; 2013:17–50. https://doi:org/10.7312/ryan16384
16. Drennan S. Constructing Takfir. *CTC Sentinel,* Jun 2008;1(7):1–4. https://ctc.usma.edu/constructing-takfir-from-abdullah-azzam-to-djamel-zitouni/
17. Ryan. Decoding, 26–50.
18. Ibid.
19. Ryan. Decoding, 51–82. Also, Kean T, Kean TH, Hamilton L. *The 9/11 Commission Report.* Pittsburgh: US Government Printing Office; 2004. https://ebookcentral.proquest.com/lib/[SITE_ID]/detail.action?docID = 4856750
20. Moghadam A. *The Globalization of Martyrdom.* Baltimore: Johns Hopkins University Press; 2008.
21. Moghadam A. Motives for martyrdom: al-Qaida, Salafi jihad, and the spread of suicide attacks. *Intl Security.* 2009; 33(3):46–78. https://doi:org/10.1162/isec.2009.33.3.46. Also, Hegghammer, Nesser. Assessing the Islamic State's commitment. https://www.bellingcat.com/news/mena/2016/02/16/tip-of-the-spear-meet-isis-special-operations-unit-katibat-al-battar/
22. https://www.investigativeproject.org/case/176/state-of-north-carolina-v-taheri-azar-2006-unc
23. Webster W. Final Report of the William H. Webster Commission on the Federal Bureau of Investigation, counterterrorism intelligence, and the events atFort Hood, Texas, on Nov 5, 2009. Jul 2012. https://www.hsdl.org/?view&did=717443
24. Chappell B. Fort Hood gunman Nidal Hasan sentenced to death for 2009 attack. NPR, 28 Aug 2013. https://www.npr.org/sections/thetwo-way/2013/08/28/216512156/fort-hood-gunman-nidal-hasan-sentenced-to-death
25. Guilty plea in airplane plot. New York Times, 4 Oct 2002. https://www.nytimes.com/2002/10/05/us/guilty-plea-in-airplane-plot.html?searchResultPosition=4
26. https://www.justice.gov/opa/pr/faisal-shahzad-indicted-attempted-car-bombing-times-square
27. https://www.justice.gov/opa/pr/faisal-shahzad-pleads-guilty-manhattan-federal-court-10-federal-crimes-arising-attempted-car
28. Fishman B. Revising the history of al-Qaida's original meeting with Abu Musab Al-Zarqawi.

CTC Sentinel. Oct 2016;9(10):28–33. https://www.ctc.usma.edu/revising-the-history-of-al-qaidas-original-meeting-with-abu-musab-al-zarqawi/

29. Sageman M. *Leaderless Jihad*. Philadelphia: University of Pennsylvania Press; 2008.

30. Hoffman B. The myth of grass-roots terrorism: Why Osama Bin Laden still matters. Foreign Affairs. 2008;87:133-138. New York: Council on Foreign Relations. https://www.jstor.org/stable/20032656

31. Hoffman B. *7/7 London Underground Bombing: Not So Homegrown: A Selection from The Evolution of the Global Terrorist Threat: From 9/11 to Osama Bin Laden's Death*. New York: Columbia University Press; 2014. http://www.vlebooks.com/vleweb/product/openreader?id=none&isbn=9780231538862&uid=none

32. Hoffman B. The myth of grass-roots terrorism: Why Osama Bin Laden still matters. Foreign Affairs. 2008;87:133–138. New York: Council on Foreign Relations. https://www.jstor.org/stable/20032656

33. Bilefsky B, De La Baume MA. French gunman seen as homegrown militant. New York Times, 21 Mar 2021. https://www.nytimes.com/2012/03/22/world/europe/mohammed-merah-france-shooting-suspect-seen-as-home-grown-militant.html

34. Ibid.

35. Dew AJ. Inspirational, aspirational and operational heroes: Recruitment, terror and heroic conflict from the perspective of armed groups. In Scheipers S, ed. *Heroism and the Changing Character of War*. London: Palgrave Macmillan; 2014:237–250. https://link.springer.com/chapter/10.1057/9781137362537_15

36. Hegghammer, Nesser. Assessing the Islamic State's commitment.

37. Ingram HJ, Whiteside C, Winter C. *The ISIS Reader*. New York: Oxford University Press; 2020.

38. On Anwar al-Awlaki's life and legacy see Shane S. *Objective Troy*. New York: Tim Duggan Books; 2016.

39. Shane S. The enduring influence of Anwar Al-Awlaki in the age of the Islamic State. *CTC Sentinel*. 2016;9(7):15–19. https://ctc.usma.edu/the-enduring-influence-of-anwar-al-awlaki-in-the-age-of-the-islamic-state/

40. Counter Extremism Project. Anwar al-Awlaki's ties to extremists. https://www.counterextremism.com/anwar-al-awlaki

41. Shane S. The lessons of Anwar al-Awlaki. New York Times, 27 Aug 2015. https://www.nytimes.com/2015/08/30/magazine/the-lessons-of-anwar-al-awlaki.html

42. Sivek, Susan. Packaging Inspiration: Al Qaeda's Digital Magazine Inspire in the Self-Radicalization Process. International Journal of Communication. 2013;7:584. https://ijoc.org/index.php/ijoc/article/view/1670

43. Ibid. For an early assessment of ISIS's connections between operations and its media campaign, see Price B, Milton D, Al-'Ubaydi M. Al-Baghdadi's blitzkrieg, Isil's psychological warfare, and what it means for Syria and Iraq. *Research Note*, Combating Terrorism Center at West Point. 2014. https://ctc.usma.edu/ctc-perspectives-al-baghdadis-blitzkrieg-isils-psychological-warfare-and-what-it-means-for-syria-and-iraq/

44. Winter C, Bach-Lombardo J. Why Isis propaganda works. *The Atlantic*, 2016. https://www.theatlantic.com/international/archive/2016/02/isis-propaganda-war/462702/

45. See Schori Liang C. Unveiling the "United Cyber Caliphate" and the birth of the e-terrorist. Georgetown J Intl Affairs. 2017 Oct 1;18(3):11–20. https://doi.org/10.1353/gia.2017.0032; Winter C. Redefining "propaganda": The media strategy of the Islamic State. RUSI J. 2020 Jan 2;165(1):38–42. https://doi.org/10.1080/03071847.2020.1734321; Winter C. Documenting the virtual "caliphate." Quilliam Foundation, 2015. https://search.informit.org/documentSummary;res=APO;dn=57763; Brangetto P, Veenendaal MA. Influence cyber operations: The use of cyberattacks in support of influence operations. 2016:113–126. https://doi.org/10.1109/CYCON.2016.7529430

46. Winter C, Bach-Lombardo J. Why Isis propaganda works. *The Atlantic*, 2016. referenced in Dew AJ. Fighting for influence in open societies: The role of resilience and transparency. Fletcher Forum World Affairs. 2019 Summer;42:2. http://www.fletcherforum.org/archives/2019/6/7/432-summer-2019

47. Vidino, Marone, and Entenmann, *Fear Thy Neighbor*.

48. Ibid., 45.

49. Winter, Documenting the Virtual "Caliphate."

50. Discussed in Shane, The Enduring Influence of Anwar Al-Awlaki in the Age of the Islamic State. Al-Adnani quoted from Cruickshank P. Orlando shooting follows ISIS call for US Ramadan attacks. CNN, 13 Jun 2016.

51. https://www.nytimes.com/2020/09/22/us/politics/isis-beatles.html

52. "Indeed your Lord is ever watchful," speech by Shaykh Abu Muhammad Al-Adnani Ashshami, Al Hayat Media, quoted more extensively in Vidino, Marone, and Entenmann, 30–32.

53. Vidino, Marone, and Entenmann, *Fear Thy Neighbor*.

54. Hegghammer, Nesser Assessing the Islamic State's commitment.

55. Paris attacks: Coulibaly "given orders by email." *BBC News*, 13 Oct 2015. https://www.bbc.com/news/world-europe-34514244

56. Allemandou S. Questions remain over Champs-Élysées attacker's links to IS group, *France 24*, 22 Apr 2017. https://www.france24.com/en/20170422-questions-remain-champs-elysees-attacker-links-islamic-state-group

57. Lyman R. After attack on German Train, fears over refugees, and from them, too. *New York Times*, 20 Jul 2016. https://www.nytimes.com/2016/07/21/world/europe/germany-train-attack-refugees.html

58. https://www.counterextremism.com/about

59. Munich shooting: David Sonboly "planned attack for year." *BBC News*, 24 Jul 2016. https://www.bbc.com/news/world-europe-36878436

60. https://www.nytimes.com/2016/07/26/world/europe/ansbach-germany-music-festival-explosion.html

61. Eddy M. Suicide bomber in Ansbach, Germany, pledged loyalty to ISIS, officials say. *New York Times*, 25 Jul, 2016. https://www.nytimes.com/2016/08/05/world/europe/germany-refugees-terrorism.html

62. https://www.counterextremism.com/extremists/esteban-santiago, and, https://www.nbcboston.com/news/national-international/plea-deal-planned-during-wednesday-hearing-for-fort-lauderdale-airport-shooter/112062/

63. https://www.justice.gov/opa/pr/akayed-ullah-convicted-detonation-bomb-new-york-city

64. https://www.justice.gov/opa/pr/chelsea-bomber-ahmad-khan-rahimi-sentenced-life-prison-executing-september-2016-bombing-and

65. Parsons Green Tube bombing: Teenager Ahmed Hassan jailed for life. *BBC News*, 23 Mar 2018. https://www.bbc.com/news/uk-43519540

66. Her Majesty's Government. Prevent Strategy, 2011. https://assets.publishing.service.gov.uk/government/uploads/system/uploads/attachment_data/file/97976/prevent-strategy-review.pdf

67. https://www.counterextremism.com/extremists/salman-abedi

68. Dearden L. Manchester Arena attack: Isis claims responsibility for suicide bombing that killed at least 22 people. *Independent* (London), 23 May 2017. http://www.independent.co.uk/news/uk/home-news/manchester-arena-attack-isis-responsible-claim-suicide-bombing-islamic-state-ariana-grande-concert-a7751221.html

69. Callimachi R, Schmitt E. Manchester bomber met with ISIS unit in Libya, officials say. *New York Times*, 3 Jun 2017. https://www.nytimes.com/2017/06/03/world/middleeast/manchester-bombing-salman-abedi-islamic-state-libya.html

70. Colquhoun C. Tip of the spear? Meet ISIS' special operations unit, Katibat al-Battar. 16 Feb 2016. https://www.bellingcat.com/news/mena/2016/02/16/tip-of-the-spear-meet-isis-special-operations-unit-katibat-al-battar/

71. Ibid.

72. https://www.start.umd.edu/gtd/search/IncidentSummary.aspx?gtdid=201705180022

73. Milan station knife attacker gets seven years. *Redazione Ansa*, 2 Mar 2018. https://www.ansa.it/english/news/2018/03/02/milan-station-knife-attacker-gets-seven-years-2_f0676de0-49fb-4b95-b655-cd7cfce20a84.html

74. https://www.dw.com/en/italy-police-probe-milan-train-station-attacker-for-terrorist-links/a-38912413

75. https://www.counterextremism.com/digital-disruption

76. Goldman A. Domestic terrorism threat is "metastasizing" in US, F.B.I. Director says. *New York Times*, 2 Mar 2021. https://www.nytimes.com/2021/03/02/us/politics/wray-domestic-terrorism-capitol.html

10

The Internet and Social Media as an Enabling Force

PATRICIA R. RECUPERO AND SAMARA E. RAINEY

INTRODUCTION

Numerous researchers and commentators have identified the internet and social media as critical enabling forces in the development of lone-actor terrorists today.[1–3] As early as 1985, long before most people had access to the world wide web, the Anti-Defamation League warned of the likelihood that hate groups would exploit the internet,[4] and, indeed, hate groups have cultivated a significant online presence since its very earliest days.[5,6] Just as information and communications technology (ICT) has become a central feature of our lives, its use is now the norm in cases of terrorism.[7,8] Gill notes that although the rise of the internet has not been matched by increasing lone-actor terrorist activity, the use of the internet for social interactions and learning does seem to be increasing among lone actors.[9] Unfortunately, empirical research on the subject of the internet and radicalization among lone-actor terrorists is limited.[10]

Researchers for the Rand Institute tested five hypotheses regarding the internet and radicalization and found support for two: that "[t]he internet creates more opportunities to become radicalised" and that "[t]he internet acts as an 'echo chamber.'"[8] They did not find support for claims that the internet increases self-radicalization, allows radicalization without any face-to-face interactions, or *accelerates* radicalization, although there was some evidence that the internet may *facilitate* the process,[8] a finding supported by other researchers.[10] Several different models proposed by scholars in the field (see Table 10.1) can help to frame the clinical or forensic professional's understanding of how the internet and social media may function as enabling forces in the development of lone-actor terrorists. For the purposes of this chapter, we apply a similar model that shares elements with each of the models proposed by Gill,[9] Neumann,[11] and Weimann and von Knop.[12] In this context, we discuss the roles of information access; logistics and planning; social needs and reinforcement; propaganda, misinformation, and escalation; and leakage. To illustrate these concepts, we utilize several hypothetical case vignettes; these vignettes and their characters are fictional, composite cases drawn from factors in numerous past incidents and investigations of lone-actor terrorism.

TABLE 10.1 DIFFERENT MODELS FOR UNDERSTANDING RADICALIZATION AND THE INTERNET

Gill[a]	Neumann[b]	Weimann and von Knop[c]
Reinforcing of prior beliefs	Mortality salience	Searching phase
Seeking legitimization for future actions	Sense of moral outrage	Seduction phase
Disseminating propaganda and providing material support for others	Extremist forums as criminogenic environments	Captivation phase
Attack signaling	Online disinhibition	Persuasion phase
Attempting to recruit others	Mobilization through role-playing	Operative phase
	Links into terrorist structures	

[a]Gill.[9]
[b]Neumann.[11]
[c]Weimann and von Knop.[12]

CASE 1: THE WHITE SUPREMACIST

Mr. John Doe is referred for evaluation through a prison diversion program for mandatory counseling following his recent arrest for violating a no-contact order that the city's mayor had obtained against him. The mayor, Mike Smith, is an attorney of African American descent who was recently voted into office. He had obtained the restraining order after Mr. Doe was found prowling outside the Smith family home carrying a handgun. Mr. Doe's pre-sentencing report contained the following information about his internet and social media activity:

Investigators determined that Mr. Doe has registered accounts at several white supremacist forums, including Stormfront. Mr. Doe first became involved with these groups online following the election of Barack Obama to the US Presidency in 2008. Although he does not consider himself to be a member of any established groups, Mr. Doe follows a number of alt-right groups on Facebook, Twitter, and YouTube, and his Facebook profile photograph features the logo for the Proud Boys group. Mr. Doe also follows several prominent right-wing conspiracy theorists and regularly shares links to their blogs on his Facebook timeline and Twitter feed, which contains a number of extreme right-wing hashtags.

Mr. Doe has posted numerous photographs of firearms and other weapons in his collection to his Facebook profile as well as to the Facebook page for an independent militia to which he belongs. In addition to its public page, the militia has a secret Facebook group in which members discuss "resistance strategies"; Doe is one of the group's administrators. Others in the group have uploaded several videos, including step-by-step instructions for assembling firearms from untracked individual components available for purchase online. The group also routinely shares links to other videos and articles elsewhere on the web, such as video footage of conflicts between white nationalist groups and anti-fascist counter-protesters. A recently uploaded video, believed to have been filmed by Mr. Doe, follows an altercation with Black Lives Matter activists demonstrating outside a police station several states away. Although Mr. Doe does not appear in the video, his voice can be heard narrating, rambling about a "Racial Holy War," and taunting the activists with racist epithets.

A search of Mr. Doe's web browser activity revealed several recent searches with troubling content, including "how to make a pipe bomb," "Mayor Mike Smith address," "West Main AME church" (the congregation where Mr. Smith and his family attend services), and "fingerprint removal." Mr. Doe had downloaded and saved to his computer several digital files containing detailed instructions for making pipe bombs.

In addition to counseling Mr. Doe, the clinical evaluator was asked whether they believed, to the best of their professional judgment, that the court should restrict Mr. Doe's internet access as a condition of his sentence and, if so, what restrictions or limitations might be appropriate.

INFORMATION ACCESS

As the preceding vignette illustrates, information access is a critical factor in the appeal of the internet for extremists and would-be lone-actor terrorists. Although bomb-making instructions, for example, existed long before the world wide web went public, they were far less easily accessible in the past. To obtain a manual, the lone actor of earlier decades might have needed to travel to a distant library and hunt down obscure publications in the darkened stacks, a process that involves considerably more planning and time than required to obtain this type of information today. Now, internet-facilitated anonymity enables the distribution and acquisition of such information with minimal risk of detection or arrest.[13,14] Groups such as al-Qaeda and the Islamic State, as well as independent extremists and other content distributors, have made instructional manuals like *The Terrorist's Handbook* and *The Anarchist's Cookbook* easily accessible online.[15,16] In a sample of terrorist offenders from the United Kingdom, Gill and colleagues found that a growing percentage of cases over time involved the perpetrator (or would-be attacker) using the internet to learn about things relevant to their attack plans; 76% of cases since 2012 featured internet-based learning.[10]

Video-sharing websites and applications like YouTube and Vimeo, and the vast data storage capacity and instant searching tools afforded by the internet, provide fast access to multimedia, step-by-step instructions and far more detailed demonstrations than what might be found through traditional printed materials and search methods of the past. In several cases, lone-actor terrorists have located multiple sources online for learning how to assemble weapons such as bombs.[9] When an initial attempt failed, the determined actor was often able to obtain more feasible instructions online; the perpetrator of the attacks in Oslo and Utøya, Norway, for example, found "a viable alternative solution that he tested successfully" from a video on YouTube.[9 (p. 96)] The availability of such information to lone-actor terrorists may be analogous to the existence of detailed suicide method descriptions on the internet, in that the proliferation of such information is all but impossible to control. By the time content has been removed from one website, often it has already been reposted on several others, one reason for the persistence of literature like al-Qaeda's *Inspire* magazine on the web.[11]

Through the web and social media, individuals also have access to a variety of different worldviews, including radical ideology rarely encountered in face-to-face settings. Literature from extremist groups and publications like *Mein Kampf* are freely shared online,[6] and advances in translation technology and video subtitling have further broadened the reach of extremist multimedia.[17] Electronic self-publishing has also enabled hate groups and extremists to reach a wider audience.[18,19] Content producers, including radicals, no longer need intermediaries such as mass media or publishing firms to disseminate their views.[20] Specialized and academic knowledge is also more easily accessible online. Sites such as WikiLeaks release classified documents,[14] enabling widespread distribution of knowledge that was formerly reserved for only well-screened professionals with a security clearance; for example, "[m]any of the extreme right's sophisticated and coordinated media disruption techniques and psy-ops are based on military guides such as leaked GCHQ and NATO's strategic communication documents."[14 (p.19)] Similarly, academic research and theory are also accessible online, and a number of loosely connected extremist communities have appropriated ideas from academic fields, such as evolutionary psychology, and adapted them to a radical message.[21]

LOGISTICS AND PLANNING

Closely related to information access are logistics and planning. Gill and colleagues found that 32% of terrorism offenders in a UK sample used resources online to prepare for an attack.[10] In addition to information-access issues such as bomb-making instructions, these preparations included surveillance, obtaining blueprints or plans for public transportation and symbolic landmarks, and reviewing the voting records of public officials.[3,9,10] Lone actors may research many aspects of potential targets online, such as vehicle traffic patterns, building security, escape routes, proximity to first responders, locations of closed-circuit video cameras, and even times of peak activity so as to maximize (or minimize) casualties. The internet may also inform the lone actor's choice of method; for example, vehicle-ramming attacks were recommended by Hamas in 2015.[22] In our preceding hypothetical case vignette, John Doe appears to be in the initial stages of logistics and planning activities online.

The Unite the Right rally in Charlottesville, Virginia, in August 2017 illustrates the key role played by social media in logistics and planning.[23] A Facebook page and the Facebook Messenger application were used to organize the event,[18] ostensibly a freedom-of-speech protest prompted by the planned removal of a statue of Confederate General Robert E. Lee.[14] The event was also promoted on less mainstream forums, such as 4chan's /pol/message board, social networking site Reddit's /The_Donald subreddit (a discussion thread), and the white-supremacist forum Stormfront, where extremist groups such as the Nationalist Socialist Movement and the Ku Klux Klan urged their members to attend.[14] Racist and xenophobic groups in Europe have also used social media to organize, plan, and mobilize anti-refugee activity.[24]

Technology has also lessened logistical hurdles for would-be lone-actor terrorists for activities such as fundraising, purchasing weapons, and obtaining fake documents. Many of these exchanges take place through black markets on the dark web, a hidden portion of the internet popular for criminal activity that is only accessible through specialized knowledge.[15,25] Extremist groups have seized on cryptocurrency like Bitcoin as a way to raise funds and purchase weapons and other items on the dark web with enhanced anonymity.[15,26] Social media have also facilitated fundraising through crowdfunding campaigns on platforms like WeSearchr, Patreon, and even PayPal.[14,18,26]

CASE 2: THE POTENTIAL JIHADIST

Mr. Richard Roe is a 28-year-old resident of Chicago who works as an electrician and handyman. He lives in an apartment that he rents with a roommate. Although Mr. Roe's parents were both Muslim, his father left the family when Richard was 7 years old, and Mrs. Roe did not attend services regularly. Until recently, Mr. Roe was not especially observant; the family followed some customs, such as observing major holidays and adhering to dietary restrictions, but prayed inconsistently. Nonetheless, Mr. Roe was isolated and bullied by his classmates in school. By the time he was a teenager, Mr. Roe had withdrawn into the world of fantasy football online and had no close friends "in the real world."

Approximately 6 months ago, Mr. Roe moved out of his mother's house and began attending services at a local mosque and meeting privately with the imam for instruction and guidance. This continued for several weeks, after which Mr. Roe, driven by the desire to learn more about Islam, began reading religious texts and watching prominent Muslim clerics on YouTube. Inspired by one of these figures, Mr. Roe reached out to the preacher via email, and they began corresponding regularly through email and text messages. Following links to outside content-hosting services such as Dump.to, Mr. Roe also came across videos of armed conflicts overseas and several jihadist propaganda videos that had been removed from YouTube. Mr. Roe also became active within an IRC-style chat room devoted to the study of Islam and began chatting directly with several of the room's members through kik, a direct-messaging app.

Mr. Roe recently came to the attention of the FBI for making a donation through a Patreon crowdfunding campaign to a "relief charity" suspected to be an affiliate of the Islamic State of Iraq and the Levant (ISIL). It is not clear whether Mr. Roe was aware that the donation might be used in connection with ISIL. Investigators monitored Mr. Roe's internet activity for several weeks but did not find any evidence that he had downloaded bomb-making manuals or similarly troubling files. With minimal evidence to support an arrest or property seizure, law enforcement authorities have requested a risk assessment to determine whether continued surveillance of Mr. Roe's internet and social media activity is warranted.

SOCIAL NEEDS AND REINFORCEMENT

Social aspects of the internet in the Web 2.0 era are a major reason that many scholars argue for the increasing importance of the internet and social media in radicalization.[7] Like Mr. Roe in the preceding vignette, many isolated young people today turn to social media to form friendships and interact with others: "virtual communities can be seen as important social arenas for the formation of interpersonal bonds."[6 (p.1003)] Through these communities, the alienated individual is afforded an opportunity for identity development and social belonging.[13,27,28] Internet communities may serve as substitutes for the sense of community or belonging that has eluded the disconnected individual in the real world.[16,29,30] Social withdrawal and isolation offline are common among lone-actor terrorists prior to the commission of an attack,[31] but many so-called lone actors today are well connected with others online.[32] Virtual communities and social media often lead to the formation of real-world friendships and face-to-face gatherings, as seen in the case of "book clubs" among extremists,[26] niche dating forums in radical communities,[6] and social events to distribute propaganda in person.[23]

Researchers have described "toxic technocultures" that have developed on the web and which rely on shared slang, memes, and inside jokes to define and enforce boundaries between the "in group" and outsiders,[33] as exemplified by forums like 4chan. While some commentators dismiss such cultures as harmless trolling, it bears noting that the Daily Stormer was founded by a man who had frequented 4chan as a teenager.[34] There are also fandom subcultures on the internet devoted to the celebration of school shootings and past incidents of terrorism and mass violence. Troll culture has also shaped the landscape of radical content online through plausible deniability and irony. Early memes and other instances of racist content, for example, were often created and shared ironically as satire for humorous purposes by trolls without any intent to radicalize others.[34] Thus, when similar memes and content are disseminated as propaganda by extremist groups or radicalized individuals, their malicious intent or "serious" nature often go initially unrecognized, thus encouraging wider distribution.[26]

Interacting with others within these subcultures online often fulfills significant social needs for the loner, and extreme views may serve to enhance a person's status within the community.

The *online disinhibition effect*, first described by Suler in 2004[35] and identified by Neumann as a mechanism of online radicalization, "leads to groups becoming more hostile and polarized and . . . may spill over into aggressive behavior offline."[11 (p. 437)] Perceived anonymity may embolden individuals with radical views or socially proscribed interests to act on these beliefs or inclinations online and to network and correspond with like-minded others[36]; subsequent social rewards may serve to reinforce more extreme beliefs. The interactive and algorithmic structures of social media contribute to a critical aspect of internet culture from the perspective of radicalization.[37,38] Threatening, abusive, and even violent behavior online is typically rewarded through social media tools such as "likes," increased follower counts, upvoting, and social interaction. These rewards may be embedded into the algorithms themselves: "Facebook's news feed, for instance, runs on an algorithm that promotes whatever content wins the most engagement. Studies find that negative, primal emotions—fear, anger—draw the most engagement. So posts that provoke those emotions rise naturally. Tribalism—a universal human tendency—also draws heavy engagement. Posts that affirm your group identity by attacking another group tend to perform well."[39]

YouTube's recommendation algorithms have been found to direct viewers to increasingly more radical content online, and users who comment on a channel's videos often reward content creators for espousing and promoting more extreme beliefs.[38] Cross-pollination among different radical worldviews is also common online; this has been seen recently in the overlap between some racist and misogynistic groups and their adherents.[27,32]

PROPAGANDA, MISINFORMATION, AND ESCALATION

The internet and social media play a key role in the spread of propaganda and misinformation today. A basic web search for a term such as "the Holocaust," for example, is likely to yield, within the top results, propaganda and misinformation promulgated by hate groups, such as Holocaust-denial conspiracy theories.[40] Such searches and their path to radical content online (such as conspiracy-theory blogs) have been implicated in lone-actor terrorist incidents, such as the

Charleston church shooting in 2015.[41] Scholars and commentators have described the internet as an "echo chamber" that can reinforce radical ideas and minimize exposure to opposing viewpoints and moderation.[8,11,27,42] As Yang and Self have noted, "[c]ontrary to the expectation that blogs and other new media would expose people to different ideas and form a marketplace of opinions, the literature is rife with studies reporting a pattern of polarization on the blogosphere and across different new media platforms."[43 (p. 49)] This phenomenon has led to the formation of political "bubbles" in social media, wherein one may avoid civil interaction with persons holding opposing viewpoints.

Members of far-right extremist groups have adopted a strategy that involves shifting the *Overton window* (i.e., "the consensus boundaries of what constitutes acceptable public discourse)"[14 (p. 15)] further to the right. Political commentary and public debates leading up to and following the 2016 US elections serve to illustrate this strategy and its sequelae: "Suddenly it was okay to talk about banning Muslims or to cast Mexican immigrants as criminals and parasites—which meant . . . even-more-extreme views weren't as far outside the mainstream as they once had been."[26]

Social media-based propaganda often uses moral outrage to promote an extremist worldview; for example, xenophobic and anti-immigration groups have used the hypothetical threat of sexual violence against women by refugees to advance nationalist views.[24] Those who espouse radical beliefs are frequently portrayed as victims through internet propaganda. This can lead to others identifying and sympathizing with the perpetrators of violent attacks, as was seen in the wake of the 1999 Columbine school shooting.[44] In his video manifestos and writings, the perpetrator of the Isla Vista, California, killings in 2014 portrayed himself as the victim of an unfair system, characterizing his attack as rebellion or uprising against perceived oppressors,[27] thus echoing the views of perpetrators of previous incidents of mass violence.

Today, radical beliefs and conspiracy theories migrate quickly from the internet's fringes to mainstream platforms such as Facebook, Twitter, and YouTube. For example, alt-right groups that began in white supremacist forums like Stormfront and the Daily Stormer have built a visible presence on Reddit and Facebook.[33] Fringe groups have also used more mainstream movements and channels to reach a wider audience and amplify their messages, intentionally "using less extreme groups as strategic mouthpieces."[14] (p. 6) In addition to the use of moral outrage, extremist groups in the West owe much of their success to the entertainment value found in some of the content they create and share. Memes and humor help to make radical propaganda more effective,[14] and the resulting entertainment value recalls the influence of the White Power music scene in spreading neo-Nazi beliefs in earlier decades.[6]

Social media may facilitate the rapid escalation of outrage and open conflict. In several regions, software applications such as WhatsApp and Facebook have been implicated in inciting lynch mobs and other forms of mob-based violence.[45-47] Modern advances in technology have enabled sophisticated editing of images and videos that can be exploited for misinformation campaigns. As exemplified by the Pizzagate fiasco in 2016,[48] conspiracy theories have thrived online, and their adherents frequently use such theories to justify aggressive and sometimes violent behavior toward others. Survivors of mass violence and those bereaved through such acts have been targeted for cyber-harassment campaigns by conspiracy theorists influenced by websites like Infowars.[49] These conspiracy theories often allege that a past violent incident (such as the school shootings in Parkland, Florida, or Sandy Hook, Connecticut) was a hoax and did not really take place.[26]

CASE 3: THE INCEL

James Stiles is a 21-year-old college student whose social media and internet activity have aroused concern among his fellow classmates. On discussion boards at 4chan, 8chan, and Reddit, Mr. Stiles goes by "TwstdWrld," a reference to the manifesto written by Elliott Rodger, the perpetrator of the mass murder in Isla Vista, California, in 2014. On these sites, Mr. Stiles participates in several "incel" ("involuntarily celibate") forums and posts regularly to an anti-feminist Men's Rights Activists discussion thread and the /pol/board on 4chan. In his posts, he has shared variations of popular incel memes, such as the "aborted girlfriend" comic and "several millimeters of bone," as well as quotations from Rodger's manifesto and final video and screenshots of news stories about the Toronto van attack in 2018. Stiles frequently hails Rodger and the alleged driver in the Toronto attack as heroes.

Up until recently, Mr. Stiles restricted most of his social media activity to interactions with other lonely young men, particularly in the incel community, and friends from online gaming communities. However, within the past few months, following the loss of a female friend who rejected his sexual advances, Mr. Stiles began posting public status updates on Twitter and Tumblr in which he complained about his classmates, particularly "Stacys," (i.e., popular, physically attractive young women, in incel slang). (Table 10.2 lists several resources for clinicians, investigators, law enforcement, and forensic professionals to research unfamiliar terms and images that one may encounter in an evaluee's internet and social media activity.) Over time, Stiles's posts grew more hostile and explicit, prompting two classmates to report the messages to the university. Stiles also began direct-messaging his former friend, Rebecca Moore, with longer, rambling commentaries about his loneliness and frustration and the perceived unfairness of his situation. In several direct messages to Ms. Moore on WhatsApp, he made what she took to be vague threats of mass violence on the campus (e.g., "Life is short, they will see how short soon enough"). Additionally, Ms. Moore's boyfriend, Jason Collins, has received a number of strange and threatening messages from multiple anonymous senders; Ms. Moore suspects that these "troll attacks" were instigated by Mr. Stiles.

Mr. Stiles recently had his Tumblr account suspended as a result of abusive and threatening messages that he and others from an 8chan forum had sent to a prominent feminist online. In addition to insulting comments, Stiles posted image files in which he had superimposed her face onto the bodies of women in pornographic and graphically violent photos, as well as other disturbing images (e.g., an empty jail cell with the caption "this is where u belong [expletive]"). Mr. Stiles maintains that he never meant the threats seriously and insists that he was "only joking around."

LEAKAGE

Leakage of violent intent (similar to Gill's concept of attack signalling[9]) prior to the commission of an offense is common and represents an important area for focus in conducting a threat assessment: "Leakage is the communication to a third

TABLE 10.2 RESOURCES FOR CASE RESEARCH

Resource	Description
Hate Symbols Database (of the Anti-Defamation League) (https://www.adl.org/education-and-resources/resource-knowledge-base/hate-symbols)	Contains images and descriptions of a wide variety of symbols used by hate groups, including numerical symbols (e.g., 88 for "Heil Hitler"), slang, and logos of known hate groups
Extremist Files (of the Southern Poverty Law Center [SPLC]) (https://www.splcenter.org/fighting-hate/extremist-files)	Database of prominent extremists and extremist organizations; the SPLC also has a blog ("Hatewatch") that tracks events and developments in hate groups in the United States and a searchable "Hate Map" that identifies known hate groups operating in the United States, organized by state
Internet Meme Database ("Know Your Meme") (https://knowyourmeme.com/)	Searchable database of popular internet memes and related internet phenomena (e.g., viral videos, web celebrities); can sort by subculture and memes that are currently trending
Emoji Meanings (http://www.emojimeanings.org/)	Known meanings of commonly used emojis, particularly in combination (e.g., white square followed by building = the White House)
Emojipedia (https://emojipedia.org/)	Displays the common name and Unicode for all current emojis; also has a blog that discusses famous uses of emojis and the common meanings of some emojis
NetLingo (https://www.netlingo.com/)	Internet dictionary; contains meanings, common usage, and other information about terms, abbreviations, acronyms, and symbols used in information and communications technology, including emoticons/smileys (other than emoji), ASCII art (e.g., @>--;---- for rose), texting terms, and chat acronyms
Tech Terms Computer Dictionary (https://techterms.com/)	Internet dictionary; contains meanings, common usage, and detailed descriptions about technical terms relating to information and communications technology (e.g., hashtag, meme)
PC Mag Encyclopedia (https://www.pcmag.com/encyclopedia)	Searchable encyclopedia of computer-, internet-, and technology-related terms (e.g., "Twitter feed")
Urban Dictionary (https://www.urbandictionary.com/)	Searchable database of pop-culture terms and slang, including hate symbols (e.g., searching for "88" will yield the "Heil Hitler" connotation but also alternative meanings)
Web Cultures Web Archive (of the Library of Congress) (https://www.loc.gov/collections/web-cultures-web-archive/about-this-collection/)	History of memes, GIFs, and emoji, among other internet-culture phenomena; contains archived content of several helpful sources of information on the web (e.g., Urban Dictionary)

party of an intent to do harm to a target. Third parties are typically other people, but the means of communication could vary widely, from planned or spontaneous utterances, to letters, diaries, emails, voice mails, blogs, journals, internet postings, tweets, text messages, video postings, and future means of social communication that are yet to be invented."[50] [(p. 514)]

Like the characters of John Doe, Richard Roe, and James Stiles in the preceding vignettes, lone-actor terrorists and other perpetrators of mass violence often leave behind a digital footprint that contains leakage of violent plans.[28,50] Ellis and colleagues found that among lone-actor terrorists, right-wing actors were more likely than religiously motivated terrorists to leave warning messages and other forms of leakage online.[51] The social media profiles of lone-actor terrorists often include multimedia propaganda,[9] such as videos endorsing radical beliefs or hate-mongering memes. Such leakage may provoke concern in others who then report the content to law enforcement or other authorities. The perpetrator of the Isla Vista killings, for example, had been reported to police by his mother after she found disturbing videos he had posted on YouTube.[52] However, as in the hypothetical case of James Stiles, often the content is dismissed as "joking" or otherwise protected free speech, particularly in the United States, where First Amendment concerns arise. The serious nature of such content and internet activity may only become clear in hindsight, after the commission of a violent offense. Leakage in and of itself may not rise to the level of a criminal offense or a violation of rules.

The individual allegedly behind a series of mail bombs sent to prominent Democrats in the fall of 2018 (nicknamed the "MAGAbomber" for his idolization of Donald Trump[53]) left behind a troubling digital footprint, making threats on Twitter against Democratic politicians and sharing right-wing conspiracy theories on Facebook,[54] some of them quite bizarre (e.g., that former President Barack Obama was the antichrist).[19,55] Prior to his arrest, he had been reported to Twitter for making violent threats against a political commentator.[53,55] Following arrest, a picture emerged of growing radicalization and increasingly violent ideation as it played out through social media: "In recent months, [his] behavior changed. His posts took on a darker, more obsessive tone, often accompanied by threats of violence and gory images of bloody animal carcasses. No longer mistakable as an everyday internet partisan, he posted repeatedly about 'unconquered Seminoles,' a reference to the tribe that he appears to have adopted. (It also appeared on his van.) And on Twitter, his messages turned dark and sinister. He directed a tweet at Ms. Waters, the California Democrat, with a photo of what appeared to be her house. The message read: 'see you soon.' "[55]

Such escalating warning signs may signal increasing risk. Neumann,[11] Bouhana and colleagues,[28] and Meloy and Gill[56] have identified internet- and social media-based leakage as critical targets for the detection of lone-actor terrorists prior to an attack.

A number of lone-actor terrorists and other perpetrators of mass violence (such as school shooters with no political or religious motive) have left behind manifestos in the form of written documents or, increasingly, recorded videos. Often, these materials are distributed prior to the commission of an offense, potentially enabling prevention of an attack. In New York, a state Senator introduced two bills (S. 9197 and S. 9191) which, if passed into legislation, would give police access to 3 years of social media activity and 1 year of internet searches for any applicants for gun permits, potentially enabling the detection of leaked plans or intent prior to the acquisition of weapons. When discovered after an attack, written or multimedia manifestos may

serve to inform future counterterrorism efforts. Manifestos of previous lone-actor terrorists (such as the Unabomber) and other mass-violence offenders (such as the Columbine shooters) are available online, have inspired subsequent lone-actor terrorists, and may influence violent extremists in the future.

RECENT TRENDS

A recent trend that bears noting is the growth of right-wing extremism in the West.[57,58] The threat posed by right-wing radicals has exceeded that posed by left-wing extremism and Muslim extremism in recent years, but funding for researching and addressing right-wing threats has been meagre in comparison to the resources devoted to counterterrorism efforts targeting Islamic radicals.[23,59-61] As Lowry notes: "White supremacists historically account for a majority of terrorism and hate crimes in the United States."[58 (p. 35)] Attacks by right-wing extremists have increased significantly since 2010, and the number of right-wing attacks today exceeds the number of Islamic terrorist attacks.[19] Within the past decade, more Americans have been killed by right-wing radicals than by Islamic or left-wing extremists.[59] Most of the perpetrators of these attacks are white supremacists, as described in our first vignette, or anti-government sovereign citizens.[19] Right-wing extremist groups' follower counts on social media have increased dramatically in recent years.[62]

A series of violent incidents within the span of 2 weeks in October–November 2018, all of which were allegedly perpetrated by right-wing lone actors, underscores the scope of the problem.[60] In the first incident, two African American individuals were killed at a Kroger store in Jeffersontown, Kentucky; witness reports suggest that the crime was motivated by racial hate and that the shooter had originally intended to attack a black church nearby.[63] Two days later, police arrested a man alleged to be the so-called MAGAbomber whose attempted mail bombings and social media-based leakage were described earlier.[19] The following day (October 27, 2018), a shooting at a synagogue in Pittsburgh claimed the lives of 11 people[19]; the suspected perpetrator had communicated with other right-wing extremists on social media site Gab,[55] voicing anti-immigrant and anti-Semitic views and conspiracy theories online before the attack.[64] Six days later, an individual believed to be connected to incel ideology opened fire in a yoga studio in Tallahassee, killing two and injuring five others before shooting himself; he had posted videos of misogynistic and racist rants online before the attack.[65]

It bears noting that the rise in right-wing extremism and its visibility in the United States and Europe has inspired some growth in anti-fascist ("antifa") and left-wing extremist groups.[66] As with the rise of right-wing extremism, left-wing radicals rely heavily on the internet and social media for information access, logistics, social needs, and propaganda.[67]

Another recent trend is the practice of *livestreaming*, the practice of broadcasting live video feeds in real time through social media, and related attempts to contain such problematic content. During the attack on two mosques in Christchurch, New Zealand, in March 2019, that claimed the lives of 51 people, an individual believed to be responsible for the incident livestreamed video of the attack on Facebook.[68] Although Facebook removed the video after being alerted to it by police, it was too late—the notorious "whack-a-mole" problem faced by content moderators and counterextremism professionals once again made containment of the video (already saved and reposted by others elsewhere online) all but impossible.[69] Media coverage of the incident characterized the shooting as "a massacre made to go viral"[70] and "a shooting disturbingly rooted in the internet."[71] Following the attack, several individuals who had shared the video online were charged under a New Zealand law prohibiting the possession or distribution of terrorist and extreme violence materials.[72] First Amendment concerns limit similar corrective responses in the United States. The Christchurch massacre is believed to have inspired a lone-actor mass shooting in El Paso, Texas, in August 2019; a manifesto posted on the 8chan website shortly before the incident references the Christchurch shooter's manifesto and anti-immigrant ideology. At the time of this writing, both of these manifestos are easily accessible online through basic searches on public sites such as Google or Bing.

Historically, most social-media firms have adopted a laissez-faire approach to content management, granting free rein to independent content creators. More recently, and in response to events like the Christchurch shooting and public outrage, technology companies like Alphabet (which owns Google and YouTube) and Facebook have begun removing hate speech content and limiting problematic use of their services, blocking users whose content is flagged for violating the site's Terms of Service, including several prominent extremist commentators and controversial figures.[73] In May 2019, New Zealand and France hosted a political summit resulting in the Christchurch Call to Action (https://www.christchurchcall.com/), a pledge by world leaders and technology companies to work together to eliminate terrorist and violent extremist content online. Under the Trump administration, the United States has thus far declined to join other countries and organizations in adopting the pledge.[74]

An encouraging future trend is the growth of artificial intelligence (AI) and its potential applications for counterterrorism and early intervention. Researchers are developing algorithms to facilitate automated electronic detection of hate speech online,[75] and larger media companies already use machine learning to identify and remove problematic content.[76] New forms of search technology are under development that may enable better penetration of the Dark Web by investigative agencies,[15] and technologically savvy activists within groups such as the Anonymous collective have assisted in the takedown of extremists' websites and social media accounts through distributed denial of service (DDoS) attacks.[11,77] Recent developments in behavioral medicine, such as the study of digital phenotyping, may help to inform counterterrorism efforts and investigations by law enforcement and homeland security agencies in the years to come.

CONCLUSION, RECOMMENDATIONS FOR RISK ASSESSMENT

Mental health clinicians, law enforcement or security personnel, investigators, or forensic professionals may be asked to perform violence risk assessments of individuals who have been identified as potential lone-actor terrorists. In conducting such assessments today, reviewing the potential offender's internet and social media activity is necessary. The referral source (e.g., court, attorney, school) should provide the evaluator with any relevant electronic communications, including social media feeds, video recordings posted by the evaluee, chat transcripts containing potential leakage of violent intent, lists of screen names or nicknames used on social networking sites, screenshots of the evaluee's profiles on social media, logs of web-search queries from engines such as Google or Bing, information from any apps that the evaluee had installed on their smartphone(s) and tablet computer(s), and so forth. Standardized and structured assessment tools, such as the Terrorist Assessment Protocol (TRAP-18; see Chapters 24 and 25), can be especially helpful. Within the TRAP-18, "dependence

BOX 10.1
FEATURES OF INTERNET AND SOCIAL MEDIA USE
AND AREAS FOR INQUIRY

INFORMATION ACCESS
- What search queries has the evaluee entered within the past month (6 months, year, etc.)?
- Who and what does the evaluee follow on [Facebook/Twitter/YouTube/Instagram]?

LOGISTICS AND PLANNING
- What application(s) does the evaluee use for travel planning? Is there a record of past entries? (e.g., Have they sought directions or street-view images of any government buildings?)
- Does the evaluee have any cloud-based file storage? Have you reviewed its contents?
- Does the evaluee's digital calendar have any cryptic or unusual entries for calendar dates that correspond with the anniversaries of past terror attacks or mass-violence incidents, or other dates significant among extremists (e.g., Hitler's birthday)?
- Does the evaluee value anonymity online? If so, how do they secure their anonymity (e.g., VPNs, encrypted messaging/browsing applications)?

SOCIAL NEEDS AND REINFORCEMENT
- What is the nature of the evaluee's interactions on social media? Do their friends "like" political content that they post?
- To what Facebook [or other social media] groups and forums does the evaluee belong?
- Does the evaluee use any fringe or lesser-known social networking sites, such as Discord or Gab?
- Does the evaluee have friends online with whom they feel close? Closer than to their offline acquaintances?

PROPAGANDA, MISINFORMATION, AND ESCALATION
- Does the evaluee's web history include visits to white supremacist websites such as the Daily Stormer?
- Do you have access to the evaluee's [Facebook/Twitter] news feed? Have they shared or retweeted many political posts?
- Does the evaluee follow any prominent conspiracy theorists, such as Alex Jones/Infowars?
- Does the evaluee perceive more freedom to express unpopular or "politically incorrect" beliefs online?

LEAKAGE
- Do any symbols you do not recognize appear on the evaluee's social media profile(s)? (If yes: see resources in Table 10.2.)
- Does the evaluee reference any past incidents of mass violence or the perpetrators of these incidents in their news feed, profile, discussion-board posts, status updates, or tweets?
- Does the evaluee's social media activity include text, images, or other media depicting animal cruelty? Violence? Hate?
- Has the evaluee ever had their [Twitter/Facebook/YouTube] account suspended as a result of violating the site's Terms of Service or in response to complaints from another user?

on the virtual community" comprises one of the 10 distal characteristics of the lone-actor terrorist,[56] but many of the other proximal and distal risk factors identified in the TRAP-18 model may find expression through the lone actor's internet and social media activity. Box 10.1 presents some initial suggested questions to help guide the clinician's or forensic professional's inquiries.

NOTES AND REFERENCES

1. Barnes BD. Confronting the one-man wolf pack: Adapting law enforcement and prosecution responses to the threat of lone wolf terrorism. *Boston Univ Law Rev.* 2012;92:1613–1662.
2. Pantucci R. What have we learned about lone wolves from Anders Behring Breivik? *Perspect Terrorism.* 2011;5(5–6):27–42.
3. Simon JD. *Lone Wolf Terrorism: Understanding the Growing Threat.* Amherst, NY: Prometheus Books; 2016.
4. Anti-Defamation League. *Computerized Networks of Hate: An ADL Fact Finding Report.* New York: Anti-Defamation League of B'nai B'rith; 1985.
5. Hawdon J, Oksanen A, Räsänen P. Exposure to online hate in four nations: A cross-national consideration. *Deviant Behav.* 2017;38(3):254–266.
6. Bowman-Grieve L. Exploring "Stormfront": A virtual community of the radical right. *Stud Conflict Terrorism.* 2009;32:989–1007.
7. Conway M. Determining the role of the internet in violent extremism and terrorism: Six suggestions for progressing research. *Stud Conflict Terrorism.* 2017;40(1):77–98.
8. von Behr I, Reding A, Edwards C, Gribbon L. *Radicalisation in the Digital Era: The Use of the Internet in 15 Cases of Terrorism and Extremism.* Cambridge: Rand; 2013.
9. Gill P. *Lone-Actor Terrorists: A Behavioural Analysis.* New York: Routledge; 2015.
10. Gill P, Corner E, Conway M, Thornton A, Bloom M, Horgan J. Terrorist use of the internet by the numbers: Quantifying behaviors, patterns, and processes. *Criminol Public Policy.* 2017;16(1):99–117.
11. Neumann PR. Options and strategies for countering online radicalization in the United States. *Stud Conflict Terrorism.* 2013;36:431–459.
12. Weimann G, von Knop K. Applying the notion of noise to countering online terrorism. *Stud Conflict Terrorism.* 2008;31:883–902.
13. McCoy J, Knight WA. Homegrown terrorism in Canada: Local patterns, global trends. *Stud Conflict Terrorism.* 2015;38:253–274.
14. Davey J, Ebner J. *The Fringe Insurgency: Connectivity, Convergence and Mainstreaming of the Extreme Right.* London: Institute for Strategic Dialogue; 2017.
15. Weimann G. Going dark: Terrorism on the dark web. *Stud Conflict Terrorism.* 2016;39(3):195–206.
16. Pantucci R. *A Typology of Lone Wolves: Preliminary Analysis of Lone Islamist Terrorists.* London: International Centre for the Study of Radicalisation and Political Violence; 2011.
17. Conway M. From al-Zarqawi to al-Awlaki: The emergence and development of an online radical milieu. *CTX: Combating Terrorism Exchange.* 2012;2(4):12–22.
18. Center for American Progress. *Change the Terms: Reducing Hate Online* (discussion forum). Washington, D.C., 25 Oct 2018. https://www.americanprogress.org/events/2018/10/15/459376/change-terms-reducing-hate-online/
19. Jones SG. *The Rise of Far-Right Extremism in the United States.* Washington, DC: Center for Strategic and International Studies; 2018.
20. Seo H, Ebrahim H. Visual propaganda on Facebook: A comparative analysis of Syrian conflicts. *Media War Conflict* 2016;9(3):227–251.
21. van Valkenburgh SP. Digesting the red pill: Masculinity and neoliberalism in the manosphere. *Men Masc.* 2018 [ePub online ahead of print, 4 Dec 2018] doi:10.1177/1097184X18816118.
22. Perry S, Hasisi B, Perry G. Lone terrorists: A study of run-over attacks in Israel. *Eur J Criminol.* 2019;16(1):102–123.
23. Anti-Defamation League. *Murder and Extremism in the United States in 2017: An ADL Center on Extremism Report.* New York: Anti-Defamation League, 2017.
24. Ekman M. Anti-refugee mobilization on social media: The case of Soldiers of Odin. *Soc Media Soc.* 2018;4(1):1–11.
25. Mörch CM, Côté LP, Corthésy-Blondin L, Plourde-Léveillé L, Dargis L, Mishara BL. The Darknet and suicide. *J Affect Disord.* 2018;241:127–132.
26. O'Brien L. The making of an American Nazi. *The Atlantic,* 14 Nov 2017. https://www.theatlantic.com/magazine/archive/2017/12/the-making-of-an-american-nazi/544119/
27. Taub A. On social media's fringes, growing extremism targets women. *New York Times,* 9 May 2018. https://www.nytimes.com/2018/05/09/world/americas/incels-toronto-attack.html
28. Bouhana N, Corner E, Gill P, Schuurman B. Background and preparatory behaviours of right-wing extremist lone actors: A comparative study. *Perspect Terrorism.* 2018;12(6):150–163.
29. Huey L. This is not your mother's terrorism: Social media, online radicalization and the practice of political jamming. *J Terrorism Res.* 2015;6(2):1–16.
30. Huey L, Witmer E. #IS_Fangirl: Exploring a new role for women in terrorism. *J Terrorism Res.* 2016;7(1):1–10.

31. Spaaij R. The enigma of lone wolf terrorism: An assessment. *Stud Conflict Terrorism*. 2010;33:854–870.

32. Tait A. Why we should stop using the phrase "lone wolf." *New Statesman*, 31 Jan 2017. https://www.newstatesman.com/science-tech/social-media/2017/01/why-we-should-stop-using-phrase-lone-wolf

33. Massanari AL. Rethinking research ethics, power, and the risk of visibility in the era of the "alt-right" gaze. *Soc Media Soc*. 2018;4(2):1–9.

34. Phillips W. In their own words: Trolling, meme culture, and journalists' reflections on the 2016 US presidential election. In *The Oxygen of Amplification: Better Practices for Reporting on Extremists, Antagonists, and Manipulators Online*. New York: Data & Society Research Institute; 2018:16–60.

35. Suler J. The online disinhibition effect. *Cyberpsychol Behav*. 2004;7(3):321–326.

36. Bargh JA, McKenna KYA. The internet and social life. *Annu Rev Psychol*. 2004;55:573–590.

37. Taub A, Fisher M. Facebook fueled anti-refugee attacks in Germany, new research suggests. *New York Times*, 21 Aug 2018. https://www.nytimes.com/2018/08/21/world/europe/facebook-refugee-attacks-germany.html

38. Lewis R. *Alternative Influence: Broadcasting the Reactionary Right on YouTube*. New York: Data & Society; 2018.

39. Fisher M, Taub A. How everyday social media users become real-world extremists. *New York Times*, 25 Apr 2018. https://www.nytimes.com/2018/04/25/world/asia/facebook-extremism.html

40. Klein A. *Fanaticism, Racism, and Rage Online: Corrupting the Digital Sphere*. Cham: Palgrave Macmillan; 2017.

41. Roof D. Untitled manifesto, originally published at http://lastrhodesian.com/data/documents/rtf88.txt, 20 Jun 2015. Republished under "Here's what appears to be Dylann Roof's racist manifesto." *Mother Jones*, 20 Jun 2015. https://www.motherjones.com/politics/2015/06/alleged-charleston-shooter-dylann-roof-manifesto-racist/

42. Sageman M. *Leaderless Jihad: Terror Networks in the Twenty-First Century*. Philadelphia: University of Pennsylvania Press; 2008.

43. Yang A, Self C. Anti-Muslim prejudice in the virtual space: A case study of blog network structure and message features of the "Ground Zero mosque controversy." *Media War Conflict* 2015;8(1):46–69.

44. Langman P. Different types of role model influence and fame seeking among mass killers and copycat offenders. *Am Behav Sci*. 2018;62(2):210–228.

45. Goel V, Raj S, Ravichandran P. How WhatsApp leads mobs to murder in India. *New York Times*, 18 Jul 2018. https://www.nytimes.com/interactive/2018/11/23/technology/whatsapp-india-killings-ES.html

46. Taub A, Fisher M. Where countries are tinderboxes and Facebook is a match. *New York Times*, 21 Apr 2018. https://www.nytimes.com/2018/04/21/world/asia/facebook-sri-lanka-riots.html

47. Mozur P. A genocide incited on Facebook, with posts from Myanmar's military. *New York Times*, 15 Oct 2018. https://www.nytimes.com/2018/10/15/technology/myanmar-facebook-genocide.html

48. Aisch G, Huang J, Kang C. Dissecting the #PizzaGate conspiracy theories. *New York Times*, 10 Dec 2016. https://www.nytimes.com/interactive/2016/12/10/business/media/pizzagate.html

49. Ryser R. Father of Sandy Hook victim sues extremists on defamation charges. *The News-Times*, 4 Dec 2018. https://www.newstimes.com/local/article/Father-of-Sandy-Hook-victim-sues-extremists-on-13442286.php

50. Meloy JR, O'Toole ME. The concept of leakage in threat assessment. *Behav Sci Law*. 2011;29:513–527.

51. Ellis C, Pantucci R, van Zuijdewijn JdR, et al. Analysing the processes of lone-actor terrorism: Research findings. *Perspect Terrorism*. 2016;10(2):33–41.

52. Lovett I, Nagourney A. Video rant, then deadly rampage in California town. *New York Times*, 24 May 2014. https://www.nytimes.com/2014/05/25/us/california-drive-by-shooting.html

53. Harriot M. A black woman reported the MAGA-Bomber to Twitter. Twitter did nothing . . . again. *The Root*, 28 Oct 2018. https://www.theroot.com/a-black-woman-reported-the-magabomber-to-twitter-twitt-1830054451

54. Goldman D. Big tech made the social media mess. It has to fix it. *CNN.com*, 29 Oct 2018. https://www.cnn.com/2018/10/29/tech/social-media-hate-speech/index.html

55. Roose K. Cesar Sayoc's path on social media: From food photos to partisan fury. *New York Times*, 27 Oct 2018. https://www.nytimes.com/2018/10/27/technology/cesar-sayoc-facebook-twitter.html

56. Meloy JR, Gill P. The lone actor terrorist and the TRAP-18. *J Threat Assess Manage*. 2016;3(1):37–52.

57. Koch A. The new crusaders: Contemporary extreme right symbolism and rhetoric. *Perspect Terrorism*. 2017;11(5):13–24.

58. Lowry KD. Responding to the challenges of violent extremism/terrorism cases for United States probation and pretrial services. *J Deradicalization*. 2018/2019;17:28–88.

59. Singer PW. National security pros, it's time to talk about right-wing extremism. *Defense One*, 28 Feb 2018. https://www.defenseone.com/threats/2018/02/national-security-pros-its-time-talk-about-right-wing-extremism/146319/

60. Reitman J. US law enforcement failed to see the threat of white nationalism. Now they don't know how to stop it. *New York Times Magazine*, 3 Nov 2018. https://www.nytimes.com/2018/11/03/magazine/FBI-charlottesville-white-nationalism-far-right.html

61. Meleagrou-Hitchens A, Kaderbhai N. *Research Perspectives on Online Radicalisation: A Literature Review, 2006–2016*. London: International Centre for the Study of Radicalisation; 2017.

62. Berger JM. *Nazis vs. ISIS on Twitter: A Comparative Study of White Nationalist and ISIS Online Social Media Networks*. Washington, DC: George Washington University Program on Extremism; 2016.

63. Zraick K, Stevens M. Kroger shooting suspect tried to enter black church before killing 2 in Kentucky, police say. *New York Times*, 25 Oct 2018. https://www.nytimes.com/2018/10/25/us/louisville-kroger-shooting.html

64. Gabriel T, Healy J, Turkewitz J. Pittsburgh synagogue massacre suspect was "pretty much a ghost." *New York Times*, 28 Oct 2018. https://www.nytimes.com/2018/10/28/us/pittsburgh-shooting-robert-bowers.html

65. Zaveri M, Jacobs J, Mervosh S. Gunman in yoga studio shooting recorded misogynistic videos and faced battery charges. *New York Times*, 3 Nov 2018. https://www.nytimes.com/2018/11/03/us/yoga-studio-shooting-florida.html

66. Beinart P. The rise of the violent left. *The Atlantic*, Sep 2017. https://www.theatlantic.com/magazine/archive/2017/09/the-rise-of-the-violent-left/534192/

67. Koch A. Trends in anti-fascist and anarchist recruitment and mobilization. *J Deradicalization*. 2018;14:1–51.

68. Osnos E. How to talk about the New Zealand massacre: More sunlight, less oxygen. *The New Yorker*, 15 Mar 2019. https://www.newyorker.com/news/daily comment/how-to-talk-about-the-new-zealand-massacre-more-sunlight-less-oxygen

69. Dwoskin E, Timberg C. Inside YouTube's struggles to shut down video of the New Zealand shooting—and the humans who outsmarted its systems. *Washington Post*), 18 Mar 2019. https://www.washingtonpost.com/technology/2019/03/18/inside-youtubes-struggles-shut-down-video-new-zealand-shooting-humans-who-outsmarted-its-systems/

70. Warzel C. A massacre made to go viral. *New York Times*, 15 Mar 2019. https://www.nytimes.com/2019/03/15/opinion/new-zealand-shooting.html

71. Roose K. A shooting disturbingly rooted in the internet. *New York Times*, 16 Mar 2019:A.1.

72. Graham-McLay C. Where sharing violent videos is against law. *New York Times*, 22 Mar 2019:A1.

73. Isaac M, Roose K. Facebook bars Alex Jones, Louis Farrakhan and others from its services. *New York Times*, 2 May 2019. https://www.nytimes.com/2019/05/02/technology/facebook-alex-jones-louis-farrakhan-ban.html

74. Klein B. Trump administration declines to join Christchurch Call to Action. *CNN*, 15 May 2019. https://edition.cnn.com/2019/05/15/politics/trump-administration-christchurch-call-to-action/index.html

75. Miró-Llinares F, Moneva A, Esteve M. Hate is in the air! But where? Introducing an algorithm to detect hate speech in digital microenvironments. *Crime Sci*. 2018;7:15.doi:10.1186/s40163-018-0089-1.

76. Editorial Board. The new radicalization of the internet. *New York Times*, 24 Nov 2018. https://www.nytimes.com/2018/11/24/opinion/sunday/facebook-twitter-terrorism-extremism.html

77. Shehabat A, Mitew T. Black-boxing the black flag: Anonymous sharing platforms and ISIS content distribution tactics. *Perspect Terrorism* 2018;12(1):81–99.

11

Geographic Context

Domestic Versus International Lone Actors

CHRISTOPHER JASPARRO AND SUZANNE LEVI-SANCHEZ[*]

INTRODUCTION

From 1980 through 2012, the target geography of jihadist attacks (by all cell types) in and against the US homeland was largely consistent in terms of locale and target spaces and types. The emergence of the Islamic State of Iraq and al-Sham (ISIS) in 2013 raised the question of whether or not new jihadist geographic and spatial targeting patterns would emerge in general and by lone actors. This chapter builds on and updates previous research by the authors[1-7] to examine that question, add to the geographic literature on terrorism, and raise questions for further research. This chapter sheds some light on the trajectory of lone-jihadist targeting in order to better understand the evolution of the threat. This, in turn, could help inform the development of proactive counterterrorism strategies and identify future research questions.

BACKGROUND

Prior to 2013, lone-jihadist attackers in the United States had a proclivity for symbolic targets mostly in line with prevailing jihadist targeting norms, particularly relating to military and Jewish targets.[8] Furthermore, in terms of locale, lone actors similarly shared a preference for New York and Washington, DC.[9] However, after 2002, within a still broad consistency of jihadist target geography, a discernable but slow trend toward more diverse target locales and types emerged.[10] Much of this was accounted for by lone attackers (and weakly connected cells) who targeted a wider array of geographic locales, with the majority

of attacks outside major urban areas as well as most of those against non-Jewish civilian targets.[11] Lone-actor jihadist attacks in the United States also showed a distinct pattern compared to those in Europe, where attackers preferred symbolic individual media or political personalities. In both regions, however, attacks produced only limited casualties and physical damage.[12]

With 5 years of data now available, lone-actor jihadist attack geography in the United States after the emergence of ISIS has become clearer. Most notably there has been an increased "vernacularization" and "individualization" of targeting, method, and ideology. The term "vernacularization" as used here is derived from what geographers refer to as "vernacular landscapes" (i.e., everyday), those where "evidences of political organization of space are largely or entirely absent."[13] Non-political, non-symbolic, and more random civilian public spaces have become prominent targets in a way that they were not in the past. Attacks have also become more geographically dispersed, increasing in localities with little symbolic or political meaning (as opposed to, say, Washington, DC). Non–high-profile individuals (such as individual police officers and ordinary citizens) have become specific and common targets, too. Similarly, the use of everyday objects as weapons, such as vehicles and knives, became more common, although firearms remained the most prevalent and effective weapon employed. Attacks also increased significantly in frequency, driving overall fatalities up, but the casualty rate per attack changed minimally. This may in part

[*] The views expressed in this chapter are those of the authors and do not represent the official views or policies of the Naval War College, US Navy, or Department of Defense.

reflect the ease of accessing everyday targets along with the limitations imposed by using commonplace weapons.

Ascertaining lone-actor motives has long been a challenge for analysts because it is a difficult and subjective task to identify whether an attack was motivated primarily by ideology or an individual grievance wrapped in a cause.[14,15] Since 2013 however, individuals are radicalizing more quickly and the conflation of personal and ideological motives seems more pronounced. The combination of ISIS's more permissive targeting ideology with personal grievances is likely a driver of target vernacularization, along with the hardening of more traditional governmental and symbolic targets and places.

The attack geography of US and European lone-jihadist actors (the majority of whom appear to have been inspired by ISIS rather than core al-Qaeda) have become more similar in several ways. In particular, the trend in the US toward vernacularization parallels existing and emerging trends in Europe, especially the focus on public spaces, increased attacks against individuals, and the use of everyday weapons (such as firearms, knives, and vehicles). US and European lone-jihadist attacks increased in both frequency and geographic scope.

On the other hand, some notable geographic concentrations have emerged in Europe, with Paris in particular becoming a more prominent target locale for lone-actor jihadists. Also, while public spaces and individuals have been commonly targeted in both the United States and Europe, the types of individuals targeted by European lone actors has changed, with a pronounced singling out of police officers and military personnel. Conversely, in the United States, non-symbolic civilians were the main individual targets, but, as in Europe, there was a notable increase in attacks against police officers. In Europe, attacks shifted more toward government and military targets, while in the United States the main focus of lone-actor jihadist attacks shifted away from them.

Lone-actor attacks by US right-wing extremists (such as white nationalists and white supremacists) appear to be following a similar trajectory as jihadist ones. Past attacks by right-wing extremists focused mainly on government facilities or abortion clinics and key leaders in African American communities. The attacks of the past were driven primarily by ideological convictions and beliefs with the geographic locations mirroring these ideologies. Today's right-wing extremist attackers adhere to similar ideologies

as their predecessors but their attacks are more geographically dispersed. The unifying feature of recent attacks appears to be that the individual attackers themselves (similar to many of their US jihadist counterparts) are loners driven by diverse personal grievances (often fueled by conspiracy theories) which in turn drive ideological adherence or attack justification.

These ideologies range more widely than jihadist ones, from neo-Nazi and white supremacist ones, to anti-Semitic and racist beliefs, to homosexual and transgender hatred. The attacks have occurred across the United States, with no clear geographic patterning. Similar to their jihadist counterparts, attacks have been conducted mainly using commonplace weapons such as small arms, knives, and vehicles. Targets have, similarly, shifted from government, military, and high-casualty targets to smaller civilian ones and individuals.

What these pattern shifts may mean in terms of countering and preventing attacks in the near term, as well as the questions they raise for future research and analysis, will be addressed in this chapter's Conclusion. Now, however, this chapter will review key themes in and the utility of geographic approaches for terrorism research and analysis. The terms, data, and methodology employed in this chapter will be discussed before proceeding to an analysis comparing post-2013 lone-actor jihadist attacks in the United States with their ideological counterparts in Europe and their domestic right-wing counterparts in the United States.

GEOGRAPHY AND TERRORISM

Geographical and spatial considerations have traditionally received little attention in terrorism research and the literature is underdeveloped.[16-19] Moreover, there is "little systematic understanding of local variability in terrorist events and the dynamics of change in targets, perpetrators, frequency and location."[19] Few attempts have been made to systematically analyze the operational geography of jihadists[20] and even less so that of US lone actors specifically.

Ultimately, terrorists must still act in physical space.[21] Therefore, examining target geography can provide insights into the motivations of terrorists.[22] How terrorists perceive and value places may also reflect why and how they target them (or not).[23] Since attack geography changes over time, analyses of current and past geographic patterns can be used as baselines against which emergent patterns can be spotted[24] and to potentially model future events.[25] In turn, if the spatiality of attack planning, targeting, and impacts can be identified, they can potentially be better policed and mitigated.[26] Geographic gaps in preparedness and at-risk populations can be identified, thus improving risk reduction measures.[27]

DEFINITIONS, METHODS AND DATA SOURCES

For this chapter, lone actors are defined as individuals who either commit violence or who threaten/plot violence but are thwarted before execution. The violence/threat is linked either to a jihadist/Islamist or right-wing extremist ideology or belief system. The analysis in this chapter is limited to single individuals who, insofar as is known by available evidence, acted primarily of their own accord (suspects may have been influenced or encouraged by ideologues or may have loose personal connections to other extremists) and not under the formal direction, funding, or orders of a handler or organized group or command structure. This analysis also focuses on actors who plotted and operated mostly if not entirely alone, and it excludes pairs in order to ensure consistency with past research on which this analysis was built. Furthermore, the analysis looks at actual attacks and attempts where the attacker initiated or attempted to initiate an operation (even if it was foiled in execution) versus plots (defined as attacks that were aspirational or being contemplated but never actually attempted). Actual acts were chosen because they provide more tangible and quantifiable evidence than do plots in which the seriousness of the suspect's targeting choices is often unclear. Moreover, almost all lone-actor plots available in the public record were disrupted by law enforcement, often through the use of informant and sting operations. In many of these cases, the actors were not intending to act alone, making it unclear whether their target preferences were derived from their interpretation of ideologies versus being influenced by or trying to impress undercover operatives.

The primary aim of this chapter is to identify changes in jihadist lone-actor attack patterns conducted in the United States since the rise of ISIS. However, in order to provide wider context and comparison, it will also analyze the geography of lone-actor jihadist attacks in Europe and attacks by lone-actor right-wing extremists in the United States. Right-wing extremism was chosen because it has been more prevalent than left-wing extremism since the 1990s,[28] and its increase has thus roughly paralleled that of jihadist extremism (according to an FBI study of lone-actor attackers between 1972 and 2015, 54% followed ideologies that fall under right-wing extremism, as defined in this article, versus 8% following discernibly liberal ideologies).[29] This approach allows for both a *within* ideology (jihadist) comparison between different places (United States and Western Europe) and *between* ideologies (jihadist and right-wing extremism) in the same place (United States).

For this study jihadist lone actors are defined, in line with the FBI, as individuals adhering to "ideologies that justified the use of force or violence to perceived threats to Islamic nations, societies, or values"; who sought to engage in violent jihad; or who expressed support for, were inspired by, or claimed affiliation with foreign terrorist organizations such as al-Qaeda or ISIS but were not following any direction or instruction from a foreign terrorist organization to carry out their attack. Also included were offenders who attempted "to use violence as retaliation for US military action against Muslim nations or groups overseas."[30]

The third category we explore in this chapter is US right-wing lone-actor attacks. Right-wing extremists (or terrorists) can be categorized in several ways. This chapter follows a definition similar to that employed by geographers Webb and Cutter,[31] which closely aligns with the FBI's definition of right-wing extremism. This defines a terrorist as someone who adheres to a "single issue," a person with a "focus on a particular issue or agenda"[32] including white nationalism, white supremacy, neo-Nazi, or anti-abortion.

Past studies of terrorist geography[33,34] largely excluded right-wing extremist terrorism,[35] particularly white nationalist and white supremacist variants.[36,37] Moreover, as Webb and Cutter point out, "The rebirth of right-wing 'hate groups' in the 1990s, which received significant media attention at the time, actually resulted in relatively few recorded incidents. The apparent discrepancy between rhetoric and action or 'propaganda by deed' suggests either these groups were merely vocalizing their sentiments rather than acting on them or conversely, law enforcement penetration of such hate groups thwarted action. Either way, there is an interesting story to be told vis-á-vis such hate groups."[38] Today the story has changed, and it has become even more important to understand it. In fact, lone-actor attacks from white nationalist/supremacist groups and individual ideological adherents have risen dramatically, thus providing a sizeable sample for comparison. Evidence also suggests that while lone-actor white supremacist and right-wing attacks are on the rise, these lone actors belong to a "like-minded online pack,"[39] which may also be contributing to a vernacularization of their attack geographies.

Terrorists use geography (places and spaces) differently, places that Alexander Murphy calls "activity spaces."[40] Activity-space approaches have proved useful in analyzing the spatial patterns of target types and locations.[41,42] For this chapter, three categories of activity places/spaces will be utilized: "places" (target locations or locales) refer to actual geographical locations (i.e., localities such as metro-areas, cities, and towns), "spaces" (target spaces) refer to the type of area targeted (i.e., public, religious, private, etc.), and "target types" refer to the specific object attacked (i.e., a military base, church, etc.). In each of these activity places/spaces, specific subcategories will be designated. Within the space categories, the following specific designators are used: public (any place where citizens gather for leisure or business or daily life such as malls, streets, bars, concerts, etc.), workplace (businesses where the attacker is or was employed), religious (any space where worshippers gather), government/military (areas owned or used by government, military, or law enforcement), and transportation (airports, bus stations, subways, etc.).

Individuals can also be specific targets (by this we mean persons who were specifically singled out as targets and attacked or threatened execution-style, rather than people who happened to be inside a targeted space such as a government building, crowded street, mall, metro station, etc.). Two types of individuals are designated: symbolic (police/security officers, military personnel, political, and media figures—in other words individuals targeted specifically because of who they are or what they represent) and non-symbolic (such as ordinary citizens or persons with personal connections to the attacker, such as family, friends, and co-workers). In some cases, space and place categories do not necessarily match (for instance, an individual military member could be the target but was attacked in a public space such as a street versus in a government/military space). The number of spaces, targets, and weapons types may be greater than the number of incidents since some involved attacks against multiple spaces and targets using multiple weapons (such as an actor employing firearms

and explosives in several places and/or over several days against numerous targets).

The data used in this study are based on that gathered in previous research[43,44] and updated through a review of media reporting, government documents (including court documents), and scholarly literature. It was crossed-checked and compared with datasets and geographic analyses compiled by other scholars, particularly Kurzman,[45] Johnston,[46] GW Extremism Tracker,[47] European Union Terrorism and Trend Reports,[48] Nesser,[49] Cutter and Webb,[50] Nunn,[51] Southern Poverty Law,[52] and START: Global Terrorism Data Base at the University of Maryland.[53]

US JIHADISTS

Target Places

From 1980 through 2018, there were 38 jihadist lone-actor attacks in the United States (11 pre-2013 and 27 post). They occurred in 27 different localities, and only 6 of them (New York-Northern New Jersey; Seattle; Washington, DC; Philadelphia; Columbus; and Minneapolis-St. Paul) were attacked more than once. Only New York, which had six incidents, and Seattle, which had four (two of which were by the same perpetrator), had more than two incidents. These are also the only two localities that were attacked both pre- and post-2013. Nine localities were attacked prior to 2013 but 27 afterward. Nine states were struck through 2013, and 22 since 2013. Five states (New York, Washington, Virginia, California, and Florida) experienced attacks pre- and post-2013. Thus, there has been a dynamic continuity in the spatial pattern of attacks with a few clusters such as New York, on one hand, and then a more random distribution, on the other. As the number of attacks increased since 2013, the breadth of their distribution correspondingly increased.

Target Spaces and Types

While there has been dynamic continuity in the geographic pattern of places attacked over time, there has been a significant shift in target spaces and types since 2013. Prior to 2013, there were only four attacks on public spaces and single attacks on a public non-symbolic target (a quad at the University of North Carolina-Chapel Hill) and a private space/business (a financial building in Tampa, Florida). Government and military spaces and targets were hit most often, with federal and military spaces attacked five times and specific government or military targets struck six times.

Furthermore, military members were targeted in two of the five instances in which individuals were singled out for attack. The other three involved one on the police and two on Jewish figures. No non-symbolic civilian individuals were targeted. Thus, prior to 2013, the target spaces and types preferred by lone actors were largely consistent with the general jihadist preferences for military/government, transportation hubs, and Jewish-affiliated spaces.

Since 2013, there was a sharp jump in attacks in or on public spaces (17) to include eight streets and roads (whether against pedestrians or persons in vehicles), four private residences, four transportation spaces, one workplace, and one federal government/military space. Public targets included four colleges and schools, two restaurants and nightclubs, two malls, and one bike path. Three transportation facilities were directly targeted (one airport, one subway station, and one bus station) and one military recruiting station. Individuals were specifically targeted 13 times and in four instances they involved random non-symbolic citizens. In three cases persons were known to the attacker, and in six cases they were symbolic individuals (including five incidents against police/security personnel and one threat against individual military members).

Attack Methods and Impacts

In terms of physical impact, on the surface it appears that lone-actor jihadists have become deadlier. After 2013, 80 persons were killed and 114 wounded as compared to 38 killed and 20 wounded prior to that time. This higher total, however, can be accounted for by an increased frequency of attacks. The deadliness of attacks actually decreased slightly from to 2.7 fatalities per attack post-2013 from 3.5 prior to 2013. With the exception of two attacks, the 2009 Fort Hood attack and 2016 Orlando nightclub attack, which account for 78 or 63% of the total fatalities inflicted on the United States by lone-actor jihadists, the overall impact of these attacks has remained small.

Prior to 2012, firearms were used in 8 of 11 incidents and accounted for all fatalities. Vehicles were used three times as weapons (two automobiles and one light aircraft). From 2013 to 2018, firearms remained the most commonly used weapon but with edged weapons a close second (10 and 8, respectively). Vehicles were utilized in two incidents. Explosives were employed in three incidents producing no fatalities. Firearms produced 76% of fatalities (61).

EUROPEAN JIHADISTS

Target Places

Before 2013, there were few lone-actor jihadist attacks in Europe. As in the United States, they were broadly distributed spatially, with 12 incidents occurring in 12 different cities and 7 different countries. Three occurred in the United Kingdom; Italy, Germany, and Denmark had two attacks each. Between 2013 and 2018, there were 38 incidents in 10 countries and 28 localities. Similarly, the distribution of attacks in the United States widened and became more random but with a few discernable and national clusters. Five countries were struck multiple times, with France bearing the most (18 attacks). The United Kingdom and Germany each had five attacks, Belgium had four, and the Netherlands had two. Paris and London were the most targeted localities with seven and four incidents apiece, respectively. Brussels and Nice were the only other localities to experience multiple attacks at two each.

Targets Spaces and Types

Pre-2013 target selection and spaces were quite different in Europe than in the United States. Seven occurred in public spaces, two in religious spaces, and two in private spaces. Individuals figured more prominently, with five incidents against specific symbolic individual targets (three cartoonists and artists, one parliamentarian, and several soldiers). Non-symbolic civilian targets were targeted five times (eating establishments, crowds in streets). Two Jewish institutions were also specifically targeted and one US military bus.

After 2013, the majority of incidents also occurred in public spaces (25) followed by transport spaces (6) and military and government spaces (6). Symbolic individuals remained the primary target (17). However, there was a significant shift in focus from media and political figures to government ones. Police and security officers were singled out 17 times and military personnel (performing policing duties) twice. Public/civilian targets, such as crowds, shops, and pedestrians, were the second most prominent target category (12). Transportation targets included train and metro stations and cars (7). Jewish institutions were attacked three times.

Attack Methods and Impacts

The absolute death toll and deadliness exacted by lone actors increased dramatically from 2013 through 2018 with 155 persons killed, for an average of four fatalities per incident. However, 55% of fatalities were the result of the Nice Bastille Day vehicle ramming attack (86 persons were killed). Prior to 2013, lone actors had killed only 10 persons (1.2 fatalities per attack), with one incident (the Toulouse/Montaubon shootings of 2012) accounting for 70% of deaths.

Prior to 2013, explosives were used in six incidents (albeit killing no one), edged weapons in three (also producing no fatalities), and firearms in three incidents. Between 2013 and 2018, edged weapons (and a hammer) were employed in 24 incidents and firearms in 7. Vehicles were used in seven incidents and accounted for nearly 75% of fatalities. Explosives were used the least—in only five incidents (still producing few fatalities).

US RIGHT-WING EXTREMISTS

Target Places

From 1980 through 2019, there were 55 right-wing lone-actor attacks in the United States (22 pre- and 33 post-2013). Post-2013, the attacks occurred each in a different city. Five states had multiple attacks (California, Texas, Kansas, Florida, and Oregon). Pre-2013, 14 different cities were attacked, while post-2013 there were 33 different localities. Pre-2013, 14 states were attacked, while post-2013 there were attacks in 23 states. Four states were attacked both pre- and post-2013: Florida, Kansas, Colorado, and New York. The attack distribution, like the Jihadist attacks post-2013, was more random, dispersed, and less clustered than pre-2013. Moreover, the number of overall attacks has quadrupled, and the geographic breadth has widened, too.

Target Spaces and Types

Prior to 2013, all attacks were in public spaces and the majority of target spaces were abortion clinics and civil rights leaders or symbolic targets. Eight attacks were against symbolic individuals in public spaces. The majority of the attacks were in southern states (10 out of 18 of the attacks). Prior to 1980, all of the right-wing extremist attacks were in the South.

Before 2013, all of the attacks were symbolic in nature—both individual, public, and private—meaning that no attacks were against non-symbolic spaces or individuals. There were only two attacks on government sites, which were also the only two attacks during this period (actually from 1951 to 2013) that were not religious or race-related. There were 26 total attacks from 1951 to 2013, whereas in the five subsequent years (from 2013 to 2019) there were 33 attacks. That is an increase of 4.25 times more attacks per year between 2013 and 2018 compared to between 1980 and 2013. This fourfold increase in attacks over the past 5 years and the corresponding diversity of locale and attack types clearly indicates a shift in behavior among lone-actor right-wing extremist terrorists. Post-2013, there were attacks on five religious sites (mosques and/or synagogues), seven government sites, three schools, and four transportation/highway sites (one highway, two with vehicles and two on trains). Five attacks were private, with three of these occurring after 2017.

After 2013, there were nine attacks against individuals, of which eight of these were symbolic targets including four for race, two police/government, one for religious, and one for sexual orientation. Right-wing extremists who are also white nationalists appear to choose primarily symbolic targets, whether individual or in public spaces, focusing on a specific grievance seemingly fueled by online social media or news sites.[54]

Attack Method and Impacts

Out of 20 pre-2013 (since 1980) attacks, 11 were committed with explosives and 9 with firearms. Out of the 20 attacks, 7 left more than 10 people injured or killed. After 2013, the majority of attacks were with small arms/weapons/firearms (26 out of 33), four were with vehicles, five used a knife, two committed arson, and only one used explosives (four of the attacks used more than one method). Clearly, attack weapons and targets have shifted toward those that are more easily accessible.

There were 1,095 total casualties (193 killed, 902 wounded) between 1980 and 2012. Post-2013 casualties totaled 236 (114 killed and 122 injured). Average fatalities increased from 6 per year between 1980 and 2012 to 21 per year between 2013 and 2019. This increase in fatalities is explained by the overall increase in attacks. Conversely, attacks themselves have become less deadly, with 10 or more people being killed or injured in only three of the attacks. The majority of attacks resulted in only one or two dead and/or injured per occurrence (20 attacks had 0–2 fatalities, and 21 attacks had between 0 and 2 injured).

Thus, attacks have become more frequent and widespread but less deadly.

SUMMARY OF FINDINGS

Between 2013 and the rise of ISIS and 2019, there have been five clear and notable changes in the trends of the attack geography of US lone-actor jihadists. Four of these changes appear to be accelerations of the trends and features exhibited in pre-2013 attacks that are also seen in US right-wing extremist and European jihadist attack patterns. There is a fifth trend that is highly specific to US jihadists. First, lone-actor attacks have become more frequent. Consequently, total casualties have increased (e.g., as in deaths per year), and lone actors now have demonstrated the ability to execute mass casualty events. However, on average, the deadliness and physical impact of individual attacks has not increased significantly. Second, explosive use by all three groups declined, while firearms and expedient weapons were the most commonly employed. Third, the geographic location of lone-actor jihadist attacks was more dispersed (although some cities such as New York and Seattle remained as clusters), as was the case with European jihadists and US right-wing lone actors. Fourth, there has been a significant shift toward public and individual target types and spaces, as was the case with European jihadist and US right-wing attackers. While there has been variation in the types of individuals targeted between the groups, targeting of police officers has increased all around. Fifth, US lone jihadists have exhibited a strong preference for non-symbolic targets and thus a higher degree of vernacularization. This is a significant departure from the previous patterns, as well as from their domestic right-wing and European jihadist counterparts who still prefer symbolic targets (despite some shifts in target space and types differing from the pre-2013 era).

One outstanding question that has emerged since the start of this project is whether disruptions in the security environment, particularly the COVID pandemic and domestic political unrest in the US surrounding the 2020 election, will prove to be a 2013-type inflection point and spur a shift in US lone-actor jihadist attack geography. As of final draft submission, full 2020 data were not available; however, although attacks were fewer, there seems to have been no significant departure in the geographic pattern of US lone-actor jihadist attacks from the prevailing post-2012 pattern despite an expansion of domestic right-wing attacks and targeting.

Recent events in the United States, including the attack on the US Capitol on January 6, 2021, point to an increase and broadening of "ideologically inspired" (as opposed to belonging to a defined group), non-jihadist lone actors. Out of the 257 currently known arrested participants in the attack, 142 were ideologically inspired.[55] They acted alone as they attended the event, but they joined a group once they arrived. The majority of the attackers also appear to have been radicalized, often in a matter of weeks, attaching themselves to various conspiracy theories.[56] These actors were from highly dispersed locations throughout the United States, coming from more than 180 counties.[57] As law enforcement shuts down or enforces restrictions on the social media platforms through which such attacks were coordinated, there is a likelihood that lone-actor attacks will increase since access to organized group attacks will become more difficult.[58] At present, targets appear to be particularly focused on government officials or those tied to them in some way and/or government buildings.[59] The targeting novelty here is the increased interest in legislative and non-federal local and state government targets beyond police. Overall, this points to a high likelihood of an increase in both individual attacks based on online messaging that inspires non-jihadist US lone attackers as well as on a continuing dispersion of attack methods and geographies.

Cases from 2020 strongly suggests a drop in both overall US and European jihadist lone-actor attack frequency but consistency in targeting patterns and methods. In Europe, lone-actor jihadist attacks were also fewer in previous years, though more numerous than in United States, and appeared to follow their prevailing patterns of weapon choice and target geography. For example, in Paris, a teacher was stabbed and beheaded in a street for allegedly showing cartoons of the Prophet Mohammed, while in another incident two persons were stabbed outside the offices of the magazine *Charlie Hebdo*. Three persons were stabbed outside church in Nice, France. Elsewhere in Europe, four persons were randomly targeted, shot, and killed in a public square and street (near a Jewish monument) in Vienna, Austria; two gay men were stabbed in Dresden, Germany; three persons were killed and another three wounded in a knife attack in a public garden in Reading, United Kingdom.

Data compiled by the New America Foundation show only two lone-actor jihadist attacks that produced fatalities in the United States during 2020 (in both cases the attackers were the casualties).[60] The first involved an attempted vehicle ramming at a Naval Air Station in Corpus Christi, Texas, in May, in which the suspect, allegedly inspired by al-Qaeda in the Arabic Peninsula (AQAP), was shot and killed by security forces. Also in May, a suspect, allegedly inspired by ISIS, was shot and killed while threatening police officers with a knife in Temple Terrace, Florida. In June 2021, a suspect was shot and injured after stabbing and wounding a New York City police officer with a knife. Although authorities allege the suspect was an Islamist extremist inspired by ISIS, the evidence appears inconclusive at this time.[61] At this time, the data do not indicate that jihadist lone actors have adopted an interest in state and local government targets.

The cumulative increase in attack numbers since 2013, the widened geographical dispersion of the attacks, and the prominence of everyday weapons indicate that a macro-scale vernacularization of lone-actor target geography has occurred across regions and ideologies. However, this localized everyday pattern also manifests itself differently at the meso, micro, and individual levels between regions and groups, which indicates that both ideology and place-specific factors combine to impact target selection in different areas. The final section highlights the main implications of these findings.

CONCLUSION

In an immediate practical and operational sense, the vernacularization of lone-actor attacks means that more places and spaces are at risk. The dispersion and profusion of target places, spaces, and types makes it difficult to allocate and concentrate resources and harden targets, especially since the level of risk in any single place is relatively low. Thus, the role of local communities, law enforcement, and emergency management agencies in preventing, preparing for, responding to, and recovering from attacks has and must increase in importance.

More broadly and long-term, this raises several questions and challenges for future research and policy-making, which fall into three main categories: First, what macro factors and trends (i.e., ideology, spread of social media, security measures) are accounting for the general vernacularization and dispersion of lone-actor attacks? How might these trends influence future attack patterns and preferences? Will these trends be reinforced or not by the recent revival of left-wing extremism[62] and rise of what the FBI calls "idiosyncratic" ideologies?[63]

Second, why do actors with similar ideologies or national origins exhibit different geographic targeting preferences (e.g., lone-actor jihadists surged post-2013 and were predominately influenced by ISIS, yet attack patterns differed between Europe and the United States)? How do various factors, such as virtual geographic proximity and ideological online media spaces, and individual grievances combine at different spatial scales to influence terrorist's spatial perception and target preferences?

Third, how can (or if) the answers of these questions be used to assess risk and vulnerability and inform strategic (macro) and local-level policy responses and countermeasures? These questions underscore the need for more monitoring of and research into terrorist attack geography as well as an increased relevance of geographically focused terrorism research in order to broaden understanding of terrorism and support policy-making and planning.

NOTES AND REFERENCES

1. Jasparro C. Place still matters: The operational geography of jihadist terror attacks against the US Homeland 1990–2012. *Dynamics Asymmetric Conflict.* 2013:1–17.
2. Jasparro C. Lone wolf: The threat from independent jihadists. *Jane's Intelligence Rev.* Dec 9, 2010.
3. Jasparro C. Sociocultural, economic, and demographic aspects of counterterrorism. In Forest J, ed. Countering Terrorism and Insurgency in the 21st Century. Vol. 2. Westport, CT: Praeger Security International; 2007:420–452.
4. Levi-Sanchez S. San Francisco State University (SFSU) and California State University (CSU) Online, "Introduction to Terrorism and the Problem of Definitions" [Module One—Prezi Course Material]. *In IR351/CJ461: Terrorism and Covert Political Warfare: Spring 2017*: https://tinyurl.com/yckkmkpf
5. Levi-Sanchez S. SFSU and CSU Online, "Terror in History." [Module Two—Prezi Course Material]. *In IR351/CJ461: Terrorism and Covert Political Warfare: Spring 2017*: https://tinyurl.com/ycknjvhx
6. Levi-Sanchez S. SFSU and CSU Online, "Terror in the Name of God Part I, II, III." [Modules Eight through Ten- Prezi Course Material]. *In IR351/CJ461: Terrorism and Covert Political Warfare: Spring 2017*: Part I: https://tinyurl.com/5n7mysrz; Part II: https://tinyurl.com/37xd87kw; Part III: https://tinyurl.com/yckkwdk6
7. Levi-Sanchez S. SFSU and CSU Online, "Suicide Terrorism." [Module Eleven—Prezi Course Material]. *In IR351/CJ461: Terrorism and Covert Political Warfare: Spring 2017*: https://tinyurl.com/295whbsw

8. Jasparro. Place still matters, 50, 55.
9. Ibid., 49.
10. Ibid., 50.
11. Ibid., 49.
12. Jasparro. Lone Wolf.
13. Jackson JB. *Discovering the Vernacular Landscape.* New Haven, CT: Yale University Press; 1984:150.
14. Liem M, van Buuren J, de Roy van Zuijdewijn J, Hanneke S, Bakker E. European lone actor terrorists versus "common" homicide offenders: An empirical analysis. *Homicide Stud.* 2018;22:45–69.
15. Quillen C. A historical analysis of mass casualty bombers. *Stud Conflict Terrorism.*2002;25:279–292.
16. Bahgat K, Medina R. An overview of geographical perspectives and approaches in terrorism research. *Perspect Terrorism.* 2013;7:38.
17. Braithwaite A, Li Q. Transnational terrorism hotspots: Identification and impact evaluation. *Conflict Manage Peace Sc.* 2007;24:281.
18. Nunn S. Incidents of terrorism in the United States. *Geographical Rev.* 2007;97:89.
19. Webb J, Cutter S. The geography of US terrorist incidents, 1970–2004. *Terrorism Political Violence.* 2009;21(3):429.
20. Jasparro C. Sociocultural, economic, and demographic aspects of counterterrorism. In Forest J, ed. Countering Terrorism and Insurgency in the 21st Century. Vol. 2. Westport, CT: Praeger Security International; 2007:422.
21. Hastings J. Geography, globalization, and terrorism: The plots of Jemaah Islamiyah. *Security Stud.* 2008;17:505–530.
22. Nunn. Incidents of terrorism in the United States.
23. Murphey A. The space of terror. In Cutter S, Richardson D, Wilbanks T, eds., *The Geographical Dimension of Terrorism.* New York: Routledge; 2003:47.
24. Jasparro. Place still matters, 55.
25. Webb, Cutter. The geography of US terrorist incidents, 430.
    a. Bahgat K, Medina R. An overview of geographical perspectives and approaches in terrorism research. *Perspect Terrorism.* 2013;7:38,59.
26. Webb, Cutter. The geography of US terrorist incidents, 430.
27. Bugajski J. The future of American terrorism. *The Hill*, 11 Aug 2019. https://thehill.com/opinion/national-security/456974-the-future-of-american-terrorism
28. Richards L, Molinaro P, Wyman J, Craun S. Lone offender: A study of lone offender terrorism in the United States (1972–2015). Nov 2019. https://www.fbi.gov/file-repository/lone-offender-terrorism-report-111319.pdf/view
29. Ibid.
30. Webb, Cutter. The geography of US terrorist incidents, 430.
31. "Although FBI uses the term 'Special-Interest' to classify terrorist groups who focus on a particular issue or agenda, we felt the term 'Single-Issue' is more appropriate. Recognizing that single-issue terrorism can be viewed as left-wing (animal rights and environmental groups) and right-wing (anti-abortion related) terrorism, Monaghan argues that the classification of special interest 'is not only over simplistic but it also detracts from the uniqueness of single-issue terrorism.'" Webb, Cutter S. The geography of US terrorist incidents, 443–444.
32. Ibid., 430.
33. Johnston W. Terrorist attacks and related incidents in the United States. 2019. http://www.johnstonsarchive.net/terrorism/wrjp255a.html
34. Webb, Cutter. The geography of US terrorist incidents, 436.
35. A report from the Center on Extremism: Murder and extremism in the United States in 2018. *The Anti-Defamation League*, Jan 2019. https://www.adl.org/media/12480/download
36. Far right terrorists aren't lone wolves. *Politico*, 9 Aug 2019. https://www.politico.eu/article/far-right-terrorists-not-lone-wolves-white-supremacy-racism-crime/
37. Webb, Cutter. The geography of US terrorist incidents, 436.
38. Diep F. A look into the evidence that 'lone wolf' terrorists are a pack. *Pacific Standard*, 29 Oct 2018. https://psmag.com/news/a-look-into-the-evidence-that-lone-wolf-terrorists-are-a-pack
39. Murphey A. The space of terror. In Cutter S, Richardson D, Wilbanks T, eds., *The Geographical Dimension of Terrorism.* New York: Routledge; 2003:47.
40. Jasparro. Place still matters
41. Nunn. Incidents of terrorism in the United States, 89–111.
42. Jasparro. Place still matters, 59–61.
43. Jasparro. Lone wolf.
44. Kurzman C. Muslim American involvement with violent extremism. 2019. https://sites.duke.edu/tcths/files/2019/01/2018_Kurzman_Muslim-American_Involvement_with_Violent_Extremism.pdf
45. Johnston W. Terrorist attacks and related incidents in the United States. 2019. http://www.johnstonsarchive.net/terrorism/wrjp255a.html
46. GW Extremism Tracker: Terrorism in the US. Program on Extremism. George Washington University. 2019. https://extremism.gwu.edu/gw-extremism-tracker
47. European Union Terrorism and Trend Reports. EUROPOL. 2019. https://www.europol.europa.eu/activities-services/main-reports
48. Nesser P. Individual jihadist operations in Europe: Patterns and challenges. *CTC Sentinel*, Jan 2012;5:14–17. https://ctc.usma.edu/individual-jihadist-operations-in-europe-patterns-and-challenges/
49. Webb, Cutter. The geography of US terrorist incidents, 428–449.

50. Nunn. Incidents of terrorism in the United States, 89–109.

51. Southern Poverty Law Center. Terror from the right: Archives. 2013. https://www.splcenter.org/terror-from-the-right-archives#2013

52. START: Global Terrorism Database. 2019. https://www.start.umd.edu/gtd/search/Results.aspx?page=3&casualties_type=&casualties_max=&country=217&expanded=no&charttype=line&chart=overtime&ob=GTDID&od=desc#results-table

53. Levi-Sanchez S, Toupin S. New social media and global resistance. In Shepard L, ed., *Gender Matters: A Feminist Introduction to International Relations*. London: Routledge; 2015:389–401.

54. This is our house: A preliminary assessment of the Capital Hill siege participants. Program on Extremism. George Washington University. Mar 2021:18. https://extremism.gwu.edu/sites/g/files/zaxdzs2191/f/This-Is-Our-House.pdf

55. Jensen M, Kane S. START Research Brief. University of Maryland. Feb 2021:1–3. https://www.start.umd.edu/pubs/START_PIRUS_QAnon_Feb2021_0.pdf

56. This is our house, 12–15.

57. MacFarquhar N. Far-right groups are splintering in wake of the Capitol Riot. New York Times, 3 Mar 2021. https://www.nytimes.com/2021/03/01/us/extremism-capitol-riot.html

58. Ibid.

59. Sterman D, Bergen P, Salyk-Virk M. Terrorism in America 19 years after 9/11 Sep 2020. https://www.newamerica.org/international-security/reports/terrorism-america-19-years-after-911/the-threat-at-home/

60. Bosnian national charged with robbery and firearms offenses in connection with attack on New York City police officers. 26 Aug 2020. https://www.justice.gov/opa/pr/bosnian-national-charged-robbery-and-firearms-offenses-connection-attack-new-york-city-police

61. Bugajski. The future of American Terrorism.

62. Richards et al. Lone offender.

12

Means, Mechanisms, and Trends
of Operationalizing Violence

CHRISTOPHER WINTER, RAMÓN SPAAIJ, AND MARILYN PRICE

INTRODUCTION

It is widely believed that lone actors present particular challenges to authorities due to the hidden and often "doing-yourself-in" nature of their operations.[1] In reality, the very nature of their (relative) loneness means that they face significant obstacles in turning extremist belief and intent into violent action. Comprehensive preparation and planning is a key element in launching a successful terrorist attack.[2] However, lone actors often face a disconnect between intention and capability, and this is particularly true in the procurement of weapons and training in their usage.[3] This disconnect tends to inform the lone actors' choice of targets and weapons. However, we also know that lone actors can be creative and learn to hone their skills at operationalizing violence.[4]

This chapter critically examines what is currently known about the operationalization of lone-actor terrorism, with a focus on the means and methods used to translate extremist beliefs into violent action. We first discuss the current state of scientific knowledge on the subject. This is followed by an examination of the international context based on an analysis of the Lone Actor Terrorism Micro-Sociological Database compiled by the first author. We then examine trends that are specific to the US context through an analysis of the American Lone Wolf Terrorism Database.[5] We interpret these findings in relation to current US gun legislation. In the final section, we draw together the main findings and propose some directions for future research, policy, and practice.

CURRENT STATE OF SCIENTIFIC KNOWLEDGE

In 2009, before the rise of the Islamic State of Iraq and al-Sham (ISIS) and its call for individuals to undertake violence, before the infamous July 22, 2011, attacks in Norway, and before the current "wave" of lone actor terrorist violence, Freilich and Chermak called on terrorism researchers to explore the specifics of the terrorist attack rather than narrowly focusing on the individual themselves.[6] Put differently, research on lone actors had to go beyond a narrow focus on the violent individual to their means and methods. With the rise and proliferation of lone-actor terrorism as a tactic, this has become an urgent concern. Fortunately, a decade later, significantly more is known about how lone actors perform their violence.

Generally, lone actors are considered to be less capable than group-based terrorists. In comparison, the lone actor has more limited access to sophisticated weapons, a lesser ability to conduct intelligence collection and reconnaissance, and a general inability to perform particularly complex operations due to their solo nature.[7] However, despite perceptions of lone actors as being unstable and volatile individuals, they are rarely impulsive in their violence, often planning and preparing for their attacks.[8] Anders Behring Breivik's attacks in Norway in 2011 are an example of the meticulous and thorough planning process lone actors can undergo in preparing for an attack. Breivik is not unique in this regard, with other lone actors spending months and even years in planning and gathering materials for their attacks.[9] However, lone actors are not an amorphous grouping, with significant variance shown across the population. Some individuals are emotionally volatile and rapidly enact violence after some triggering event. This results in an attack being conducted with little to no prior preparation with whatever weapons are at hand.[10] Alternatively, some lone actors, despite having undertaken significant levels of preparation, impulsively undertake an attack with only a portion of their collected arsenal.[11]

To understand how and why lone actors choose and use the weapons they do, it is thus important to consider the wider situational and societal context that lone actors operate in. *Situational crime prevention* (SCP) does exactly this. According to SCP, a lone actor will rationally assess what targets, weapons, tools, and other facilitating conditions are present for an attack—the "four pillars of terrorist opportunity."[12] Specifically, a lone actor will seek weapons that are multipurpose, undetectable, removable, destructive, enjoyable, reliable, obtainable, uncomplicated, and safe— or "MURDEROUS."[12] Put differently, lone actors are calculating and rational actors who will seek to maximize the impact of their attacks given their available resources and skills. However, as explored later in this chapter, for some lone actors, obtaining weapons can become more than a rational and utilitarian desire, instead being a symptom and operationalization of their revenge fantasies.

The social geography in which a lone actor operates is a key element in determining what kinds of weapons they will find to be accessible.[9] Lone actors will often use weapons they already possess, with one study finding that only 47% of lone actors specifically sourced a firearm for an attack.[9] This has meant that lone actors in the United States have used firearms at a higher rate than their international counterparts, owing largely to the widespread accessibility and legality of guns.[4,13] In other countries, access to firearms is more limited by gun legislation. This forces lone actors to seek other, more accessible weapons. For example, lone actor attacks in Israel see a particularly high usage of vehicles as weapons. Most of the time, the car used by the attacker was their own, again demonstrating the tendency to use what is familiar and at hand.[14] *Melee weapons* also tend to be readily accessible, often being simple kitchen knives. Explosives remain attractive to lone actors for their destructive and visceral potential. However, explosives are inherently difficult to use, both in terms of sourcing

the components and in the technical challenge of creating a working device. Indeed, one study found that only 45% of lone-actor explosive plots led to an attack, contrasting significantly to 100% of firearm plots and 92% of bladed-weapon plots resulting in an attack.[13]

Beyond access, lone actors prefer weapons that they are familiar with, perhaps through use or exposure in daily life. Indeed, governments are now facing the threat of battle-hardened returnees from the conflicts in Syria and Iraq. These individuals are threats not just because they may be ideologically inclined to carry out violence, but also because of their practical experience with handling weaponry. Familiarity also functions in the sense that other attackers have demonstrated the harmful potential of a weapon. These attacks become exemplars for others, leading to a string of copycat attacks that often resemble the initial attack. This mimetic quality can be seen in the aftermath of the 2019 Christchurch mosque shooting, which saw a series of mass shootings, with the perpetrators of these citing the mosque shooting and its perpetrator as a direct inspiration.[15] These attacks, despite being in different countries, all used similar models of firearms.

As noted earlier, the scientific literature indicates that lone actors have some distinct operational disadvantages due to their solitary nature. Research has noted the importance of social and organizational links in emotionally supporting the performance of violence, with Alakoc's comparative study of lone-actor and group-directed suicide attacks finding the latter to be more lethal.[16] Crucially, he partially ascribes this lethality to the emotional peer support shared by group-based terrorists. This social support allows attackers to be more concentrated, less fearful, and less nervous in the conduct of a terrorist operation. The impact of these inhibitors (among others) can be seen in the generally lower lethality rate ascribed to lone actors.[4]

Despite these relative weaknesses, the lone actor's capabilities seem to have little influence on how targets are selected. Somewhat paradoxically, lone actors are not necessarily inhibited by security measures around a target or the actual capabilities of the individual. Gill and Corner found that, overall, lone-actor target choice had little to do with capabilities or planning.[17] Hemmingby found that while both group-based and lone European Islamist perpetrators overwhelmingly preferred soft targets, lone actors were more than twice as likely to attack a hardened target.[18] Indeed, for many lone actors, the ideological or symbolic value of a target is a priority. Hamm and Spaaij found that, in the US, police and military officers had become the preferred target for lone actors.[19] Outside of the US, security forces have been targeted by lone actors. As a result of the long-running *Operation Sentinelle*, thousands of French soldiers have patrolled public spaces across the country with the intent of hardening these spaces against potential attacks. However, this means that French soldiers have become an easily accessible target for French lone actors. That security forces are frequently targeted despite being comparatively well-armed and trained to deal with an armed assailant speaks to the performative and symbolic importance of target selection to the lone actor.

INTERNATIONAL CONTEXT AND DATASET

Though the concept of lone-actor (or "lone-wolf") terrorism emerged in the United States during the mid-1990s amid a heightened threat of far-right violence,[20] individuals from around the globe have conducted politically motivated violence for some time. The example of the Russian noblewoman Vera Zazulich is an example of the lingering relevance of the lone-actor terrorist. During a crackdown on student activists in 1870s Imperial Russia, Zazulich resolved to kill the regional governor. Approaching him during his public audience hours, she pulled a pistol from her clothing and shot the governor, injuring him.[21] One hundred thirty-nine years later, Thomas Mair approached a British Member of Parliament, Jo Cox, as she left a local library in West Yorkshire after conducting a public audience. Like Zazulich, Mair drew a firearm and shot his target a point-blank range, though Mair killed Cox after shooting and stabbing her.

Outside of the United States, lone-actor terrorist attacks have ranged from sophisticated and carefully planned operations to simplistic acts of violence using only the most rudimentary weapons, often sourced from the household. In the former category, the 2011 Norway attacks are an exemplar. After a years-long period of preparation that saw Breivik develop a massive fertilizer bomb, prepare a disguise, and (legally) purchase several firearms, he bombed a government building in central Oslo before travelling to Utoya Island. There, over 72 minutes, he methodically shot and killed dozens of teenagers and adults attending a summer camp. This multistage attack resulted in 77 deaths and more than 300 wounded.[22] Conversely, many lone-actor attacks

are much simpler. This is particularly true in Europe, where numerous attacks have been conducted with knives. The 2015 Leytonstone Station stabbing in London is an example of this kind of low-effort, low-sophistication attack. Armed with a blunt bread knife, Muhaydin Mire targeted commuters at a train station, cutting the throat of one man and injuring another two who intervened before he was incapacitated by police officers. During the attack, he shouted that he was doing this for his brothers in Syria.[23]

Capturing the diverse attack methods used by lone actors was one of the objectives in the creation of the Lone Actor Terrorism Micro-Sociological Database (LATMD) by the first author. Specifically, the dataset focused on confrontational attacks that required the attacker to share physical space with their targets. This dataset captures 148 such lone-actor attacks in 14 countries since September 11, 2001, to December 2018. (The dataset includes attacks in Australia, Belgium, Canada, Denmark, Finland, France, Germany, Italy, Norway, Spain, Sweden, The Netherlands, the United Kingdom and the United States.) During this period, 84 lone-actor attacks occurring in countries outside of the United States were identified. These attacks resulted in 91 fatalities and 336 injuries. It is believed that this represents the majority of lone-actor terrorist attacks carried out in these countries, though the process of identifying and classifying an incident as a lone-actor terrorist attack is a challenging and contentious task exacerbated around definitional difficulties.

Outside the United States, the most common weapon type used by lone actor terrorists are melee weapons, with 56% ($n = 47$) of attacks utilizing some form of an edged blade, hammer, or, in some rare cases, the attacker's fists. In 44% ($n = 37$) of attacks, melee weapons were the only weapon used in an attack. This reflects the low level of sophistication and limited capabilities of the attackers. The previously mentioned Leytonstone attack is a good example of how these attacks are typically conducted, with an attacker targeting vulnerable civilians in a stabbing spree before being incapacitated. Other such examples of this attack type include the 2017 Edeka supermarket stabbing in Hamburg and a series of knife attacks in Australia (including the 2018 Mill Park stabbing, the 2018 Bourke Street stabbing, and the 2016 Minto stabbing), as well as several similar attacks in France. Contrary to theories around targeting, which hypothesize that low-capability attackers will avoid hardened targets, security forces have regularly been the target of knife attacks, particularly in France. While this may seem counter-productive, as police officers and soldiers are well-armed and trained, they serve as readily available symbols of the state.[17]

Despite their ubiquity, melee attacks are associated with a low lethality rate. Attacks performed with melee weapons alone were responsible for only 5% of fatalities and 15.5% of injuries in the dataset ($n = 8$ and $n = 13$, respectively). These low numbers are unsurprising given the difficulty of using a melee weapon to kill another human, but they also speak to the relatively crude nature of many of these attacks. Indeed, many melee attacks involved the lone actor simply yelling and charging at armed security forces, almost invariably resulting in the attacker's death or capture after a short struggle.

After melee weapons, firearms are the most common weapon, being used in 38.1% of all non-US attacks in the database ($n = 32$). Firearms were typically the only weapon type used, though there was a higher rate of mixed weapon type usage when firearms were involved (29.8% firearm-only, 8.3% firearms alongside other weapons). In contrast to attacks that involve only melee weapons, firearms offer a much higher degree of tactical flexibility, resulting in a wider range of event types. Breivik's attack on Utoya Island is a particularly devastating example of what could be called a "rampage shooter" or "active shooter" who actively moves around an area, searching for and engaging targets. This type of attack has been particularly common in Canada, with the 2017 Moncton shootings in which three police officers were killed and two injured, the 2014 attack on the Canadian Parliament in which a Canadian soldier was killed and other police and security guards were injured, and the 2017 Quebec City Grand Mosque attack in which six worshippers were killed, with 19 more being injured. France and Belgium have also experienced similar attacks. In 2006, an 18-year-old Belgium white supremacist by the name of Hans Van Themsche purchased a .30-30 Marlin lever-action hunting rifle and then traveled to central Antwerp. He first shot a Turkish woman as she read a book on a park bench before shooting a Malian nanny and her 2-year-old ward. Van Themsche was then shot by a police officer. He had only purchased the rifle an hour before the attack.[24]

Firearms can also be used to effectively force hostage situations. The 2018 Trèbes supermarket siege is an example of the tactical possibilities offered by a gun. Armed with a pistol, Redouana

Lakdim shot several people and held a dozen more hostage in a supermarket in southern France. This resulted in a 4-hour-long stand-off during which Lakdim delivered various demands. French special forces finally stormed the building after a police colonel was shot and killed by Lakdim.[25] Three people were killed, along with a dozen wounded. Guns have also been used in hostage situations in Australia, with three such incidents occurring: the 2001 East Melbourne Fertility clinic attack, the 2014 Lindt Café siege in Sydney, and 2017 Brighton siege.

Firearms were the single most deadly weapon in non-US lone-actor attacks in the dataset. Attacks conducted with firearms (38.1% of attacks) were responsible for 70% and 55.8% of fatalities and injuries respectively ($n = 112$ and 249). These numbers are inflated by the 2011 Utoya Island attack, and, if this attack is excluded, attacks involving firearms were responsible for 47.3% and 41.4% of fatalities and injuries respectively ($n = 43$ and 139). Even when excluding this attack, firearms represent the deadliest type of weapon used by lone actors in an international context.

One notable element concerning firearms usage outside of the United States is the relative absence of "over-arming." This concept is more fully explored in the following section on American lone actors but, simply put, describes the tendency for some lone actors to amass large arsenals of firearms—more than could be used in a single attack. Indeed, the only example of over-arming (or the collection of more than two guns) in the dataset of non-US lone actors occurred in Canada. Richard Bain, the Canadian anglophile nationalist who attacked the Parti Québécois' 2012 electoral victory party in an attempt to kill the party's leader, used two guns: a CZ-858 semi-automatic rifle and a pistol. However, Bain also had brought another two CZ-858 rifles and another pistol with him, leaving them in his SUV.[26] Investigators later found 12 guns and more than 20,000 rounds of ammunition hidden around Bain's house.[27] That Bain operated in Canada, a country where there is a relatively high availability of firearms, is not inconsequential.

Vehicles are the third most common type of weapon, with 19% of non-US attacks involving the use of a vehicle as a ramming weapon ($n = 16$). After firearms, vehicles were the deadliest weapon. Attacks involving the use of a vehicle were responsible for 21.9% of all fatalities ($n = 35$). Notably, 41% of all injuries in the dataset were the result of attacks with vehicles ($n = 183$). Contrary to the other weapon categories, vehicles are often used in conjunction with other weapons, with 10.7% of all attacks involving only a vehicle and 8.3% of all attacks using a vehicle in conjunction with a firearm, melee weapon, or explosive device. One notable aspect is the relative recency of lone actors using vehicles as weapons (with the notable exception of Israel). Outside the United States and excluding Israel, vehicular attacks by lone-actor terrorists only appear in the dataset in 2014, with the Saint-Jean-sur-Richelieu ramming attack in which a Canadian man rammed two Canadian soldiers with a car, killing one.[28] After this attack, the use of vehicles as weapons by lone actors becomes increasingly common, with a large spike in 2017, when seven such attacks occurred. These findings are consistent with other studies that have observed the "virus-like" adoption of the vehicle as a weapon among terrorists in the West, where high-profile attacks using vehicles have served as inspiration for an "imitative wave" of copycats.[29] A similar "wave" was observed in Israel which, despite experiencing low but persistent rates of lone-actor vehicular attacks since 2000, saw a sudden increase in the use of vehicles, with 53.2% of all such attacks occurring in 2015.[14]

As noted earlier, vehicles represent readily accessible and familiar weapons. In the 2017 Flinders Street ramming attack in Melbourne, Australia, Saeed Noori drove through a busy pedestrian crossing in his mother's Suzuki SUV, killing 1 and injuring 15 others.[30] Similarly, in 2018, Salih Khater drove his Ford Fiesta through a group of cyclists to hit police officers stationed outside Westminster Palace in London, injuring four.[31] Other attackers have specifically sought access to larger and thus more potentially damaging vehicles, particularly in the aftermath of the devastating 2016 Nice truck attack in which 86 were killed and more than 400 wounded. In both the 2016 Berlin Christmas market ramming attack and the 2017 Stockholm ramming attack, the perpetrators hijacked large trucks similar to the one used in the Nice attack, again demonstrating the tendency for terrorists to be inspired by the methods of others.

Finally, 4.7% of lone-actor attacks in the international dataset utilized some form of explosive. This seems like a remarkably low number, but this is more a result of the specific scope of the Lone Actor Terrorism Micro-Sociological Database, which focuses on confrontational violence. As bomb attacks tend to be non-confrontational, using some form of remote trigger or timer detonation, they are not captured in the dataset. This

also applies to arson attacks. Rather, the use of explosives alongside other methods is captured. In this context, rather than being a method to inflict harm, confrontational lone actors use explosives as a "threat enhancer" or distraction that forces responding police and military to maintain their distance from the attacker or to create a sense of confusion. Often, explosives are used as an empty threat—in both the Trèbes supermarket siege and Lindt Café siege, the perpetrators claimed they had explosives. They did not.

This is not to suggest lone actors do not use explosives as killing weapons. They not only remain attractive for their destructive potential, but also for their terrifying visceral value, with one study of European lone actors finding that 16–20% of attacks since 2000 involved explosives.[32] However, lone actors rarely create effective bombs owing to the relative difficulty of both accessing bomb-making materials and possessing the knowledge to create a working bomb. After his 1999 bombing campaign in which he detonated three home-made pipe bombs in non-white and gay communities in London, David Copeland said he "fantasize[d] about the chaos and disruption" caused by the explosions.[31] Breivik was also attracted to the chaotic potential of explosives and spent months carefully refining the materials required to make a large fertilizer bomb. In the atmosphere of confusion after the explosion, he disguised himself as a police officer and was ferried to Utoya Island, where he began his shooting.[32] The 2017 Manchester Arena bombing saw 21 concert attendees being killed and hundreds more wounded when a 23-year-old man detonated a triacetate triperoxide (TATP) bomb as people left the venue. However, the attacker had close connections and trained with radical Islamist groups in Libya, reaffirming how difficult it is for an unsupported individual to create an effective bomb. Overall, the use of bombs as a weapon of choice has been eclipsed by other more readily available weapons. In the next section, we show how this finding also holds for the US context.

US CONTEXT AND DATASET

The American Lone Wolf Terrorism Database created by Mark S. Hamm and Ramón Spaaij allows us to compare the aforementioned international patterns in the means and mechanisms of operationalizing lone-actor terrorist violence.[5] This database contains a comprehensive dataset of all known cases of lone-actor terrorism in the United States between 1940 and mid-2016. It identifies 123 cases during the period, including left-wing extremists, white supremacists, jihadists, and other anti-government extremists, and each case was examined across 21 different variables. Like the LATMD, the database is used as a basis for providing "thick descriptions" of cases of lone-actor terrorism. It includes interviews and communication with lone-actor terrorists in prison, which are mined for insights into the process of identity transformation whereby alienated young men turn into armed terrorists.[5]

The data provided in the American Lone Wolf Terrorism Database indicate a significant shift in the choice of weaponry used by lone-actor terrorists in the United States over the past two decades: from bombings to firearms. Before 2000, the most common and deadliest weapons used in lone-actor terrorist attacks were improvised explosive devices. Notable cases include the Unabomber, Theodore Kaczynski, who committed 16 bombings over 17 years; Muharem Kurbegovic, the so-called Alphabet Bomber, who launched 10 attacks in 2 years; and the Atlanta Olympics bomber Eric Rudolph. Since 2001, however, there has been only a handful of bombings by lone actors, and they have left no fatalities.[5] This decline may reflect the stringent government controls on the purchase of bomb-making materials enacted in the aftermath of the 1995 Oklahoma City bombing.

In the US context, the lone actor's preferred weaponry is now a wide range of high-velocity firearms.[5] Among lone-actor terrorists since 2001, 50% used multiple weapons in their attacks, 32% used only handguns, and 14% used only assault rifles. The 2016 Orlando nightclub attack, which killed 49 people and wounded 53 others, is a case in point. The perpetrator, Omar Mateen, used a Remington-made Sig Sauer .223-caliber assault rifle with a collapsible stock and a 9 mm Glock to murder and maim 235 people inside the Pulse nightclub in Orlando, Florida, on June 12, 2016. Even though he was formerly on the Terrorism Watch List, Mateen was nevertheless able to purchase these weapons, along with hundreds of rounds of military-grade ammunition, from a gun store in St. Lucie, Florida, just days before the attack. Mateen armed himself for the attack through over-the-counter purchases with no questions asked.

The US database shows that Mateen was not alone in this regard. The examples of lone actors using advanced firearm weaponry are overwhelming.[5] Richard Poplawski, who killed three

Pittsburgh police officers in 2009, stockpiled weapons and ammunition in anticipation of a forthcoming gun ban. He acquired a semi-automatic WASR-10 rifle (a Romanian variant of the AK-47), a 12-gauge Savage 67 shotgun, and at least two handguns, including a .357 Magnum revolver. All of these weapons were purchased legally. While most of the firearms, including the WASR-10, were bought online, at least one of the weapons was sold to Poplawski at a gun store in Wilkinsburg, Pennsylvania—the same store where the .22 caliber revolver Ronald Taylor used in his 2000 shooting rampage was purchased. Christopher Dorner used a 9 mm Glock, an AR-15 assault rifle, and a silencer-equipped Remington sniper's rifle in his 2013 Los Angeles attack. In his ambushing of Texas police, Thomas Caffall stood at his front door and fired dozens of rounds from a Vz. 58 Tactical Support rifle, a Mosin-Nagant M91/30 rifle with a bayonet, and a .40-caliber Glock pistol belonging to a slain policeman. For backup, Caffall possessed a Romanian marksman rifle.[33]

Hamm and Spaaij refer to this mechanism as "over-arming," which they argue has become a common trait of lone-actor terrorism in the United States.[5] The authors situate this mechanism with the individual's transformation to violent action, which is "a highly emotional affair allowing for a confrontation with one's enemy—the 'other'—and the circumvention of social and psychological barriers to violence." This finding is consistent with Collins's theory that perpetrators seek pathways to circumvent confrontational tension/fear in order to be able to perform violence effectively.[34] Collins regards violence as inherently emotionally difficult to engage in, even by motivated actors. Over-arming may be viewed as one such pathway to managing confrontational tension/fear in the operationalization of lone-actor terrorist violence This is not only in the sense of the physical ability to conduct an attack, but in the sense that amassing an arsenal serves as a private ritual for the lone actor, one that "has a motivating effect that deeps the spiral of clandestine plotting into a private world."[33] This private world emotionally empowers the individual, enabling them to move toward carrying out their attack. Hamm and Spaaij conclude that "because of its emotionality, the transformation may lead to a public oversharing of extremist beliefs and an obsessive preparation for violence centered on collecting an arsenal of weaponry; individuals will often over-arm themselves with far more weapons and ammunition than they eventually use. Over-arming indicates that an extremist has flipped from inspirational status to being fully operational."[5]

Finally, the American Lone Wolf Terrorism Database offers valuable insight into alternative weaponry that lone-actor terrorists have occasionally used, or attempted to use, to carry out their attacks. In his seminal book *The New Terrorism: Fanaticism and the Arms of Mass Destruction*, the late Walter Laqueur argued that lone actors are among the most likely candidates to use weapons of mass destruction in their attacks (i.e., nuclear, biological, radiological, or chemical weapons).[34] To date, this threat has not materialized to any real degree.[4] There are very few publicly known instances where lone actors have successfully operationalized or used weapons of mass destruction. Arguably the best-known attempt occurred in 1974, when Muharem Kurbegovic, dubbed the Alphabet Bomber, threatened to release sarin in populated areas and claimed that he was already conducting experiments with it. He had reportedly acquired most ingredients needed to build a nerve gas bomb.[35]

Recent years have seen a small number of similarly idiosyncratic threats, attacks, and aborted attacks.[5] Bruce Ivins, a government microbiologist, was responsible for the 2001 anthrax attacks which killed 5 and injured 17 in the deadliest instance of biological terrorism in US history.[36] Once the FBI began questioning Ivins, he displayed signs of severe stress and went into treatment for depression and suicidal ideation. He later committed suicide without ever being arrested. In a copycat of the 2001 anthrax attacks, anti-abortion activist Clayton Waagner mailed 554 letters to abortion clinics across the United States, each containing white flour and an anthrax threat. His letters disrupted clinic operations, temporarily shutting down hundreds of abortion clinics. Likewise, from a Denver jail cell, inmate Marc Ramsey single-handedly brought John McCain's 2008 Republican presidential campaign to a standstill as a result of a mailed anthrax hoax, again a copycat of the Ivins attack. Finally, the case of neo-Nazi James Cummings represented the first attempt to build a dirty bomb on American soil. Cummings purchased the radioactive materials over the Internet and planned to detonate his bomb at the presidential inauguration of Barack Obama, but the plan was aborted when Cumming's wife murdered him.[5]

PREVENTION AND DISRUPTION: FIREARMS IN LONE-ACTOR TERRORISM

The preceding analysis of international and US datasets demonstrates that firearms are a significant weapon of choice for lone-actor terrorists but more prominently within the United States than outside it. In the international database, melee weapons are the most common weapon used in an attack, reflecting the relatively low level of sophistication and limited capabilities of the attackers, including their restricted legal access to firearms. Internationally, firearms are still the second most common weapon, and they are also the deadliest weapon used in lone-actor attacks. In the United States, consistent with the relaxation of US gun laws since the early 2000s, the lone actor's preferred weaponry is a wide range of high-velocity firearms.

The vast majority (78%) of firearms used in the international (non-US) context were illegal. This is not surprising given the relatively strict restrictions on firearms in Europe. The weapons that were used were mostly sourced from various black market connections. For example, the attacker in the 2014 Jewish museum in Brussels used a fully automatic AKS-47 assault rifle supplied by an associate,[37] Van Themsche purchased the Marlin hunting rifle from a seller over the internet,[38] and the Lindt Café siege attacker purchased his sawed-off shotgun immediately before initiating the hostage crisis.[38] The reliance on black market sources for their weaponry seems to have had a perverse effect on the weapon use of French and Belgian lone actors who have been able to source and employ fully automatic Kalashnikov-type rifles not seen elsewhere in the dataset.

Other lone actors, lacking access to underworld sources, have attempted to procure firearms during their attack. This occurred during the 2014 Orly Airport attack, where the attacker almost successfully used a French soldier's FAMAS assault rifle after taking her hostage.[39] Similarly, during the 2018 Liège attack, an Islamic extremist on a day's leave from prison stabbed and killed two police officers before taking their FN 5-7 sidearms and engaging in a shoot-out with a police tactical team.[40]

The only legally owned, or legally owned but illegally modified, weapons used in the entire international dataset (12.5% and 6.3%, respectively) were all in Canada, with only two exceptions. The Orly Airport attack was initiated with the use of a possibly legal air-powered pistol. The other exception was the 2011 Utoya Island attack. Breivik attempted to purchase illegal weapons in Prague but was unable to do so.[41] Instead, he decided it was easier and less conspicuous to go through the legal requirements of purchasing a legal Mini-14 semi-automatic rifle and Glock 34 pistol. Overall, the occurrence of legally owned guns being used in lone-actor attacks outside of the United States is very rare, with the notable exceptions of Canada and Norway. What specific types of firearms are used depends heavily on the broader availability of weapons that the attacker has access to.

The US Legislative Context

That lone-actor terrorists in the United States much more often use firearms than their equivalents in other countries reflects the fact that the availability of firearms in the United States far exceeds that of other countries. Karp reports that, by the end of 2017, there were 857 million civilian-held firearms in the world, based on registration and survey data and estimates from 230 different countries and territories.[42] This represented a 32% increase since 2006. Approximately 393 million of the 857 million civilian held firearms in the world were in the United States. This represented a rate of national ownership of firearms of 120.5 firearms per 100 residents in the United States. To put this in perspective, there were more firearms in the United States than in the next 24 countries with the highest rates of firearm ownership combined.[42] Research has shown that when persons in the United States engage in violent behavior, the violence is often more lethal than in other countries, largely related to the more frequent use of firearms.[43]

Various approaches to firearm legislation have been promoted in the United States. Many have proposed a renewal of the Federal Assault Weapons Ban as a means of reducing mass violence. The Federal Assault Weapons Ban was a subsection of the Violent Crime Control and Law Enforcement Act of 1994. The Federal Assault Weapons Ban included a prohibition on the manufacture for civilian use of a defined set of automatic and semi-automatic weapons and "large capacity magazines." The ban expired in 2004.

DiMaggio et al. compared the period from 1994 to 2004 to the following 10-year period in an observational study to assess the effectiveness of this policy intervention.[44] They found that assault rifles accounted for 430 or 85.8% of the total 501 mass-shooting fatalities reported in 44 mass shooting incidents. The federal ban period was associated with a statistically significant nine fewer mass shooting related deaths per 10,000 homicides. Mass-shootings were 70% less likely to occur during the federal ban period. DiMaggio et al. concluded that "[m]ass-shooting related homicides in the United States were reduced during the years of the federal assault weapons ban of 1994 to 2004."[44] Fox and DeLateur also studied the impact of the federal assault weapons ban.[45] They found that assault rifles were used in fewer than 25% of shootings and that the initial rate of mass shootings continued to increase at the same rate both while the ban was in place and after it ended. They concluded that banning assault rifles alone would be unlikely to change the rate of mass shootings appreciably. However, a reduction in fatalities from mass shooting could be a more realistic goal.

Since the expiration of the Federal Assault Weapon Ban in 2004, sales of semi-automatic rifles have increased. By 2012, sales of semi-automatic rifles accounted for 13% of all US civilian new gun purchases.[42] A survey conducted in 2016 found that 42.3% of US hunters owned at least one AR 15 Platform (M-16 style) rifle. In 2016, 6% of adults who were surveyed responded that they had used a modern sporting rifle or semi-automatic assault weapon.[42]

The ability to pass a renewal of the Federal Assault Weapon Ban is problematic in the wake of Supreme Court decisions in *Heller* and *McDonald*. The Second Amendment to the US Constitution protects the rights of individuals to keep and bear arms. In *District of Columbia v Heller*, 554 U.S. 570 (2008), the US Supreme Court held that the Second Amendment protects an individual's right to keep and bear arms, unconnected with service in a militia, for traditionally lawful purposes such as self-defense within the home. Heller held that the District of Columbia's ban on handguns and requirement that lawfully owned rifles and shotguns be kept "unloaded and disassembled or bound by a trigger lock" violated the Second Amendment guarantees. The *Heller* decision was extended to states and municipalities through a second Supreme Court decisions, *McDonald v. Chicago* 561 U.S. 742 (2010). Heller held that Second Amendment rights are not unlimited. For example, prohibitions on the possession of guns by those convicted of a felony can still be applied. Heller held that permitted firearms are those in "common use at the time."

Many believe that *Heller* would protect the use of assault-style weapons and high-capacity magazines. By 2017, eight US states had laws banning high-capacity magazines, limiting the number of rounds to 10 or 15. In 2016, California passed Proposition 63, banning the possession of high-capacity magazines holding more than 10 rounds. On appeal, the federal courts stayed the new law because the state failed to show how this law did not violate the Second Amendment or the property rights of owners of previously legal goods.[46]

Fourteen states in the United States have enacted risk-based firearm-removal laws, variously known as red-flag, gun violence restraining order (GVRO), extreme risk protection order (ERPO), or risk-warrant laws.[47] ERPO laws are distinct from but influenced by domestic violence restraining orders. They allow family members (and in some states other persons such as mental health professionals) to petition the Court for an emergency civil order so that law enforcement can remove firearms from a person in crisis. The individual may or may not have a mental illness. The individual is a person who has a firearm(s) and is known to pose a high risk of harm to themselves or others in the near future. The Court will issue a warrant based on probable cause of imminent harm. Within a period, specified in the state statute/regulation, the Court must hold a hearing with due process protections, attended by both parties. The state must show clear and convincing evidence of ongoing risk. If the Court issues a final order, then the respondent will be restricted from purchasing or possessing a firearm for a defined period, typically about a year. Then the order expires unless renewed. Unlike many other legislative proposals for gun control, ERPO laws have support on both sides of the political aisle, even among gun owners.[48] Support for ERPO laws appears to have been growing since the Parkland shooting on February 14, 2018.[49]

As many gun-control bills,[50] risk-based firearm removal laws began as state-level responses to mass shootings. Although incidents of mass violence are statistically rare events that account for only a small percentage of overall gun-violence death rates,[51] firearm legislation passed in their wake may help to reduce firearm-related deaths overall.[52] Investigations following such tragedies often reveal that warning signs or "red flags" of likely violent behavior were known to, and sometimes even reported by, persons who interacted with the perpetrator before the event. Such was the case in the Tucson, Arizona, shooting in 2011 and the Isla Vista, California, massacre in 2014, for example. In both cases, those closest to the shooters identified dangerous behaviors, expressed concern, and took concrete actions to intervene and address a risk they correctly perceived. Importantly, in neither case did the level of dangerousness rise to a point that caused those involved to initiate involuntary commitment procedures, and, as a result, they were left with few options to intervene and no systematic mechanism to limit gun access. They did what they could with the tools available to them under the law but were ultimately unable to restrict firearm access by the two young men who went on to commit horrific acts of gun violence.[53]

Many other types of gun bills in recent years have placed a misguided focus on mental illness, which is not a reliable indicator of future violent behavior. Furthermore, laws that restrict firearm access based on a psychiatric diagnosis or mental health treatment history may have a stigmatizing and chilling effect that deters persons in need of treatment from seeking it.[54] Such a result is counterproductive to the laws' intent; among persons with mental illness, those engaged in treatment are less likely to become violent.[54]

As noted by the American Psychiatric Association (APA) in a Resource Document approved in 2018, one of the benefits of risk-based firearm seizure laws is that they do not stigmatize mental illness.[55] Under an ERPO law, the seizure of firearms is authorized due to threatening behavior, a more reliable indicator of the likelihood of violent behavior than the person's history of mental health treatment or diagnosis.[55,56] In 1999, Connecticut became the first state to enact a risk-based firearm-removal law, with Indiana following in 2005.[56] Many of these bills have been drafted and advanced within the past 5 years, informed by the findings of the Consortium for Risk-Based Firearm Policy (the Consortium), a group of epidemiologists, public health professionals, and other scientific experts that met in Baltimore for a 2-day conference in March 2013.[57] The specifics of ERPO or red-flag laws vary from state to state; some commentators feel that the first true ERPO law was passed by California in 2014.[53]

Previous gun-control initiatives, such as the Brady Act's establishment of the National Instant Criminal Background Check System (NICS) in the 1990s, have failed to achieve the desired reductions in gun-violence deaths,[50] prompting calls for legislation with an emphasis on public health and empirical data. Risk-based firearm removal laws are consistent with the evidence-based recommendations of the Consortium and the APA.[54,55]

Further research is needed to determine whether various measures that have aimed to decrease the incidence of firearm-related deaths will be effective in decreasing the incidence, lethality, and numbers of victims associated with lone-actor terrorism. Evidence-informed solutions are needed.

CONCLUSION

This chapter examined the means and methods used by lone actors to commit acts of terrorist violence. Drawing on current international and US data, we found that lone-actor terrorist attacks range from sophisticated and carefully planned operations to simplistic acts of violence using only the most rudimentary weapons. Outside the United States, the most common weapon type used by lone-actor terrorists is melee weapons. In contrast, in the US context, the lone actor's preferred weaponry is now a wide range of high-velocity firearms. In this chapter we suggested cultural and legislative factors that help to explain this difference. We then focused specifically on the US legislative context to consider how the incidence, lethality, and numbers of victims associated with lone-actor terrorism may be decreased. As noted earlier, measures such as risk-based firearm removal laws may hold promise in this regard, but their efficacy in relation to lone-actor terrorism is yet to be ascertained.

While there is now a sizeable scientific and gray literature on the factors and processes that contribute to lone-actor terrorism, research on methods of intervention and prevention of lone-actor violence is still in its infancy. The recommendations of the National Council for Behavioral Health could help inform future research and analysis on the prevention of lone-actor terrorism.[46] We would suggest that, for the US context, the Council's recommendations related to gun use may be adapted and applied to the study of the prevention and interdiction of lone-actor terrorism. For example, what is the value of enacting red flag or ERPOs laws that allow the temporary removal of guns from individuals who are known to pose a high risk of harming others? To what extent does the full implementation of existing federal background check requirements for firearm purchases affect the means and methods available to lone actors to commit violence? What (if any) has been the effectiveness of ERPO laws in states that have enacted them on lone-actor terrorism? These are just some of the questions that would advance the study (and possibly the disruption) of the means and mechanisms of operationalizing violence in lone-actor terrorism.

NOTES AND REFERENCES

1. Spaaij R. Lone actors: Challenges and opportunities for countering violent extremism. In Richman A, Sharan Y, eds. *Lone Actors: An Emerging Security Threat.* Amsterdam: IOS Press; 2015:120–131.
2. Williams C. *Terrorism Explained.* Sydney: New Holland; 2004.
3. Burton F, Stewart S. The "lone wolf" disconnect. STRATFOR Global Intelligence. 2008. http://www.stratfor.com/weekly/lone_wolf_disconnect
4. Spaaij R. *Understanding Lone Wolf Terrorism: Global Patterns, Motivations and Prevention.* 1st ed. New York: Springer; 2012.
5. Hamm MS, Spaaij R. *The Age of Lone Wolf Terrorism.* New York: Columbia University Press; 2017.
6. Freilich J, Chermak SM. Preventing deadly encounters between law enforcement and American far-rightists. *Crime Prev Stud.* 2009;Oct:141–172.
7. Becker M. Explaining lone wolf target selection in the United States. *Stud Confl Terror.* 2014;37(11):959–978. doi:10.1080/1057610X.2014.952261.
8. Gill P, Horgan J, Deckert P. Bombing alone: Tracing the motivations and antecedent behaviors of lone-actor terrorists. *J Forensic Sci.* 2014;59(2):425–435. doi:10.1111/1556-4029.12312.
9. Schuurman B, Bakker E, Gill P, Bouhana N. Lone actor terrorist attack planning and preparation: A data-driven analysis. *J Forensic Sci.* 2017. doi:10.1111/1556-4029.13676.
10. Lindekilde L, O'Connor F, Schuurman B. Radicalization patterns and modes of attack planning and preparation among lone-actor terrorists: An exploratory analysis. *Behav Sci Terror Polit Aggress.* 2017;4472(Jan 2018):1–21. doi:10.1080/19434472.2017.1407814.
11. Meloy JR, Pollard JW. Lone-actor terrorism and impulsivity. *J Forensic Sci.* 2017;62(6):1643–1646. doi:10.1111/1556-4029.13500.
12. Clarke RV, Newman GR. *Outsmarting the Terrorists.* Westport, CT: Praeger Security International; 2006.
13. Ellis C, Pantucci R, Zuijdewijn JDR Van, et al. Analysing the processes of lone-actor terrorism: Research findings. *Perspect Terror.* 2016;10(2):33–41.
14. Perry S, Hasisi B, Perry G. Lone terrorists: A study of run-over attacks in Israel. *Eur J Criminol.* 2018:1–22. doi:10.1177/1477370818769257.
15. Burke J. Norway mosque attack suspect "inspired by Christchurch and El Paso shootings." *The Guardian,* 12 Aug 2019. https://www.theguardian.com/world/2019/aug/11/

norway-mosque-attack-suspect-may-have-been-inspired-by-christchurch-and-el-paso-shootings

16. Alakoc BP. Competing to kill: Terrorist organizations versus lone wolf terrorists. *Terror Polit Violence*. 2017;29(3):509–532. doi:10.1080/09546553.2015.1050489.

17. Gill P, Corner E. Lone-actor terrorist target choice. *Behav Sci Law*. 2016;34:693–705. doi:10.1002/bsl.2268.

18. Hemmingby C. Exploring the continuum of lethality: Militant Islamists' targeting preferences in Europe. *Perspect Terror*. 2017;11(5):25–41.

19. Hamm M, Spaaij R. Lone wolf terrorism in America: Using knowledge of radicalization pathways to forge prevention strategies. US Department of Justice, 2015, https://www.ojp.gov/pdffiles1/nij/grants/248691.pdf

20. Smith BL, Gruenewald J, Roberts P, Damphousse KR. The emergence of lone wolf terrorism: Patterns of behavior and implications for intervention. *Sociol Crime Law Deviance*. 2015;20:89–110. doi:10.1108/S1521-613620150000020005.

21. Moskalenko S, McCauley C. The psychology of lone-wolf terrorism. *Couns Psychol Q*. 2011; 24(2):115–126. doi:10.1080/09515070.2011.581835.

22. Pantucci R. What have we learned about lone wolves from Anders Behring Breivik? *Perspect Terror*. 2011;5(5-6):27–42.

23. Dodd V, Addley E. Leytonstone knife attack: Man convicted of attempted murder. *The Guardian*, 9 Jun 2016. https://www.theguardian.com/uk-news/2016/jun/08/leytonstone-knife-attack-man-convicted-of-attempted

24. Graff J. Skinhead rampage highlights Belgium's race anxiety. *Time*, 12 May 2006. http://content.time.com/time/world/article/0,8599,1193952,00.html

25. France shooting: Police kill supermarket gunman. *BBC*, 23 Mar 2018.

26. Bernstein J. Richard Bain murder trial hears guns in SUV were loaded, ready to fire. *CBC*, 20 Jun 2016. https://www.cbc.ca/news/canada/montreal/richard-bain-trial-day-8-1.3643196

27. Bernstein J. Richard Cain murder trial: Police found stockpile of guns, ammo at rustic cabin. *CBC*, 22 Jun 2016. https://www.cbc.ca/news/canada/montreal/richard-bain-trial-day-10-1.3646254

28. Gollom M, Lindeman T. Who is Martin Couture-Rouleau? *CBC*, 21 Oct 2014. https://www.cbc.ca/news/canada/who-is-martin-couture-rouleau-1.2807285

29. Miller V, Hayward KJ. "I did my bit": Terrorism, Tarde and the vehicle ramming attack as an imitative event. *Br J Criminol*. 2018;59(Jun 2017):1–23. doi:10.1093/bjc/azy017.

30. Wilson A. ISIS backer drove at Flinders St crowd "in name of Allah" court hears. *The Age*, 2019. https://www.theage.com.au/national/victoria/isis-backer-drove-at-flinders-st-crowd-in-name-of-allah-court-hears-20190212-p50xa8.html

31. Westminster car crash: Salih Khater guilty of attempted murder. *BBC*, 17 Jul 2019. https://www.bbc.com/news/uk-england-london-49017105

32. Liem M, van Buuren J, de Roy van Zuijdewijn J, Schönberger H, Bakker E. European lone actor terrorists versus "common" homicide offenders: An empirical analysis. *Homicide Stud*. 2017;22(1):108876791773679. doi:10.1177/1088767917736797.

33. Police: Gunman fired more than 60 times in College Station shooting. *KLTV*, 18 Aug 2012. https://www.kltv.com/story/19308669/police-release-timeline-of-shooting-that-killed-constable-civilian/

34. Meyer S. Impeding lone-wolf attacks: Lessons derived from the 2011 Norway attacks. *Crime Sci*. 2013;2(7):13. doi:10.1186/2193-7680-2-7.

35. Collins R. Micro-sociology of mass rampage killings. *Rev Synth*. 2014;135(4):405–420. doi:10.1007/s11873-014-0250-2.

36. Frenchman convicted of Jewish museum terror murders. *SBS*, 8 Mar 2019, https://www.sbs.com.au/news/frenchman-convicted-of-jewish-museum-terror-murders/d1c37d56-176f-4150-97d8-99ed13c35e1d

37. Wapenwet: Wapen als Van Themsche? Wij kochten het via internet. *Gazet van Antwerpen*, 28 Sep 2007, https://www.gva.be/cnt/aid612039

38. Michael Barnes, *Inquest into the Deaths Arising from the Lindt Café Siege: Findings and Recommendations*. Glebe: Corners Court of New South Wales; 2017, http://www.lindtinquest.justice.nsw.gov.au/Documents/findings-and-recommendations.pdf

39. What we know about the Paris Orly airport attacker. *The Local France*, 18 Mar 2017. https://www.thelocal.fr/20170318/what-we-know-about-the-paris-orly-airport-attacker

40. Liege shootings: Gunman "had killed day before attack." *BBC*, 30 May2018, https://www.bbc.com/news/world-europe-44299952

41. Stewart S. Norway: Lessons from a successful lone-wolf attacker. Stratfor. 2011. https://worldview.stratfor.com/article/norway-lessons-successful-lone-wolf-attacker

42. Karp A. Estimating global civilian-held firearm numbers. Briefing Paper 9. Geneva: Small arms survey. 2018. http://smallarmssurvey.org/fileadmin/docs/T-Briefing-Papers/SAS-BP-Civilian-Firearms-Numbers.pdf

43. Wintemute GL. The epidemiology of firearm violence in the twenty-first century United States. *Ann Rev Pub Health* 2015;36(1):5–19.

44. DiMaggio C, Avraham J, Berry C et al. Changes in US mass shooting deaths associated with the 1994-2004 federal assault weapon ban: Analysis

of open-source data. *J Trauma Acute Care Surg.* 2019;86(1):11–19.

45. Fox J, DeLateur M. Mass shootings in America: Moving beyond Newtown. *Homicide Studies.* 2013;18(1):125–145.

46. National Council for Behavioral Health. *Mass Violence in America, Causes, Impacts and Solutions.* Washington, DC: National Council Medical Director Institute; 2019.

47. Frizell W, Chien JDO. Extreme risk protection orders to reduce firearm violence. *Psychiatr Serv.* 2019;70(1):75–77.

48. Barry CL, McGinty EE, Vernick JS, Webster DW. Two years after Newtown: Public opinion on gun policy revisited. *Prev Med.* 2015;79:55–58.

49. Astor M, Russell K. After Parkland, a new surge in state gun control laws. *New York Times,* 14 Dec 2018. https://www.nytimes.com/interactive/2018/12/14/us/politics/gun-control-laws.html

50. Price M, Norris DM. Firearm laws: A primer for psychiatrists. *Harv Rev Psychiatry.* 2010;18(6):326–335.

51. Gold LH. Gun violence: Psychiatry, risk assessment, and social policy. *J Am Acad Psychiatry Law.* 2013;41(3):337–343.

52. Ramchand R, Morral AR. Can the national call to prevent gun violence reduce suicides? *Psychiatr Serv.* 2018;69(12):1196–1997.

53. Frattaroli S, McGinty EE, Barnhorst A, Greenberg S. Gun violence restraining orders: Alternative or adjunct to mental health-based restrictions on firearms? *Behav Sci Law.* 2015;33(2–3):290–307:293.

54. Pinals DA, Appelbaum PS, Bonnie RJ, Fisher CE, Gold LH, Lee LW. Resource document on access to firearms by people with mental disorders. *Behav Sci Law.* 2015;33:186–194. doi:10.1002/bsl.2181.

55. Kapoor R, Benedek E, Bonnie RL, et al. *Resource Document on Risk-Based Gun Removal Laws.* Washington, DC: American Psychiatric Association; 2018.

56. Vernick JS, Alcorn T, Horwitz J. Background checks for all gun buyers and gun violence restraining orders: State efforts to keep guns from high-risk persons. *J Law Med Ethics.* 2017;45(S1):98–102.

57. Consortium for Risk-Based Firearm Policy. *Guns, Public Health, and Mental Illness: An Evidence-Based Approach for Federal Policy.* Washington, DC: Consortium for Risk-Based Firearm Policy; 2013.

13

Role of Forensic Mental Health in Lone-Actor Violence

ASHLEY H. VANDERCAR, RYAN C. WAGONER, PHILLIP J. RESNICK,
FRANK FARNHAM, AND EMILY CORNER

INTRODUCTION

A lone-actor terrorist is more than 13 times more likely than a group-based terrorist to have a mental health problem.[1] Mental health problems exist on a spectrum. At their most severe, they can prevent a defendant from going to trial because they are not competent, and, if tried, mental health problems can prevent them from being held criminally responsible through a not guilty by reason of insanity verdict (NGRI). Competency and sanity are legal determinations. Judges and juries rely heavily on forensic evaluations when deciding these issues. This chapter describes the role of forensic mental health professionals during the prosecution of a suspected lone-actor terrorist.

ROLE OF FORENSIC MENTAL HEALTH IN LONE-ACTOR VIOLENCE

There are several definitions of lone-actor terrorism. The nuances of these definitions are discussed elsewhere in this volume. For this chapter, we define a lone-actor terrorist as someone who engages in an act of violence on their own, in furtherance of an ideological belief.

To be tried for a criminal offense, such as a terrorist act, a defendant must be competent. *Competency* refers to a defendant's current mental state. If a lawyer or judge has concerns that a defendant's mental health problem is preventing them from assisting in their defense or understanding the charges and associated proceedings, they can ask a forensic mental health professional to perform a competency evaluation.

Forensic mental health evaluations can be done by a psychologist or psychiatrist. A psychologist has a master's or doctoral (PhD) degree. A psychiatrist has a degree as either a medical doctor (MD) or doctor of osteopathy (DO); they have completed 4 years of medical school, a 4-year psychiatry residency program, and often a 1-year forensic psychiatry fellowship. Psychologists usually have more expertise in psychological testing than do psychiatrists. Psychiatrists can prescribe medications; in most states, psychologists cannot.

If the defendant is found competent they can proceed to trial. At trial they can plead "not guilty by reason of insanity." This is rarely successful.[2] When successful, the defendant avoids criminal responsibility. Judges and juries decide whether a defendant's NGRI plea succeeds based in part on a forensic psychologist or psychiatrist's *sanity evaluation*. A sanity evaluation retrospectively looks at whether, at the time of the crime, the defendant's mental illness prevented them from appreciating that their criminal actions were "wrong" (nuances and variations of this are discussed later).

A defendant can be prosecuted for terrorism in state or federal court.[3] Some states have terrorism statutes. Others use generic criminal charges, such as murder, and apply them to terrorist behavior. Whether a defendant is tried in state or federal court is beyond the scope of this chapter. However, this decision is of great importance because different jurisdictions (state or federal court system) can vary in their procedures and standards for competency and sanity.

No matter where a case is tried, the process begins with a law enforcement investigation and ends only after all appeals have been abandoned or exhausted. Here, we present a hypothetical case describing this process in the United States.

CASE STUDY

Mr. Doe is a 48-year-old man with a long history of schizophrenia and strongly held "pro-life" beliefs. He recently mailed bombs to a number of abortion clinics; none detonated. After his last package was found and publicized, Mr. Doe sent his congressman an unsigned letter: "outlaw abortion now or the next bomb will kill the baby-murderers."

Law enforcement investigated and arrested Mr. Doe at the post office. He was preparing to mail another bomb.

POTENTIAL INVOLVEMENT OF A FORENSIC MENTAL HEALTH PROFESSIONAL IN A LONE-ACTOR TERRORIST CASE

- Psychiatric treatment at the jail
- Evaluation for competency to stand trial
- Restoration of competency at a mental health facility
- Evaluation of sanity at the time of the crime
- Evaluation of mitigating factors for purposes of sentencing
- Post-conviction evaluation of competency for appeal
- Psychiatric treatment at the prison

Jail: While in jail Mr. Doe talked to himself and repeatedly banged his head on the wall. He refused to eat. He said his food had been poisoned. A jail psychiatrist saw him, found him to be psychotic, and gave him medication.

Competency to stand trial: Mr. Doe appeared in court. The judge found a reasonable basis (probable cause) for his arrest and appointed a public defender (an attorney for Mr. Doe). Mr. Doe met with his attorney but refused to discuss the case. He believed the judge and his attorney were in cahoots with the government. The defense attorney became concerned about Mr. Doe's mental health and requested a competency evaluation.

A forensic mental health professional evaluated Mr. Doe and diagnosed him with schizophrenia. She gave the opinion that, as a result of his mental illness, Mr. Doe could not effectively assist in his defense. The judge agreed and ruled that Mr. Doe was not competent to stand trial. Mr. Doe was sent to a mental health facility for competency restoration. A forensic psychiatrist treated him, prescribing a new medication. Mr. Doe improved and a few weeks later was found "restored" to competency.

Insanity plea: Mr. Doe was brought back in front of the judge. He pleaded not guilty by reason of insanity (NGRI). He was evaluated by two forensic mental health professionals: one for the defense and one for the prosecution. Both experts wrote reports and testified in front of the jury, reaching opposite conclusions. The jury rejected the NGRI plea. They did not believe that Mr. Doe's delusions interfered with his ability at the time of the crime to understand that his actions were wrong. Mr. Doe was found guilty on all charges.

Sentencing: At the sentencing hearing the defense expert came back to testify. The defense attorney successfully used Mr. Doe's mental health condition to mitigate (reduce the severity of) his sentence. Mr. Doe was sentenced to 7 years in prison.

Appeal and post-conviction evaluation: After sentencing, Mr. Doe told his attorney: "I knew you were an agent of the devil—you set me up—you are trying to keep me from doing my God-given job of saving the babies." The defense attorney filed a motion for a new trial alleging that Mr. Doe had not been competent to stand trial. The trial court denied the motion.

The defense attorney appealed, citing a (new) forensic mental health professional's post-conviction evaluation. The appellate court rejected this argument and upheld the trial court's refusal to grant a new trial.

Prison: Mr. Doe exhausted all appellate remedies while in prison. He was placed on a mental health pod and treated by yet another forensic psychiatrist. He was given antipsychotic medications. His delusions and hallucinations improved.

Mr. Doe was a lone-actor terrorist. He happened to have a serious mental illness: schizophrenia. His mental health initially impacted his competency. However, he was restored to competency and held criminally responsible for his actions.

In this chapter, we examine the concepts of competency, sanity, and mitigation more closely. We primarily look at the United States, with brief comparisons to practices abroad.

COMPETENCY TO STAND TRIAL

For hundreds of years, common law has required that a defendant have a certain degree of mental fitness in order to be criminally prosecuted.[4] The 1960 case of *Dusky v. United States*[5] is often cited as the basis for the US standard for this mental fitness.[6] Milton Dusky was a man with schizophrenia who was charged with kidnapping.[7] He was initially found competent to stand trial. The trial court judge noted that he was "oriented as to time and place and person . . . [and] based on the limited evidence that ha[d] been presented . . . [was] able to assist counsel in his own defense."[7]

Mr. Dusky's attorneys appealed to the US Supreme Court, which reversed that ruling and sent the case back to the trial court. The Supreme Court stated that the appropriate test for Mr. Dusky's competence to stand trial was

1. Whether he has sufficient present ability to consult with his lawyer with a reasonable degree of rational understanding, and
2. Whether he has a rational as well as factual understanding of the proceedings against him.[5]

This standard has become the framework for states' competency standards. Some states add to the definition, for example by requiring that incompetence be due to a mental abnormality.[8]

Forensic mental health professionals are regularly asked to perform competency evaluations. They are asked for an opinion on a defendant's psychiatric diagnoses and how the diagnoses *currently* affect the defendant's ability to (1) consult with their attorney and (2) understand the proceedings (rationally and factually). This evaluation usually includes a clinical interview, where the mental health professional obtains information about current and past psychiatric symptoms. They ask specific questions to determine the defendant's understanding of the proceedings, such as

- What are you being charged with?
- What could happen if you are found guilty of that charge?
- What is your lawyer's role?
- What is the prosecutor's role?
- What is the judge's role?

The forensic mental health professional also assesses the defendant's decision-making ability; that is, their ability to decide between plea options and assess the importance of pieces of evidence in their case.[8] Since legal standards vary, forensic evaluators must be aware of—and apply—the standard in the defendant's jurisdiction.

After performing this evaluation, the evaluator reaches an opinion and writes a report. Then the judge holds a competency hearing, taking the contents of the report into consideration to determine if the defendant is legally competent to stand trial. If so, the trial proceeds. If not, the defendant is usually referred to a hospital competency restoration program, where they are treated and educated in an attempt to restore competency.

CASE STUDY: COMPETENCE TO STAND TRIAL—INCOMPETENT AND RESTORED

In September 2012, 18-year-old Adel Daoud was arrested and indicted on federal charges. Daoud was indicted on charges of attempting to use a weapon of mass destruction (as defined in the Federal Code section labeled "Terrorism," Title 18 Part 1 Chapter 113B) and attempting to destroy a building by means of an explosive.[9-12]

These charges came from an undercover investigation. Mr. Daoud had been posting in an extremist online forum about the need for a jihad to protect Muslims from America. Undercover FBI agents contacted him and put him in touch with someone they said was an "operational terrorist" (but who was actually another undercover FBI agent). After a number of conversations, that undercover FBI agent drove Mr. Daoud to a Jeep and told him an inert bomb inside was an explosive device. Mr. Daoud drove the Jeep to a Chicago bar, parked, and walked to an alley that was a block away. He tried to detonate the device. It did not go off. He was arrested and prosecuted in federal court.

While incarcerated, Mr. Daoud was indicted on additional charges. In 2013, he was indicted based on a "murder for hire" plot; he allegedly attempted to have one of the undercover agents (from the 2012 incident) killed. Then, in 2015, he was indicted for the assault of a fellow inmate.

In court, Mr. Daoud said he would plead guilty if "you all admit that you're part of Illuminati and that you arrested me because I'm Muslim . . . and that there's plans to kill Muslims in this country."[12] His attorneys requested a competency evaluation. The court agreed. Before the evaluation could be completed, at a status conference, Mr. Daoud told the court: "I know that my case is a hoax. My trial is a hoax . . . the jury is Freemasons hired by the judge . . . all the judges and the prosecutors who represent them, the lawyers who represent me they're all members of the government . . . and they're conspiring against me."[12]

Two mental health professionals evaluated Mr. Daoud. One said that he was competent to stand trial. The other said that he was not. Over the next few weeks, Mr. Daoud sent letters to the court, including a statement that: "I know you are part of something much bigger than you. I want you and the Illuminati to know that you can't destroy Islam."[12] The judge sent Mr. Daoud to a Federal Medical Center for further psychiatric evaluation.

Again, there were different expert opinions. The psychologist at the medical center stated that Mr. Daoud was competent to stand trial and that while his beliefs were "peculiar," they were not "delusional." The defense psychiatrist disagreed, saying that Mr. Daoud had delusional disorder and was not competent.

Mr. Daoud was sent back to the correctional center to await a competency hearing. Meanwhile, he prepared and sent a "Will" to the court, stating: "my life is under threat by the Illuminati, their machines/robots that run the [correctional center], and [Judge] Sharon Johnson Coleman who recently killed my 49th celle [sic] most probably by placing a drug in his food that made him want to kill himself."[12] The court found Mr. Daoud incompetent to stand trial and sent him to a Federal Medical Center for restoration of competency.

Mr. Daoud was diagnosed with a psychotic disorder. He was prescribed medications and attended competency restoration groups. A year later, in 2017, both the psychologist at the medical facility and the defense psychiatrist agreed that Mr. Daoud was competent. In 2018, the court found Mr. Daoud competent and scheduled his case for trial.

Ultimately, Mr. Daoud pleaded guilty, under what is called an *Alford*[13] plea. In other words, he accepted that the government's case would likely lead to his conviction but maintained his innocence (specifically: citing an entrapment defense and a potential "mental health defense"). He was sentenced to 16 years in prison, followed by 45 years of supervised release. This was much less than the 40-year sentence the prosecution had requested.

UNIQUE COMPETENCY CONSIDERATIONS IN LONE-ACTOR TERRORISM

Terrorism can have many different motivations; an oft cited one is the commitment to a belief. Ideology helps to shape the way an individual sees the world and can influence their behavior.[14] This is seen most dramatically when a terrorist justifies violence with an ideology (e.g., religious, political, or moral beliefs). This belief can influence their perception of the legal system. For instance, an accused terrorist may believe that the court has no authority over them. Alternatively, a defendant may refuse to cooperate with an attorney who does not share their ideology.

Although such a defendant might not cooperate with their defense attorney or participate in the proceedings, under a *Dusky* competency standard this does not matter. The focus is on their *ability* to do so. The choice not to follow court rules or work with their attorney is not necessarily reflective of an inability to do so. Instead, it can indicate a voluntary decision to place ideology above the law. This distinction is crucial and can determine whether a defendant is competent to stand trial. In these cases, a forensic mental health professional must evaluate whether the defendant is operating from a delusion or an extreme overvalued belief.[15]

A delusion is indicative of psychosis. It is a "false belief . . . that is firmly held despite what almost everyone else believes and despite . . . incontrovertible and obvious proof or evidence to the contrary."[16] An extreme overvalued belief is a "nondelusional, strongly held belief."[17] An example of a delusion would be a belief that Muslim babies are systematically being targeted for abortions—despite extensive evidence to the contrary. An example of an extreme overvalued belief would be a belief that abortion is a moral sin that must be stopped by whatever violence is necessary.

In general, delusions are specific to the person experiencing them. Extreme overvalued beliefs are shared by others (e.g., within a subculture).[18] An extreme overvalued belief is different from an "overvalued idea," as that term is used in the *Diagnostic and Statistical Manual of Mental Disorders* (DSM-5). According to the DSM-5, an "overvalued idea" is an "unreasonable and sustained belief that is maintained with less than delusional intensity . . . The belief is not one that is ordinarily accepted by other members of the person's culture or subculture."[16] There is controversy about the use of the term "overvalued idea" in terrorism cases; specifically, whether it should include beliefs maintained in a subculture.[15,18]

When evaluating an accused terrorist's competence to stand trial, their underlying beliefs can provide insight into whether a lack of cooperation is due to inability or choice. The delusional defendant who bombed abortion clinics because he believes Muslim babies are systematically being aborted and that his attorney is in on the conspiracy might be incompetent to stand trial. The pro-life defendant who fanatically believes in his right to use violence to stop abortion is likely competent.

CASE STUDY: COMPETENCE TO STAND TRIAL—COMPETENT

On May 9, 2003, 62-year-old Biswanath Halder broke into a building at Case Western Reserve University wearing tactical equipment and wielding two semi-automatic handguns. He killed one person and fired at a number of others. There was an 8-hour hostage standoff. He ultimately surrendered. This was in Ohio, which has its own terrorism statute. Mr. Halder was indicted on 338 charges, including terrorism.[19-22]

Mr. Halder had a personal history with Case Western Reserve University. He had received his MBA there in 1999. Afterward, unable to get work, Mr. Halder started his own online business. In 2000, he believed a Case Western Reserve University employee deleted his website. He sued that person. The civil suit was dismissed. Mr. Halder appealed and reached out to public officials and law enforcement agencies for help. The appeal was dismissed. Then Mr. Halder attacked the University. He was arrested and tried.

Mr. Halder pleaded not guilty to all charges. Before trial, his defense attorneys requested a competency evaluation. Two psychologists stated that he was not competent to stand trial, citing delusional beliefs that would prevent him from rationally assisting his attorneys (a belief that his attorney was conspiring with the prosecutors and the University). The third psychologist said that Mr. Halder was competent. The trial court adopted the opinion of the third psychologist, finding him to be the most experienced and credible of the three. That psychologist had testified:

> [Halder] understood the charges. He knows what he's charged with. He didn't particularly understand what the designation, "aggravated" meant with aggravated murder but he knows he's accused of killing someone. He knows the person's name. He knows why he's charged with attempted murder. He knows all the charges. He knows what the charges mean, what they allege. . . . He told me what plea he wanted to enter and gave me a rationale for why he wanted to enter that plea. . . . [H]e is capable of understanding the nature and significance of the charges. . . .
>
> [Halder] is capable of understanding the adversarial nature of the prosecutorial process; he is capable of participating in a meaningful manner in the process, in the courtroom while it's going on and in my opinion, he is capable of consulting with his attorneys to develop a defense.[23]

Mr. Halder attempted to have his (second set) of attorneys disqualified—he did not feel they were working in his best interest. He asked to represent himself *pro se*. The trial court refused these requests.

Under Ohio Revised Code, § 2909.24, terrorism requires an attempt to:

1. Intimidate or coerce a civilian population;
2. Influence the policy of any government by intimidation or coercion; [or]
3. Affect the conduct of any government by the specified offense.

The trial court dismissed the terrorism charges, finding Mr. Halder did not meet any of these criteria. Mr. Halder was found guilty on a number of other charges, including capital murder. He was sentenced to life in prison without parole. He appealed on several issues, including his competence to stand trial.

Ohio's 8th Appellate District Court of Appeals upheld the trial court's ruling. They noted that when experts disagree, the trial judge is given great latitude to decide which expert is the most credible. They distinguished between a defendant's unwillingness and inability to cooperate with their attorneys. They noted that Mr. Halder had a severe personality disorder and had been *unwilling* to assist his attorneys.

INTERNATIONAL PERSPECTIVES ON COMPETENCY TO STAND TRIAL

The United States (except for Louisiana) is a "common law" system, derived from English law.[24] In the US common law system, state and federal legislative bodies create statutes. These must comply with the state and federal constitutions. Statutes tend to be fairly broad. When specific cases arise, they are brought to a judge in state or federal court. The judge makes factual findings and applies the relevant statute. The judge has broad leeway to interpret the statute and their interpretation creates a different type of law: "common law." When a higher-ranking court creates common law, it is binding on lower courts who—in the future—face the same factual situation.

In civil law countries (such as France or Germany), the judge is primarily a finder of fact. The statutes are frequently updated and more specific. Unlike in the United States, in civil law, a judge's ruling on a case does not typically create broadly applicable law.

Countries that were initially British colonies have, for the most part, retained the British concept of common law and many of their legal theories.[24] England, Australia, and the United States thus have strikingly similar standards for competency to stand trial and NGRI. There are also fundamental differences.

The US Supreme Court case *Dusky* was a judicial decision. It was based on the US Code, which applies to defendants in federal court. Over the years, US courts have interpreted *Dusky* to be the minimum constitutional requirement for competency to stand trial.[8] In England and Wales, the legal standard is based on the case of *Regina v. Pritchard* (1836).[25,26] In Australia, it is based on *Regina v. Presser* (1958)[27] (modeled on *Pritchard*).[28] In these countries, competence to stand trial is part of a concept referred to as "fitness to plead."[26,28]

ENGLAND'S *PRITCHARD* CRITERIA
England's *Pritchard* criteria requires consideration of the following:
First, whether the prisoner is mute of malice or not; secondly, whether he can plead to the indictment or not; thirdly, whether he is of sufficient intellect to comprehend the course of proceedings on the trial, so as to make a proper defen[s]e—to know that he might challenge any of [the jurors] to whom he may object—and to comprehend the details of the evidence.[25]

AUSTRALIA'S *PRESSER* CRITERIA
Austrialia's Presser *criteria* requires the ability
(1) [T]o understand the nature of the charge; (2) to plead to the charge and to exercise the right of challenge; (3) to understand the nature of the proceedings, namely, that it is an inquiry as to whether the accused committed the offence charged; (4) to follow the course of the proceedings; (5) to understand the substantial effect of any evidence that may be given in support of the prosecution; and (6) to make a defen[s]e or answer the charge.[29]

As in the United States, over the years, courts have added to and refined their interpretation of the *Pritchard* and *Presser* criteria. The underlying concept remains one of fairness: the state should not criminally try someone who is unable to sufficiently understand and participate in the legal process. If you take this concept to its extreme, with a man who has profound intellectual disability and is a deaf mute, the concept is straightforward. If you look at a man with schizophrenia and paranoid delusions about his defense attorney, the issue becomes more nuanced.

For example, in England, these criteria have been interpreted to mean that a defendant is "unfit" if he is incapable of "(1) understanding the charges; (2) deciding whether to plead guilty or not; (3) exercising his right to challenge jurors; (4) instructing solicitors and counsel; (5) following the course of the proceedings; [or] (6) giving evidence in his own defen[s]e."[30]

It is in this gray area that you see the differences between the three countries. In England, Wales, and Australia, a fitness evaluation focuses on cognitive ability far more than decision-making capacity. This framework has been heavily criticized; opponents argue that it places too much emphasis on intellectual ability and shows little concern for decision-making skills.[26,28,31] A defendant with high intellectual functioning can be found fit despite impairing paranoia and delusions.

In England and Wales, very few defendants are found unfit to stand trial: approximately 100 a year.[26] Statistics are not readily available for Australia. Although definitive statistics are unavailable in the United States, it is estimated that 60,000 competency evaluations are completed each year, 20–30% of which result in an opinion that the defendant is incompetent to stand trial.[32] Twenty percent of 60,000 is 12,000—more than a hundred times greater numbers than in England and Wales. This difference is partly definitional and partly philosophical.

The criminal justice system's treatment of mentally ill defendants has generally been less adversarial in the United Kingdom than in the United States. The United Kingdom places more of an emphasis on treatment rather than retribution based on the notion that a mentally ill defendant is a victim of their mental illness.[33] In the United Kingdom, prosecutors can overtly consider whether prosecution of an accused criminal is in the "public interest."[34] They can consider hospital commitment as an alternative to prosecution.[34] When a crime is serious, public interest tends to favor prosecution even if a defendant is severely mentally ill. The defense and prosecution can then obtain independent experts to evaluate the defendant's mental illness, and the atmosphere becomes more adversarial.

Terrorism cases are serious and usually high-profile. There are political considerations and public expectations. In the United Kingdom, this can influence the decision to prosecute and the disposition of the case. Fitness to plead remains relevant, but much less so than in the United States.

CRIMINAL RESPONSIBILITY

One of the goals of prosecuting terrorists is to hold them responsible for their crime. Usually, this means sending them to prison. But what if the defendant's terrorist offense was a direct result of a severe mental illness? On rare occasions, this can mean that even though the defendant committed an illegal act, they are not criminally punished; they either lacked the legally required mental state (*mens rea*), or their behavior is legally excused through an NGRI verdict.

The United States

When a defendant is tried for a crime, the prosecutor has the burden of proving the prima facie case beyond a reasonable doubt. In general, a prosecutor must prove that the defendant committed an illegal act (*actus reus*) with a specific mental state (*mens rea*). If a first-degree murder charge requires "the death of another human being with intent to kill that person,"[35] the killing of "another human being" is the illegal act and "intent to kill" is the required mental state.

In rare instances, a defendant's mental illness can prevent them from forming the required *mens rea*.[36] If a defendant lacks the required *mens rea* they cannot be found guilty (at least not of that particular crime). For example, a delusional defendant who thought he was destroying a robot but was actually killing a person would not have the *mens rea* required for first-degree murder.[37] He might, however, be guilty of a lesser offense such as negligent homicide.[38]

In contrast, in a classic NGRI plea, the defendant acknowledges having committed the crime with the required *mens rea*. However, they argue that they should not be held criminally responsible because of the effect of their mental illness. For example, one may argue that it prevented them from appreciating that their actions were wrong.

Kansas uses a *mens rea* approach, rather than an affirmative insanity defense. The US Supreme Court case of *Kahler v. Kansas*, 580 U.S.(2020) recently noted that it did not mean that Kansas had abolished the insanity defense. For purposes

of this chapter, the *mens rea* approach is clearly distinguished from a classic, affirmative, NGRI defense. This is necessary in order to understand the concepts and their academic and legal significance. In light of *Kahler v. Kansas*, this distinction might—over time—become more nuanced than it already is.

CASE EXAMPLE: MENS REA—SPECIFIC INTENT

In October 2012, Raulie Wayne Casteel engaged in a "three-day random shooting spree." He shot at moving cars and caused public panic. He was arrested and charged in the Michigan state court system.[39] Charges included assault with intent to commit murder and terrorism. Michigan has its own terrorism statute.[40]

At trial, Mr. Casteel argued that because of his mental illness he lacked the specific intent to commit these crimes. He tried to present mental health testimony that he had a "persecutory type delusional disorder." This testimony was not allowed. The court cited a 2001 Michigan Supreme Court case[41] which had interpreted Michigan statutes as prohibiting this type of mental health evidence to reduce criminal responsibility except when used for an insanity defense.

Mr. Casteel was, however, permitted to testify about his delusions and intentions. He testified "that he did not intend to shoot at people, that he only intended to shoot at cars."[39] He described his past delusions and paranoia: "government-controlled advanced technologies . . . caused his wife to miscarry twice [and] killed one of his cats . . . [and the] people in the vehicles he shot at were part of a government conspiracy and that they were monitoring him."[39]

The jury found Mr. Casteel guilty of the lesser-included offense of felonious assault, instead of assault with *intent* to commit murder. They still found him guilty of terrorism. In Michigan, a charge of terrorism requires a "willful and deliberate act . . . [that is] a violent felony . . . *intended* to intimidate or coerce a civilian population or influence or affect the conduct of government . . . through intimidation or coercion."[42]

Mr. Casteel appealed. The appellate court upheld the trial court's ruling that Mr. Casteel had the required *intent* for the charge of terrorism. Many of Mr. Casteel's paranoid delusions related to the government. He believed people in the vehicles he shot at were "part of a government conspiracy."[39] He testified that he "may have wanted to send the driver of a vehicle a message to 'back off.'"[39] The appellate court thus found the defendant's mental state, even if delusional, was sufficient for the required *intent* in the state's terrorism statute.

NOT GUILTY BY REASON OF INSANITY

An NGRI defense is typically an affirmative defense (like duress) that excuses a defendant's behavior. In an affirmative defense, the defendant admits having committed the criminal conduct but states that society should excuse him because he is not morally blameworthy. The NGRI defense is commonly misunderstood. The lay public, and even members of the criminal bar, grossly overestimate its success and view it as a quick and easy way for guilty defendants to avoid being punished.[43] In reality, the NGRI defense is infrequently used, rarely succeeds, and usually leads to incarceration (in a hospital) for as long or longer than if found criminally responsible.[44,45]

It is not the presence of a mental illness alone that allows an insanity defense to succeed. Rather,

it is the effect of that illness on the defendant's ability to control and/or understand their criminal behavior. When a forensic mental health professional conducts a sanity evaluation, they assess the defendant's mental state at the time of the crime and the impact of that mental state on the defendant's perception of their criminal activity.

Imagine two defendants—Defendant A and Defendant B. They are both charged with 12 counts of first-degree murder after fatally driving a truck into a group of individuals of Hispanic descent at a local market. Both defendants have schizophrenia and were in an acute psychotic episode at the time of the incident. Defendant A acted in response to a personal grudge against people of Hispanic descent; two Hispanic men had mugged him. Defendant B acted in response to a delusion that Hispanic individuals are demons sent to subjugate the human race; he drove his truck into the crowd while hearing auditory hallucinations telling him to "kill the Hispanics, save the world." Defendant B might succeed with an insanity defense. Defendant A would not.

Whether someone like Defendant B qualifies for an insanity defense depends on when and where they are tried. Over the years, the stringency of NGRI laws have shifted like a pendulum, often by legislators in response to highly publicized cases involving an NGRI acquittee.

Types of Insanity Defenses

A defendant can be eligible for an insanity defense if they have a mental defect or disease that, at the time of the crime, prevented them from engaging in a "mental process defined as necessary for sanity."[37] A defect is permanent, like intellectual disability; a disease can fluctuate in intensity, like bipolar disorder.[46] Severe conditions, such as profound intellectual disability or psychotic disorders (e.g., schizophrenia), are most likely to be considered eligible.[47] On rare occasions, diagnoses such as PTSD have been found sufficient.[47]

In organized group-based terrorism, the authors argue that the recruitment process seems to try to avoid selecting prospective terrorists with mental illness, likely due to their lack of predictability.[48] Lone-actor terrorists do not undergo that same form of screening. Lone-actor terrorists have a higher likelihood of having a mental illness that would be considered in an NGRI defense.[1]

Four states have functionally abolished the NGRI defense.[49] For the rest, most require that a defendant, in order to be eligible for an NGRI acquittal, committed their crime while lacking cognitive, volitional, or moral capacity.[37] There are many nuances to this.

Cognitive capacity refers to a defendant's ability to understand the nature and quality of their acts. If an acutely psychotic defendant stabs his wife—believing that she has been possessed by a demon and will be "purged" and returned to normalcy (and not die) if he puts a knife through her heart—he might lack cognitive capacity. There is an overlap between the concept of *mens rea* and cognitive capacity[50]; a discussion of that area of law is outside the scope of this chapter.

Volitional capacity refers to a defendant's ability to control their actions. If an acutely psychotic defendant stabs his wife in response to command auditory hallucinations ("kill your wife, she deserves it"), he might lack volitional capacity.

Moral capacity refers to a defendant's ability to recognize that their actions are "wrong." If an acutely psychotic defendant stabs his wife believing she is possessed by a demon and will burn in hell unless he kills her, he might lack moral capacity. Depending on the state, wrongfulness can be assessed in several ways: *legal wrongfulness* (knowledge that the conduct is illegal), *subjective wrongfulness* (the defendant's personal belief of what is right or wrong), or *objective wrongfulness* (the defendant's belief about society's standards of what is right or wrong).[51]

Most of the United States has an insanity standard based on M'Naghten (cognitive or moral capacity) or the American Law Institute (ALI)'s Model Penal Code (moral or volitional capacity).[47] The M'Naghten rule was named after Daniel McNaughton (his name has been spelled many ways over the years; we will use the "M'Naghten" spelling here, for clarity).

In 1843, Mr. M'Naghten shot and killed the private secretary of England's Prime Minister.[52] At trial, he presented evidence of persecutory delusions. He was found "not guilty, on the ground of insanity."[52] There was a public outcry. This resulted in England's M'Naghten rule, which clarified that defendants can only be acquitted based on insanity if, at the time of the crime, they lacked cognitive or moral capacity.[37] Variations of this test spread across the United States.

Then, in 1962, the ALI published the Model Penal Code's insanity standard.[53] A defendant could meet this test if they lacked moral or volitional capacity. Over the next 20 years, many states adopted the ALI standard.[54] In 1981, John Hinckley Jr. attempted to assassinate President Reagan. His defense attorney argued that Mr. Hinckley was mentally ill, infatuated with Jodie Foster (an actress), and shot the president to impress her.[55] The defense further argued that Mr. Hinckley was detached from reality in a way that made him unable to appreciate the wrongfulness of his actions.[56] Mr. Hinckley was acquitted by reason of insanity under the ALI standard.[56] There was a public outcry. Many states and the federal government changed their insanity standards, making the insanity test more stringent, substantively and/or procedurally.[57]

The Insanity Evaluation

When a forensic mental health professional performs a sanity evaluation, they are assessing two main issues: (1) whether the defendant had a qualifying mental disease or defect at the time of the alleged crime and (2) whether that mental disease or defect resulted in a specific type of incapacity.

To answer these questions, the forensic mental health professional must know the jurisdiction's standard for sanity. They then review records from the crime (e.g., victim and witness statements, interrogation interviews, photos and videos of the crime scene, detective reports, etc.), records about the defendant (e.g., school and psychiatric records), and collateral information

(e.g., interviews of friends and family). They usually interview the defendant, asking questions about their life history and psychiatric condition, as well as thoughts and behaviors before, during, and after the crime. Historical details are critical; for instance, whether the defendant attempted to conceal the crime or avoid being caught. Based on this information the forensic mental health professional develops an opinion about the defendant's mental state at the time of the crime and whether they fulfill the criteria of that jurisdiction's insanity standard.

CASE EXAMPLE: MR. DOE'S INSANITY PLEA

In the hypothetical case at the start of our chapter, Mr. Doe bombed abortion clinics to influence the government's policy on abortion. Though he had schizophrenia, his insanity plea was rejected.

Sanity evaluations frequently revolve around a defendant's moral capacity: whether their mental illness prevented them from appreciating the wrongfulness of their criminal actions. Although Mr. Doe delusionally believed that he had a God-given duty to stop abortion, he knew that murder was illegal and viewed by society as wrong. In a subjective moral wrongfulness jurisdiction, he could theoretically qualify for an insanity verdict if he had delusionally believed his actions were morally right (e.g., he was hearing God's voice telling him "bomb the clinics, stop abortion"). Juries would likely be skeptical because this is very close to an ideological belief rather than a delusional one.

To have a stronger argument for an insanity verdict, there would need to be some key changes to the fact pattern. For the sake of comparison, let us examine a different hypothetical defendant: Mr. Jones. Mr. Jones delusionally believed that abortion clinics were delivering live babies and then killing them. He believed he was saving lives.

Mr. Jones could theoretically succeed in a jurisdiction with a subjective *or* objective moral wrongfulness standard, although the facts would need to support his story (e.g., his pre-offense postings online, scene investigations by law enforcement, collateral interviews with his friends, his description of what happened). Subjectively, it would need to look like Mr. Jones truly believed that he was doing the right thing due to his delusional belief system. Objectively, society (and the jury) would need to agree with this perception: that his delusion, if true, would justify his conduct.

INTERNATIONAL PERSPECTIVE ON CRIMINAL RESPONSIBILITY

Australian and US insanity laws draw heavily from the 1843 M'Naghten case. In both countries there are jurisdictional differences. In Australia, for instance, New South Wales explicitly follows England's M'Naghten doctrine,[58] while Queensland adds a volitional capacity prong.[59] Similarly, in the United States, North Carolina explicitly follows the M'Naghten doctrine,[60] while New Mexico adds a volitional capacity prong.[61] Both countries allow states or provinces to determine the standard for insanity defenses.

In England and Wales, the insanity standard continues to be based on M'Naghten; it requires

that a defendant lack cognitive or moral capacity.[62] While a defendant's volitional capacity is relevant, it is channeled into the diminished responsibility doctrine.[63] This is a partial defense that allows a defendant to reduce a murder charge to manslaughter if they have a mental abnormality that substantially impaired their ability to "understand the nature of [their] conduct; to form a rational judgment; [or] to exercise self-control."[63] In practice, the diminished responsibility defense always requires psychiatric testimony, but it is distinct from the insanity defense (which, if successful, fully absolves a defendant of criminal responsibility). Both approaches allow a judge in England or Wales to send a defendant to a hospital instead of prison.[62,64]

In 2018, only 76 people were hospitalized in England and Wales for an NGRI acquittal—1.3 per million people.[65,66] In comparison, in the United States, according to a 2014 survey of state psychiatric hospitals, there were an average of 140 people *per state*—roughly 22 per million people.[67,68] There are many possible reasons for this disparity, including differences in procedure and in prosecutorial discretion.

The majority of mentally disordered offenders in England who require hospital admission are admitted to a hospital for treatment (e.g., in lieu of other sentence) via "sections." These are contained within Part III of the Mental Health Act of 1983, as amended in 2007.[69] This is usually through a "Hospital Order," which can be done irrespective of the nature of an offense or the capacity of an offender. In England, in 2015–2016, which is the last year with an adequate dataset, 1,696 people were admitted to the hospital utilizing forensic sections (sections found are under Part III of the Mental Health Act, as opposed to the similarly named civil "sections").[70] Of those, 638 were Section 37 "Hospital Orders," meaning that the court opted to use hospital admission as a means of sentencing.

It may also be relevant that the United Kingdom has abolished the death penalty, and "defendants often prefer the certainty of a prison term to the uncertainty of a release date from hospital"—especially given the availability of the diminished responsibility defense for murder.[62] Despite these examples of legal and procedural differences, forensic mental health professionals play many of the same roles in England, Wales, and Australia as in the United States. They evaluate and treat defendants' psychiatric symptoms in jails, prisons, and hospitals. They also help to assess the impact of a defendant's psychiatric symptoms on their ability to participate in criminal proceedings and their culpability.

SENTENCE MITIGATION

When the public thinks about mental illness and criminal behavior, they often jump to the idea of insanity. However, as we have seen, there are very strict criteria for an insanity acquittal. In an insanity defense, the focus is on the defendant's mental state at the time of the offense. If the defendant is found guilty, information about their long-term mental illness becomes much more relevant for sentence mitigation.[47]

States and the federal government often delineate specific factors that can be considered in sentencing. These factors can be *mitigating*, to decrease a defendant's sentence, or *aggravating*, to increase their sentence. Emotional or mental distress can be considered a mitigating factor.[71] On the other hand, it can also act as an aggravating factor if the judge or jury is concerned that the defendant's mental illness increases their likelihood of future violence.

The motivation, background, and mental illness of an accused terrorist can play an important role in sentencing.[72] Details, such as whether the defendant's mental illness made them more susceptible to extremist ideology or otherwise affected their motivation, can affect perceived culpability and sentencing.[73]

CONCLUSION

When a lone-actor terrorist is arrested, they are criminally prosecuted just as any other criminal. Like other defendants, if there are concerns about their mental health, they are treated and evaluated by mental health professionals. The mental health professional can be in a treatment role (prescribing medications at a jail or prison) or an evaluator role (evaluating the defendant for competency or sanity). The nature of a forensic evaluation, for competency or sanity, differs depending on the jurisdiction. The legal framework and procedure for these evaluations vary from state to state and country to country.

NOTES AND REFERENCES

1. Corner E, Gill P. A false dichotomy? Mental illness and lone-actor terrorism. *Law Hum Behav.* 2015;39(1):23–34. doi:10.1037/lhb0000102.
2. Cirincione C, Steadman HJ, McGreevy MA. Rates of insanity acquittals and the factors associated with successful insanity pleas. *Bull Am Acad Psychiatry Law.* 1995;23(3):399–409.
3. Sinnar S. Separate and unequal: The law of "domestic" and "international" terrorism. *Mich Law Rev.* 2019;117(7):1333–1404.
4. Hale M. *The History of the Pleas of the Crown.* 1. London: 1735.
5. *Dusky v. United States,* 362 U.S. 402 (1960).
6. *Indiana v. Edwards,* 554 U.S. 164 (2008).
7. *Dusky v. United States,* 271 F.2d 385 (8th Cir. 1959).
8. Wall BW, Ash P, Keram E, Pinals DA, Thompson CR. AAPL Practice resource for the forensic psychiatrist evaluation of competence to stand trial. *J Am Acad Psychiatry Law.* 2018;46(3):S4–S79. doi:10.29158/JAAPL.003781-18.
9. Criminal Complaint, *United States of America v. Adel Daoud,* No. 12 CR 723 (N.D. Ill. Sep. 15, 2012).
10. Indictment, *United States of America v. Adel Daoud,* No. 12 CR 723 (N.D. Ill. Sep. 20, 2012).
11. *United States v. Daoud,* 755 F.3d 479 (7th Cir. 2014).

12. Defendant Adel Daoud's Sentencing Memorandum, *United States of America v. Adel Daoud*, No. 12 CR 723 (N.D. Ill. Apr 26, 2019).
13. *North Carolina v. Alford*, 400 U.S. 25 (1970).
14. Drake CJM. The role of ideology in terrorists' target selection. *Terrorism Political Violence*. 1998;10(2):53–85. doi:10.1080/09546559808427457.
15. Rahman T. Extreme overvalued beliefs: How violent extremist beliefs become "normalized." *Behav Sci*. 2018;8(1):10–21. doi:10.3390/bs8010010.
16. American Psychiatric Association. Glossary of technical terms. In *Diagnostic and Statistical Manual of Mental Disorders*. 5th ed. Arlington, VA: American Psychiatric Association, 2013: 817–831.
17. Rahman T, Resnick PJ, Harry B. Anders Breivik: Extreme beliefs mistaken for psychosis. *J Am Acad Psychiatry Law*. 2016;44(1):28–35.
18. Rahman T, Meloy JR, Bauer R. Extreme overvalued belief and the legacy of Carl Wernicke. *J Am Acad Psychiatry Law*. 2019:47(2):180–187. doi:10.29158/JAAPL.003847-19.
19. *State v. Halder*, No. 87874, 2007 Ohio App. LEXIS 5258 (Ohio Ct. App. Eighth Dist. Nov. 8, 2007).
20. *Halder v. Tibals*, Case No. 1:09CV1701 (N.D. Ohio Sep. 14, 2012).
21. Memorandum in Support of Jurisdiction of Appellant Brian Wallace, Administrator of Estate of Norman E. Wallace, *Wallace v. Halder*, Case No. 11-0708 (Ohio Apr 28, 2011).
22. McIntyre TE. Protecting against terrorism or symbolic politics: Fatal flaws in Ohio's criminal terrorism statute. *Case W Res L Rev*. 2005;56(1):203–246.
23. *Halder v. Tibals*, Case No. 12-4244, at 3-4 (6th Cir. 2014).
24. Tetley W. Mixed jurisdictions: Common law v. civil law (codified and uncodified). *La L Rev*. 2000;60(3):678–737.
25. *Rex v. Pritchard*, 7 Car & P 303 (1836).
26. Law Commission (England and Wales). *Unfitness to Plead, Volume 1: Report*, Report No. 364, 2016.
27. *Regina v. Presser*, VR 45 (1958).
28. McSherry B, Baldry E, Arstein-Kerslake A, Gooding P, McCausland R, Arabena K. *Unfitness to Plead and Indefinite Detention of Persons with Cognitive Disabilities*. Melbourne: Melbourne Social Equity Institute, University of Melbourne; 2017.
29. *Kesavarajah v. The Queen*, 181 CLR 230 (1994).
30. *Regina v. John M*, EWCA Crim 3452 (2003).
31. Freckelton I. Rationality and flexibility in assessment of fitness to stand trial. *Int'l J L Psychiatry*. 1996;19(1):39–59.
32. Pirelli G, Gottdiener WH. A meta-analytic review of competency to stand trial research. *Psychol Public Policy Law*. 2011;17(1):1–53.
33. Badger D, Vaughan P, Woodward M, Williams P. Planning to meet the needs of offenders with mental disorders in the United Kingdom. *Psychiatric Serv*. 1999;50(12):1624–1627.
34. Crown Prosecution Service. *Mental Health Conditions and Disorders: Draft Prosecution Guidance*. 12 Mar 2019. https://www.cps.gov.uk/publication/mental-health-conditions-and-disorders-draft-prosecution-guidance
35. Wis. Stat. § 940.01.
36. *United States v. Pohlot*, 827 F.2d 889 (3d Cir. 1987).
37. *Clark v. Arizona*, 548 U.S. 735 (2006).
38. Morse SJ, Hoffman MB. The uneasy entrente between legal insanity and mens rea: Beyond *Clark v. Arizona*. *J Crim L Criminol*. 2007;97(4):1071–1149.
39. People of Michigan v. Raulie Wayne Casteel, 321340 (Mich. Ct. App. Sept 15, 2015).
40. Michigan Penal Code, MCL 750.543(f).
41. People v. Carpenter, 627 N.W.2d 276 (Mich. 2001)
42. Michigan Penal Code, MCL 750.543b(a).
43. Perlin ML. The insanity defense: Nine myths that will not go away. In White MD, ed. *The Insanity Defense: Multidisciplinary Views on Its History, Trends, and Controversies*. Santa Barbara, CA: Praeger; 2017:3–22.
44. Peters AJ, Lex, IA. Improving insanity aftercare. *Mitchell Hamline L Rev*. 2016;42(2):564–601.
45. *Jones v. United States*, 463 U.S. 354 (1983).
46. *Durham v. United States*, 214 F.2d 862 (D.C. Cir. 1954).
47. American Academy of Psychiatry and the Law. AAPL Practice guidelines for forensic psychiatric evaluation of defendants raising the insanity defense. *J Am Acad Psychiatry Law*. 2014;42(4):S3–S76.
48. Federal Research Division, Library of Congress. *The Sociology and Psychology of Terrorism: Who Becomes a Terrorist and Why?* Sep 1999. https://www.loc.gov/rr/frd/pdf-files/Soc_Psych_of_Terrorism.pdf
49. *State v. Jorrick*, 4 P.3d 610 (Kan. 2000).
50. *Kahler v. Kansas*, 580 U.S._(2020).
51. *United States v. Ewing*, 494 F.3d 607 (7th Cir. 2007).
52. Dalby JT. The case of Daniel McNaughton: Let's get the story straight. *Am J Forensic Psychiatry*. 2006;27(4):17–32.
53. ALI, Model Penal Code § 4.01(1) (Proposed Official Draft 1962).
54. *State v. Johnson*, 121 R.I. 254 (R.I. 1979).
55. Caplan L. Annals of Law: The Insanity Defense. *The New Yorker*, 2 Jul 1984. https://www.newyorker.com/magazine/1984/07/02/the-insanity-defense
56. Fuller VJ. United States v. John W. Hinckley Jr. (1982). *Loy LA L Rev*. 2000;33(2):699–704.
57. Callahan L, Mayer C, Steadman HJ. Insanity defense reform in the United States: Post-Hinckley. *Mental Physical Disability L Rep*. 1987;11(1):54–59.
58. *Regina v. Southon*, NSWSC 255 (2002).
59. *Criminal Code Act* 1899, § 27 (Queensland).
60. *State v. Thompson*, 328 N.C. 477 (N.C. 1991).
61. *State v. Hartley*, 565 P.2d 658 (N.M. 1977).
62. Law Commission (England and Wales). Criminal liability: Insanity and automatism, a discussion

paper. 23 Jul 2013. http://lawcommission.justice.gov.uk/areas/insanity.htm

63. Coroners and Justice Act 2009, § 52 (England and Wales).

64. Sentencing Council. Manslaughter by reason of diminished responsibility. 1 Nov 2018. https://www.sentencingcouncil.org.uk/offences/crown-court/item/manslaughter-by-reason-of-diminished-responsibility/

65. Office for National Statistics. Population estimates for the UK, England and Wales, Scotland and Northern Ireland: Mid-2018. 26 Jun 2019. https://www.ons.gov.uk/peoplepopulationandcommunity/ populationandmigration/populationestimates/bulletins/annualmidyearpopulationestimates/mid2018

66. Ministry of Justice. Restricted patients statistical bulletin: 2018. 25 Apr 2019. https://www.gov.uk/government/collections/offender-management-statistics-quarterly-october-to-december-2018

67. National Association of State Mental Health Program Directors. Forensic patients in state psychiatric hospitals: 1999-2016. Aug 2017. https://www.nasmhpd.org/sites/default/files/TACPaper10.Forensic-Patients-in-State-Hospitals_508C_v2.pdf

68. United States Census Bureau. Monthly population estimates for the United States: Apr 1, 2010 to Dec 1, 2019. www2.census.gov/programs-surveys/popest/tables/2010-2018/national/totals/na-est2018-01.xlsx.

69. Mental Health Act 1983 (as amended by the Mental Health Act of 2007), Part III (England and Wales).

70. NHS Digital. Mental Health Act Statistics, Annual Figures 2017-18. 9 Oct 2018. https://digital.nhs.uk/data-and-information/publications/statistical/mental-health-act-statistics-annual-figures/2017-18-annual-figures

71. Hessick CB, Berman DA. Towards a theory of mitigation. *B U L Rev.* 2016;96(3):162–217.

72. Hong N. Disabled man sentenced in Kansas terrorism case. *Wall Street Journal.* 18 Oct 2016. https://www.wsj.com/articles/disabled-man-sentenced-in-kansas-terrorism-case-1476822526

73. Term M. Would-be bomber gets 16-year term: Judge cites mental health. *U.S. News,* 6 May 2019. https://www.usnews.com/news/us/articles/2019-05-05/judge-to-announce-sentence-in-chicago-terrorism-case

14

An Ethics Analysis of Lone-Actor Terror and Society's Response

DANIELLE B. KUSHNER AND PHILIP J. CANDILIS

INTRODUCTION

Terrorism by lone actors is a more complex issue than world governments and the media portray. It is not simply a conflict between good and evil, but one of complicated ethnic, political, and social tensions. In today's political climate, nations and political groups cannot arrive at a consensus on the definition of terrorism, let alone its ethical nuances. Lone actors themselves have been shown to espouse similar grievances as group terrorists, so that even experienced observers struggle to distinguish them. In this chapter, we explore the complementary structural and narrative ethics frameworks that provide the context for lone-actor terror.

ETHICS OF DEFINING TERRORISM

The development of an ethics analysis of terrorism has a fatal flaw: there is no consensus definition. Indeed, researchers have counted more than 100 definitions of terrorism.[1,2] At first glance it would appear that crafting a universal definition for such a well-known phenomenon would be simple and mandatory. The problem is that diverse political interests have made the process of uniting terrorism's complex elements even more complex. The expected components of any definition appear to include rogue actors, states, and civilian victims, but nations and organizations continue to differ on what truly constitutes any of these terms.

In theory, the word "terrorism" refers to a violent extra-military tactic in times of conflict, usually aimed at civilians. It has traditionally referred to actions by well-known rebel groups such as al-Qaeda, Islamic State of Iraq and al-Sham (ISIS), the Red Brigades, and the Irish Republican Army (IRA), among others. Recently, a focus on so-called lone-actor terrorism has resurfaced because

of events as disparate as the Fort Hood shootings and the Norwegian summer camp massacre.

In media coverage, commentators and governments alike cloud the issue by using the term to identify certain ideas or politics as unacceptable, evoking public emotion to support their particular perspective. US President Trump is among those criticized for his reticence in identifying domestic acts of violence perpetrated by white extremists as terrorism while using the word more readily for Islamic individuals.[3] Both fragile and established governments can be quick to judge new or oppositional ideologies without taking the time to explore the behavior they condemn. One-sided interpretations consequently stereotype foreign-born individuals while ignoring violent actions from other racial groups or minorities that are better known or tolerated.

Recent Middle East violence exemplifies this problem. A painful irony is that Osama bin Laden and the Taliban were once called "freedom fighters" and backed by the US Central Intelligence Agency (CIA) when they opposed the Soviet occupation of Afghanistan.[4] Now the Taliban may be the most familiar example of terrorism in the Western world.

Indeed, the idea of the freedom fighter has been controversial from the days of the Irgun battling for Israeli independence (i.e., the British identified Menachem Begin, Irgun leader and future Israeli prime minister, as a terrorist) to the Nicaraguan Contras championed by US President Ronald Reagan. During the height of the Northern Ireland conflict in the 1970s, IRA operatives insisted on being called "prisoners of war" when they were treated like terrorists by the British government.[5] Fundamental struggles over national liberation and self-determination show that reaching a consensus remains difficult because the value of the term shifts easily to match political and social interests.

Consequently, academics, nations, and world organizations have put forward their own definitions. The United States defines terrorism in Title 22, Chapter 38 (2656f) of the US Code[6] as "premeditated, politically motivated violence perpetrated against noncombatant targets by subnational groups or clandestine agents." Other countries focus on people and ideas that question their government. Saudi Arabia's 2017 Penal Law for Terrorism and Its Financing defines terrorists as those who question the government or Islam and does not restrict the definition to violent acts.[7] China's 2016 legislation is broad enough to encompass political thought or speech and punishes government dissidents. China defines terrorism as "Any advocacy or activity that by means of violence, sabotage, or threat, aims to create social panic, undermine public safety, infringe on person or property rights, or coerce a state organ or an international organization, in order to achieve political, ideological, or other objectives."[8] The government removed the term "thought" from its original definition, but human rights advocates contend that the word "advocacy" is still vague enough to punish dissenting thinkers.

Although the United Nations has provided terminologies more consistent with Western approaches, it remains unable to promote one specific definition due to the lack of consensus between member states, especially about self-determination and state violence. Nonetheless, one helpful example is the 2004 UN Security Council Resolution 1566 (2004)[9] that defines terrorist acts as

> criminal acts, including against civilians, committed with the intent to cause death or serious bodily injury, or taking of hostages, with the purpose to provoke a state of terror in the general public or in a group of persons or particular persons, intimidate a population or compel a government or an international organization to do or to abstain from doing any act, which constitute offences within the scope of and as defined in the international conventions and protocols relating to terrorism, are under no circumstances justifiable by considerations of a political, philosophical, ideological, racial, ethnic, religious or other similar nature.

Lone-actor terrorism suffers the same definition problem: some commentators allow for an element of group involvement, while others even allow an accomplice.[10] The motivation for some attacks, often against schools or other large groups, may not be political or philosophical, yet they clearly provoke terror in the general public.[11,12]

Recent work with Iraqi terrorists has not yet yielded meaningful distinctions between those identifying themselves as working alone or working with others. Features often thought to distinguish lone actors, like mental illness, marital status, unemployment, affiliation of family members with a terror group, or loss of a family member, may not necessarily identify the lone actor.[13]

The unsettled nature of these definitions motivates the exploration of the ethical characteristics and principles that lead nations and organizations to use and apply these terms, including the subset identified as lone actors.

AN ETHICAL ANALYSIS OF TERRORISM

The lack of consensus on fundamental definitions has important consequences for the ethical understanding of terrorism itself. Labeling acts as terrorism rather than warfare affects ethical judgments about them. Governments, popular culture, and media portray a stark difference between the two, emphasizing the destructive effects of terrorism while idealizing state-sponsored conflict. This is exemplified by the recent positive portrayal of the Syrian government in its civil war, despite indiscriminate violence that likely included the use of chemical weapons against civilians. One of the ways Syria's President Assad was able to retain local support against heavy odds was by presenting his government as the secular defender of religious pluralism and characterizing protesters as violent, foreign, sectarian Islamists.[14]

State-sponsored warfare that is legitimized by international conventions often runs through subversive processes like coups, "fifth columns" (a group that undermines from within), and rigged elections, all of which may result in support by the international community. Western involvement in the overthrow of governments in Chile, Congo, and others are examples of controversial interventions with legitimized outcomes. Nor are nation-states a stranger to proxy wars, revolutions, assassinations, and military rebellions that change governments, borders, and international affiliations. Russia invaded Crimea after fomenting unrest in 2014, while Egypt, Turkey, and Sudan all provide recent examples of military coups within established nations.

Although it may be difficult to appreciate terrorism's conceptual relationship to more accepted uses of military power, it is important to consider that there may be experiences or thought experiments that result in a more clear-eyed assessment of what truly characterizes terrorism. When British journalist Gerald Seymour wrote, "One man's terrorist is another man's freedom-fighter," he was underscoring the importance of perspective in assessing the legitimacy of violence. This moral ambiguity, found in Seymour's novel *Harry's Game*[15] was situated during the height of the Northern Ireland conflict and threw the brutality of both sides into stark relief. Other well-known examples of the importance of perspective include the Israeli and Palestinian outlooks on the Middle East conflict, the Greek and Turkish struggle over Cyprus, and the Sino-Japanese disagreement over off-shore islands, all of which underscore the frank importance of one's outlook.

Other viewpoints can be much more difficult to cast as a matter of perspective. White nationalist attacks, generally defined as those espousing white supremacist or white separatist ideologies, including the recent Wal-Mart shooting in El Paso, Texas, are more easily seen as terrorist acts by the general public, while those who adhere to these racist philosophies portray the violence as necessary to preserve their values and heritage.[16]

Consequently, a moral assessment depends not only on structural conditions that lead to action, but on one's beliefs about the world one lives in. Two dominant ethical approaches are therefore useful for understanding terrorism: a structural-functional understanding that centers on the means and effects of terrorism and a genealogical-narrative understanding that takes its causes into account.

Structural-Functional Theories

Structural-functional arguments include consequentialist ideas, just war theory, and rights-based ethics. These define the structures and parameters that justify the moral legitimacy or impermissibility of terrorism. *Consequentialist* arguments, for example, have been made both for and against terrorism. They judge events and practices solely based on their outcomes, utility, or consequences, most often positing that the goals of terrorism can never outweigh the consequences of violence and terror.[17]

Others counter that even terrorist acts are justifiable if they lead to better alternatives, such as preventing a full-scale war, for example, or overthrowing tyranny.[18] How far one goes to justify violence is a problem for such arguments: the danger of slippery slopes is inherent to consequentialism, especially because it relies on subjective cutoffs and thresholds to determine right and wrong. Where the cutoffs lie may slip further down the slope of permissibility given the ambiguity of definitions, motives, and outcomes.

Even more important, a *utilitarian* calculus generally ignores non-consequentialist arguments that assess the innate value of an action or the intrinsic duties of persons to one another. These so-called *deontologic* or *Kantian approaches* commonly reject both terrorism and violence no matter the specifics. Since it remains difficult to predict the results of either war or terrorism, the power of consequentialist approaches remains uncertain.

Just war theory supports violence if the right to go to war (*jus ad bellum*) and the conduct in war (*jus in bello*) meet certain standards. The justifying principles of war include being declared by a proper authority, having just cause, and possessing right intention—ideas which have been codified into the well-known Geneva and Hague Conventions.[19] This approach necessarily excludes terrorism, since terrorism does not generally involve governments or group conventions.

At the same time, just war theory subordinates citizen movements that may be more populist or representative but that do not achieve sufficient standing within the governance of a recognized state. Indeed, describing groups who cannot stand up to armies as conducting "asymmetric" warfare is one way of attempting to discriminate one violent activity from another.[20]

Under just war theory, terrorism violates the principles of conduct regarding discrimination and proportionality by targeting civilians and intending, rather than avoiding, "collateral" damage.[21] Despite concerns that the distinction between terrorism and traditional warfare has weakened in modern conflicts, it remains an important distinction for many who oppose a simple consequentialist calculus. Just war theory relies implicitly on the inherent value of societies, collectives that are established for communal purposes like self-protection and commerce.

Complaints of *state-sponsored terrorism*, however, underscore the imperfect nature of these approaches. Indeed, even the American Revolutionary War, often described as a just war with unconventional or asymmetric tactics, is an example that tests the parameters of this theory. George Washington, for example, acted under civilian authority and refused to engage the British under established rules of warfare. Nor did he avoid attacks on civilians, including Loyalists and Native Americans.[22]

Rights-based theories argue, more cogently in our view, against terrorism because terrorist violence violates individual human rights of self-rule, liberty, opportunity, and the right to be left alone. Political violence that targets civilians affects life, health, and freedom of speech, movement, assembly, and related rights—all identified as fundamental by important international theorists and conventions (e.g., the US Declaration of Independence of 1776, the French Declaration of the Rights of Man of 1789, the UN Universal Declaration of Human Rights of 1948, the African Charter on Human Rights of 1986).[23]

The more complex question for the rights-based approach that dominates contemporary ethics is whether it is morally justifiable to violate some rights for the rights of others, or whether there is truly any calculus that can resolve the question. This is the problem of *incommensurability*—the inability to measure different rights, outcomes, or perspectives on the same scale.

Finally, whose right is it to decide how or whether the rights of one group outweigh those of another? The UN, the World Court, the International Criminal Court, and other similar bodies struggle with these questions daily.

Genealogical-Narrative Theories

Separately, genealogical-narrative theories, such as root cause theory and liberation theory, explore the social and cultural underpinnings of terrorism. *Root cause theory* recognizes the underlying sociocultural and economic conditions that give rise to anti-state violence, while *liberation theory* argues that severe political oppression might be legitimately countered by terrorist means. Individual rights, such as life and liberty, remain prominent and may justifiably require violence to achieve their goals.

Such theories help explain how racial discrimination, class divides, and poverty have played a major role in the rising Islamic radicalization and extremism of modern Europe and the United States. A recent Internet study, for example, suggests that minority groups may be more susceptible to radicalization if they experience discrimination in isolated settings or compete for limited financial resources.[24] This provides insight into cases like that of the Mississippi couple arrested for attempting to travel to Syria to join ISIS; they lived in a part of the state with

some of the greatest ethnic homogeneity and anti-Muslim sentiment in the United States.[24]

Justifying violence to overcome oppression is a common theme for ethical analyses, especially within frameworks that recognize certain conflicts as legitimate (e.g., revolutions, democratic uprisings, independence movements). Such approaches generally ignore pacifism and non-violence—which for many are the ideal means of social resistance. The problem for mainstream approaches that justify violence based on oppression narratives is that they come up against the narrative of neighboring peoples and cultures. If narratives are ethically legitimate on their own, there can be no resolution between them when they conflict. Moral relativism rules the day.

Ethicist John Arras has described a use of narrative ethics that helps makes sense of this problem.[25] A narrative, he writes, may enrich the discussion of right and wrong but should not take the place of the entire moral enterprise (i.e., judging what is right). Arras is among those who recognize the need for some kind of criteria for assessing the force of each story, rules that determine which version is most compelling.[26] These might be criteria, for example, that minimize distortions, eschew violence, and generally avoid destructive, divisive alternatives.

Narrative strengthened by structural rules may consequently provide a rich model for deciding the legitimacy of violence. Principled choices of peace over war, diplomacy over conflict, and collaboration over division can only fortify the varied perspectives that clash over land, liberty, and culture.

Lone-Actor Terrorism and Combined Models

For lone actors, both structural and narrative approaches are similarly useful. Lone actors are only individuals in their mode of action, not their ideology. Their endeavors only make sense within the set of beliefs of a particular community, but they enjoy a freedom that is unrestrained by actions or words that alienate supporters or trigger government crackdowns.[27] One such example is the San Bernardino, California, attack in which the perpetrators were a married couple who were homegrown extremists inspired by ISIS, not actors directed by a terrorist cell or network.

Indeed, for Sageman (2008),[28] terrorists are not necessarily aggrieved themselves, often coming from middle-class roots and taking on the injustices experienced by others. Interceding in distressed communities to address criminogenic factors (e.g., poverty, lack of opportunity, lack of education)[29] is another way in which combining structural and narrative approaches fortifies the understanding of lone and group actors alike.

ETHICS OF COUNTERTERRORISM

Society's response to terror often invokes extremist positions of its own. High-profile terror attacks ignite political rhetoric that describes terrorism as one of the great threats to civilization.[30] Statistics are clear, however, that the risks of murder, suicide, accidents, flu, and even air pollution are far greater.[31] Inflating terror risk to deflect attention from other societal or political ills has become an identifiable political strategy. Russian President Vladimir Putin, for example, famously used the threat of terrorism in Chechnya to centralize political control at home and advance Russian interests in neighboring regions. Mobilization against the threat of terrorism has served as recognizable a function for Putin as the threat of "imperialist aggression" did for Stalin's murderous regime.[32] This ease of manipulation and lack of proportionality is a core problem for ethics theories that already struggle to balance rights, outcomes, and methods.

The volume of media coverage following terrorist events usually focuses attention on the identity and characteristics of the perpetrator. This often results in the elevation of the individual and his political causes to his followers—usually one of the terrorist's objectives. Such media coverage may also inspire copycat behavior even among lone actors who do not have a specific terrorist organization to train and direct them. This occurred in the involuntary celibate or "incel" community when the 2014 Isla Vista killer became an Incel hero, leading to more mass violence like the 2018 Toronto van attack.[33]

At the same time, news agencies have been severely criticized for covering killings in detail, including the posting of video from the Christchurch, New Zealand, massacre. Such coverage ignores the role of all elements of society in combating terror. Some media outlets recognize this ethical lapse and have reported that they will not post photographs of terrorists to avoid "posthumous glorification."

For both structural and narrative ethics, intense emotional responses toward those perceived as potential terrorists (e.g., foreigners, immigrants, persons of color, those of non-dominant faiths) prevent a just and fair response to common societal grievances that affect far more people. These intense reactions in turn rationalize repressive measures that frequently shape modern counterterrorism.

Modern counterterrorism incorporates strategies, tactics, and techniques that governments, militaries, law enforcement agencies, businesses, and intelligence agencies alike can use to combat or prevent terrorism. Yet, since September 11, 2001, militarized counterterrorism efforts have developed preferentially in a number of countries, including the United States and United Kingdom. Such methods have included the use of "enhanced interrogation," "rendition" to "black sites" that torture detainees, the assassination of radicalized US citizens overseas by drone strike, heightened data surveillance, and legislation that restricts immigration, civil liberties, and human rights (e.g., the US Patriot Act).[34]

In a classic consequentialist rebuke to such approaches, the 2014 US Senate Committee Study of the CIA's Detention and Interrogation Program concluded that "enhanced interrogation techniques" on detainees between 2001 and 2006 during the "War on Terror" did not help acquire actionable intelligence or gain cooperation from detainees, while simultaneously damaging the United States' international standing.[35]

Dating back to the 1798 Alien and Sedition Acts, a common US response to outside threats is restricting liberty, which trades the protection of rights for security. This then alienates minority communities who, in some analyses, become less likely to collaborate with law enforcement.[36] Community-based prevention programs can be affected as well because immigrants feel these programs are geared more toward gathering intelligence than offering support.[37]

Increased surveillance has not just been limited to minority communities, as the US National Security Agency's (NSA) broad data collection programs have shown. These were gradually implemented on a massive scale through a series of legislative changes and laws following the September 11, 2001, attacks. They included the PRISM program that collected email, Facebook, and instant messages for an unknown number of people and the Verizon metadata collection order, among others.[38] Following scrutiny from the Obama administration, Congress, and a national security court in 2009, the Justice Department acknowledged that the NSA had collected emails and phone calls that exceeded legal limitations.[39]

Another poignant illustration of the overreach of just war thinking is the medical support for interrogations during the administration of US

President George W. Bush. The US Department of Justice and the Pentagon initially crafted policies supporting healthcare professionals' participation in interrogations in Iraq, Afghanistan, and Guantanamo Bay. Providers were allowed to operate in an exceptional role—in a consultative rather than treatment role so that traditional medical ethics did not apply. Allegations included force-feeding of hunger strikers (even anally), developing and monitoring water-boarding, stress positions, sleep deprivation protocols, and advising interrogators of ways to increase psychological stress. It was a painful compromise of traditional structural and narrative ethics in an effort to combat terrorism.[40,41]

The United Kingdom's counter-terrorism efforts have included detaining suspected terrorists indefinitely without trial since the Troubles in Northern Ireland in the 1970s and 1980s. Under the Prevention of Terrorism (Temporary Provisions) Act of 1984, officials could authorize detention for up to 7 days—a breach of article 5(3) of the European Convention on Human Rights. As a result, the British government exempted itself from this article, leading to even greater civil disturbance and diminished respect for the rule of law. With the updated Terrorism Act of 2006, the United Kingdom extended pre-charge detention of terrorist suspects for up to 28 days without charge.[42]

In a similar tradeoff, alleged terrorists have not consistently been afforded trials commensurate with common criminal or military models; they are not considered traditional criminals or prisoners of war. In the United States, cases against alleged terrorists have been tried in both civilian criminal courts and military tribunals established by President Bush's well-known November 2001 executive order.

Military tribunals have been controversial because they can convict by a two-thirds majority, rather than by the more common unanimous agreement. Moreover, the exclusionary rule that keeps illegally seized evidence out of a civilian criminal trial does not apply. These exceptions may be considered direct threats to common human rights and the ideas of fairness often espoused by deontologic writers.

The Military Commissions Act of 2009 helped to address some basic concerns surrounding the US military commissions,[43] such as excluding from trial any statements made under torture. But problematic distinctions remain. Commissions continue, for example, to permit coerced testimony obtained at the point of capture or during combat itself. This varies from the trial rights routinely provided to US service members in courts martial. Moreover, commissions still include an overbroad definition of who can be tried and permit defendants to be tried *ex-post facto* for conduct not considered a war crime at the time it was committed. This is a seminal problem for Western law, which is not typically retroactive. Supporters posit that these laws balance the demands for fairness and due process against a need for flexibility, while opponents argue that this second-tier system is designed merely to facilitate quick convictions.[44]

At the same time, states and agencies have developed less controversial counterterrorism responses that are more consistent with sound structural and narrative ethics. Programs such as the US National Strategy for Counterterrorism and the UK Counter-Terrorism Strategy (CONTEST) program are well-known examples that guide national responses.

The CONTEST program, for example, was first developed in 2003 and has four arms: protecting targets (Protect), preparing against (Prepare), and stopping terrorist attacks (Pursue), while simultaneously working to prevent people from becoming terrorists or supporting terrorism (Prevent). The Prevent agenda includes countering terrorist ideology and supporting individuals at risk of radicalization through a specific program called Channel. Channel was first piloted in 2007, with the goal of identifying individuals at risk of radicalization, assessing the nature of that risk, and developing an appropriate individualized support plan. These plans addressed vulnerabilities surrounding health, education, employment, or housing as well as providing mentoring specialists and diversionary activities.

Despite their alignment with important principles of acculturation and engagement, Prevent and Channel have nonetheless raised controversy because they identify at-risk individuals with a newly developed assessment tool, the Extremist Risk Guidance 22+ (ERG 22+). The instrument was not published initially, did not follow a credible peer-review process, and extended beyond its scope into a domain imprecisely called "pre-radicalization."[45]

The UK Counter Terrorism and Security Act of 2015[46] further expanded the Prevent program to require teachers, physicians, and social workers to become mandated reporters—but it conducted trainings to identify those at risk using the controversial ERG 22+. While most aspects of CONTEST have been publicly supported, the

Prevent strategy has invoked alarm due to concerns of stigmatizing and alienating Islamic and other non-dominant youth.[45]

Given the challenges of such interventions, programs in the Netherlands, Denmark, and Sweden, among others, have shifted their focus to violent radicalization rather than broader extremism, improving communication and assessment and emphasizing assessment of the effectiveness of these programs. For example, the Netherlands Polarisation and Radicalisation Action Plan 2007–2011 was initially conceived as a national strategy to prevent the "processes of isolation, polarization, and radicalization by the (re-) inclusion of people." It targeted those at risk of separating from Dutch society and democratic legal order. This approach has been criticized for being too broad and not relying on sufficient empirical evidence, so authorities have narrowed their focus on forms of radicalization more closely linked to violence.[47]

There is concern that political commentary and restrictive legislation have led to increased anti-immigrant rhetoric and further marginalization of the immigrant and minority communities. For example in the American Southwest, the passage of Arizona's S.B.1070 "Show Me Your Papers" law (that was weakened after an outcry) and other anti-immigrant laws has coincided with the startling growth of white supremacist and neo-Nazi groups throughout the region.[48]

In Europe, Danish lawmakers have proposed a woefully named "Ghetto Package" that mandates immigrant children living in certain neighborhoods be sent to school to learn Danish language and values. How children are chosen is related to a government-defined "particularly vulnerable public housing area," also formally known as a "ghetto" (*ghettoområde*). This is legally identified as a neighborhood where more than a thousand people meet certain criteria, including at least 50% being non-Western immigrants, at least 40% being unemployed, and those having a criminal record at least three times the national average over the past 2 years.[49] The choice of these cutoffs is heavily imbued with discriminatory cultural values and underscores the slippery slope dangers of consequentialist approaches. The Package also mandates harsher punishments for those convicted of crimes within a "ghetto" than those committed elsewhere, raising substantial questions of fairness and social justice.[50]

The reinforcement of existing social biases, the absence of culturally sensitive integration, and the increased potential for future attacks violates basic preventive principles that are central to many ethics approaches. Acting to improve future human interactions by preventing problems is critical to both improved group outcomes as well as to the efficacy of individual ethics and policy initiatives, whether in decreasing terrorism or improving common criminogenic risks.

For many commentators, policies that accentuate rather than moderate cultural and ethnic differences have contributed to the recent rise of right-wing parties in Europe. Hungary, Poland, Sweden, Germany, and France have all experienced a backlash against permissive immigrant policies.[51] Other observers trace Brexit to the same divisive considerations.

APPLICATION OF ETHICAL THEORIES

Just war theory, human rights, and consequentialism have accordingly been used to analyze society's counterterrorism efforts in the same way they do terrorism. The central question is whether counterterrorist activities are justified or whether they simply add to the problem itself.

The challenge for counterterrorism efforts is that the human rights theories that legitimately dominate the ethics landscape assert that all people, civilians and terrorists alike, are entitled to similar—and humane—treatment. All violence is equivalent in this analysis, undermining the suggestion that one form of violence is qualitatively different from another. In this view, violence directed at civilians walking a promenade in Nice, France, or attending a Pittsburgh synagogue is not qualitatively different from torturing detainees or accepting a certain number of civilian deaths from traditional military operations. Consequently, a state's warcraft, criminal investigations, incarceration, and legal proceedings must keep to human rights standards: one cannot justify the sober, considered rights abuses by a state without undermining the principles of a humane society and perpetuating the destructive cycle.

The principles of self-governance and religious freedom that many terrorists themselves espouse cannot withstand the scrutiny of this analysis. Terrorists do not honor the human rights of those they terrorize. Indeed, counterterrorism often uses self-defense or the emergency exception to justify itself, underscoring the special nature of efforts to protect a community from outside threats.

Consequentialist or utilitarian arguments, on the other hand (as opposed to narratives or rights), justify counterterrorism by balancing the greater potential for saving lives against the rights of terrorists.[21] Military counterterrorism is perceived as the better calculation. Even with this freedom, however, US officials have been criticized for their lack of transparency, especially for not providing an accurate account of deaths from drone strikes.[52] Legitimate state actors still have responsibilities to international rules and principles, even when dealing with those who do not follow them. This is among the cardinal characteristics that legitimize societies and delegitimize terrorists.

Narrative theorists exercise a broader scope of argumentation by moving beyond ascribing responsibility to the terrorist or counterterrorist directly. Instead, some assign responsibility to all who contribute to creating harms—those creating the hateful breeding-ground along with those overtly supporting either terrorism or oppressive counter-efforts.[52] Simply prioritizing one bad choice over another is not the traditional exercise of ethical decision-making.

The ideal balance is more likely one that maintains human rights while advocating more sensitive exercises of state power; namely, improving social welfare, educating home and immigrant communities, developing relationships with immigrant groups, teaching tolerance, and conducting more evidence-based monitoring and intervention. This approach is in keeping with ethics models that minimize the negative effects of competing values and intrude least on other principles.[53]

In one particularly egregious violation of such an integrated approach—and a classic misuse of consequentialist arguments—the "ticking-time-bomb scenario" permits torture of a terrorist to extract information that can save others. This unfortunate tradeoff not only ignores the questionable information obtained by torture (a consequentialist concern), but also the principled and human rights objections to torture and the militarization of civil defense. Duties to captives and to international agreements like the Geneva Convention are generally considered to enrich the ethical discussion of such scenarios.

There is a common rebuttal to such human rights objections from the perspective of one's standing in the conflict, a form of status ethics or exceptionalism.[54,55] This is an attempt to categorize terrorists (or interrogators) as exceptional—outside the reach of societal agreements. Terrorists are not seen as formal combatants and

are therefore outside the usual conventions. They do not become prisoners of war, but military detainees.

So-called *asymmetrical warfare* conjures the same exception: where insurgencies do not have the resources of nations and resort to tactics outside the rules, nations are historically allowed to create new rules in response. Those individuals who act outside the rules must renounce the usual rights afforded to traditional combatants, while nations can decline to respond to the UN and World Court while continuing their abuses. This may be the more ironic asymmetry. Indeed, the ethical discomfort with these approaches is often signaled by the very need for terms like "asymmetrical warfare" and "military detainee."

We recommend a thought experiment that considers both a hunger strike and a roadside bombing as asymmetrical warfare, and we invite the reader to apply consequences and exceptionalism to both situations.

Both the hunger strike and the roadside bomb are commonly considered asymmetrical warfare, yet each carries a different moral valence. For many, the hunger strike is more tolerable and less harmful; consequently, it is more deserving of legitimacy. Nonetheless, UK Prime Minister Margaret Thatcher did not think so when IRA leader Bobby Sands died from his well-known fast. She said simply, "Mr. Sands was a convicted criminal. He chose to take his own life. It was a choice that his organization did not allow to many of its victims."[56]

For most, however, the nature of a hunger strike makes it qualitatively different. Its individual nature and its use by historically oppressed groups or beloved leaders like Mahatma Gandhi and Alice Paul lends it legitimacy. But what if the hunger strike incites violence or disrupts a legitimate security organization like a prison?

Conversely, what if the roadside bombing protests the verified inhumane treatment of a non-dominant group? What if the perpetrator is Menachem Begin or Nelson Mandela, revered leaders of non-dominant groups who were accused of terrorism by their oppressors? Is one's perspective or agreement with the actor enough to alter the analysis?

Consequentialist arguments generally favor these individuals because their actions led to a better society, while narrative ethics also supports their redress of injustice and economic conditions. Although these individuals conducted asymmetrical warfare and terrorized the group in power, they may have found a kind of grudging balance for those gauging the legitimacy of their violence.

Finding this balance is not always easy, however. The white supremacist shooters of Christchurch, New Zealand, and Charleston, South Carolina, believed that they were bringing about a better society, too. Although genealogical arguments can outline the socioeconomic factors that led to their attacks, their worldview does not stand up to either consequentalist, narrative, or human rights scrutiny. As we have seen, narratives matter, but so do the rules used to gauge them; namely, championing oppressed minorities, undertaking diplomacy, not targeting civilians, and favoring non-violence.

The ultimate standard for human rights theorists like Thomas Jefferson, Immanuel Kant, and John Stuart Mill is that certain rights like life and liberty are inalienable and un-renounceable: they cannot be taken away and they cannot be given up (e.g., the US Declaration of Independence).[57] Trading off fundamental obligations between persons is the path of relativism and nihilism that even terrorism exploits. It cannot be the path of established nations in a global community.

Ultimately, our objection to the tradeoff or balancing approach of many ethical theories is that no individual or act can withstand the weight of society. Individuals can never outweigh the community; community rights are unfailingly more numerous and therefore more worthy of protection. Consequently, the balancing approach is unhelpful because it cannot distinguish the ethical elements that matter to any exploration of either structural or narrative ethics; it simply counts bodies.

In analyses of *forensic ethics*—the closely related ethics of experts who serve institutions like courts, employers, or the military—scholars have integrated structural and narrative ideologies to emphasize the importance of protecting vulnerable persons and values.[58] This is a fundamental position that calls for identifying where the vulnerabilities arise and then behaving to provide a "structurally stabilizing, morally protective force." Communities and analysts must decide two things: first, which is more vulnerable, the society or the individual who breaks violently with it. And second, what protections for both society and individuals are required to provide structural stability and moral protection.

CONCLUSION

Since terrorism is an existential threat to the social order, the impulse to put traditional rules aside is as tempting to governments as it is to terrorists. To counter this impulse, we have explored the structural and narrative tools that assess the acceptance or rejection of terrorism, from just war and root cause theories, to consequentialism and human rights. Similar ethical arguments are available for counterterrorism efforts as well. Overall, we are among those who believe that damage to fundamental rights from any source—government or insurgency, group or lone actor—is more problematic for society than even the threat of terrorism itself.

NOTES AND REFERENCES

1. Laqueur W. *The New Terrorism: Fanaticism and the Arms of Mass Destruction*. New York: Oxford University Press; 1999.
2. Kruglanski AW, Fishman S. Terrorism between "syndrome" and "tool." *Curr Dir Psychol Sci.* 2006;15(1):45–48. doi:org/10.1111/j.0963-7214.2006.00404.x.
3. Corbin CM. Terrorists are always Muslim but never white: At the intersection of critical race theory and propaganda. *Fordham L Rev.* 2017;86(2):455–485.
4. Cook R. The struggle against terrorism cannot be won by military means. The Guardian, 8 Jul 2005. https://www.theguardian.com/uk/2005/jul/08/july7.development
5. Caesar SA. Captive or criminal? Reappraising the legal status of IRA prisoners at the height of the troubles under international law. *Duke J Comp Intl L.* 2016;27:323–348.
6. 22 United States Code Ch. 38. 2656f. Annual country reports on terrorism. https://uscode.house.gov/view.xhtml?path=/prelim@title22/chapter38&edition=prelim
7. Human Rights Watch, Saudi Arabia: New counterterrorism law enables abuse. Refworld. 23 Nov 2017. https://www.refworld.org/docid/5a1803644.html
8. Zhou Z. China's comprehensive counterterrorism law. The Diplomat, 23 Jan 2016. https://thediplomat.com/2016/01/chinas-comprehensive-counter-terrorism-law/
9. United Nations Security Council. Resolution 1566. 8 Oct 2005. https://www.un.org/ruleoflaw/files/n0454282.pdf
10. Borum R. Loner attacks and domestic extremism. *Criminol Public Policy.* 2013;12(1):103–112.
11. Borum R, Knoll JK. The "pseudocommando" mass murderer: Part I, the psychology of revenge and obliteration. *J Am Acad Psychiatry Law.* 2010;38(1):87–94.
12. Borum R, Knoll JK. The "pseudocommando" mass murderer: Part II, the language of revenge. *J Am Acad Psychiatry Law.* 2010;38(2):263–272.
13. Dhumad S, Candilis P, Dyer A, Cleary S, Khalifa N. Risk factors for terrorism: A comparison

of family, childhood, and personality factors among Iraqi terrorists, murderers, and controls [Published online ahead of print Mar 17, 2019]. *Behavioral Sciences of Terrorism and Pol.* 2019. doi:10.1080/19434472.2019.1591481.

14. Phillips C. The world abetted Assad's victory in Syria. The Atlantic, 4 Aug 2019. https://www.theatlantic.com/international/archive/2018/08/assad-victory-syria/566522/

15. Seymour G. *Harry's Game.* New York: Random House; 1975.

16. Andone D, Levenson E, Chavez N, Vera A. The El Paso shooter faces the death penalty in a "domestic terrorism: case. CNN, 4 Aug 2019. https://www.cnn.com/2019/08/04/us/el-paso-shooting-sunday/index.html

17. Fotion N. The burdens of terrorism. In Leiser BM, ed. *Values in Conflict: Life, Liberty, and the Rule of Law.* New York: Macmillan;1981:463–470.

18. Coser LA. Some social functions of violence. *Ann Am Academy Political and Soc Sci.* 1966;364(1):8–18. doi:org/10.1177/000271626636400102.

19. Taylor I. Just war theory and the military response to terrorism. Soc Theory Pract. 2017;43(4):717–740. doi:10.5840/soctheorpract2017103020.

20. Boot M. The evolution of irregular war. Foreign Affairs. Mar/Apr 2013. https://www.foreignaffairs.com/articles/2013-02-05/evolution-irregular-war

21. Hersh MA. Terrorism, human rights and ethics: A modeling approach. *IFAC Proc Volumes.* 2006;39(23):8–19. doi:10.1016/S1474-6670(17)30087-3.

22. Hoock H. *Scars of Independence.* New York: Crown Publishing; 2017.

23. Shelton DL. An introduction to the history of international human rights law. GW Law Faculty Pub Other Works. 2007;1052. doi:10.2139/ssrn.1010489.

24. Bail CA, Merhout F, Ding P. Using internet search data to examine the relationship between anti-Muslim and pro-ISIS sentiment in US counties. *Sci Adv.* 2018;4 (6):1–9. doi:10.1126/sciadv.aao5948.

25. Arras JD. Nice story, but so what? In Nelson HL, ed. *Stories and Their Limits, Narrative Approaches to Bioethics.* New York: Routledge; 1997:65–90.

26. Burrell D, Hauerwas S. From system to story: An alternative pattern for rationality in ethics. In Englehardt HT, Callahan D, eds. *Knowledge, Value, and Belief.* Hastings-on-Hudson, NY: Hastings Center; 1977:115–152.

27. Hamilton M. Threat assessment framework for lone-actor terrorists. *Fla Law Rev.* 2018;70(6):1319–1356.

28. Sageman M. *Leaderless Jihad.* Philadelphia: University of Pennsylvania Press; 2008.

29. Smith AG. Risk factor and indicators associated with radicalization to terrorism in the United States: What research sponsored by the National

Institute of Justice tells us. National Institute of Justice, US Dept. of Justice, Jun 2018. https://www.ncjrs.gov/pdffiles1/nij/251789.pdf

30. Chainey R. Narendra Modi: These are the 3 greatest threats to civilization. World Economic Forum, 23 Jan 2018. https://www.weforum.org/agenda/2018/01/narendra-modi-davos-these-are-the-3-greatest-threats-to-civilization/

31. Ritchie H, Roser M. Causes of death. OurWorldInData.org, Feb 2018. Updated Apr 2019. https://ourworldindata.org/causes-of-death

32. Baev PK. Counter-terrorism as a building block for Putin's regime. In Hedenskog J, Konnander V, Nygren B, Oldberg I, Pursiainen C, eds. *Russia as a Great Power: Dimensions of Security Under Putin.* New York: Routledge; 2005:323–344.

33. Robertson A. Should we treat incels as terrorists? The Verge, 5 Oct 2019. https://www.theverge.com/2019/10/5/20899388/incel-movement-blueprint-toronto-attack-confession-gender-terrorism

34. Public Law 107-56. United and strengthening America by providing appropriate tools required intercept and obstruct terrorism (USA Patriot Act) Act of 2011. https://www.sec.gov/about/offices/ocie/aml/patriotact2001.pdf

35. United States Senate. Report of the Senate Select Committee on intelligence. Committee study of the Central Intelligence Agency's Detention and Interrogation Program. Forward by Chairman Feinstein and additional and minority views. 2014. https://www.intelligence.senate.gov/sites/default/files/publications/CRPT-113srpt288.pdf

36. Kirk DS, et al. The paradox of law enforcement in immigrant communities: Does tough immigration enforcement undermine public safety? *Ann Am Acad Political Soc Sci* 2012;641(1):79–98. doi:org/10.1177/0002716211431818.

37. Weine SM, et al. Violent extremism, community-based violence prevention and mental health professionals. *J Nerv Ment Dis.* 2017;205 (1):54–57. doi:10.1097/NMD.0000000000000634.

38. FAQ: What you need to know about the NSA's surveillance programs. Propublica, 5 Aug 2013. https://www.propublica.org/article/nsa-data-collection-faq

39. Lichtblau E, Risen J. Officials said US wiretaps exceeded law. New York Times, 15 Apr 2009. https://www.nytimes.com/2009/04/16/us/16nsa.html

40. Keram EA. Will medical ethics be a casualty of the war on terror? *J Am Acad Psychiatry Law.* 2006;34(1):6–8.

41. McCarthy M. US health professionals helped in the torture of detainees, report says. *BMJ.* 2013;347 (7932):1–2. doi:10.1136/bmj.f6680.

42. The Law Library of Congress, Global Legal Research Center. United Kingdom: Pre-charge detention for terrorist suspects. Oct 2008. https://www.loc.gov/law/help/uk-pre-charge-detention/uk-pre-charge-detention.pdf

43. United States Congress. Military Commission Act 2009. https://www.mc.mil/Portals/0/MCA-20Pub20Law200920.pdf

44. Human Rights First. Myth vs. Fact: Trying Terror Suspects in Federal Court. Feb 2018. https://www.humanrightsfirst.org/sites/default/files/Federal-Court-Myth-vs-Fact.pdf

45. Qureshi A. CAGE Advocacy UK Ltd. The 'science': of pre-crime. The secret 'radicalisation' study underpinning Prevent. 2016. https://www.cage.ngo/product/the-science-of-pre-crime-report

46. UK Public General Acts. Counter Terrorism and Security Act 2015. http://www.legislation.gov.uk/ukpga/2015/6/contents/enacted

47. Vidino L, Brandon J. Countering Radicalization in Europe. The International Centre for the Study of Radicalisation and Political Violence. 2012. https://icsr.info/wp-content/uploads/2012/12/ICSR-Report-Countering-Radicalization-in-Europe-1.pdf

48. Van Zeller M. Anti-Latino hate crimes rise as immigration debate intensifies. Huffington Post, 18 Oct 2011, updated 6 Dec 2017. www.huffpost.com/entry/anti-latino-hate-crimes-rise-immigration_n_1015668

49. Ghettolisten 2018. Ministry of Transport and Housing. 1 Dec 2018. (In Danish.) https://www.trm.dk/media/3680/ghettolisten-2018.pdf

50. Rutten, R. Assimilation, or alienation? Denmark mulls "ghetto" laws targeting immigrants. World Politics Review, 13 Nov 2018. https://www.worldpoliticsreview.com/articles/26741/assimilation-or-alienation-denmark-mulls-ghetto-laws-targeting-immigrants

51. Green-Pedersen C, Otjes S. A hot topic? Immigration on the agenda in Western Europe. *Party Politics*. 2019;25 (3):424–434.

52. Eckenwiler L, Hunt M. Counterterrorism, ethics and global health. *Party Politics*. 2014;44(3):12–13. doi:org/10.1002/hast.308.

53. Childress J. *Practical Reasoning in Bioethics*. Bloomington: Indiana University Press; 1997.

54. Phillips RTM. Expanding the role of the forensic consultant. *Am Acad Psychiatry Law Newsl*. 2005;30(1):4–5.

55. Schafer JR. The ethical use of psychology in criminal investigations. *J Am Acad Psychiatry Law*. 2001;29(4):445–446.

56. Margaret Thatcher House of Common PQs. Margaret Thatcher Foundation. 5 May 1981. https://www.margaretthatcher.org/document/104641

57. Kant I. *The Metaphysics of Morals*. Frankfurt: Suhrkamp; 1979.

58. Wynia MK, Latham SR, Kao AC, Berg J, Emanuel L. Medical professionalism in society. *N Engl J Med*. 1999;341:1612–1616. doi:10.1056/NEJM199911183412112.

15

Law Enforcement Response to Lone-Actor Incidents at the Local Through Federal Levels

*DOUGLAS BRENNAN, MARK CONCORDIA, AND MICHAEL MADDEN** *

INTRODUCTION

This chapter outlines the law enforcement role when responding to an event involving lone-actor violence. This role can be proactive and preventive, as described in the first part of this chapter, with federal, state and local agencies forming partnerships to facilitate communication and intelligence-sharing. This is an ongoing process to enhance cross-systems collaboration to assess, intervene, and manage individuals of concern before an act of violence occurs. In the second part of this chapter, the reactive nature of the law enforcement response is covered, starting with the immediate response to an event with a discussion regarding tactics used to locate and neutralize threats and arrange for a medical response. General concepts such as incident management and notification/incorporation of outside agencies are discussed, as well as the emotional toll that first responders experience. The early stages of the criminal investigation are then covered, highlighting the need for both a central overarching investigative organization as well as robust local participation.

LAW ENFORCEMENT INTELLIGENCE GATHERING AND ASSESSMENT

Here we examine the use of threat assessment and protective intelligence gathering to prevent an attack from occurring. The role of local and state law enforcement agencies in the prevention of lone-actor terrorism and mass casualty attacks is increasing. Traditionally, local and state police agencies emphasized response protocols

centering on active shooter incidents. Active shooter response protocols dictate that responding officers, as soon as tactically possible, take immediate steps to locate the active shooter, fix the shooter's location, and, if necessary, eliminate the shooter through the use of deadly physical force. Active shooter training and response protocols are an essential aspect of readiness; however, when combined with prevention-based protocols, they represent the future of law enforcement responses to lone-actor terrorism and mass casualty attacks.

The threat of a terrorist attack in the United States has evolved and expanded. The large-scale coordinated attack plans of al-Qaeda and its affiliates have given way to ideologically inspired attacks by Islamic State of Iraq and al-Sham (ISIS) supporters with no actual connection to the terror group. The threat has further morphed to loosely affiliated or non-affiliated violent extremists. Many at-risk individuals identify with the unifying agents of anger and frustration enhanced in the dark corners of the jihadist, white supremacists, Columbiners, and involuntary celibates' online communities.

Between 2011 and 2014, mass shootings, a form of targeted violence in the United States involving the murder of four or more people, tripled in frequency.[1] During this period, a mass shooting occurred on average every 64 days, compared to every 200 days in the previous 29 years.[1] In a recent publication by the Department of Justice, Federal Bureau of Investigation on active shooters in the United States, it was noted that 2017 saw the highest number of active shooter

---

* The opinions expressed in this chapter are the chapter authors' and not those of the Federal Bureau of Investigation.

incidents recorded by the FBI in 1 year. Based on the FBI analysis, in 2017, an active shooter incident occurred on average every 12 days and every 13.5 days in 2018.[2]

The transformation of the terrorist threat can be described as a hyper-decentralization, which poses problems for the collecting and analyzing of threat intelligence.[3] This amalgam of threats has complicated counterterrorism investigative strategies. The FBI is the lead agency charged with preventing and investigating acts of terrorism constituting violations of federal law. The Behavioral Analysis Unit (BAU), nested in the National Center for the Analysis of Violent Crime, leads the FBI's efforts at countering the challenge of hyper-decentralization by advancing the use of a behavioral threat assessment (BTA) and management by local and state law enforcement professionals.[4] The BAU focuses on the behavior of a subject of concern to better understand what is motivating him or her to choose violence as an acceptable resolution to a personal, ideological, or political grievance.

BTA is defined as a "set of investigative and operational techniques that can be used by law enforcement professionals to identify, assess, and manage the risks of targeted violence and its potential perpetrators."[5] Randy Borum, one of the leading contributors to contemporary scholarship in the field of threat assessment and management, identifies three main principles of threat assessment:

> First, targeted violence, at times, referred to as intended violence, is the result of an understandable and often discernible process of thinking and behavior; second, violence stems from an interaction among the potential attacker, past stressful events, a current situation, and the target; third, the key to investigation and resolution of threat assessment cases is identification of the subject's "attack related" behaviors.[6]

Targeted or intended violence differs from impromptu violence in that the act of violence is not the result of a spontaneous or impulsive act by the perpetrator but instead the final stop on a systematic process of rationalizing violence.[7] The pathway to intended violence model is a widely accepted, useful tool for local and state law enforcement agencies to guide intelligence gathering and assessment protocols to respond to threats of targeted violence because it addresses the question of "why?"[4]

Local and state law enforcement agencies are in a unique position as first responders to aid in the early identification of possible lone offenders. Recent studies by the FBI Behavioral Threat Assessment Center on lone-offender terrorism in the United States identified that "many of the offenders had personal experiences, motives, and life stressors that co-mingled with their violent ideologies and their reasons for carrying out an attack."[8] It is a well-known construct in targeted violence prevention that offenders exhibit pre-attack behaviors that are often recognized by people, commonly referred to as "bystanders," in the offenders' social network.[8,9,10] Bystanders are likely to report to police, or the police may come in pre-attack contact with the would-be lone offender based on concerning behaviors manifesting from life stressors such as mental health, financial, family, marital, and criminal activity.[8]

Conceptualizing the "why" in a model that identifies behavior and thinking patterns at each step of the pathway provides police with a framework to gather risk-relevant data. When correctly assessed by a certified threat manager or a trained multidisciplinary team, it can inform investigative strategies to prevent attacks by lone-actor terrorists and others committed to targeted violence. However, the challenge of integrating law enforcement first-responders into an intelligence-driven multidisciplinary investigative protocol that prioritizes prevention instead of reaction is significant. One problem is the lack of police training and awareness of BTA and management as a viable threat response paradigm. The Federal Bureau of Investigation's National Center for the Analysis of Violent Crime (NCAVC) acknowledged the challenge facing law enforcement in its publication "Making Prevention a Reality":

> Traditional law enforcement techniques historically have focused on the apprehension and prosecution of violent offenders after violent crimes are committed. When police are given information that someone may potentially commit a crime or become violent in the future, their responsibilities, authorities, and available investigative tools are suddenly less clear.[4]

Federal law enforcement agencies such as the US Secret Service, FBI, and the US Capitol Police have operationalized BTA into their protective intelligence and assessment protocols. Likewise, major metropolitan police departments, such as the Los Angeles Police Department Threat Management

Unit, have been using BTA protocols for decades.[11] However, there exists a significant gap in research on the use of BTA protocols by local and state law enforcement agencies.[12] The methodologies are in place for local and state law enforcement agencies to integrate threat response protocols (TRPs) into police operations.

BUILDING LAW ENFORCEMENT THREAT RESPONSE PROTOCOL

The creation of law enforcement TRPs represents local and state law enforcement's attempt to emphasize preventative responses and threat assessment and management protocols. When appropriately applied, threat assessment and management protocols can mitigate the risk of targeted acts of violence such as lone-actor terrorism, mass shootings, and lethal intimate partner violence. The US Secret Service is one of the federal law enforcement agencies advocating the use of threat assessment by state and local law enforcement agencies. The Service defines the threat assessment process as follows:

> Threat assessment or protective intelligence is the process of gathering and assessing information about persons who may have the interest, motive, intention, and capability of mounting attacks against public officials and figures. Gauging the potential threat to and vulnerability of a targeted individual is key to preventing violence. Among criminal justice functions, threat assessment holds great promise for determining vulnerability and guiding interventions in potentially lethal situations.[13]

A TRP encompasses reactive aspects of current threat-response investigative protocols and formalizes enhanced review processes, preventative interventions, and case-management strategies using threat assessment. A TRP addresses the threat holistically, with an emphasis on collecting the necessary protective intelligence to inform intervention and case management strategies that

consider the needs of the subject making the threat as well as the target of the threat. Collaboration across disciplines and agencies is an essential element of preventative strategies, providing the necessary vehicle for integrated systemic intervention as well as case management protocols to help lower risks of targeted violence incidents. In short, adopting a threat response model allows first responders to comprehensively respond, intervene, and manage cases with heightened or accelerating static and dynamic risk factors for targeted violence.

The creation of a structured TRP to address allegations or concerns of targeted violence includes the following implementation stages:

- *Building awareness and "buy-in"* by providing briefings and training on risk factors and warning behaviors related to targeted violence, consistent with research from the professional threat-assessment community
- *Adopting investigative protocols and reporting tools* to increase efficacy in identifying cases with heightened or accelerating static and dynamic risk factors for targeted violence
- *Articulating policies to guide reporting requirements*, developing systematic triage review of targeted violence threat incidents to identify cases that require additional investigation, and developing methods to engage multiple stakeholders in designing intervention and case-management strategies
- *Identifying a threat coordinator* to conduct comprehensive follow-up investigations of substantive threat or stalking cases and to coordinate interagency collaboration and intervention actions
- *Emphasizing community intervention* by increasing community willingness to identify, report, and respond to concerns before an individual engages in criminal activity by establishing protocols that prioritize the prevention of targeted violence over response to acts of targeted violence and restorative principles of assistance and support over criminalization and incarceration.

CASE STUDY: ROCHESTER, NEW YORK: AN ANALYSIS OF THREAT RESPONSES BY THE GREATER ROCHESTER PUBLIC SAFETY COMMUNITY AND THE ESTABLISHMENT OF THE ROCHESTER THREAT ADVISORY COMMITTEE

In 2017, a project was initiated in Rochester, New York, by the Justice and Security Institute at Roberts Wesleyan College to understand efforts by multiple systems to address the threat of lone-actor terrorists and other violent extremists. The focus of the Threat Assessment and Management

Project (TAMP) was to gather information about targeted violence threat responses and assess the overall state of adult threat assessment and management protocols in use by the Greater Rochester Public Safety Community.[14] The project intended to advance public safety in Monroe County by raising awareness of recommended threat response paradigms that promote prevention through therapeutic intervention, not violence prediction, and that balance public safety concerns with the needs of individuals who present as threats of targeted violence. One such paradigm is the Behavioral Threat Assessment and Management (BTAM) team model, which, according to the FBI Behavioral Analysis Unit-National Center for the Analysis of Violent Crime, "is a viable and effective method for assessing violence potential and disrupting planned attacks of targeted violence."[14]

The project identified that agencies and organizations that comprise the Greater Rochester Public Safety Community and various support organizations lacked the benefit of formalized adult threat assessment and management teams as a resource for responding to allegations or concerns across the targeted violence continuum. Law enforcement agencies commonly used preexisting programs operated by the County Office of Mental Health as a response to crisis cases involving suspected mental illness and apparent threats to self or others; however, these programs are not explicitly designed to serve as systemic threat-mitigation and case-management responses across the threat continuum.

A review of services provided or supported by the Monroe County Department of Mental Health indicated the agency's commitment to crisis intervention, ensuring coordination of services across levels of care and among an array of community providers.[15] The Consortium for Trauma, Illness & Grief in Schools (TIG) is a countywide, multiagency effort that attempts to support threat assessment in K–12 school districts by providing clinically appropriate training, support, and resource services.[16] Training sessions on the Virginia Model for Student Threat Assessment and the adoption of structured assessment tools are available through the TIG for school districts that want to adopt a threat assessment and management approach.

Programs such as the mobile crisis team offer mobile psychiatric emergency department services for individuals and families within Monroe County who are experiencing a crisis in mental health.[15] Led by the Monroe County Office of Mental Health and the Law Enforcement Council, multijurisdictional coordination and strategy groups such as the Criminal Justice Mental Health Committee and Multijurisdictional Crisis Intervention Task Force meet to discuss and coordinate crisis intervention strategies and advance enhanced community response protocols. The Monroe County Multijurisdictional Crisis Intervention Task Force is co-chaired by the Monroe County Office of Mental Health and the Law Enforcement Council. The council represents a consortium of law enforcement and mental health professionals who meet bi-monthly to discuss mental hygiene procedures. Their goal is to establish sound policies and improve law enforcement practices when assisting individuals experiencing mental illness or emotional disturbance.[17] The Office of Mental Health also adopted the use of forensic intervention teams (FIT). The FIT program partners mental health clinicians with law enforcement agencies to assist individuals with mental health needs and who have frequent contact with law enforcement.[18]

Enhanced coordination among stakeholders for threat and stalking cases did exist in Monroe County; however, coordination lacked the benefit of cross-systems engagement and did not conform to recommended paradigms and best-practices identified by most of the threat assessment and management community. Through the efforts of the FBI Rochester Joint Terrorism Task Force (RJTTF), an off-ramping model was implemented to respond to task force cases involving individuals with a possible mental or emotional disorder who make direct, indirect, or veiled threats to commit targeted violence. Once these cases are determined to have no nexus to international or domestic terrorism, the individual's identity and the background of the incident are provided to the Monroe County Office of Mental Health to assist in determining the most appropriate mental health intervention strategy.[14]

The RJTTF adopted a collaborative referral model to coordinate mental health services across levels of care and among an array of community providers when appropriate for individuals making threats or when concerns existed related to targeted violence. Subjects in this category were not under investigation for committing a serious violation of federal or local criminal statutes, nor was there a nexus to a designated terrorist group. These subjects were not agents of a foreign power and were experiencing mental health symptoms that contributed to the threatening communication or behavior. The Office of Mental Health designee acted as a point of coordination and access to services addressing the needs of the at-risk individual. The model was based more on diagnosis and access to care, versus ongoing BTA and long-term case management directed by a law enforcement agency or a threat assessment and management team.

The Rochester JTTF adopted this approach out of necessity due to the exponential increase in referrals by various sectors of the community dealing with specific types of targeted violence. The RJTTF response served to triage individuals with clear and convincing signs of mental illness who, in many cases, had made threats to commit mass shootings, bombings, ideologically inspired attacks, or who threatened public figures. The RJTTF and Office of Mental Health collaboration remains an effective response to threat cases involving mentally disordered individuals who make specific types of threats that are perceived to fall within the RJTTF investigative priorities. However, cases referred to the RJTTF represented only a portion of the threat cases in Monroe County. Cases manifesting from domestic incidents or workplace violence and individuals not experiencing a mental health crisis were not likely to receive the same comprehensive intervention efforts.

Beyond Crisis Intervention and the RJTTF Model

While crisis intervention and coordination of mental health services for individuals who present as a threat are critical aspects of threat response, they do not and should not represent the breadth of systemic threat response and management. It is unrealistic to expect any county mental health system or mental health providers to lead comprehensive fact-gathering strategies and coordinate long-term case management of persons presenting as a risk to commit targeted violence. Also, the current paradigm of intervention does not account for the exponential increase in threatening situations that do not come to the attention of law enforcement or county health departments. The relationship between serious mental disorder and targeted violence risk is "small but significant" and must be a consideration when developing targeted violence-threat response strategies, but not the primary consideration.[4]

Given the small correlative relationship between a serious mental disorder and risk for targeted violence, it is logical to assume that most events that necessitate threat assessment and management protocols will fall outside of a mental health crisis. Predicating events could include a "threat or inappropriate communication, a report of concerning or threatening behavior, issuance of a protective order, or recognition of warning behaviors."[4] These events are likely to be reported to various authorities beyond the FBI, including local law enforcement, private security, human resources personnel, teachers, faculty, staff, or supervisors.

The assumption that a referral to the FBI, the county's mental health office, or involuntary transports to a psychiatric emergency room will initiate intervention protocols is not reliable when developing comprehensive threat assessment and management policies. The FBI RJTTF initiative and the Multijurisdictional Crisis Intervention Task Force may represent the building blocks for a future county-wide threat assessment and management; however, that model does not conform to the recommended paradigm for addressing threats of targeted violence.[4]

The FBI National Center for the Analysis of Violent Crime (NCAVC) released a report completed by its Behavioral Threat Assessment Center, "Making Prevention a Reality: Identifying, Assessing, and Managing the Threat of Targeted Attacks" (2017). In the section of the report labeled, "Mental health is not 'the answer'—threat management is the key," a collaborative group of targeted violence and threat assessment experts concluded, "The mental health system is no longer able to be the primary response mechanism in dealing with a mentally ill person of concern. . . . The mental health system is simply not in a position to be responsible for long-term threat management."[4]

It is common for news media to conflate targeted violence with the existence of mental illness or mental health crisis; however, outcome studies of targeted violence incidents often reveal that, proximal to the attack, the perpetrator was not involved in emergency crisis services provided or coordinated by a public mental health system or provider. Post-incident review and assessment may reveal a distal history of mental hygiene incidents, mental health treatment, or the likely presence of a mental disorder; however, this is not a guarantee. Response strategies focusing on threats of targeted violence from subjects who are involved in involuntary psychiatric treatment or who present as an imminent threat to self or others create vulnerabilities in comprehensive and wide-ranging policies to address targeted violence. The "loophole" created by approaches focusing on mental healthcare excludes persons who do not meet the criteria for involuntary treatment and do not seek out treatment, or cases that manifest in the form of intimate-partner violence, familial homicide, mass shootings, honor-based violence, or workplace violence.[19] An example of a perpetrator of targeted violence who, at the time of his attack, was not involved in mental health crisis intervention is Elliot Rodger.

On May 23, 2014, Rodger, a 22-year-old college student in Isla Vista, California, killed 6 people and wounded 14 others before taking his own life. Much is known about the life of Rodger due to a 137-page autobiographical manifesto entitled, *My Twisted World*.[20] Stephen White published a known-outcome case study on the Isla Vista mass murders in the *Journal of Threat Assessment and Management* (2017). The article noted that Rodger's psychological problems were "both serious and complex," but, while undergoing past voluntary mental health treatment, Rodger "was very conscious of keeping his secret."[20] Rodger was the subject of a law enforcement welfare check a month before the attack in which, following a brief interview, deputies from the sheriff's office had determined that Rodger was not a threat to himself or others and warranted no further investigation.[20] The event caused Rodger to write in his manifesto, "I tactfully told them it was a misunderstanding, and they finally left . . . for a few horrible seconds, I thought it was all over."[20] White notes in reference to the welfare check, "one lesson, in this case, is the reminder that not all who are suspected of lethality risk are either psychotic or overtly despondent."[20]

Since the 2017 completion of the Justice and Security Institute project, significant developments occurred in Rochester, New York, related to the awareness and adoption of behavioral threat assessment and management protocols by local and state law enforcement agencies. One of the most significant developments was the establishment of the Rochester Threat Advisory Committee (ROCTAC).

Explanation of ROCTAC
Community-Based Responses

In 2019, the ROCTAC was established in Rochester, New York. ROCTAC represents a consortium of stakeholders with diverse expertise and access to resources dedicated to the prevention of targeted acts of violence. ROCTAC's objective is to act as a central clearinghouse of information flow and consultation on the development of balanced intervention and case management strategies specific to cases where there is a high need for interventions to mitigate the risk of targeted violence.

ROCTAC represents a new initiative for New York state and is considered to be a valuable tool for advancing a balanced approach to mitigating threats to public safety. However, ROCTAC as a concept is not new. Much of the structure and philosophy of ROCTAC is derived from the Marion County (Oregon) Threat Advisory Team, which has been in existence for nearly two decades.[21] ROCTAC's core philosophy synthesizes therapeutic intervention and case management strategies to meet the needs of the individual posing a danger while simultaneously balancing the safety needs of the threatened subject and the community at large. ROCTAC serves as a resource for the law enforcement community to improve targeted violence TRPs by providing multidisciplinary expert advice and seamless sharing of threat information across systems.

ROCTAC is comprised of select representatives from participating member agencies across systems. ROCTAC acts as a central clearinghouse of information flow specific to situations, herein referred to as *threat cases*, where the risk of violence is assessed to be substantive and clustered risk factors and warning behaviors commonly associated with targeted violence are present. ROCTAC assists agencies with the development of balanced intervention and case management strategies for threat cases presented to ROCTAC and, if warranted, facilitates expedited and timely intervention actions. ROCTAC has no authority to mandate that presenting agencies implement or act on suggested intervention and case management strategies and solely acts as an advisory group.

Presentation of Threat Cases

Any agency with personnel assigned to ROCTAC may bring a case for presentation or facilitate the introduction of a threat case by a non-member agency with a determined critical need. ROCTAC hears the initial presentation and makes recommendations to the presenting agency. To facilitate a case presentation, a "Threat Assessment Investigative Guide" is provided to the presenting agency. The assessment guide acts as a tool to collect risk-relevant data and behaviors associated with targeted violence. All the responsibilities related to case ownership, determination of case status, documentation, and custody of case files remain with the presenting agency.

ROCTAC recommendations rely on the collective expertise, education, and training of its members, along with case management and intervention strategies commonly agreed upon and utilized by the majority of the threat assessment community. ROCTAC recommendations aim to improve information sharing, intervention, and care coordination between providers, families, and other systems involved in the threat case.

ROCTAC also serves as a committee of dedicated stakeholders in a position to make recommendations to improve systems protocols relating to threat response, risk mitigation, and timely intervention strategies. By the nature of ROCTAC's mission, it serves as a leader in promoting threat assessment training and innovative community-based responses to threats or concerning behavior with a nexus to targeted violence.

Conclusion

If the various campaigns and uprisings which have taken place in Italy have given the appearance that the military ability has become extinct, the true reason is that old methods of warfare were not good and no one has been able to find new ones. A man newly risen to power cannot acquire greater reputation than by discovering new rules and methods. Machiavelli, *The Prince* [21]

Law enforcement mitigation of threats posed by lone-actor terrorists and other violent extremists is incumbent on the ability to identify and be open to new rules and methods to collect intelligence and prevent attacks. The collection and sharing of intelligence to assess and mitigate a threat must not remain solely in law enforcement silos. Traditional counterterrorism sources and methods for intelligence gathering operate in strict information-controlled classified environments. Classified counterterrorism investigations will remain a staple for investigating threats to US national security coming from designated foreign terrorist organizations and state sponsors of terrorism. However, the hyper-decentralization of domestic threats from lone-actor terrorists and other violent extremists necessitates a multidisciplinary community approach to intelligence

gathering, assessment of the danger, and holistic interventions that integrate a myriad of responses other than arrest. The decision to commit to lone-actor violence is not a spontaneous one; it is a process that is recognizable and discernible. Local and state law enforcement, mental health clinicians, teachers, co-workers, and family members are the ones likely to recognize concerning pre-incident behaviors and attitudes. The prioritization of new rules and methods such as behavioral threat assessment and management that foster a culture of shared responsibility, information sharing, and early identification of threats will dictate the efficacy of strategies to combat the threat of lone-actor terrorism.

LAW ENFORCEMENT RESPONSE TO AN EVENT

The second part of this chapter covers the law enforcement response to a terrorist event incorporating the personal experience of San Bernardino Police Lieutenant Michael Madden. Lieutenant Madden was the first officer to respond to the scene of a terrorist attack at an office Christmas party in San Bernardino, California, in 2015. During this attack by Syed Farook and his wife Tashfeen Malik, 14 people were killed and 22 were seriously injured. Lieutenant Madden made the initial entry into the building complex to search for shooters and coordinated subsequent search efforts.

It is difficult to characterize a single law enforcement response to all potential lone-actor terrorism scenarios in the United States. Not only is the United States a large and diverse country, with densely populated cities, sparsely populated rural tracts, and suburban areas ranging somewhere in between, but there are almost 18,000 different departments or agencies tasked with providing a local law enforcement response with varying levels of resources available. These organizations range from the New York Police Department (with 35,000 sworn officers) to more than 8,000 departments with 10 or fewer employees.[22] Complicating matters further, these departments operate within differing legal frameworks that involve local ordinances and county, state, territorial, federal, and even tribal laws.

It is also important to note that terror attacks can take many forms. The weapons used during a terrorist attack in 2013 in Great Britain were a knife and meat cleaver, and a similar attack there a year later involved a hammer and a knife. There have been truck attacks in Nice, France, and in

Barcelona, Spain; the September 11 attackers used box cutters and, ultimately, airliners; the Unabomber, the Shoe Bomber, and others used improvised explosive devices (IEDs); and many others have used firearms to wreak havoc. The San Bernardino attackers used firearms and unsuccessfully attempted to use IEDs. Despite these differences in the weapons used and other factors, there are certain features that are common to lone-actor terrorist events that can guide first responders in their approach to these situations.

Training the Responders

From a study of 84 active shooter events from 2000 to 2010, it was noted that, more than half the time, an attack will still be in progress when the first law enforcement officers arrive.[23] Another key finding was that, of the incidents still in progress when officers arrive, 56% of the time police were required to use force to stop the attack. Most law enforcement agencies put a significant amount of time and money into training their tactical response units, who are the best equipped to effectively deal with these events with enhanced training, weaponry, tools, and safety equipment. However, the initial response to a terror event will almost always come from the nearest law enforcement officers in the field, which generally consist of non-tactical patrol units.

Lieutenant Michael Madden shares his experience from the terrorist attack in San Bernardino, California:

> Such was the case for me on December 2, 2015. This was a day in which two individuals armed with AR-15 assault rifles stormed into a conference room at the Inland Regional Center in San Bernardino, California. Prior to entering the conference room they shot and killed two victims outside and upon making entry, they unleashed a barrage of gunfire upon the 80 plus attendees of the workplace training session for Health Department workers from the San Bernardino County Department of Public Health. One of the attackers was an employee of the Health Department who just moments before had been attending the training session prior to leaving abruptly. He went to his vehicle, which was parked outside, and changed into black military-looking gear, and he armed himself with an automatic rifle and a 9 mm handgun and hundreds of rounds of ammunition. There was a second suspect in the car dressed identically and equipped

identically to him and that suspect was later learned to be his wife. Once the two entered, they opened fire, and in less than three minutes they shot 36 people, fatally wounding 14. Following the attack, the suspects returned to their vehicle and fled the scene. Fourteen minutes later they would take to social media and pledge their allegiance to ISIS.

> The attack occurred on Wednesday morning at 10:58 AM. This was a day like many others, and there was nothing that arose suspicion in our community that a senseless act of violence of this magnitude was about to unfold. At the time, I had just left a meeting. I had driven through a McDonalds to grab a quick bite to eat and I decided to put gas in my unmarked department-issued vehicle at our city yard, which was less than 2 miles away from the Inland Regional Center. At the time, I had been a law enforcement officer for 25 years, and I worked in a city which was no stranger to violence-related crimes. Throughout the course of my career I had seen and dealt with my fair share of action. Now though, I was a lieutenant for the San Bernardino Police Department, and my current assignment was managing the Department's Dispatch and Records Units. Although both are very vital to the daily operations of any law enforcement agency, this was not a position that anyone would deem as being high-risk or even remotely dangerous. I was a manager of primarily civilian personnel. The biggest threat that I now was faced with daily was papercuts. I was, however, still a cop. I wore a uniform and carried a gun, and I still had peace officer powers. When that initial call went out at 10:58 AM, I could hear that we had a possible active shooter event taking place and I responded toward the location. After all, I was a manager and we would need "bosses" there to manage the situation.

> I arrived at the location less than 2 minutes after the initial calls. I quickly came to the realization that I was the first one there. I parked my unmarked unit approximately 100 yards south of the building where I believed the attack was occurring. As I stopped and exited, it was eerily quiet. I did not hear gunshots, nor could I hear screams. I observed people running from the building, but all were fleeing in the opposite direction of my location from doors which were approximately 200 yards away. I took a

position behind the trunk of my car to serve as cover and concealment as I began assessing what was taking place and my next course of action. The adrenaline was pumping heavily, and I quickly had to make some decisions about my next course of action. Should I begin establishing a command post and directing in the large response of other officers who were on their way with lights and sirens? Or should I go rushing in to search for the shooter?

The lessons learned from tragic events such as the Columbine School shootings in Littleton, Colorado, in 1999, and more recently at Stoneman Douglas High School in Parkland, Florida, in 2019, have changed law enforcement tactics significantly. Instead of having the first officers on scene setting up a perimeter and waiting for designated tactical units to make first contact with the attackers, the current recommended approach involves five-person or less entry or contact teams. This approach has been promoted through the FBI's Officer Robert Wilson III Preventing Violence Against Law Enforcement Officers and Ensuring Officer Resilience and Survivability (VALOR) initiative, which has provided funding to train more than 56,000 local police officers in an active-shooter training program using these tactics.[24,25]

Lieutenant Madden described the training he had received and how he applied it to the situation before him:

Reflecting back on this and my prior active shooter training that I had received, I decided that we needed to get in there as quickly as possible to locate, isolate, and stop the threat. I requested the next three first officers on scene to come to my location to formulate an entry team. The wait seemed as if it took forever. I still could not hear gunshots nor did I have any of the fleeing subjects come in my direction. I did however see a single subject in the parking lot just east of my location. I was able to get him to come to me and discovered that he was a nonuniformed unarmed security guard for the complex. He informed me that one suspect had possibly fled in a black-colored SUV and there were potentially as many as two more suspects still inside. Both he and the other callers who were reporting the incident to Dispatch advised that the suspects had automatic rifles. While kneeling behind the trunk of my car, I thought about the engagement with the suspects which was

likely about to occur. I was in uniform but was not wearing my vest. It was in the truck of my unit rather than on me where it belonged. I had an AR-15 assigned to me, but it was back in the armory at the station rather than with me where it should have been. I was a manager of personnel and our day-to-day operations. I was no longer the guy who would be in these types of situations. After all, an active shooter incident will not occur in my city and if it were to happen, it would not be me who would be first on scene. I had allowed complacency to override my judgment and duties as an officer sworn to protect the safety of others. This is something that none of us in the profession of serving as a first responder can allow ourselves to fall victim to.

Although it seemed like an eternity waiting for the other officers to arrive at my location, the reality was that the next three were there with me in less than two and half minutes. The first officer on scene was a patrol officer. He was a 9-year veteran and a good cop. Like me, though, he had no prior tactical training assignments such as SWAT [Special Weapons and Tactics]. He had his handgun and shotgun when we made entry. The third officer on scene was a motor officer. He was a 7-year veteran, and he, too, was a good cop but had no prior SWAT experience. He had his handgun. The fourth officer was a detective. This detective was a 16-year veteran and had had a very exemplary career. He had served in a variety of assignments and duties during his career, but, like the rest of us, he had no prior SWAT experience. His current assignment was as a homicide detective. In the 4 years prior to December 2, he rarely if ever put on a uniform. He was only wearing one that day to help fill in shortages that we were having in staffing our patrol division following the municipal bankruptcy which the City of San Bernardino was going through and which had caused the loss of approximately one-third of our sworn officer positions. The detective, too, had only his handgun. Over the next 15 to 20 seconds, I quickly briefed the officers and informed them that we were going to utilize that diamond formation that we had all been previously trained on during our prior active shooter training that we had received. Assignments were given, and we approached and entered.

If you were looking for a team of first responders for an event of this magnitude, the four of us would not have been on your roster. Although we were all capable and experienced officers, none of us had prior SWAT training and none of us had the proper equipment or weaponry to confront the threat that we were about to go in search of. This, however, is the team that we had. This was the team that most any other agencies under similar circumstances will have to be first on scene and first to enter. This reality underlies the importance of agencies across the nation to continue to focus upon the value of training and equipping all officers within their organizations for events of this magnitude.

Upon entry, the situation was surreal. None of us were immune to bloodshed but this was like nothing any of us had ever experienced. There were victims everywhere. Many in great amounts of pain and many others unfortunately deceased. The fire alarms were blaring, and we could barely hear one another. The lights were flickering and the fire sprinklers were going off, given the heavy amount of fresh gun smoke in the air. One of the rounds the suspects had fired struck a water line in the ceiling, and it was causing water to gush out and saturate the ceiling tiles, which were falling to the floor. This added to the chaos which was taking place.

In the time since Columbine, I had gone through our in-house active shooter training a total of three times prior to that date. It was put on by our Department's SWAT officers, and I remember the training getting more and more elaborate. They would play loud recordings of sirens and people screaming. They would introduce smoke and flash-bang grenades. They would put trip wires out for the entry teams and have what appeared to be improvised explosive devices in various locations to heighten the threat, awareness, and senses of the trainees. The last time I had gone through the training 5 years before, I was a sergeant. I remember talking with one of my fellow sergeants about how the SWAT guys had gone overboard and were getting carried away. The reality was that what we were then experiencing was all of that and more. It was overwhelming to the senses but had we not received the prior training, we would not have been as prepared for what we were now experiencing.

Training their first responders is a major expense for law enforcement agencies. There is the cost of the training itself, which can be substantial. However, in addition to this, there is an associated opportunity cost. Most departments across the country face shortages in staffing, so to allow personnel to attend training, there is often a need to backfill shortages in patrol or other divisions, which leads to overtime expenditure. If the training is not within close proximity to the department, there will be associated costs of travel, lodging, and meals. The governing body for most local law enforcement agencies across the country are state-specific peace officer standards and training (POST) organizations. Any curriculum created by individual agencies will first require the review and approval of that department's POST governing body, which can cause delay in implementation and additional expense. One resource available for both reducing the financial burden on police and for increasing standardization of tactical response is the federal government's VALOR initiative, funded by a grant through the Bureau of Justice Assistance, a component of the US Department of Justice's Office of Justice Programs.[25] The VALOR initiative pays for training and equipment for various aspects of law enforcement, including that specific to active shooter events.

Addressing the Wounded

The current fire department and/or emergency medical service (EMS) approach to active shooter events is to stage responding units in an area nearby that allows quick access yet is relatively safe. This approach by fire/EMS has largely remained unchanged over the years despite the change in law enforcement response, but it is important to note that these responders are not only unarmed, they also do not generally have access to protective equipment such as Kevlar vests. However, due to the chaotic nature of these events, often with conflicting or incorrect reports regarding the location of the shooter(s), the medical response can be overly delayed while law enforcement methodically clears the scene. One way to address this delay in care is to train law enforcement officers in first aid or other life-saving measures, including additional equipment.[26]

Lieutenant Madden discusses how the challenge of caring for the injured was addressed during the San Bernardino incident.

> The two suspects in our attack fired 117 rounds from their AR-15 assault rifles. Fourteen people were killed in the attack and another 22 were wounded, with 18 of

those being deemed as critical. The attack was contained to the Conference Room facility at the Inland Regional Center, but we had reason to believe upon our initial entry that the suspects had likely penetrated further into the building in search of additional victims. This created a hard choice to have to make. The initial inclination is to assist the injured but our goal as the initial entry team had to be to locate, isolate, and stop the threat. As such, we were forced to have to move past the wounded and go deeper into the facility.

It becomes the responsibility of other officers arriving on scene to address the needs of the injured. I was not hearing gunfire but because the alarms were so loud in the building, it could have been muffling the sounds of them. I also was seeing that many of the rounds that were fired by the suspects had penetrated several layers of drywall. I was concerned that the suspects' rounds could still strike others entering behind or penetrate through the ceiling if they had made their way to the second floor above the conference room. As such, I did not deem the conference room to be safe.

The common vernacular used to describe zones in active shooter training is hot, warm, and cold zones. Hot zones are those where the threat is actively occurring. Civilian and medical personnel are not allowed in this zone except for those victims in need of extraction. Warm zones are those where the threat is nearby but there is not an imminent threat present. It will be the decision of the incident commander or other on-scene tactical supervisors to determine if medical personnel can or should enter the warm zone. Cold zones are those that are considered safe from the threat, and civilian and medical personnel can generally have access.

Within 12 minutes of our initial entry into the building, the first SWAT team from the San Bernardino Police Department arrived on scene. This was an extraordinarily quick response and only occurred because our SWAT team happened to be conducting training that morning in another part of the City, and they responded as soon as the first call went out. I relinquished my search team coordinating duties to the SWAT sergeant who brought a team of his officers into my location, and I then returned to the Conference Room to address the needs of the wounded.

The scene was dramatically different from what I had left just minutes before. There were uniformed and non-uniformed personnel in the room from both my agency as well as several other surrounding jurisdictions. Officers were actively trying to bandage and apply pressure to gunshot wounds, and several were picking up and carrying other victims out to safety and the triage area. Another SWAT team sergeant from my agency approached me and told me that one of our tactical medics was there and ready to take a lead role. That medic was a member of the San Bernardino City Fire Department, and he was also a reserve police officer for the San Bernardino Police Department. As such, he had peace officer powers and the ability to carry a weapon. He was dressed in the same tactical uniform that the other SWAT team members wore and was armed with a semi-automatic handgun and an AR-15. He was prepared and trained to engage suspects if need, but his primary role was to provide medical aid to wounded victims, officers, and potentially to the suspects as well. I asked the medic to triage the wounded and tell us who was the next one that needed to go. His role was critical in the quick extraction of the wounded.

The wounded were carried out to the triage zone, which had been established across the street, and loaded into awaiting ambulances. We were fortunate that we had two Level One trauma centers within 5 miles of the location of the Regional Center. The last of the wounded were in one of those centers within 58 minutes of having been shot, and, as such, none of those that were transported from the scene died as a result of the wounds they had received.

Scene Coordination

During the early and more acute stages of an active shooter event, questions of jurisdiction are less important than is the need to gain early control of the situation. The top priority is safety (for both the public and the responding units), although coordination between responding departments is crucial to prevent friendly-fire situations or lapses in coverage. As events continue to unfold and the scene becomes more stable, the need to establish more formal command and control begins to take precedence. Depending on the event, this can occur quickly, in minutes, or, as in the case of the San Bernardino shooters, take more than an hour to fully crystallize. A lot depends on the nature of the event since events categorized as terrorist attacks will entail a much different response than workplace violence or gang shootings.

Lieutenant Madden describes how the San Bernardino investigation was coordinated by the various federal, state, and local entities.

> Our event occurred in an urban city environment with a population of 215,000. There are several other surrounding jurisdictions, each with their own law enforcement personnel. Within a matter of 30 minutes, there were more than 300 law enforcement officers on scene. This may not be the case in all instances, where the event occurs in a more rural jurisdiction where resources are not so readily available.
>
> After our entry into the building, one of the first supervisors on scene was a sergeant from my agency who was still in his personal vehicle, in plain clothes, and on his way to work. He heard what was happening, and he responded to the scene. He immediately began asking for road closures from other responding units to only allow police and medical personnel access. He established a command post and a triage zone and started directing in responding units. He continued acting as the Scene Incident Commander until he was relieved by other higher-ranking officers from our department who assumed command.

INCIDENT INVESTIGATION

Once control of the scene has been established with a command structure in place, the law enforcement response then undergoes a retooling to enter an investigative phase. Similar to earlier in the chapter, where we identified the potential for a wide variety of responses to an attack that is under way, there are many approaches to conducting an investigation based on the scope of the attack, number of suspects involved, the geographic location of the event, and, most importantly, any continuing risk to public safety.

> The location of our event was 60 miles east of Los Angeles, which is the second largest media market in the Country. Within a short period of time, the scene was swarmed by media and the situation was now being viewed across the nation. Handling and coordination of that information also became a critical component of successfully controlling the scene. Our suspects had fled just prior to our arrival and the world knew that we had heavily armed, extremely violent suspects on the loose. In addition, there were early indicators that there could potentially be other factors involved in the attack. This was a well-coordinated attack with at least two heavily armed and somewhat trained and equipped suspects. An improvised explosive device had been left behind in the conference room, and fortunately it did not activate despite being an operable device with a remote detonator. These factors led many to believe that this was likely something more than an isolated workplace violence incident.

The primary investigative entity for any terrorist attack on US soil is the FBI.[27] Although the FBI may have overall jurisdiction, its agents cannot operate in a vacuum and must rely on local and state law enforcement agencies. As to be expected, there are localities where this partnership works well and there is good communication and coordination between agencies, but there are also regions where this relationship is rocky at best. The advantage of having a federal agency with nationwide jurisdiction in charge of the investigation is that it streamlines the flow of information and creates a central repository, which is particularly valuable for events that have multiple locations of investigative interest, including across state lines or even internationally. A downside, however, is that the FBI often does not have the local knowledge or close relationship with each community that local police departments have. To address this, the FBI has established numerous Joint Terrorism Task Forces (JTTFs) throughout the United States to incorporate local officers as investigators alongside federal agents. In addition to improving information collection and dissemination, the JTTF is a manpower magnifier, adding experienced investigators and broadening the FBI's reach.

> The FBI responded and were on scene within 90 minutes of the attack. There was a massive response from law enforcement, and it is vital in these types of situations that the highest

ranking person from each agency responding to the scene reports directly to the command post. It is there that they will be given the most current and accurate information and then be given assignments which they can in turn provide to their personnel. Individual departments have their own radio frequencies, and not all departments have access or the ability to monitor other agencies' communications. This can create a void and a need for someone to be readily available at the command post to successfully convey information to their officers in a timely manner.

The attack at the Inland Regional Center in San Bernardino, California was determined to have been a terrorist event. This, however, represents only one example of potential threats that local, state, and national law enforcement agencies must concern themselves with. Terrorism itself, whether it be international or domestic, is something that we have traditionally viewed as being a role of the federal government to investigate. Domestic terrorism, however, particularly when addressing the issue of homegrown violent extremists, will most likely first come to the attention of local law enforcement before ultimately being forwarded on to federal authorities.

From a law enforcement perspective, the initial response to an active shooter and/or mass casualty event is only the beginning. The event itself will likely be over within a matter of minutes, but the subsequent investigation will take days, weeks, and even months. The sheer scope of an event can quickly deplete the resources of smaller policing agencies, and it is likely that mutual aid and a sharing of resources will be required to see an investigation to its successful conclusion.

In the San Bernardino event, there were multiple crime scenes that had to be locked down, protected, and investigated, the first being the conference room where the attack had taken place. The surrounding office space/buildings had to be included in that as well, at least during the initial investigation. Although the attack was discovered to have been limited to the conference room, it was not initially known whether the suspects had penetrated deeper into the building and into the adjoining offices and buildings. In addition to the 84 attendees at the training event, there were another 488 employees in the adjacent offices/buildings who needed to be accounted for and interviewed. The initial primary investigative

agency for this crime scene was the San Bernardino Police Department. Within 2 days of the attack, the event was determined to have been an act of terrorism, and the FBI at that time assumed responsibility for the investigation.

The second crime scene was a city street 1.6 miles away from the Inland Regional Center. This was the location where law enforcement officers from several different agencies engaged the suspects in a prolonged gun battle, causing the wounding of two officers and the ultimate death of the two suspects. In the engagement, the suspects fired 97 rounds at officers, with 22 officers from several different agencies returning over 450 rounds. Both suspects were pronounced [dead] at the scene. The crime scene stretched nearly a half mile. Given that the resources of the San Bernardino Police Department were depleted at that point, the San Bernardino County Sheriff's Department offered their assistance and took over as the lead investigative agency for this scene.

The third crime scene was the suspects' residence, which was in a neighboring city 7 miles from the Inland Regional Center. This scene consisted of the townhome in which they resided and the detached garage, which was found to have multiple improvised explosive devices in various stages of completion. The FBI's investigators and their bomb technicians assumed command of this scene.

The resources of the San Bernardino Police Department and several surrounding assisting agencies were stressed for weeks to come. Another important note is that although this was drawing a tremendous amount of attention and resources, there was still a community to be policed and calls to be answered. Unrelated to the attack that took place at the Inland Regional Center, the City of San Bernardino had five separate homicides in the 8 days following the attack.

CONCLUSION

The violence seen in terrorist attacks results in a chaotic situation that can both monopolize and exhaust local resources. However, a review of recent events over the past few years shows that first responder departments can, to a certain extent, train for and ameliorate some of this uncertainty by having an established protocol to follow. This training is offered through the federal government. Once the scene has stabilized and the response becomes more investigative in nature, there is a shifting of responsibility and jurisdiction. As with the initial response, this change can be facilitated through close partnerships among local, state, and federal law enforcement agencies. Communication and trust are imperative for this partnership to work, and trust in particular can only be achieved through working and training together.

The following link takes the readers who are interested in more information on community-based prevention strategies and want to view the guide to a webpage located on the industry resource page for AT-RISK International: https://at-riskinternational.com/sta-guide/

NOTES AND REFERENCES

1. Follman M, Follman M, Follman M, et al. Rate of mass shootings has tripled since 2011, new research from Harvard shows. *Mother Jones*, 2020. https://www.motherjones.com/politics/2014/10/mass-shootings-increasing-harvard-research/
2. Texas State University, Federal Bureau of Investigation (2014). *A Study of Active Shooter Incidents, 2000-2013*. Washington, DC: US Department of Justice.
3. Pillar P. Beyond al Qaeda: Countering a decentralized terrorist threat. In Howard R, Hoffman B, eds., *Terrorism and Counterterrorism: Understanding the New Security Environment*. 4th ed. New York: McGraw-Hill; 2004:522.
4. Federal Bureau of Investigation. *Making a Prevention a Reality: Identifying, Assessing, and Managing the Threat of Targeted Attacks*. Washington DC: Behavioral Analysis Unit—National Center for the Analysis of Violent Crime; 2018.
5. Fein R, Vossekuil B, Holden G. Threat assessment. Ppcta.unl.edu, 1995. http://ppcta.unl.edu/
6. Borum R, Fein R, Vossekuil B, Berglund J. Threat assessment: Defining an approach for evaluating risk of targeted violence. Behav Sci Law. 1999;17(3):323–337.
7. Calhoun F, Weston S. *Contemporary Threat Management*. San Diego, CA: Specialized Training Services; 2003.
8. US Department of Justice Federal Bureau of Investigation Behavioral Analysis Unit. *A Study of Lone Offender Terrorism in the United States (1972-2015)*. Quantico, VA: National Center for the Analysis of Violent Crime; 2019:29–35.
9. Silver J, Simons A, Craun S. *A Study of the Pre-Attack Behaviors of Active Shooters in the United States Between 2000-2013*. Washington, DC: Federal Bureau of Investigation, US Department of Justice; 2018.
10. Borum R. Operationally relevant research and practice in terrorism threat assessments. J Threat Assess Manage. 2015;2(3–4):192–194. doi:10.1037/tam0000046
11. Dunn J. The Los Angeles Police Department Threat Management Unit. In Meloy J, Hoffmann J, eds., *International Handbook of Threat Assessment*. New York: Oxford Press; 2014:285.
12. Malone R. Protective intelligence: Applying the intelligence cycle model to threat assessment. J Threat Assess Manage. 2014;2(1):53–62. doi:10.1037/tam0000034
13. US Department of Justice. *Protective Intelligence and Threat Assessment Investigations: A Guide for State and Local Law Enforcement Officials*. Washington, DC: National Institute of Justice; 1988:3.
14. Concordia M. *Roberts Wesleyan College Justice and Security Institute: Threat Assessment and Management Project (TAMP) Summary Report*. Rochester, NY; 2017.
15. Monroe County. Emergency-crisis services. Monroe County, NY, 2020. Www2.monroecounty.gov. https://www2.monroecounty.gov/mh-emergency-resources|
16. Training–TIG. Tigconsortium.org, 2020. https://tigconsortium.org/training/
17. Monroe County. FIT Page Monroe County, NY, 2020. https://www2.monroecounty.gov/mh-fit.php
18. Hall K. Monroe County Community College Home. Monroeccc.edu, 2015 https://www.monroeccc.edu/
19. Meloy J, Mohandie K. Mass casualty homicides on elementary school campuses: Threat management lessons learned from Bath, Michigan, to Newtown, Connecticut. In Meloy J, Hofmann J, eds., *International Handbook of Threat Assessment*. New York: Oxford Press; 2014:148–159.
20. White S. Case study: The Isla Vista campus community mass murder. J Threat Assess Manage. 2017;4(1):20–47. doi:10.1037/tam0000078
21. Van Dreal J, Okada D, Swinehart R, Rainwater A, Byrd R. Threat assessment and adults: Adult threat advisory team. In Van Dreal J, ed., *Assessing Student Threats: Implementing the Salem-Keizer System*. 2nd ed. Lanham, MD: Rowan and Littlefield; 2017:147.
22. Reaves B. Census of State and Local Law Enforcement Agencies (CSLLEA), 2008. ICPSR Data Holdings, Mar 2011. doi:10.3886/icpsr27681.v1.
23. Blair JP, Martaindale MH. Active shooter events in the United States from 2000 to 2010. *Active Shooter Events Response*. May 2013:49–64. doi:10.1201/b14996-4.

24. Schweit K. Addressing the problem of the active shooter. FBI, 7 May 2013. https://leb.fbi.gov/articles/featured-articles/addressing-the-problem-of-the-active-shooter

25. VALOR. Officer safety is paramount. Home. VALOR for Blue. https://www.valorforblue.org/

26. Smith ER. Supporting paradigm change in EMS' operation medical response to active shooter events. J Emerg Med Serv. 2013;38(12).

27. US Government. National Security Decision Directive Number 30, Federation of American Scientists. https://fas.org/irp/offdocs/nsdd/nsdd-30.pdf

16

Post-9/11 US Military and Intelligence Approaches to Lone Actors

CORRI ZOLI

INTRODUCTION

Drawing on two-decades of US involvement in the post-9/11 wars, this chapter examines the transformation of US counterterrorism policy, with a focus on the complex phenomenon of lone-actor terrorism. The chapter further addresses this species of political violence from the security policy perspective, with emphasis on the role of US military and intelligence communities in counterterrorism innovation. The security lens is critical as it captures the concerns of governments, particularly democratic and representative governments, when dealing with destabilizing forces like lone-actor terrorism and the challenge of building measured (not excessive) risk assessment and threat identification processes. This lens also captures policy priorities not necessarily urgent for other approaches to terrorism (i.e., history, economics) because the ability of governments to manage lone-actor terrorism often goes to the core of questions of legitimacy.

Although there are many ways to describe the counterterrorism security policy process over the past 20 years, two features dominate US efforts to manage the homeland component of the terrorist threat as developed by the US military, defense, law enforcement, and intelligence communities: an interagency "whole of government" approach[1] and an applied understanding of the nature of the threat gleaned from hard-won and often crisis-driven lessons on irregular battlefields, particularly Afghanistan, but also Iraq, Syria, and sub-Saharan African theaters. Combined, these features have gone some distance in shaping innovation in US counterterrorism policy at home, as this chapter describes, but also in framing multilateral efforts for affected states worldwide.[2] US Department of Defense (DoD) counterterrorism partner training programs, for instance, stretch across the world.[3]

In the US homeland security setting, lone-actor terrorism poses, as the Introduction describes, a complex challenge, as both the agents of this form of political violence and the phenomenon itself involve multiple factors and forces to which governments must respond.[4] While the term "lone-actor terrorism," like much of the canon of modern terrorism research, is the subject of debate, this chapter, consistent with the co-editor's (Holzer et al.) Introduction, understands lone-actor terrorism as multidimensional, involving a spectrum of actors with a range of types and levels of organization, motivation, and especially tactical capabilities.[5] Yet what distinguishes lone-actor terrorism from other forms of violent extremism and what makes it complex to manage is the lone actor's self-sufficiency. This terrorist actor above all is relatively independent from existing terrorist infrastructures, whether state or organizational. The lone actor plans, prepares, and executes violent acts in ways removed from existing terrorist organizations and command structures, proceeding largely without material assistance from a group, cell, or network engaged in violence. The dilemma for terrorism research and mitigation efforts alike, then, is to understand how and why these lone agents choose violence as their preferred mode of political mobilization and messaging—whether they are inspired by extremist ideologies, for instance, or intend to give sympathy and support, however virtual or attenuated, for extremist agendas. Despite the complexity of the lone-actor phenomenon, as Holzer et al. emphasize, the outcome is straightforward: to instigate calculated harm to victims and to society.

Recent critiques of the concepts of "lone wolf," "known wolves," "lone offender," or "lone actor" dispute whether these agents can really be seen as independent, including this author,[6] or as acting without coordination from terrorist groups and their often loosely coupled and dispersed networks. Leaderless warriors, for instance, tactically advocated for by the Islamic State of Iraq and al-Sham (ISIS) and al-Qaeda, are well-known in the literature.[7] In many cases, these relatively independent actors deploy social and political violence for unidentifiable ends and are shaped by hard-to-identify vectors of influence. In that sense, lone-actor terrorism is recognized as generally less knowable than other forms of violent extremism and highly contextual, responsive at once to local and transnational triggers and conditions while frequently ideologically inspired, including by online mechanisms of radicalization. Accordingly, increasingly sophisticated analysis seeks to find correlations in multiple variables (i.e., level of commitment, opinion, crime, identity, social networks, etc.).[8]

For governments especially, this lack of group participation or a traceable nexus between individual and group makes for the complexity of the lone-actor phenomenon, as compared to other terrorist agents—including those engaged in designated terrorist organizations, social and political movements, or irregular forces. Law enforcement often scrambles to make sense of the nature of this threat without the usual red flags, group and network connections, or galvanizing ideology to trace. Modern democratic governments, which prize open societies and value restraint in intruding into citizens' lives, find these actors not only logistically difficult to preempt, but view their unpredictable style of attack as corrosive to democratic norms.[9] In the United States, specifically, counterterrorism policy must be nested in a rule of law system that is at once agile and forward-leaning while respectful of the range and forms of dissent, opposition, outrage, protest, and grievances common in free-speech democracies.[10] Open and resilient governments must balance security and civil liberties in counterterrorism responses without doing damage to the open and inclusive nature of democratic societies. This requires a robust and adaptive policy response that can see "around the corner" to predict unpredictable attacks while at the same time uncovering root causes in lawful ways when multiple causal factors are at play.

Despite the intensity of US federal investment in counterterrorism efforts at home and abroad

(i.e., in revenue, human capital, capabilities) in the post-9/11 period, results have been uneven at best, especially when it comes to anti-terrorism outcomes. Most observers, whether academic or military, are far from happy with the results of the post-9/11 wars.[11] In addition to valid critiques of military strategy, tactics, and national policy, these unsatisfying results are due in large part to the complex asymmetric nature of contemporary terrorism in which largely jihadist organizations have evolved highly adaptive tactics to evade and exploit to their advantage modern government's military, rule of law, and law enforcement strengths.[12] Such violent actors' asymmetric "success," such as it is, depends on the use of calculated violence against "soft targets," unsuspecting noncombatants, civilian property, and public infrastructure. It also depends on targeting the gaps in existing governance policies and systems—the invariable lateness of legislation or an incoherent or naïve grand strategy.[13] Targeting these gaps occurs alike in low-governance areas of the world where irregular armed groups can succeed in becoming shadow or parallel governments, as in Iraq, Somalia, Syria, Mali, and Afghanistan, and in developed nations in which "soft" targets and the undefended assets of open societies multiply in the eyes of terrorist actors. In especially the latter case, lone actors can "fall through the cracks" of the interagency net, eluding shifting law and policy initiatives or the lawful restrictions placed on federal and local authorities. As lone actors increasingly take advantage of multiple settings, preying on missing or deliberately restrained security responses, they can do significant damage in a brief period, increase copycats, and hide in plain sight, even achieving strategic impact.

From the security policy perspective, the rising role of information saturation and politicized disinformation campaigns used by any number of internal and external conflict actors, whether competitive foreign governments or nonstate armed groups, is exacerbating the existing "fog of war" surrounding the hard-to-identify lone actor, including domestic terrorist agents, homegrown extremists, and other violent groups at work in the domestic context. What makes this development especially hard for government response is that information operations often exploit the blurry line, the difficulty in separating lawful protest and political expression from unlawful, violence-directed activity, including at its edges terrorist recruitment activity, anarchist rioting, property destruction, and the systemic denial of the civil rights of others.

From this broad view of the contemporary security policy landscape that frames the rise of the lone-actor phenomenon, we turn, first, to academic research on lone-actor trends and, second, to US intelligence and military influence in counterterrorism policy innovation.

LIMITED ACADEMIC-POLICY ENGAGEMENT IN THE STUDY OF LONE ACTOR TERRORISM

Much of the US counterterrorism policy response has proceeded with only limited or episodic engagement with the academic terrorism research community, including its methods and findings. Despite Gunning (2007a), Jackson (2012a) and Ranstorp's (2007) observation[14] that terrorism research is too strongly tied to states' interests and the latest threat, robust dialogue between academics and US government officials, including the military and law enforcement, is limited, including engagement with experts at the Departments of Homeland Security (DHS), Justice, and Defense. When episodic engagement and collaboration does occur, it is largely through federal research and development (grant) programs, government sponsored research, and convened expert conferences. With some exceptions like RAND, what has not been developed are durable mechanisms for collaboration (i.e., under the purview of the National Academies of Science, for instance) in which findings or even methods and paradigmatic questions helpful for crafting terrorism-related public policies can be engaged by both government practitioners and academics alike, as well as the public. One notable exception in international public affairs is the United Nations Security Council Counter-Terrorism Committee (CTC) and Counterterrorism Executive Directorate (CTED), which regularly convene shared research events for experts and governments on issues from foreign terrorist fighters to international humanitarian law in combating terrorism.[15] In the eyes of many policymakers, however, academic research does not readily provide actionable policy advice.

All of this indicates significant daylight between scholars of terrorism and US policymakers, themselves constrained by the labyrinthine national security and intelligence apparatus in which antiterrorism measures are negotiated across multiple agencies, each with its own specific remits, budgets, and authorities.[16] It is also true that, along with the demands of their "day jobs," government officials are hard pressed to absorb the cross-disciplinary literatures (i.e., in public affairs, international relations, sociology, anthropology, political science, public health) and the often narrow terms of debate in which terrorism research is anchored. The problem of standpoint, however, cuts both ways, as academics, too, live inside institutional cultures and constraints (some would say "bubbles") in which, as Schuurman (2019; 2020) recently noted, most of the field's 2007–2016 articles in leading journals overly focused on only some terrorist groups (al-Qaeda, ISIS), terrorist types (jihadism), and regions (broad Mideast), as the field as a whole remains event-driven (neglecting state terrorism; e.g., left- and right-wing non-jihadist extremism)—even as data and collection techniques improve.[17] If there is little "meeting of the minds" between the academy and the national security state, a third, pivotal interlocutor also remains "missing in action" from these important public conversations—too few concerted efforts are made to inform and involve ordinary Americans who bear the burden of counterterrorism policies.[18]

Despite these limits, and given recent intensive lone-actor research in separate academic and policy spheres, three emergent areas of scholarly inquiry offer promise for bridging the academic–public policy gap. These include (1) the role of organizational theory, organizational culture, and behavior, including network pressures and formalist approaches, to explain individual lone-actor conduct and cases of attenuated relationships to organizations, networks, or galvanizing ideologies[19]; (2) research into the increasing sophistication of extremist radicalization processes and information operations, including the role of internet, algorithmic, and communication technologies for online violent communities; and (3) the rising interest in social psychological and cognitive behavioral approaches to violent extremism for individuals but also in group dynamics. Because these are detailed elsewhere,[20] I do not address them here, but each area helps to explain the layered factors and contexts for lone-actor behavior, including interdependencies (i.e., extremist ideology delivered online as part of the radicalization process with social-psychological dimensions). Each area also underscores the "thick" interdisciplinary landscape of lone-actor terrorism studies, with recent contributions from criminology, organizational management, legal research, sociology and anthropology, public health, psychology and psychiatry, and media and communications, in addition to long-standing studies in politics, science, history, international relations, and strategic and security studies.

We turn next to the more forward-leaning domains for US counterterrorism policy innovation organized around the lone actor, particularly in its legislative-intelligence and military-operational dimensions.

POST-9/11 COUNTERTERRORISM ARCHITECTURE: CODIFYING THE "LONE WOLF" IN INTELLIGENCE AUTHORITIES

The post-9/11 institutional architecture for the US counterterrorism response emerges from the scathing critique of preparedness by the bipartisan National Commission on Terrorist Attacks upon the United States, known as the 9/11 Commission, established by Congress from November 27, 2002 to August 21, 2004.[21] Activating Congress's oversight role and prioritizing public understanding of the al-Qaeda attacks on the homeland, the 9/11 Commission was both matter of fact and specific in its criticisms of government performance: information-sharing failures ("to connect the dots") on the part of the US intelligence community; multilevel "failures in imagination" across federal agencies; "deep institutional failings" across all sectors of government; and the failure by both Clinton and Bush administrations to comprehend the nature of the al-Qaeda threat—understood as a "lone-wolf" phenomenon in al-Qaeda's difference from typical state-supported terrorist groups like Hezbollah, Hamas, Shining Path in Peru, etc.[22] After providing a "complete account" of the September 11, 2001 attacks, the *9/11 Commission Final Report* issued 41 recommendations, including 14 specific steps to prevent future terrorist attacks. For the first time in US law and policy, the concept of the lone actor, or "lone wolf" as it was known in the federal statute, became expressly part of the US intelligence-based counterterrorism arsenal.

In addition to intelligence gathering, law enforcement, and border, airport, and aviation security, most of the federal government came under scrutiny, from the National Security Agency, Federal Aviation Administration, Immigration and Naturalization Service, Justice Department, Customs, the State Department, to the White House and Congress itself.[23] New legislation, much of it initiated by the Senate Committee on Homeland Security and Governmental Affairs,

included the USA PATRIOT Act, signed into law on October 26, 2001, and the Homeland Security Act of 2002, which merged 22 separate federal entities (i.e., FEMA, the Coast Guard, US Immigration and Customs Enforcement) into a unified mission to protect the homeland. It also included the hefty eight-title Intelligence Reform and Terrorism Prevention Act (IRTPA) of 2004, designed to "reform the intelligence community" and the "intelligence-related activities" of the US government. For our purposes, the IRTPA changed the structure of terrorist response, with tectonic shifts for the US Intelligence Community (IC), including the new cabinet-level Director of National Intelligence (DNI), with oversight over the FBI, CIA, and whole IC. The 9/11 Commission also recommended a merging of the National Counterterrorism Center (NCTC) under DNI authority with the Bush administration's Terrorist Threat Integration Center (TTIC), established, May 1, 2003, to aggregate all threat information so that the White House would no longer need to synthesize data from 17 (now 18, with the newest addition in 2021 of the US Space Force) IC elements. Through Executive Order 13354 and the IRTPA, the NCTC added additional responsibilities beyond terrorist analysis integration and information sharing: it became the agency site for "strategic operational planning in direct support of the President"[24] and, as such, took on a formative, forward-learning operational role in US counterterrorism policy. We return to this operational emphasis shortly.

On the legislative side, "lone-wolf" provisions, as they are known, appeared for the first time in this period of intensive reform in the Intelligence Reform and Terrorism Prevention Act of 2004, which amended the 1978 Foreign Intelligence Surveillance Act (FISA) to expand its definition of an "agent of a foreign power" to include a non-US person engaged in international terrorism activities but who lacks obvious or traditional connections to a terrorist group or foreign power.[25] Section 6001 of the IRTPA, known as the "lone-wolf amendment," expanded the legal authority for government to surveil suspected terrorists unconnected to any organization (i.e., lone wolves) without requiring evidence of those links.[26] The lone-wolf provision itself, again, like much evolving counterterrorism policy, bore the imprint of the 9/11 crucible: the so-called missing hijacker, French citizen Zacarias Moussaoui, believed to be part of the United Airlines Flight 93 team out of Newark (forced down in rural Pennsylvania), was deemed a "missed opportunity" in the *9/11 Commission Final Report*.[27] Moussaoui was detained on August 16, 2001 for a visa waiver violation by FBI and Immigration and Naturalization Service (INS) agents in Minneapolis who learned he was an "Islamic extremist preparing for some future act in furtherance of radical fundamentalist goals" somehow related to his flight training.[28] It was the flight instructors at Pan Am International Flight Academy in Eagan, Minnesota, who tipped off FBI field officers about his suspicious behavior. While working with the Radical Fundamentalist Unit at FBI Headquarters, Minneapolis FBI agents were stymied in their request for a court order under FISA to authorize a search of Moussaoui's computer and possessions—FBI Headquarters declined to proceed with the FISA process, believing the evidence insufficient. The Moussaoui episode prompted the "lone-wolf" legislative response, and advocates for FISA authorities to this day continue to argue that, without it, the government cannot expeditiously respond to lone-wolf threats.

There is no doubt that the lone-wolf amendment recognized the evolution of national security threats beyond Cold War state actors, thus adding another lawful tool in dealing with the lone actor as unaffiliated foreign agent: "any person other than a United States person who engages in international terrorism or activities in preparation."[29] To obtain a secret FISA surveillance warrant, the government would not need to show probable cause that a suspect was linked to a foreign power or organization so long as the individual was a non-US person and preparing or engaging in international terrorism—an essential tool that lowered the evidentiary bar needed for an emergent era of decentralized, leaderless networks inspiring individuals to violence. The "lone-wolf" actor at this time was equated with rising nonstate armed groups, as reflected in the post-9/11 legal authorities—rather than the way we use the term today to mean far more independent terrorist agents.

More importantly, this tool revealed—from the perspective of the federal legislative and executive branches—that the US intelligence apparatus, the bureaucratically complex multiagency ecosystem of the IC, would become the "go to" place to take the fight against a new form of transnational terrorism. The United States is distinctive among nations in codifying in law its intelligence authorities so that even covert, clandestine, and secret operations are subject to rules and restraint (e.g., Moussaoui was not permitted

to be surveilled). But it is also true that this default intelligence institutional locus for innovation in counterterrorism policy, no matter how lawful, can easily become a governance weakness as well as an adaptive strength. The most obvious problem is secrecy, including the secret court (FISC) and associated intelligence surveillance processes, when applied in overbroad ways in the domestic security context. Critics note two decades of overreach in surveillance tools and authorities involving US persons.[30]

But problems of effective governance, public management, and counterterrorism outcomes are more widespread. In the case of lone actors, in concentrating a significant portion of the counterterrorist policy response in the IC, from expanding foreign intelligence surveillance powers to expanding "black budgets," a weighty institutional realignment has occurred in which the IC becomes tasked with all aspects of US security governance, even overseas kinetics (as we shall see) while the public remains outside these secret processes—all of which works against the grain of traditional US constitutional national security norms designed to defend "liberty as well as physical security."[31] When the lone-wolf counterterrorism response remains tucked away in the IC and secret processes, the public has little understanding of the nature of the threat or the policy response, which then creates difficulties when citizens ask for proactive help (as per the infamous "see something, say something" missive on the part of the FBI) or when renewing or supporting such authorities.[32]

Some observers find even greater systemic issues with the US counterterrorism policy response beyond this lack of public participation in self-governance. National security law and policy scholars have long raised concerns about the rising presence of intelligence and military assets and authorities in the homeland in ways that upset the balance between national security authorities abroad and at home and sideline the local law enforcement role in protecting domestic security. As William Banks notes, "After September 11, the military presence in the homeland increased literally overnight" despite the fact that "for more than 200 years, our laws and traditions have made military presence in the homeland exceptional."[33] Stephen Dycus likewise observes the "unprecedented effort to organize and harmonize this nation's homeland security activities," bringing together the DOD and the IC after 9/11 against "the background of a deep-seated American tradition of avoiding military entanglement in civilian affairs." Two decades later, the balance is arguably still off, as the recent extension (until May 2021) of 5,000 National Guard troops at the US Capital Building indicates, with rising calls for a permanent "quick reaction force" in DC— all for the express purpose of defending against domestic and lone-actor terrorism. Under the rubric of domestic counterterrorism policy, the nation has moved considerably from expanded "lone-wolf" legislative authorities in 2004 to a durable counterterrorism military force stationed in Washington, DC in 2021[34] These events, in addition to the broadened definition of lone-actor terrorism to encompass mass criminal activity,[35] indicate a "normalization" of the intelligence and military counterterrorism infrastructure in the homeland setting.

It is perhaps then ironic that in recent Congressional debate over whether to extend the lone-wolf amendment among other FISA authorities (set to expire by December 15, 2019, but delayed by Congress due to COVID until March 15, 2020), the public learned for the first time that in the 15-plus years since the statute's implementation, the lone-wolf amendment has never been used—not once—in the course of an investigation, despite many domestic lone-actor attacks since its enactment in 2004. As captured in Congressional testimony from FBI and National Security Agency (NSA) officials, many wished this authority to remain "in the government's toolkit for the future," especially as international terrorist groups increasingly seek to inspire individuals to carry out domestic attacks without evidence of coordination or support.[36] The lone-wolf amendment, as well as additional FISA authorities, expired on March 15, 2020.

In the aftermath of 9/11, transformative reform was on the menu at a level not undertaken since the National Security Act of 1947. At the core of this reorganization was the increased role of the military and intelligence agencies in domestic security and defense, with a special focus on counterterrorism policy and the lone actor. The "whole of government" approach—imposing collaboration or "jointness" on diverse public agency boundaries to manage complex, cross-cutting, even wicked problems like lone-actor terrorism— was designed to implement this new integrated homeland defense posture, given stove-piped agencies, the separation of powers structure, and the long-standing "wall" between foreign intelligence and military capabilities from domestic law enforcement.[37] In the context of the military, that whole of government approach, also known

as "unity of effort" in the *9/11 Commission Final Report*, has increasingly informed DoD attempts to bring more than kinetic tools to the counterterrorism fight abroad, by using all instruments of national power (so-called DIME-FIL or diplomatic, international, military, and economic plus finance, intelligence, and law enforcement) for counterterrorism (CT) and even counterinsurgency (COIN) missions.[38]

We turn to these and their homeland effects for lone-actor counterterrorism policy next.

OPERATIONAL COUNTERTERRORISM AND LONE ACTORS: LESSONS FROM THE IRREGULAR BATTLESPACE

Thus far we have emphasized the role of the political branches, Congress and the President, legislation and executive orders, in the US interagency story of counterterrorism policy transformation, hinged on an enlarged IC institutional role and expanded authorities pertaining to lone actors. What is thus far missing in this account is counterterrorism policy innovation driven by the US military and defense policy communities, particularly in their activities abroad. Unlike the prior section, this portion of the story is an international one, as both IC and DoD operations adapted to nonstate adversaries in irregular battlespaces. The "lessons learned," in turn, came to influence counterterrorism policy at home in myriad ways—not the least in changing perceptions and approaches to lone-actor terrorism.

Traditionally, the US national security law and policy structure is split into international and national security components reflective of the US Constitutional framework, as mentioned, but new post-9/11 pressures have sparked an increased military and intelligence presence in homeland defense and removed "the wall" between intelligence, the military, and law enforcement.[39] DHS, ODNI, and especially the new combatant command, US Northern Command (NORTHCOM), established on October 1, 2002, brought new capabilities to combat terrorism into the homeland. NORTHCOM in particular represented the first time since the Civil War that a military entity was made responsible for military activities inside the domestic United States by providing command and control for DoD homeland defense efforts and defense support for civil authorities. Both the first "National Strategy for Homeland Security" (2002), whose purpose was "to mobilize and organize our Nation to secure the US homeland from terrorist attacks," and the 2001 "Quadrennial Defense Review Report" (known as the National Defense Strategy after 2017) made the defense of the homeland the DoD's primary mission.[40]

However, a world away, the task of developing new approaches to confront transnational terrorism was occurring apace as deployed intelligence officers and, later, uniformed military service members, eager to deploy a kinetic response to the 9/11 attacks, brought the fight to a new type of terrorist actor, understood at the time as "lone wolves" or "terrorist entrepreneurs" insofar as they were not aligned with foreign states or their paramilitaries.[41] On September 26, 2001, a small seven-man CIA team, including a special operator and three pilots, known as the Northern Alliance Liaison Team (NALT), led by long-term CIA field officer and Near East Division Deputy Chief Gary Schroen was inserted by helicopter into northern Afghanistan to prepare the battlespace for follow-on special operation forces. The CIA's covert team's first task was to secure support from the Northern Alliance, the "only army left on the ground in Afghanistan" to oppose Taliban leader Mullah Omar, who had hosted Osama bin Laden.[42] From late September through November 2001, intelligence, special operations, and regular military task forces increasingly joined the fight and together on the ground began to invent new counterterrorism modalities to deal with highly committed, transnational, dispersed organizations—very different from the 1970s and 1980s terrorist militants like the Palestine Liberation Organization or Hamas, sponsored by governments or trying to form their own government.

Schroen's description of his experiences offers a window into this innovative process. CIA covert operations units had prior "connections to the Northern Alliance and Ahmed Shah Massoud's group of Tajik fighters up in the north," Schroen noted, as the CIA had been "sending teams into northern Afghanistan from [19]97 up until about 2000 to meet with Massoud's people, to try to get them involved" in opposing the Taliban and growing jihadist forms of extremism in the region.[43] The al-Qaeda 1998 American embassy attacks in Nairobi, Kenya, and Dar es Salaam, Tanzania, and the group's suspected role in the 2000 *USS Cole* bombing had strengthened CIA commitment to operational counterterrorism, evident in the work of CIA's multiregional CTC, prompting focus on Osama bin Laden himself in the still-new Bin Laden Issue Station established in 1996 at the CTC. Still, CIA direct action capabilities had atrophied with lack of leadership, funding, and commitment during the Clinton years. Nevertheless, days after 9/11, on September 13, 2001, Schroen found himself confronted by CIA CTC Director Cofer Black who asked him: "Will you take a team into Afghanistan . . . link up with Massoud's guys in the Northern Alliance and prepare the battlefield, bring the special forces in, and let's get the war started."[44] Such was the crisis-driven beginning of a deployed CIA, a military role that would increasingly characterize IC "joint" operations with the DOD in the many post-9/11 military theaters, heightening the role of Special Operations Command (SOCOM) and Joint Special Operations Command (JSOC) over the next two decades.

This original CIA "light footprint" approach, with its mission scope that depended on in-country relationship-building, cultural and language knowledge, and field-based operational leadership pushed down to the lowest "strategic corporal" levels, would come to define a sustainable counterterrorism policy in and beyond Afghanistan.[45] As Schroen explained, "We traveled so light and so small that we didn't need a whole lot of infrastructure" and "once [special forces] got on the ground, the relationship between CIA and those special forces A-teams was superb; it was seamless," even while "it was clear to us that the US military really struggled to come up with a plan as to how to deal with this one."[46] It would take more than a decade, with intermittent neglect of the Afghan mission, the subsequent Iraq invasion in 2003, and the 2007 troop surge to salvage the US–Iraq War (itself a far more conventional war than Afghanistan), before national security policy would catch up to the operational realities of the counterterrorism mission. In fact, Schroen recalled his "surprise" at "how slow the US military was to get themselves in a position where they could come and join us" more than a month later on October 20, 2001, when the first special forces arrived.[47] "Big army" delays, he notes, included the "heavy and cumbersome" plan by Central Command (CENTCOM) head Tommy Franks, disputes over which special operations group gets "to take the lead," and the need to stand up a large-footprint military facility in an Uzbekistan airfield at Karshi Khanabad (K2) "with tons and tons of equipment and miles of tents."[48] Ultimately, four combined or joint "task forces" (i.e., Combined Joint Task Force Mountain) mobilized for Operation Enduring Freedom (OEF) would join the CIA team in theater, including Australian and British forces.[49]

While there are many hard lessons learned in theater, essential features helped in the slow but steady US counterterrorism policy transformation: the emphasis on integrated counterterrorism operational planning, as encapsulated in the central role of the ODNI's NCTC from 2004 forward.[50] That planning expertise depended on a new intensive level of information sharing and situational awareness in all terrorism matters, which the NCTC provided for the whole IC in a 24/7 operations center, which also included CIA, FBI, and military personnel. Second, and most important, as the DHS 2019 "Strategic Framework for Countering Terrorism and Targeted Violence" makes clear, no success in countering terrorism is possible without the recognition of an evolving, highly dynamic threat.

CONCLUSION

Gregory Treverton's *Intelligence for an Age of Terrorism* notes that September 11, 2001 "marked a sea change for US intelligence," one widely acknowledged but not fully grasped: it marked a "reversal in the priority of targets" from large nation-states (with addresses and stories) to smaller, harder-to-track transnational groups and lone-actor individuals, a change which "goes to the heart of how intelligence does its business: from collection to analysis to dissemination."[51] The quest for and defeat of bin Laden also illustrates not only how much targets have changed after 9/11, but also "what has become the intensely operational nature of the counterterrorism intelligence task," one necessarily integrated with military capabilities.[52]

But the most significant difference between state and terrorist targets is how demanding the latter are from an intelligence perspective—and, hence, for governments and effective security policies. As Treverton explains:

If preventing a terrorist attack is the name of the game, the pressure on intelligence is extraordinary. The dominant strategy of the Cold War—deterrence—was less sensitive to the specifics of intelligence. It rested on the assumption that, for all its differences in goals and ideology, the Soviet Union was like us: modern, rational (in our terms), and not self-destructive. In contrast to deterrence, the prevention of suicidal attacks—whether by preemption, disruption, or simply defending vulnerabilities—requires enormous precision in intelligence, even to the point of understanding individual intentions.

Whether the actor is a near or distant lone wolf—a US Army Major Nidal Hassan, the Fort Hood killer of 2009, or bin Laden—these are "small targets" whose stories are hard to divine. Even a single suicide bomber can cause major damage—all while presenting US intelligence with insurmountable challenges simply in describing their story (without inducing governments to collect endless information on citizens in ways that also damage civil liberties).

These challenges will only grow as lone actors increase and as counterterrorism efforts must collaboratively manage the sheer volume of data accompanying the dynamic nature of a changing threat—in addition to making sense of "the lack of a story with parameters," which most nations possess.

NOTES AND REFERENCES

1. Peña-López I. Taking a whole-of-government approach. UN e-Government Survey 2012. *E-Government for the People*, 2012:55–60; Christensen T, Lægreid P. The whole-of-government approach to public sector reform. *Publ Admin Rev.* 2007;67(6):1059–1066. https://publicadministration.un.org/egovkb/Portals/egovkb/Documents/un/2012-Survey/Chapter-3-Taking-a-whole-of-government-approach.pdf
2. Romaniuk P. *Multilateral Counter-terrorism: The Global Politics of Cooperation and Contestation.* New York and London: Routledge; 2010.
3. For a recent example, see Strengthening partner networks and capacity. US Department of Defense, Lead Inspector General for East Africa, North, and West Africa Counterterrorism Operations, Quarterly Report to US Congress, Apr. 1. 2020–Jun. 30. 2020:11. https://www.dodig.mil/reports.html/Article/2331453/lead-inspector-general-for-east-africa-and-north-and-west-africa-counterterrori/
4. US Department of Homeland Security. *Strategic Framework for Countering Terrorism and Targeted Violence.* Sept. 2019; Hamm MS, Spaaij R. *The Age of Lone Wolf Terrorism.* New York: Columbia University Press; 2017:17, 35–37..
5. The range of actors, conditions, motivations, and different weapons and tactics is clear across recent attacks in and outside the United States, such as the 2009 Fort Hood shooting by Army psychiatrist Nidal Hasan; the San Bernardino multi-weapons attack in 2015 by married couple Syed Rizwan Farook and Tashfeen Malik; the Orlando Pulse nightclub massacre by security guard Omar Mateen; the Charleston, South Carolina, church attack by Dylan Storm Roof in 2015; the synagogue attack in Pittsburgh by Robert Gregory Bowers in 2018 (alleged, pre-trial at time of this writing); the Anders Breivik summer camp attack in Norway in

2011; the Mohamed Salmene Lahouaiej-Bouhlel cargo truck attack in Nice, France in 2016; and the Christchurch, New Zealand, shootings by Brenton Tarrant in 2019.

6. Zoli C. Lone-wolf or low-tech terrorism? Emergent patterns of global terrorism in recent French and European attacks. *Lawfare*. 8 Jun 2016:17–05; Hofmann D. How alone are lone-actors? Exploring the ideological, signaling, and support networks of lone-actor terrorists, *Studies in Conflict & Terrorism*. 2020;43(7):657–678.

7. One example of many is Sageman M. *Leaderless Jihad: Terror Networks in the Twenty-First Century*. Philadelphia: University of Pennsylvania Press; 2011.

8. See, for instance, Singh P, Sreenivasan S, Szymanski SK, Korniss G. Accelerating consensus on co-evolving networks: the effect of committed individuals. *Phys Rev E*. 2012;85(4):046104; Xie J, Emenheiser J, Kirby M, Sreenivasan S, Szymanski BK, Korniss G. Evolution of opinions on social networks in the presence of competing committed groups, *PLoS ONE*. 2012;7(3):e33215; Lu Q, Korniss G, Szymanski BK. The naming game on social networks: Community formation and consensus engineering. *J Econ Interact Coord*. 2012;4(2):221–235; Sambanis N, Shayo M. Social identification and ethnic conflict. *Am Pol Sci Rev*. 2013;107(2):294–325; Sanín FG, Wood EJ. Ideology in civil war: Instrumental adoption and beyond. *J Peace Res*. 2014;51(2):213–226; and Szymanski BK, Lizardo O, Doyle C, Karampourniotis P, Singh P, Korniss G, Bakdash J. The spread of opinions in societies. In *Modeling Sociocultural Influences on Decision Making: Understanding Conflict, Enabling Stability*. New York: CRC Press: Taylor & Francis; 2016:61–84.

9. One of the strongest voices for this issue was Paul Wilkinson in *Terrorism and the Liberal State* (New York: Macmillan International Higher Education; 2015) and *Terrorism Versus Democracy: The Liberal State Response*. 3rd ed. (New York: Routledge; 2011).

10. See Dycus S, Banks WC, Raven-Hansen P, Vladeck SI. *Counterterrorism Law*. Philadelphia: Wolters Kluwer Law & Business; 2016.

11. Bolger DP. *Why We Lost: A General's Inside Account of the Iraq and Afghanistan Wars*. New York: Houghton Mifflin Harcourt/Eamon Dolan Books; 2014.

12. Zoli C. Asymmetric warfare. In Moghaddam F, ed., *Sage Encyclopedia of Political Behavior*. Thousand Oaks, CA: Sage; 2016.

13. See Arreguin-Toft I. Tunnel at the end of the light: A critique of US counter-terrorist grand strategy. *Cambr Rev Intl Aff*. 2002;15(3):549–563; and Rothstein H, Arquilla J, eds. *Afghan Endgames: Strategy and Policy Choices for America's Longest War*. Washington, DC: Georgetown University Press; 2012.

14. Gunning J. Babies and bathwaters: Reflecting on the pitfalls of critical terrorism studies. *Eur Pol Sci*. 2007a;6(3):236–243; Jackson R. The study of terrorism 10 years after 9/11: Successes, issues, challenges. *Uluslararasi Iliskiler*. 2012a;8(32):1–16; and Ranstorp M. Introduction: Mapping terrorism research –challenges and priorities. In Ranstorp M, ed., *Mapping Terrorism Research: State of Art, Gaps and Future Direction*. London/New York: Routledge, 2007:1–28).

15. See Lewis DA, Modirzadeh NK, Burniske JS. Legal briefing March 2020: The CTED and International Humanitarian Law: Preliminary considerations for states. 2020. http://blogs.harvard.edu/pilac/files/2020/03/CTED-and-IHL.pdf

16. For a journalistic anatomy of the growth of the post-9/11 US security architecture, its lawful authorities, public private partnerships, defense contractors, and law enforcement and policing domains, see Priest D, Arkin W. *Top Secret America: The Rise of the New American Security State*. New York: Little, Brown; 2011; and Gellman B, Miller G. "Black budget" summary details US spy network's successes, failures and objectives. *Washington Post*, 29 Aug 2013..

17. Schuurman B. Topics in terrorism research: Reviewing trends and gaps, 2007–2016. *Crit Stud Terrorism*. 2019;12:(3):463–480; and Schuurman B. Research on terrorism, 2007–2016: A review of data, methods, and authorship. *Terrorism Pol Viol*. 2020;32(5):1011–1026.

18. A lack of public understanding of the post-9/11 military efforts has remained a palpable concern. See Zoli C, Maury R, Fay D. *Missing Perspectives: Servicemembers' Transition from Service to Civilian Life*. Syracuse, NY: Syracuse University, Institute for Veterans and Military Families; 2015.

19. Some examples include Parkinson SE. Organizing rebellion: Rethinking high-risk mobilization and social networks in war. *Am Pol Sci Rev*. 2013;107(3):418–432; and Shapiro J. *The Terrorist's Dilemma: Managing Violent Covert Organizations*. Princeton, NJ: Princeton University Press; 2013.

20. Chenoweth E, English R, Gofas A, Kalyvas SN. Approaches and methods. In *The Oxford Handbook of Terrorism*. New York: Oxford University Press; 2019.

21. Commission Chair Kean and Vice Chair Hamilton found the FBI and CIA in particular did not serve Presidents Clinton or Bush well in their security missions, that our failures took place over many years and many administrations, and none of the measures adopted by the US government before 9/11 disturbed or even delayed the progress of the al-Qaeda plot. See Shovelan J. 9/11 commission finds "deep institutional failings." Australian Broadcasting Corporation, 23 Jul 2004; and Kranes M. Our government failed us: All agencies

left the door open to evil, probers say. *New York Post*, 23 Jul 2004. https://nypost.com/2004/07/23/our-govt-failed-us-all-agencies-left-the-door-open-to-evil-probers-say/

22. *The 9/11 Commission Report: Final Report of the National Commission on Terrorist Attacks Upon the United States*. New York: Norton; 2004; US General Accounting Office. *Combating Terrorism: Selected Challenges and Related Recommendations*, GAO-01-822. Washington, DC: General Accounting Office; 20 Sep 2001).

23. The USA PATRIOT Act of 2001 (Uniting and Strengthening America by Providing Appropriate Tools Required to Intercept and Obstruct Terrorism), Public L. 107-56, Oct. 26, 2001, 115 Stat. 272) and the Homeland Security Act of 2002 (Pub. L. 107-296, Nov. 25, 2002, 116 Stat. 2135).

24. US Director of National Intelligence. Today's NCTC:5. https://www.dni.gov/files/NCTC/documents/features_documents/NCTC-Primer_FINAL.pdf

25. Bellia PL. The Lone Wolf Amendment and the future of foreign intelligence surveillance law. *Villanova L Rev.* 2005;50(3):425–478.

26. Congressional Research Service (CRS). Foreign Intelligence Surveillance Act (FISA): An overview. 10 Mar 2020. https://fas.org/sgp/crs/intel/IF11451.pdf. See, also *United States v. Moalin*; US Department of Justice, Office of the Inspector General. *Review of Four FISA Applications and Other Aspects of the FBI's Crossfire Hurricane Investigation*. Dec 2019. https://www.justice.gov/storage/120919-examination.pdf

27. Moussaoui was seen as a lone actor in the context of the rise of nonstate armed groups, reflected in the post-9/11 legal authorities (IRTPA, the PATRIOT Act, FISA amendments); today lone actors work far more independently.

28. *9/11 Commission Report*, 273.

29. See 50 USC. § 1801(b)(1)(C). The legislative history of FISA indicates that surveillance targets at the time were associated with a foreign state or organization, including international terrorist groups like Black September; domestic terrorist groups are excluded. H.R. REP. NO. 95-1283, pt. 1, at 30 (1978), https://fas.org/irp/agency/doj/fisa/hspci1978.pdf

30. US Department of Justice, Office of the Inspector General. *Review of Four FISA Applications and Other Aspects of the FBI's Crossfire Hurricane Investigation*, Oversight and Review Division 20-012. Dec 2019.

31. Baker JE. *In the Common Defense: National Security Law for Perilous Times*. New York: Cambridge University Press; 2007:2.

32. Minopoli S. An illusion of safety: Why Congress should let FISA's Lone Wolf amendment expire. *Natl Sec L Brief.* 2020;10:197.

33. Banks WC. The normalization of homeland security after September 11: The role of the military in counterterrorism preparedness and response. *Louisiana L Rev.* 2003;64(4):735–778, at 738; Dycus S. The role of military intelligence in homeland security. *Louisiana L Rev.* 2004;64(4):779–808, at 780. Dycus asked these prescient questions: "Before we agree that military intelligence services should play a more expansive role in our domestic life, several practical questions need to be addressed . . . [including] whether such a change would actually make us more secure. Would a more aggressive use of military intelligence at home make a uniquely valuable contribution to current counterterrorism efforts of the FBI, local law enforcement, and other civilian agencies? Or would it be merely redundant, wasteful, and perhaps even counterproductive?"

34. More than 26,000 National Guard troops were originally activated on January 6, 2021, in response to the riots that breached the US Capitol Building. See Beynon S. Task force calls for permanent National Guard force to protect DC. 8 Mar 2021. https://www.military.com/daily news/2021/03/08/task-force-calls-permanent-national-guard-force-protect-dc.html

35. Deloughery K, King RD, Asal V. *Understanding Lone-Actor Terrorism: A Comparative Analysis with Violent Hate Crimes and Group-Based Terrorism*. Final Report to the Resilient Systems Division, Science and Technology Directorate, US Department of Homeland Security. College Park, MD: START; 2013.

36. Orlando MJ. Deputy Assistant Director, Federal Bureau of Investigation, Reauthorizing the USA Freedom Act of 2015, Joint Statement for the Record, Joint Statement with Department of Justice Deputy Assistant Attorney General J. Bradford Wiegmann and Susan Morgan, National Security Agency, Before the Senate Judiciary Committee, Washington, DC. 6 Nov 2019. https://www.fbi.gov/news/testimony/reauthorizing-the-usa-freedom-act-of-2015-110619

37. Garamone J. Dempsey talks caution, whole-of-government approach. *DoD News*, 24 Sep 2015. ; Halligan J, Buick F, O'Flynn J. Experiments with joined-up, horizontal and whole-of-government in Anglophone countries. In *The International Handbook on Civil Service Systems*. 2011. (greater collaboration and coordination across department boundaries is emphasized to eliminate resource waste and optimize effort and synergies).

38. Joint Doctrine Note 1-18, Strategy; Joint Publication (JP) 1, Doctrine for the Armed Forces of the United States; JP 3-08, Interorganizational Cooperation; and the Joint Concept for Integrated Campaigning. See, also, *9/11 Commission Final Report*, treating unity of effort recommendations across all of government, at 399–422.

39. *9/11 Commission Final Report*, 8–80; 271; 424.

40. US Office of the Secretary of Defense. *2001 Quadrennial Defense Review* (QDR), Sep 2001; US Office of Homeland Security. *National Strategy for Homeland Security*, 16 Jul 2002:4: This is an exceedingly complex mission that requires coordinated and focused effort from our entire society—the federal government, state and local governments, the private sector, and the American people.

41. See de Mesquita EB. Regime change and revolutionary entrepreneurs. *Am Pol Sci Rev.* 2010;104(3); *9/11 Commission Final Report*, 5.1 Terrorist Entrepreneurs, at 145.

42. Schroen PBS interview (2006).

43. Frontline. Interview with Gary C. Schroen. 20 Jan 2006. https://www.pbs.org/wgbh/pages/frontline/darkside/interviews/schroen.html. "Our whole reason for being was to take on the main enemy, the KGB, to fight these communist regimes. . . . When it all fell apart, it took the agency several years to really recover and try to get a new focus. We have enemies that are out there, actively working against the United States, but they're so different. It's not a huge government; it's these tiny cells of individuals who are out there." See also CIA. *Devotion to Duty: Responding to the Terrorist Attacks of September 11th.* Langley, VA: Central Intelligence Agency; 2010.

44. See J. Cofer Black, Testimony (Unclassified), US Congressional Hearings, Joint Investigation into September 11th: Fifth Public Hearing, 26 Sept. 2002, Joint House/Senate Intelligence Committee Hearing. https://fas.org/irp/congress/2002_hr/092602black.html

45. Morris J. *Strategic Corporal, 2025: Operationalizing Small-Unit Leaders for Theater-Level Operations.* Quantico, VA: United States Marine Corps School of Advanced Warfighting Marine Corps University.

46. Ibid.

47. Ibid.

48. Ibid.

49. For a description of this early period, see, *The United States Army in Afghanistan: Operation Enduring Freedom*, Oct 2001–Mar. 2002:5–14. https://history.army.mil/html/books/070/70-83/cmhPub_70-83.pdf

50. Recommendation 32 of the *9/11 Commission Final Report* (p. 415) states, "Lead responsibility for directing and executing paramilitary operations, whether clandestine or covert, should shift to the Defense Department, and consolidated with the capabilities for training, direction, and execution of such operations already being developed in the Special Operations Command." The concern was little robust capability to conduct paramilitary operations by CIA personnel prior to 9/11, relying on proxies and resulting in poor outcomes and resource issues in building two separate secret forces. See, also, Carney JT Jr., Schemmer BF. *No Room for Error: The Covert Operations of America's Special Tactics Units from Iran to Afghanistan.* 2002:ix– x.

51. Jenkins BM, Godges JP. *The Long Shadow of 9/11: America's Response to Terrorism.* Santa Monica, CA: RAND; 2011:163–164; see also Treverton GF. *Intelligence for an Age of Terror.* Cambridge: Cambridge University Press; 2009.

52. Ibid.

17

US Legal Perspectives

Legislative, Intelligence, and Law Enforcement Aspects

JEFFREY H. SMITH, AMY JEFFRESS,
*CHRISTOPHER E. BEELER, AND TIAN TIAN XIN**

INTRODUCTION AND OVERVIEW

From the earliest days of the American Republic, lone individuals have engaged in violent acts motivated by politics, racism, or religion. Most notably, four US presidents (Lincoln, Garfield, McKinley, and Kennedy) have been assassinated by lone gunmen. In addition, individuals acting alone have committed countless other acts of violence directed at ordinary Americans or institutions for the same reasons. Until relatively recently, these were generally regarded merely as criminal acts, and US criminal laws seemed adequate to prosecute those who could be apprehended.[1] Today, these acts would widely be regarded as "terrorism."

The advent of widespread political violence in the 1970s—much of it arising out of the Israeli–Palestinian conflict (e.g., the Black September attack on the Israeli team at the 1972 Munich Olympics), radical leftists in Europe (e.g., the Baader-Meinhof Gang kidnappings and murders in Germany), and numerous aircraft hijackings[2,3]—led to the characterization of such acts as "international terrorism."

Because these acts occurred largely outside the United States, "terrorism" was not a high priority for domestic US law enforcement or intelligence agencies. However, as American installations and officials became targets of these acts, "international terrorism" increasingly became a national priority. Congress promulgated new laws, such as 18 USC § 2339A, which was enacted in 1994, making the provision of "material support to terrorism" a crime. In addition, Congress enacted other laws that extend the extraterritorial jurisdiction of the United States to cover attacks on American citizens and interests occurring outside of the United States.[4,5]

The attacks on September 11, 2001 ushered in vast changes in US policy, specifically its approach to terrorism. "Combatting terrorism" became a watchword. New laws were passed and new institutions created. The Department of Homeland Security (DHS) and the Director of National Intelligence were established on the recommendation of the 9/11 Commission.[6] Existing agencies were reorganized, refocused, and given additional funding and authority.[7] The PATRIOT Act[8] expanded the power of the federal government to collect intelligence on potential terrorists. Greater emphasis was placed on international cooperation in both intelligence collection and counterterrorism operations.

On a broader front, the United States marshaled a coalition that attacked the Taliban-led

* Authors Smith, Jeffress, and Xin have previously served in several positions in the US government, including in the Department of Justice, Department of State, Staff of the Senate Armed Services Committee, Central Intelligence Agency, and the US Army. Author Beeler, who was an attorney at Arnold and Porter when he participated in the preparation of this chapter, had previously served in the US Army and is now an Assistant US Attorney in the Office of the US Attorney in San Diego, California. The views expressed in this chapter are entirely those of the authors and do not represent the views of the US government or any department or agency in which the authors previously served or, in the case of Mr. Beeler, is now serving.

government of Afghanistan, which had sheltered Osama bin Laden and al-Qaeda, which carried out the attacks of 9/11. Subsequently, the United States led a different coalition that invaded Iraq in 2002, on grounds that Saddam Hussein possessed weapons of mass destruction (WMDs) and was supporting terrorism directed against the United States, although no WMDs were found, and there was no evidence that Hussein was responsible for the 9/11 attacks.

Those wars are not within the scope of this chapter, much less this volume. But it must be acknowledged that some Muslims regard the wars (and the treatment of detainees at the Abu Ghraib prison and Guantánamo Bay detention facility) as attacks on Islam by the West. This view has spawned deep anger that, in turn, has motivated many acts of terrorism by groups and lone individuals directed against the United States and its European allies. More recently, the United States has seen a growth in acts of violence by individuals motivated by hate against minority racial or religious groups. For instance, the FBI's Hate Crime Statistics Program accounts for 7,120 hate crime incidents in 2018, with 1,550 offenses motivated by religious bias.[9] These are regarded as "hate crimes" under US law, but to the victims and the public they may equally be regarded as acts of terrorism.

Until the 1970s, "terrorism" had little significance as a legal term. However, it now appears in several US criminal and related statutes. Although these statutes define terrorism, they do not define "lone wolf terrorist" or "lone-actor terrorist."[10,11,12] "Domestic terrorism" is defined as activities that involve acts "dangerous to human life" that violate US or state criminal laws and "appear to be intended (i) to intimidate or coerce a civilian population; (ii) to influence the policy of a government by intimidation or coercion; or (iii) to affect the conduct of a government by mass destruction, assassination, or kidnapping."[13] Thus, for purposes of this chapter, we will regard a lone-actor terrorist as an individual, acting alone, who engages in domestic terrorism, as defined. Notably, the definition is focused on the actor's *intended outcome* rather than the actor's *motivation*. That is, whether a person is a terrorist depends not on the beliefs that motivate them to act, but rather whether they intend the action to intimidate or coerce the government or the civilian population.

Any analysis of terrorism also requires discussion of the line between "terrorist acts" and "hate crimes"—a line that is not always clear.[14] As discussed later, the federal criminal code has provisions addressing both "terrorism" and "hate crimes." Hate crimes are beyond the scope of this chapter, although they have many similar characteristics to acts of terrorism. Victims of terrorism and hate crimes committed by a lone individual may care little how the acts are treated in the law. That said, law enforcement and intelligence officials have the responsibility to identify individuals before they act and stop them. If that fails, they have the responsibility to prosecute them to the full extent of the law.

The discussion that follows covers two broad areas. The first main section summarizes the laws applicable to lone-actor terrorists and prosecutions of such individuals that have occurred. Later sections discuss the far more complex issue of how, in our democracy, to identify lone-actor terrorists before they strike.

It is not possible in the span of a single chapter to discuss these issues in any great depth. In the following pages, we attempt to convey to the reader the complexity of the applicable laws and challenges as US authorities and judges struggle to keep their fellow citizens safe while remaining true to the principles of civil liberties and due process of law enshrined in the US Constitution. Their task is daunting, but getting it right is essential.

APPLICABLE LAWS AND PROSECUTIONS

The Department of Justice has been remarkably successful in prosecuting lone-actor terrorists in federal courts.[15] Ordinary federal criminal statutes adequately cover nearly all of the acts of "terror" and may be prosecuted under a more general charge, such as murder, attempted murder, arson, or assault. The addition of federal criminal statutes focused on terrorism—such as the prohibition on harboring or financing terrorists and the expanded authority to collect information, including by electronic surveillance—has assisted in identifying and prosecuting terrorists.

In addition, various states have enacted anti-terrorism statutes that criminalize terrorist acts.[16] But most state-level prosecutions of lone-actor terrorists proceed under criminal laws that are broadly applicable; for instance, murder, attempted murder, assault, and felony possession of firearms.[17]

STATE AND FEDERAL LAWS ON TERRORISM

Federal Laws

The US Attorney's Manual identifies 23 statutes as "International Terrorism Statutes."[18,19] It further contains a separate section on WMDs and notes the potential connection that WMD statutes may have to terrorism.[20] The US Attorney's Manual does not list specific statutes for domestic terrorism.[21]

In brief, the following are federal criminal charges that have been or could be brought against lone-actor terrorists for completed or attempted criminal offenses or conspiracies to commit those offenses.[22]

- The use of biological, nuclear, chemical, or other WMDs[23];
- Possession of a "biological agent, toxin, or delivery system" that is not reasonably justified by certain peaceful purposes[24];
- Providing material support to terrorists or designated terrorist organizations[25];
- Attacks on foreign officials, official guests, or internationally protected persons[26];
- Attacks on federal officers or employees, members of the US Congress, Justices of the Supreme Court, or the President[27,28,29,30,31];
- Murder or attempted murder of a federal officer or employee while that person is on duty[32];
- Attacks on certain federally protected activities or associated facilities, such as voting and enjoying benefits provided by the US government[33];
- Damage of religious properties and obstruction of a person's free exercise of religious beliefs[34];
- Hindrance of free access to clinic entrances[35];
- Failure to register a firearm or felony possession of firearms[36,37];
- Transportation, receipt, or distribution of explosive materials without a license[38]; and
- Commission of violence at international airports.[39]

A wide array of other criminal statutes that lack direct relation to terrorism may also apply to a terrorist's conduct, such as murder,[40] attempted murder,[41] mailing threatening communications,[42] receiving the proceeds of extortion,[43] committing fraud,[44] falsifying information and committing hoaxes,[45] and selling or receiving stolen vehicles.[46]

In addition, many statutes that criminalize hate crimes also apply to acts of terrorism.[47]

State Laws on Terrorism

After the September 11, 2001, attacks, many states enacted anti-terrorism statutes.[48] Like federal statutes, some prohibit providing material support to terrorists or terrorist organizations.[49] Some states have also enacted statutes on WMDs.[50]

Prosecution of Lone-Actor Terrorists

Our research has reviewed 125 lone-actor terrorist acts in the United States between September 11, 2001 and June 2019.[51] These include acts of terror that garnered national attention as well as planned attacks stopped before the act. Criminal charges—in both federal and state courts—brought against suspects for these acts are summarized here.

- Thirty-one individual perpetrators were killed or died by suicide during the attack
- Fifty-three individuals were charged with violations of federal law only
- Thirty-three individuals were charged with violations of state law only
- Six individuals were charged with violations of both federal and state laws
- One individual is a fugitive who was never formally charged and has been missing since June 2011[52]

The charged individuals have faced varying outcomes. Approximately one-third of them were charged with violations of terrorism statutes. Seventy-eight of those individuals were convicted of at least one count, two individuals were found not fit to stand trial,[53] two cases were dismissed, one individual was acquitted by reason of insanity, one individual died while awaiting a competency evaluation,[54] and nine individuals had not been tried as of June 28, 2019. In addition, one individual was initially found incompetent to stand trial, but the court later found him competent, and his case remains pending.[55]

Prosecutions Under Federal Law

Lone-actor terrorism cases are charged under federal law where the alleged act targets federal entities, individuals or entities protected by federal law, or interstate commerce. Our research identified 59 individuals charged by federal prosecutors, including four prosecutions that involved both federal and state or District of Columbia laws. Forty-four were convicted of at least one count. In the majority of the cases identified, the alleged perpetrator was charged under general criminal statutes only and not under a terrorism statute.[56] There were only four instances of reliance on a terrorism statute alone, three of which related to bombings or bomb threats.[57]

Federally charged lone-actor terrorism often involves events related to bombings, bomb threats, or conspiracies. Accordingly, the federal terrorism statutes most frequently used to prosecute lone-actor terrorists are those prohibiting the use or possession of WMD[58] and material support of terrorism charges.

Prosecutions Under State Law
Our research identified 39 state prosecutions of lone-actor terrorists since September 11, 2001. Of these cases, 33 resulted in a conviction on at least one count. State prosecutions of lone-actor terrorists rarely involve terrorism statutes, in large part because many states do not have such statutes—only four cases involved charges under anti-terrorism statutes enacted following 9/11 in those states (i.e., Michigan, New Jersey, New York, and Pennsylvania). Instead, state prosecutions of terrorism typically rely on the respective state's general criminal statutes. The most common charges filed for state prosecutions of lone-actor terrorism are various state murder and assault charges, as well as charges related to discharging firearms or disorderly conduct.

Comparison Between Federal and State Prosecutions
Federal and state prosecution of lone-actor terrorism has differed in terms of the types of crime prosecuted, and, for convicted lone-actor terrorists, sentences imposed. The types of crimes that are considered state crimes versus federal crimes underlie these differences: our research shows that federal prosecutors bring more prosecutions of bombing or bomb plot cases than their state counterparts.[59] This difference arises because of the *targets* of the bomb threats: the federal cases were brought where the targets were federal land or personnel, or involved a federal instrumentality, such as use of the US Postal Service, to commit a crime.

The differences in sentencing between state and federal courts have similar explanations. Although it appears that state courts impose harsher sentences than federal courts,[60] that is in part because the lone-actor terrorism cases

brought and tried by state prosecutors often involved murder charges, while many of the federal crimes for which lone-actor terrorists were convicted involved planned, but not realized, attacks.

Acquittal and Dismissal of Charges
Although most of the lone-actor terrorists who have been charged have been convicted, not all have been. In federal court, one defendant was found not fit to stand trial,[61] while another died waiting for a competency evaluation.[62] Another case was dismissed without prejudice in light of a commitment order in a second case against the same defendant.[63] Only one defendant was acquitted. In that case, the defendant was found not guilty by reason of insanity.[64,65]

As for state prosecutions, one case was dismissed on the state's motion, suggesting it lacked sufficient evidence to support a conviction.[66,67] In another case, the defendant has remained in a psychiatric hospital after being declared legally incompetent in 2016; as a result, his case remains pending.[68]

Legislative Responses to Terrorism
Since the September 11, 2001, attacks, Congress has proposed various laws relating to lone-actor terrorists. In particular, Congress added the "lone-wolf provision" to the USA PATRIOT Act as part of the Intelligence Reform and Terrorism Prevent Act of 2004.[69,70] The language authorizes the wiretapping of a non-US person who "engages in international terrorism or activities in preparation therefore."[71] The provision was originally enacted to respond to the belief that the FBI could have caught 9/11 perpetrator Zacarias Moussaoui if such a provision had existed prior to the attack.[72] Congress adopted the "lone-wolf provision" with a "sunset" clause, meaning that it will expire at a date designated in the law. That date has passed, but Congress has repeatedly extended it.[73,74] However, despite reauthorization of the provision, it has apparently never been used.[75,76]

Many bills have been introduced in Congress that explicitly address lone-actor terrorism, although as of the time of this writing none has been adopted. Some have sought to establish a commission to examine and report on violent radicalization and homegrown terrorism as well as the motives underlying it.[77,78,79] In addition, there have been proposals to increase protection of members of Congress in light of the recent lone-actor terrorist acts.[80,81] Such efforts increased following an attack by a solitary gunman against the Republican Congressional baseball team in the summer of 2017.[82]

Recent mass shootings have renewed the call for additional criminal statutes (e.g., "A domestic terrorism statute doesn't exist. Congress must pass one—now," said former federal prosecutor Harry Litman, *Washington Post*, August 5, 2019). As discussed later, some changes may be necessary, for example, to enhance the ability of law enforcement agencies to monitor social media. But so far, Congress has been reluctant to adopt additional criminal statutes to combat lone-actor terrorists because current laws have proved adequate to prosecute individuals who commit such acts of terror.

INTELLIGENCE COLLECTION AND CIVIL LIBERTIES

As discussed in the preceding section, prosecution of lone-actor terrorists—at both the state and federal level—has been quite successful. The more formidable challenge is identifying individuals before they act.

Post-9/11 Surveillance and Infiltration Programs

In the wake of the 9/11 attacks, federal and state law enforcement and intelligence agencies began aggressive electronic surveillance and "human intelligence activities"[83] directed toward possible terrorist groups and individuals operating domestically. Congress passed the USA PATRIOT Act giving federal agencies increased authority to collect and share information among federal agencies and with state and local law enforcement agencies. Many of the provisions were controversial, particularly those that raised concern about possible infringement of civil liberties of US citizens. As a result, the law contained a "sunset" provision requiring its reauthorization; most recently, the law was renewed in 2015. It was set to expire in December 2019,[84] but as of this writing, was again extended by Congress.

Among the more controversial measures was the "Terrorist Surveillance Program," approved secretly by President George W. Bush, which authorized the government to collect, without a warrant from the Foreign Intelligence Surveillance Act (FISA) Court, massive amounts of data from public electronic communications, including those of US citizens. The program was briefed to only a handful of members of Congress who were sworn to secrecy. When it was disclosed by the *New York Times* in December 2005,[85] a

furor arose. Congress eventually adopted revisions of the law restricting the program and requiring a warrant from the FISA court to collect such data.[86,87]

The use of informants in religious organizations has also generated much criticism. For example, in Irvine, California, the FBI's use of undercover informants to investigate Ahmadullah Niazi caused national concern over law enforcement's respect for American Muslims' civil liberties.[88,89,90,91,92,93] Likewise, the FBI's undercover involvement in the arrest of the "Newburgh Four" called into question the appropriate role of law enforcement where the undercover informants facilitate potential terrorist plots.[94,95,96,97] In addition to federal activities, following 9/11, state and local governments became more aggressive in their investigations, as demonstrated by the New York City Police Department (NYPD)'s "demographics unit."[98,99,100,101,102,103,104,105]

These techniques have caused rising tensions between American Muslims and law enforcement agencies. In response to these tensions, the FBI, under the Obama administration, enacted a series of community-based initiatives as part of the DHS's Countering Violent Extremism (CVE) program.

The FBI's use of undercover agents and operatives is primarily governed by the US Attorney General Guidelines. The Guidelines "were intended . . . to diminish the perceived need for legislation to regulate and restrict the FBI's use of informants."[106] But the Guidelines may be changed at the discretion of any Attorney General. Since the 9/11 attacks, two such significant changes occurred. First, in 2002, former Attorney General John Ashcroft released Guidelines that provided the FBI with greater flexibility in the use of undercover operations.[107] Second, in 2008, former Attorney General Michael Mukasey's Guidelines granted the FBI greater freedom to engage in undercover operations in a new "assessment" stage of investigation.[108] Under the Trump administration, the FBI's surveillance and infiltration of mosques likely continued, if not increased, in scope.

For individuals arrested and charged as a result of the FBI's surveillance and infiltration activities, few defenses are available to challenge the government's conduct. The most commonly asserted is "entrapment." To be successful in this defense, a defendant must establish that the government induced the criminal act and that the defendant lacked a criminal predisposition. Juries have been reticent to find entrapment as a valid defense in federal terrorism prosecutions.[109] Defendants in terrorism cases also often assert that the government's conduct is so "outrageous" that the charges must be dismissed. To be successful, the defendant must establish that the government's conduct is "shocking to the universal sense of justice." This argument likewise rarely, if ever, succeeds.

Law enforcement agencies have often targeted local religious and political organizations to identify potential terrorists.[110,111] According to multiple studies, informants played a significant role in nearly half of the more than 500 domestic terrorism-based convictions between 2002 and 2011.[110] Additionally, almost one-third of those cases involved a sting operation, where the informant played an active role in the underlying criminal plot.[110] Not everyone views the use of informants favorably. These activities appear to have disproportionately targeted Muslim organizations, including mosques.[112]

Understandably, this is a major source of distrust between American Muslims and law enforcement.[113,114,115] Various civil rights and faith-based organizations have actively condemned the presence of informants in mosques as a violation of civil liberties.[116,117]

Responses to Post-9/11 Surveillance and Infiltration Programs

Reports of the use of undercover informants have severed long-standing collaborative ties between American Muslims and law enforcement.[89] For example, many leading national Muslim organizations suspended contacts with the FBI.[89] According to the Muslim Public Affairs Council, the FBI's targeting of the Islamic Center undermines years of relationship-building with American Muslims and "sends a devastating message to community leaders and imams who have worked diligently to foster greater understanding between law enforcement and their communities."[114] Echoing this sentiment, Ingrid Mattson, former president of the Islamic Society of North America, argues that the presence of undercover informants in mosques creates "a sense that law enforcement is viewing [Muslim] communities not as partners but as objects of suspicion."[115]

Others accuse the FBI and local law enforcement's surveillance and infiltration activities of perpetuating the perceived association between Islam and terrorism. These critics argue that the widespread use of undercover informants in Muslim communities and institutions sends a message that terrorism is an Islamic phenomenon.[114,117] In a report to the US Committee on the Elimination of Racial Discrimination, multiple US civil rights and community groups assert that "[b]y subjecting Muslims to law enforcement scrutiny that isn't visited upon any other community, the [FBI's] surveillance program stigmatizes all people of that faith."[102] This focus on American Muslims as the targets of surveillance and infiltration reinforces the notion that terrorism "has now become essentially synonymous with being [M]uslim and little else," according to the ACLU's Matthew Harwood.[117]

American Muslims have reported feeling pressure to avoid being perceived as overly religious and, in some cases, have stopped attending mosque services entirely to prevent attracting the attention of an undercover informant.[118] The potential entry of an undercover informant to surveil and report to law enforcement has produced an atmosphere of fear and mistrust within mosques and the larger Muslim community.[119] Congregants and community members often view newcomers with caution—unsure if they will be arbitrarily targeted for surveillance purposes.[110] American Muslims have reported that the potential presence of an undercover informant discourages them from engaging in political speech out of concern that what they say will be taken out of context as part of a criminal proceeding.[120] Some religious leaders have gone so far as to welcome potential NYPD and FBI informants at the beginning of every sermon—both to let potential informants know that the leaders are aware of their presence and to remind congregants that they are being watched.

The FBI has endeavored to learn from the widespread condemnation of its surveillance and infiltration activities. The FBI clearly must use informants, but also must collaborate with American Muslim communities.[120,121,122] The FBI and Department of Justice officials, including former Attorney General Eric Holder, have met frequently with the Muslim community.

In 2011, the Obama administration launched the DHS CVE program,[113] which is a community-based approach to surveillance and infiltration. It has become a cornerstone of DHS's domestic terrorism prevention efforts.[123,124] The stated goal of CVE is to "empower local partners to prevent violent extremists and their supporters from inspiring, radicalizing, financing, or recruiting individuals or groups in the United States to commit acts of violence."[124] Although neutral in name, CVE appears to have focused almost exclusively on American Muslim communities.[125]

While CVE receives praise for its successful implementation in some communities, others question the program's approach.[126] According to these critics, CVE merely substitutes the FBI's use of outside undercover informants with community members—further deepening a culture of distrust. These critics caution that "[b]y deputizing Muslims to spy on Muslims, CVE strategy policing brings with it the perils of dividing communities, intensifying the sectarian tension, and carrying forward baseless investigations and prosecutions."[113] Additionally, these critics further note that CVE's targeting of solely Muslim communities has done nothing to counter the perception that terrorism is primarily a Muslim problem.[113]

While in the immediate aftermath of 9/11 federal and state law enforcement priorities may have focused on Muslim communities, evidence is mounting that violence from racially motivated groups,[127] many fueled by white supremacist ideology, has escalated in recent years.[128] In February 2020, the FBI identified racially/ethnically motivated violent extremists as a major source of domestic terrorism.[129] The threat from racially motivated extremists tends to be decentralized and is often perpetrated by lone actors. Some experts argue that even though many attacks motivated by white supremacist ideology are perpetrated by isolated individuals, the crimes are better understood as a group phenomenon, rooted in a shared "mission, kinship, and acceptance" and facilitated by the internet and social media platforms.[130] Regardless, white supremacists and other far-right extremists have been responsible for almost three times as many attacks on US soil as Islamic terrorists.[131] Such violent extremists are often radicalized online and pursue minorities and easy targets, creating unique challenges for law enforcement to identify the individuals and disrupt the violence.

The Trump Administration

While the Trump administration did not take an official position on the surveillance and infiltration of religious or political organizations, it hinted that it was willing to engage in such activities—particularly targeting American Muslims. For example, in November 2015[132] and again in June 2016,[133] then-presidential candidate Trump called for an increase in the surveillance of mosques. Furthermore, in December 2016, *Politico* reported that a prominent member of the then-president-elect's transition team told DHS officials that CVE "is likely to be renamed Countering Radical Islam or Countering Violent Jihad."[134] Finally, during his Senate confirmation hearings, FBI Director Christopher A. Wray repeatedly declined to answer questions regarding the surveillance of mosques.[135]

SOCIAL MEDIA AND ELECTRONIC COMMUNICATIONS: LAW ENFORCEMENT AND CIVIL LIBERTIES DIMENSIONS

The pervasive use of social media raises new tensions between the responsibility of the government to protect its citizens and the right of those citizens to privacy. Among the most thoughtful voices on this subject is Judge Richard Posner, recently retired from the US Court of Appeals for the Seventh Circuit. Judge Posner sums up this issue thusly, "protected communications are valuable to the persons communicating, whether they are good people or bad people, and this duality is the source of both the costs and the benefits of intercepting communications for intelligence purposes."[136]

The recent roles that Facebook and other online social media platforms have played in the spread of misinformation and extremist ideology have focused the spotlight on the dangers to democratic systems and public health if malign influences are left unchecked.[137] However, government regulations of electronic communications for the purposes of combating misinformation, similar to government intervention to combat terrorism, can carry significant consequences for free speech and civil liberties.

Curbing Terrorism Versus Ensuring Privacy on Social Media

The complete eradication of terrorism is impossible. Even to embark on such a mission would require drastic changes to American law and society; the "cure would be much worse than the disease [because] [s]uch heavy-handed tactics would undoubtedly violate the Constitution."[138] Courts have grappled with these issues, principally in criminal cases, and we summarize these cases in the following paragraphs.

Some clarity is emerging in criminal law, but the explosion of social media—and its use by terrorist organizations and individuals—presents even more difficult issues with which courts, legislatures, and government agencies must struggle. For example:

- How can intelligence and law enforcement agencies identify potential lone-actor terrorists using social media before they act?
- What criteria should be used, and what level of approval is required, to monitor the social media activity of individuals?
- As social media is global, how can government agencies coordinate and share information about potential terrorist organizations and individuals given the widely divergent legal and political regimes in the world?
- Can democratic countries believe information on potential terrorists provided by authoritarian governments who may be seeking to punish their political opponents?

The United States and its European allies are struggling with the issues of privacy in social media and the outsize role played by the global corporations who provide social media platforms. Will steps to regulate these industries take into account the need for law enforcement and intelligence agencies to be able to monitor potential threats? Will increased efforts to monitor or regulate social media lead to the development of more sophisticated encryption available to individuals to shield their social media activity from government surveillance?

These are all very difficult legal and policy questions and beyond the scope of this chapter, but hopefully the precedents being developed by US courts in criminal cases will be of value as democratic states collectively struggle with how to keep us safe as technology marches on.

First Amendment Implications

The First Amendment to the US Constitution protects "freedom of speech" and the right to "peacefully assemble." Over the years, courts have considered countless cases that addressed the interplay between technology and these freedoms. The advent of social media presents fresh challenges to both legislatures and courts.

Described as a "critical cornerstone of American culture and democracy[,]"[139] the freedom to associate promotes open discussions, tolerance, new ideas, and individuality.[140] Most importantly, the First Amendment freedom of association ensures that groups can remain autonomous and free from government intrusion.[141] Individuals need "intellectual privacy," the freedom to think, read, and communicate with others without government oversight.[142] This theory suggests that new and meaningful ideas often

come about outside the public's and government's watchful eye. This type of privacy is threatened by the fact that constant surveillance can have a "chilling effect" on such free thoughts because it "inclines us to the mainstream and boring."[143] For example, forcing a group to reveal the identities of its members may reduce membership because people fear retaliation after their beliefs have been exposed.

The very technological communications that allow people to "associate" also provide ways for these associations to be exposed to the public when they are in the earlier stages of organization, thereby threatening their existence.[144] Targeted "link analysis," in which a suspicious person and their web of relationships are analyzed, inevitably leads to surveilling innocent people and associations "solely on the basis of their communications with the targeted individual or even solely based on communications with those who communicate with the targeted individual."[139]

Pattern-based social network analysis can reveal non-mainstream and disfavored groups or ideas to the government. While this analysis can be a tool to target would-be lone-actor terrorists before they strike, the government may not always be successful in distinguishing between the malevolent groups or individuals and innocent groups or individuals that do not possess violent intentions. This struggle can (and does) chill free speech.[145,146] There is evidence that pattern-based social network analysis has chilled involvement in Muslim communities, causing fewer people to attend political demonstrations, donate to Muslim charities, and speak out against the government.[147] Pattern-based social network analysis could also chill academics and journalism, as both scholars and journalists interact with terrorist groups online and in person to study and report on them.[148]

Intelligence collection tactics may be discriminatorily implemented, burdening minority groups and raising equal protection concerns. In a post-9/11 world, investigative decisions are often based on one's "race, ethnicity, national origin, or religion."[149] The FBI policy promotes collecting and storing data about particular ethnic communities and has exposed a large population of persons to government scrutiny,[150] including, most recently, the government surveillance of the #blacklivesmatter movement to identify potentially threatening individuals.[151] This type of intelligence collection could be tantamount to racial profiling and have a chilling effect on First

Amendment freedom of speech and freedom of association.

In contrast, Judge Posner describes privacy protections in technology as a "terrorist's best friend" that has been enhanced with developments in technology, allowing terrorists to hide behind anonymity while conspiring to commit violent attacks.[132] Because people voluntarily disclose personal information on a daily basis to both private and public entities,[152] Judge Posner argues that the government should be allowed to digitize, pool, and search electronically that information to be better able to identify and track terrorists and their support organizations, with a firewall in place to prohibit criminal prosecutions based on that information.[132] Thus, privacy protections at home exist in tension with the growth of terrorism both at home and abroad.[132]

Fourth Amendment Implications

Technology's threat to privacy rights is best understood in the context of the Fourth Amendment, which protects against unreasonable searches and seizures. As technology has evolved over the past two centuries, courts have developed a distinction between truly personal information stored on or transmitted through technology, and non-personal or "non-content" information.

Courts recognize that the Fourth Amendment's bar on unreasonable search constrains the government's ability to collect the contents in communications or data without a warrant; thus, the government cannot tap a phone without a warrant. On the other hand, courts have held that non-content information (e.g., bulk data—account or subscriber information or transaction history records) about individuals can be collected and shared, so the government does not need a warrant to find out that an individual placed a call.[153,154] Under the "Third-Party Doctrine," Courts have distinguished between the *contents of the phone call* and the *fact that the call took place* because telephone subscribers willingly share call information with third parties (e.g., the telephone company that facilitates each call).[155,156,157]

Modern surveillance technologies used by the government collect vast amounts of information, the majority of which is perfectly innocent.[158] Courts recognize this distinction. For instance, the Southern District of Texas denied a search warrant authorizing the use of data extraction technology where the government could not ensure that an unrelated person would not be surveilled in the government's execution of the warrant.[159] This is especially important because once the personal data is collected, the Fourth Amendment provides few, if any, protections on how the information is stored or used.[147]

Like the non-content information shared with the phone company, anything posted on a public website, including social media profiles with public settings, is not afforded Fourth Amendment protection. Today, law enforcement can also gain access to privately held content through cooperating "friends" and fake undercover accounts.[160] However, the courts have yet to rule on whether the government needs a warrant before monitoring, as opposed to merely viewing, the content of an individual's social media activity.

US courts have recognized privacy as a fundamental right enjoyed by individuals who are US citizens or reside in jurisdictions under US control,[161] including undocumented immigrants[162] and detainees at Guantánamo Bay.[163] But American society is still grappling with the tension between the right to privacy and the role of transparency in social media. For instance, the revelations in the investigations of Russian "sweeping and systematic" meddling in the 2016 presidential election demonstrate the impact of social media on American political life—reaching "millions of US persons" on social media.[164] This has generated much debate in Congress and the public about whether, and if so how, to regulate social media to assure it cannot be used for purposes that undermine our electoral system.[165,166] Following these revelations, there is wide consensus that more disclosure about the identity of the persons or organizations who post is necessary.[167] There is growing support among some in Congress that regulation may be necessary, although the form and reach of such regulation has much less agreement.[168]

In the context of American democracy, government infringement of its citizens' privacy rights has even more profound implications.[169] For example, the Chairman of the Homeland Security Committee Bennie G. Thompson (D-MS) has argued that by surveilling Americans after 9/11, the National Security Administration (NSA) had started to blur the line between domestic and foreign intelligence operations. In doing so, the government put at risk privacy protections preserved by the US Constitution and legal framework, causing Americans to distrust their government.[160] Stated more ominously, in "fail[ing] to respect the rights of our citizens, however, we risk winning the war on terror without their cooperation, confidence, or commitment—a hollow victory indeed."[160]

Courts' Rulings on Social Media Privacy

Current case law provides little protection against the government monitoring an individual's public social media postings.[170] Beginning with the Third-Party Doctrine, courts have extended this principle to network accounts, subscriber information,[171] and non-content information provided to internet service providers (ISPs).[172] In *Forrester*, the court held that a pen register, which is a device that monitors a defendant's internet usage, did not require a search warrant because the defendant had no reasonable expectation of privacy in source or destination addresses of email or IP addresses of websites visited.[167] In *Guest*, the court held that users of an electronic bulletin board system seized in an obscenity investigation had no reasonable expectation of privacy in their subscriber information.[166] Citing *United States v. Miller*,[173] the court compared communicating subscriber information to a systems operator with a bank customer conveying their information to a bank.[166] In handing over the information to a third party and putting it under its control, one assumed the risk that the bank (or systems operator) could convey it to the government. A similar reasoning has also been applied to emails forwarded to "lists" created by chat room members because once the recipient receives it, the sender has no control over the fate of the message; any privacy expectation had been diminished.[174,175]

There have been a few cases upholding a person's reasonable expectation of privacy in content stored on a third-party server when they take active steps to keep the content private. In *State v. Reid*, a New Jersey court held the defendant had a reasonable expectation of privacy in her ISP account information under the New Jersey state constitution because she had used an anonymous IP address, which the court likened to a coded screen name, manifesting her intent to keep her identity anonymous.[176] Two military courts have also found a reasonable expectation of privacy in stored email messages.[177,178] Courts have also held that social media users may have a higher expectation of privacy when messages are sent through a private messenger system, such as direct user-to-user Facebook messages.[179]

Courts have held that one who makes their social media content available to the public has no reasonable expectation of privacy; when the government views this public information, no "search" has occurred for Fourth Amendment purposes.[180,181,182] In *Harris*, the court granted a subpoena ordering Twitter to provide the prosecutor with the user information, including email addresses and posted tweets, of the defendant's Twitter account.[175] The court held that the non-content subscriber information and public postings were not protected by the Fourth Amendment because "[i]f you post a tweet, just like if you scream it out the window, there is no reasonable expectation of privacy. There is no proprietary interest in your tweets, which you have now gifted to the world."[175] Courts have therefore declared that information disclosed on the public internet—as opposed to through a private internet message—is not protected by the Fourth Amendment and no search warrant is required.[183,184,185]

A search warrant is also not needed when a social media friend shares the received information with the government.[186] In *Meregildo*, the government applied for a search warrant for the content of the defendant's Facebook account, which the government had been able to view with the cooperation of a Facebook "friend" of the defendant.[181] The Facebook profile content provided the evidence of probable cause supporting the warrant application.[181] The court rejected the defendant's claim that the government had violated the Fourth Amendment when it accessed his profile because when he posted to his profile for all of his Facebook "friends" to see, his legitimate expectation of privacy ended. Despite the fact that the defendant likely believed that his profile would not be shared with police, his Facebook "friends" were free to share that information with whomever they wanted, including law enforcement. Several other courts have come to the same conclusion regarding disclosure of third-party social media connections' data.[187,188] Therefore, "courts have consistently held that agents do not need a search warrant before looking through social network data provided by a cooperating private party with access to a protected network."[178]

The government can also access social media data by creating fake accounts and "friending" individuals whose profiles they want to access. Under traditional Supreme Court precedent, one assumes the risk that any friend with whom they speak may tell a third party about the conversation. If that friend later goes to the police, or happens to be an undercover agent, the speaker does not have a Fourth Amendment claim.[189] Under the same structure, evidence obtained through an undercover Instagram account created by police officers is admissible.[190] If an individual accepts a friend request on a social media account from an undercover agent, "that acceptance provides the same access as if the individual knowingly exposed their private social media publications to the government agent."[178] In accepting the request, the holder of the content assumes the risk that their private information will be shared with a third party. This same reasoning has also been applied when a defendant befriends an undercover agent and shares materials with the agent over a "closed" peer-to-peer file sharing program.[191]

Courts have yet to address whether monitoring the content of social media communication implicates a reasonable expectation of privacy.[192] Case law regarding content has largely addressed emails. For example, the Sixth Circuit has held that a person has a reasonable expectation of privacy in the contents of emails stored with or transmitted through an ISP.[193] The *Warshak* court came to its conclusion by distinguishing *Miller* on the grounds that the seminal third-party case dealt with bank records transmitted to a bank in the ordinary course of bank business, whereas the defendant in the case at hand had received confidential emails through an intermediary ISP that was not the intended recipient.

Given that courts have yet to decide, scholars have taken different approaches to determining how Fourth Amendment doctrine applies to the government monitoring the content of one's social media activity. Some consider the constant monitoring of social media accounts "deeply invasive" and have questioned whether more protection is necessary than courts have previously held.[178] Few have also proposed that the Third-Party Doctrine needs to be reevaluated and should not apply to the content of social media or electronic data because "a reasonable expectation of privacy should not require secrecy as a requisite condition."[194] Others have proposed applying the "mosaic theory,"[195,196]— which is the idea that significant amounts of data collected about a person over a long length of time is qualitatively better than a single occasion of observation—to social media posts in order to preserve privacy interests and protect a person's ability to develop online relationships without altering Fourth Amendment doctrine.

Courts' Rulings on Cell Phone Location Privacy: *Carpenter* and Its Implications

The Supreme Court's 2018 *Carpenter v. United States* decision will likely impact this analysis.[197]

In *Carpenter*, after a man was arrested in connection with armed robberies of a number of electronics stores, he provided the police with the telephone numbers of his co-conspirators.[194] The government applied for and was granted an order to produce the cell site location information (CSLI identifies the location of a cell tower that has been used by a particulate cell phone, thus disclosing the user was within close proximity to that tower) for 159 days of the defendant's cell phone number. The issue before the Court was whether a warrant is required to access CSLI. The Court held that an "individual maintains a legitimate expectation of privacy in the record of his physical movements as captured through CSLI."[194] Obtaining this information now constitutes a "search" under the Fourth Amendment and requires a warrant. Chief Justice Roberts, writing for the majority, declined to extend the Third-Party Doctrine to CSLI and reasoned that one had a reasonable expectation of privacy in such data because it "provides an intimate window into a person's life, revealing not only his particular movements, but through them his 'familial, political, professional, religious, and sexual associations.' "[194]

A few academics have already commented on what they believe to be *Carpenter*'s impact on governmental surveillance. David Kris, a national security specialist, believes the Supreme Court has now applied the Fourth Amendment to the Twenty-First Century because CSLI is a new and unique type of digital technology that is necessary for modern-day life.[198] In his article, Kris notes, however, that *Carpenter* leaves many questions unanswered; nevertheless, Kris reflects that its holding implies that if the government uses Twenty-First-Century technology, such surveillance will likely be a search. Under this theory, bulk collection of non-location data under the FISA could require a warrant.

Similarly, digital privacy lawyers have argued that since the government now needs a search warrant to obtain cell tower location information, under the same reasoning, authorities should have to seek a warrant for other kinds of digital data that provide extensive personal information, such as internet searches.[199]

Orin Kerr, a renowned criminal procedure and computer crime law professor, has reflected on how *Carpenter* leaves unanswered the question of when a search officially begins and ends for purposes of the Fourth Amendment "search."[200] The Fourth Amendment provides no protection where a "search" has not begun, and data collection has many different stages. Thus, defining the stage at which a Fourth Amendment search begins in data collection is critical to determine the constitutionality of surveillance.

Even when the Fourth Amendment allows courts to give authorization for law enforcement to search certain devices, strong, end-to-end, "warrant-proof" encryption may prevent the government from carrying out the warrant and accessing the digital information.[201] The "going dark" debate has sparked tension between law enforcement agencies seeking to access evidence necessary to detect, investigate, and prosecute criminal activity and the technology companies competing to have more secure products in order to meet consumer demands.

The friction between law enforcement and technology companies reached a fever pitch in the wake of the San Bernardino attack.[202] When the FBI couldn't unlock the iPhone of one of the suspected shooters, the government sought a court order demanding Apple create a "backdoor" to its operating software which would bypass Apple's own security measures and give the government the information it wanted from the iPhone. Eventually, the government was able to unlock the San Bernardino iPhone with help from a third party.[203] But the same issue resurfaced and the FBI obtained a search warrant and again sought Apple's help to access the iPhone belonging to the lone actor who opened fire at the Naval Air Station in Pensacola in December 2020.[204] Again, the FBI managed to unlock the iPhone without support from Apple.[205]

The "going dark" debate remains unresolved, and, even if the government overcomes the Fourth Amendment legal hurdles to obtain a search warrant, there is no guarantee law enforcement can actually access the encrypted information it needs to fully investigate and prosecute lone actor attacks.

CONCLUSION

Individuals acting alone who commit violence for political or religious purposes have been part of the human experience for as long as we know. Over time, nations have adopted laws that punish such conduct. In the United States, which is the focus of this chapter, those laws are adequate to deal with lone actor acts of terror as ordinary criminal acts. In the past few decades the federal government and states have added criminal provisions that seek to address the increasingly global aspect of terrorism.

As we have seen, those laws enable both federal and state authorities to successfully prosecute solitary individuals who commit acts of terror.

They are also a predicate that permits law enforcement authorities to investigate individuals who reasonably pose a threat of committing acts of terror, regardless of the motivation. For example, electronic communications and use of computers can be monitored by law enforcement and intelligence agencies if the requisite statutory threshold is met and a court order is obtained.

However, the world is now connected electronically in ways that enable individuals to communicate with and/or be inspired by acts of terror committed by other individuals anywhere in the world. For example, the murderous rampage by an individual in Pittsburgh at the Tree of Life Synagogue directly inspired recent murders by lone-actor terrorists of Muslims attending services in New Zealand and Jews attending services in San Diego. As noted by the *New York Times* these "[l]one actors who come out of the blue present a daunting challenge for law enforcement."[206]

Democracies are struggling with the impact of the interconnected world on many aspects of our lives, ranging from protecting privacy to preventing covert foreign interference in elections. Those are difficult problems to solve. But among the most urgent challenges is to find ways to identify potential lone-actor terrorists and stop them before they can act.

ACKNOWLEDGMENTS
The authors are grateful for the invaluable research assistance of our colleagues at Arnold & Porter, including Junghyun Baek, Alexandra Barbee-Garrett, Elizabeth Carney, Trevor Schmitt, and Stesha Turney.

NOTES AND REFERENCES
1. Peterson RE, Manning JE, Congressional Research Services. Violence against members of congress and their staff: selected examples and congressional responses. 2017:11. https://fas.org/sgp/crs/misc/R41609.pdf
2. Among the best known are the four Puerto Rican "nationalists" who, in 1954, fired shots from the public gallery onto the floor of the House of Representatives, wounding five members of Congress in a bid for Puerto Rican independence. See Peterson et al. Violence against members of Congress. Also well-known is the Sacco-Vanzetti case in the 1920s, where Italian-born US citizens regarded as "anarchists" were convicted of murdering two men in an armed robbery in Boston.
3. Office of the Historian, US Department of State. Significant terrorist incidents, 1961–2003. Mar 2004. https://2001-2009.state.gov/r/pa/ho/pubs/fs/5902.htm

4. See, e.g., 18 USC § 2332f.
5. See, e.g., Ibid. (bombing places of public use is a US federal crime where US nationals are among the victims).
6. National Commission on Terrorist Attacks Upon the United States. The 9/11 commission report: Final report of the National Commission on Terrorist Attacks Upon the United States (9/11 report). 22 Jul 2004. https://www.govinfo.gov/app/details/GPO-911REPORT/
7. Structural changes to enhance counter-terrorism efforts. Department of Justice Archives website. https://www.justice.gov/archive/911/counterterrorism.html
8. Uniting And Strengthening America by Providing Appropriate Tools Required to Intercept and Obstruct Terrorism Act (USA PATRIOT Act) of 2001, Pub. L. 107-56 (Oct. 26, 2001), 115 Stat. 272 (2001), codified at scattered sections of Titles 18, 31, 42, 47, 49, and 50 of the US Code.
9. Federal Bureau of Investigation. 2018 Hate Crime Statistics. https://ucr.fbi.gov/hate-crime/2018/topic-pages/incidents-and-offenses
10. Southern Poverty Law Center. Age of the Wolf. Montgomery, AL: Southern Poverty Law Center; 2015.
11. Hamm M, Spaaij R. Lone Wolf Terrorism in America: Using Knowledge of Radicalization Pathways to Forge Prevention Strategies. Washington, DC: National Institute of Justice; 2015.
12. Hamm MS, Spaaij R. The Age of Lone Wolf Terrorism. Columbia University Press; 2017.
13. 18 USC. § 2331(5).
14. Federal hate crime statutes include the Matthew Shepard and James Byrd Jr. Hate Crimes Prevention Act of 2009, 18 USC. § 249; Criminal Interference with Right to Fair Housing, 42 USC. § 3631; Damage to Religious Property, Church Arson Prevention Act, 18 USC. § 247; Violent Interference with Federally Protected Rights, 18 USC. § 245; Conspiracy Against Rights, 18 USC. § 241.
15. We have not evaluated the cases currently underway in the US military commissions in Guantánamo.
16. The US Legal Survey of Lone Actor Incidents and State Laws chart is hosted by Syracuse University at https://cbzoli.expressions.syr.edu/wp-content/uploads/2020/12/Survey-of-Lone-Wolf-Incidents-and-State-Laws-120120.xlsx
17. Ibid.
18. Dep't of Justice. US Attorney's Manual 9-2.136 (1997) (hereinafter, USA.M.). https://www.justice.gov/jm/jm-9-2000-authority-us-attorney-criminal-division-mattersprior-approvals#9-2.136
19. Specifically, the US Attorney's Manual lists the following as international terrorism statutes: 18 USC. § 2332 (Terrorist Acts Abroad Against United States Nationals); 18 USC. § 2332b (Terrorism Transcending National Boundaries); 49 USC. §

46502 (Aircraft Piracy); 18 USC. § 32 (Aircraft Sabotage); 18 USC. § 956 (Conspiracy Within the United States to Murder, Kidnap, or Maim Persons or to Damage Certain Property Overseas); 18 USC. § 2339A (Providing Material Support to Terrorists); 18 USC. § 2339B (Providing Material Support to Designated Terrorist Organizations); 18 USC. § 2339C (Prohibition Against Financing of Terrorism); 50 USC. § 1705(b) (Violations of IEEPA involving E.O. 12947 (Terrorists Who Threaten to Disrupt the Middle East Peace Process), E.O. 13224 (Blocking Property and Prohibiting Transactions with Persons who Commit, or Support Terrorism or Global Terrorism List), and E.O. 13129 (Blocking Property and Prohibiting Transactions with the Taliban)); 18 USC. § 2339 (Harboring Terrorists); 18 USC. § 1993 (Terrorist Attacks Against Mass Transportation Systems); 18 USC. §§ 175, 175b, 229, 831, 2332a (Use of Biological, Nuclear, Chemical or Other Weapons of Mass Destruction); 42 USC. § 2284 (Sabotage of Nuclear Facilities or Fuel); 18 USC. §§ 112, 878, 1116, 1201(a)(4) (Crimes Against Internationally Protected Persons); 18 USC. § 2332f (Bombings of Places of Public Use, Government Facilities, Public Transportation Systems and Infrastructure Facilities); 18 USC. § 175c (Production, Transfer, or Possession of Variola Virus (Small Pox)); 18 USC. § 832 (Participation in Nuclear and WMD Threats to the United States); 18 USC. § 2332g (Missile Systems Designed to Destroy Aircraft); 18 USC. § 2332h (Production, Transfer, or Possession of Radiological Dispersal Devices); 18 USC. § 2339D (Receiving Military-Type Training from an FTO); 21 USC. § 960A (Narco-Terrorism); 18 USC. § 43 (Animal Enterprise Terrorism). Ibid.
20. USA.M. at 9-2.138
21. USA.M. at 9-2.137.
22. Ibid.
23. 18 USC. § 175(a).
24. 18 USC. § 175(b).
25. See 18 USC. §§ 2339A, 2339B.
26. 18 USC. § 112.
27. 18 USC. § 111.
28. 18 USC. § 351.
29. 18 USC. § 1114.
30. 18 USC. § 1751.
31. 18 USC. § 111 (Assaulting, Resisting, or Impeding Certain Officers or Employees); 18 USC. § 351 (Congressional, Cabinet, and Supreme Court Assassination, Kidnapping, and Assault); 18 USC. § 871 (Threats Against President and Successors to the Presidency); 18 USC. § 1114 (Protection of Officers and Employees of the United States); 18 USC. § 1751 (Presidential and Presidential Staff Assassination, Kidnapping, and Assault).
32. 18 USC. § 1114.
33. 18 USC. § 245.
34. 18 USC. § 247.

35. 18 USC. § 248.
36. 18 USC. §§ 922, 930.
37. 26 USC. §§ 5841, 5861.
38. 18 USC. § 842(a)(3).
39. 18 USC. § 37.
40. 18 USC. § 1111.
41. 18 USC. § 1113.
42. 18 USC. § 876.
43. 18 USC. § 880.
44. 18 USC. § 914.
45. 18 USC. § 1038.
46. 18 USC. § 2313.
47. 18 USC. § 249.
48. Most of these state laws are identified in the attached spreadsheet. See, e.g., Ariz. Rev. Stat. § 13-2308.01 *et seq*; Conn. Gen. Stat. § 53a-300 *et seq*.
49. See, e.g., Mo. Rev. Stat. § 576.080.
50. See, e.g., S.C. Code § 16-23-710 *et seq*.
51. The lone-actor terrorists identified in this chapter and attached spreadsheet were pulled from the following sources: Southern Poverty Law Center. *Age of the Wolf*; Hamm, Spaaj. *Lone Wolf Terrorism* Hamm, Spaaij. *The Age of Lone Wolf Terrorism*.
52. Meili H. Montana forest still holds mystery of vanished militia organizer. *NBC Montana*, 5 Nov 2018. https://nbcmontana.com/news/local/montana-forest-still-holds-mystery-of-vanished-militia-organizer-and-notorious-gunman
53. Mesiner J. Suburban man facing trial over terrorism bomb plot wants to enter unusual guilty plea. *Chicago Tribune*, 14 Nov 2018. https://www.chicagotribune.com/news/local/breaking/ct-met-chicago-terrorism-plot-guilty-lea-20181114-story.html
54. Robbins LJW. von Brunn, accused museum gunman, dies at 89. *New York Times*, 6 Jan 2010. https://www.nytimes.com/2010/01/07/us/07vonbrunn.html
55. Adel Daoud: *US v. Daoud*, 1:12-cr-00723 (N.D. Ill.).
56. Thirty-two such individuals were charged under general criminal statutes only and no terrorism statute.
57. These three cases were brought under 18 USC. § 2232a (use of WMD) against the following individuals: Mohamed Osman Mohamud for attempting to set off a bomb at a Christmas tree lighting ceremony, although the bomb was a decoy that Mohamud received from undercover FBI agents after years of correspondence and meetings concerning his terror plots; Khalid Aldawsari for plotting to bomb residences of military service members and former President George W. Bush; and Amine el Khalifi for a plot to carry out a suicide bomb attack on the US Capitol. The fourth individual charged solely under a terrorism statute was Steven Kim, who was charged under 18 USC. § 112 (protection of foreign officials, official guests, and internationally protected persons)

58. for firing shots at the United Nations building in New York.
58. The relevant statute, 18 USC. § 2332a, defines WMD very broadly to include "any destructive device," such as bombs and grenades.
59. Of 28 bomb-related prosecutions total, only two were prosecuted under state law.
60. Of the 33 defendants convicted under state law, 14 were sentenced to life (or longer) in prison. Four defendants were sentenced to death. In contrast, federal sentences comprise mostly of term sentences. Of the 44 defendants convicted in federal court, only 4 were sentenced to prison sentences of life or longer and one was sentenced to death.
61. Minnesotan in 2002's 'smiley face bomber' case could finally face trial. *Twin Cities Pioneer Press*. 15 May 2013. https://www.twincities.com/2013/05/15/minnesotan-in-2002s-smiley-face-bomber-case-could-finally-face-trial/
62. James von Brunn: *US v. von Brunn*, 1:09-cr-00184-RBW (D.D.C.).
63. Matthew Ryan Buquet: *US v. Buquet*, 2:13-cr-00085-MAH (E.D. Wa.).
64. Gregory Weiler: *US v. Weiler*, 4:13-cr-00018-CVE (N.D. Okla.).
65. Suburban man in Okla. bombing plot ruled insane. *Chicago Tribune*, 19 Jan 2014. https://www.chicagotribune.com/suburbs/ct-xpm-2014-01-19-ct-gregory-weiler-met-0119-20140119-story.html
66. Leslie Allen Merritt Jr.: *People v. Merritt*, S-0700-CR-2015144211 (Ariz. Maricopa Cty. Sup. Ct.).
67. Tulumello K, Anglen R. State moves to drop charges against Phoenix freeway shooting suspect. *AZ Central*, 23 Apr 2016. https://www.azcentral.com/story/news/local/phoenix-breaking/2016/04/22/accused-phoenix-freeway-shooter-charges-dismissed/83415724/
68. Associated Press. Judge: Planned Parenthood shooter still mentally incompetent. *Denver Channel*, 26 Jan 2019. https://www.thedenverchannel.com/news/crime/judge-planned-parenthood-shooter-still-mentally-incompetent
69. Intelligence Reform and Terrorism Prevention Act of 2004, Pub. L. No. 108-458, § 6001(a), 118 Stat. 3638, 3742 (2004).
70. H.R. Rep. 108-72, pt. 5, at 170–71 (2004) ("Today, the 'lone wolfs' often are not formal members of any group. . . . This new definition reaches unaffiliated individuals who engage in international terrorism, i.e. 'lone wolf' terrorists.").
71. 50 USC. § 1801(b)(1)(C).
72. Cordero C. Orlando, The lone wolf & FISA. *Lawfare*, 3 Jun 2015. https://www.lawfareblog.com/orlando-lone-wolf-fisa
73. USA Freedom ACT of 2015, Pub. L. 114-23, § 705, 129 Stat. 268, 300 (2015).
74. USA PATRIOT Improvement and Reauthorization Act of 2005, Pub. L. 109-177, § 103, 120 Stat. 192, 195 (2006).

75. Harris S. The Patriot Act may be dead forever. *Daily Beast*, 28 May 2015. https://www.thedaily-beast.com/the-patriot-act-may-be-dead-forever

76. Chesney R. Why is the lone wolf FISA provision never used? And just how broad is the FISC understanding of group agency? *Lawfare*, 3 Jun 2015. https://www.lawfareblog.com/why-lone-wolf-fisa-provision-never-used-and-just-how-broad-fisc-understanding-group-agency

77. H.R. 5911, 114th Cong. (2016).

78. H.R. 1955, 110th Cong. (2007).

79. S. 1858, 110th Cong. (2007).

80. H.R. 2945, 11th Cong. (2017).

81. H.R. 2940, 115th Cong. (2017).

82. Peterson et al. Violence against members of congress.

83. These include recruitment of informants and infiltration of domestic religious and ethnic groups.

84. USA FREEDOM Act, Pub. Law 114-23, 129 STAT. 268.

85. Risen J, Lichtblau E. Spying program snared US calls. *New York Times*, 21 Dec 2005.

86. FISA Amendments Act of 2008, Pub. L. 110-261, § 702 (2008).

87. Risen J. Administration pulls back on surveillance agreement. *New York Times*, 2 May 2007:A18. https://www.nytimes.com/2007/05/02/washington/02intel.html

88. Markon J. Mosque infiltration feeds Muslims' distrust of FBI. *Washington Post*, 5 Dec 2010. http://www.washingtonpost.com/wp-dyn/content/article/2010/12/04/AR2010120403720.html

89. Adams G. FBI plant banned by mosque because he was too extreme. *Independent*, 7 Dec 2010. https://www.independent.co.uk/news/world/americas/fbi-plant-banned-by-mosque-ndash-because-he-was-too-extreme-2153057.html

90. See Notice of Motion to Set Aside Restraining Order Points and Authorities in Support and Declaration of Craig F. Monteilh, Islamic Ctr. of *Irvine v. Monteilh*, No. 07HL02626 (Cal. Super. Ct. filed Feb. 25, 2009).

91. *United States v. Niazi*, No. 0:09-cr-00028-CJC (C.D. Cal. Filed Feb. 11, 2009).

92. Government's Unopposed Ex Parte Application for Leave of the Court to Dismiss Indictment Without Prejudice Pursuant to Fed. R. Crim. P. 48(a), *United States v. Niazi*, No. SA CR 09-28-CJC (C.D. Cal. filed Sept. 9, 2010), https://www.courtlistener.com/recap/gov.uscourts.cacd.437115.39.0.pdf

93. FBI informant Craig Monteilh spent more than 15 months attending daily prayers at a mosque as part of an FBI operation to record conversations with Abmadullah Niazi, a suspected terrorist, to build a case against him. In May 2007, Monteilh reported a conversation with Niazi in which Monteilh suggested an operation to blow up buildings.

Niazi, alarmed by Monteilh's jihadist suggestion, reported this conversation to local community leaders, who, in turn, reported Monteilh to the FBI. In June 2007, community leaders—believing he was a danger to the congregation—obtained a restraining order against Monteilh. Though the FBI cut ties with Monteilh shortly after the restraining order was filed, it continued to pursue its case against Niazi, and in February 2009, a federal grand jury indicted Niazi on charges of lying about his connections with terrorists on immigration documents. Citing a lack of overseas witnesses and "evidentiary issues," the US Attorney's Office in Los Angeles ultimately dropped all charges against Niazi.

94. The Newburgh Four carried out attempted attacks on two synagogues in the Bronx using fake bombs and stinger missiles given to them by an undercover FBI informant named Shaheed Hussain. According to court records, Hussain even instructed the men how "to launch the missiles and how to wire the detonating devices for the bombs." Most controversially, Hussain offered the men extravagant incentives to complete the mission and for recruiting coconspirators. The Newburgh Four were convicted of various terrorism-related crimes and each was sentenced to a minimum of 25 years in prison. Though the trial court criticized that "the Government recruited persons who (as far as the record shows) had never before expressed any interest in jihad, and gave them the opportunity to become terrorists," the jury rejected the Newburgh Four's entrapment defense, the Second Circuit affirmed, and the Supreme Court declined review.

95. *United States v. Cromitie*, 727 F.3d 194, 201-03 (2nd Cir. 2013).

96. *United States v. Cromitie*, No. 09-Cr-558(CM), 2011 WL 1842219, at *23 (S.D.N.Y. May 10, 2011).

97. *Cromitie v. United States*, 135 S.Ct. 53 (2014).

98. Goldman A, Apuzzo M. With cameras, informants, NYPD eyed mosques. Associated Press, 23 Feb 2012. https://www.ap.org/ap-in-the-news/2012/with-cameras-informants-nypd-eyed-mosques

99. Apuzzo M, Goldstein J. New York drops unit that spied on Muslims. *New York Times*, 15 Apr 2004. https://www.nytimes.com/2014/04/16/nyregion/police-unit-that-spied-on-muslims-is-disbanded.html

100. *Hassan v. City of New York*, 804 F.3d 277 (3rd Cir. 2015); *Raza v. City of New York*, 998 F. Supp. 2d 70 (E.D.N.Y. 2013).

101. Ctr. For Constitutional Rights et al., Suspicionless Surveillance of Muslim Communities and the Increased Use and Abuse of Muslim Informants, NGO Shadow Report Before the UN Committee on the Elimination of Racial Discrimination (2014).

102. Apuzzo M, Goldman A. After spying on Muslims, New York police agree to greater oversight. *New York Times*, 6 Mar 2017.

103. Letter to the Department of Justice seeking an investigation into the NYPD's suspicionless surveillance of Muslims. 24 Oct 2013. https://www.aclu.org/sites/default/files/assets/2013-10-24_doj_investigation_letter_combined.pdf

104. Pilkington E. NYPD settles lawsuit after illegally spying on Muslims. *The Guardian*, 5 Apr 2018. https://www.theguardian.com/world/2018/apr/05/nypd-muslim-surveillance-settlement.

105. Following the 9/11 attacks, the NYPD extensively surveilled and infiltrated mosques and other Muslim community centers, often without prior evidence of criminal operations. This surveillance program was part of a larger "demographics unit" and planned to have a source inside every mosque within a 250-mile radius of New York City. After becoming the subject of two federal lawsuits and drawing international criticism for its religion-based surveillance strategies, the NYPD disbanded the controversial "demographics unit."

106. Department of Justice Office of the Inspector General. The Federal Bureau of Investigation's Compliance with the Attorney General's Investigative Guidelines. Sep 2005. https://oig.justice.gov/special/0509/chapter2.htm

107. Ashcroft J, US Dep't of Justice. The Attorney General's Guidelines on General Crimes, Racketeering Enterprise and Terrorism Enterprise Investigations II.A. 2002.

108. Mukasey MB, US Dep't of Justice. The Attorney General's Guidelines For Domestic FBI Operations II.A.4. 2008.

109. Human Rights Watch. Illusion of justice: Human rights abuses in US terrorism prosecutions. 2014. https://www.hrw.org/report/2014/07/21/illusion-justice/human-rights-abuses-us-terrorism-prosecutions

110. Bartosiewicz P. Deploying informants, the FBI stings Muslims. *The Nation*, 14 Jun 2012. https://www.thenation.com/article/deploying-informants-fbi-stings-muslims/

111. Lichtblau E. FBI watched activist groups, new files show. *New York Times*, 20 Dec 2005. https://www.nytimes.com/2005/12/20/politics/fbi-watched-activist-groups-new-files-show.html

112. Beydown KA. Lone wolf terrorism: Types, stripes, and double standards. *Nw U L Rev.* 2018;112(5):1213.

113. FBI losing partnership with American Muslim community. Muslim Public Affairs Council website. 25 Feb 2009. https://www.mpac.org/programs/government-relations/fbi-losing-partnership-with-american-muslim-community.php

114. Vitello P, Semple K. Muslims say F.B.I. tactics sow anger and fear. *New York Times*, 17 Dec 2019. https://www.nytimes.com/2009/12/18/us/18muslims.html

115. Hirsh M. Inside the FBI's secret Muslim network. *Politico*, 24 Mar 2016. https://www.politico.com/magazine/story/2016/03/fbi-muslim-outreach-terrorism-213765

116. Harwood M. The lone-wolf terror trap: Why the cure will be worse than the disease. American Civil Liberties Union website. 5 Feb 2015. https://www.aclu.org/blog/national-security/lone-wolf-terror-trap-why-cure-will-be-worse-disease

117. Berman E. *Domestic Intelligence: New Powers, New Risks.* New York: Brennan Center for Justice; 2011:26.

118. *Mapping Muslims: NYPD Spying and Its Impact on American Muslims.* New York: Muslim American Civil Liberties Coalition/CLEAR; 2013: 12–15.

119. Factsheet: The NYPD Muslim surveillance program. American Civil Liberties Union website. https://www.aclu.org/other/factsheet-nypd-muslim-surveillance-program

120. Morgan C. Feds work to build trust with Muslim community. *McClatchy*, 6 May 2011. http://www.mcclatchydc.com/2011/05/16/114255/feds-work-to-build-trust-with.html

121. Markoe L. To fight ISIS, West Point cadets secretly build Facebook page. *Washington Post*, 3 Feb 2016. https://www.washingtonpost.com/national/religion/to-fight-isis-west-point-cadets-secretly-build-facebook-page/2016/02/03/b1dabfaa-cac5-11e5-b9ab-26591104bb19_story.html

122. The government has also engaged in alternative tactics in an attempt to combat terrorist ideology. For example, as part of an international contest sponsored by the State Department and the DHS, 16 West Point cadets created a fake Facebook page to persuade young Muslims not to join terrorist groups.

123. FBI Nat'l Sec. Branch. A new approach to countering violent extremism: Sharing expertise and empowering local communities. *L Enforcement Bull.* 7 Oct 2014. https://leb.fbi.gov/articles/featured-articles/a-new-approach-to-countering-violent-extremism-sharing-expertise-and-empowering-local-communities

124. Rascoff SJ. Establishing official Islam? The law and strategy of counter-radicalization. *Stan L Rev.* 2012;64:125, 127.

125. Patel F, Koushik M. Brennan Center for Justice. Countering violent extremism. 2017. https://www.brennancenter.org/sites/default/files/publications/Brennan%20Center%20CVE%20Report.pdf

126. Abdollah T, Marcelo P. "It sets people off": Some Muslims see profiling in US anti-terror program. *NBC Los Angeles*, 20 Apr 2015. https://www.nbclosangeles.com/news/local/Obama-Muslims-Countering-Violent-Extremism-SoCal-civil-liberties-300678641.html

127. Wray C, Director FBI. Statement before the House Judiciary Committee: FBI oversight. 5 Feb 2020. https://www.fbi.gov/news/testimony/fbi-oversight-020520

128. Donaghue E. Racially motivated violence elevated to "national threat priority," FBI director says. CBS News, 5 Feb 2020. https://www.cbsnews.com/news/racially motivated-violent-extremism-isis-national-threat-priority-fbi-director-christopher-wray/

129. Wray. Statement before the House Judiciary Committee.

130. Kayyem J. There are no lone wolves. Washington Post, 4 Aug 2019. https://www.washingtonpost.com/opinions/2019/08/04/there-are-no-lone-wolves/

131. Bergengruen V, Hennigan WJ. "We are being eaten from within": Why America is losing the battle against white nationalist terrorism. Time, 8 Aug 2019. https://time.com/5647304/white-nationalist-terrorism-united-states/

132. Gerstein J. Court mulls FBI mosque surveillance. Politico, 8 Dec 2015. https://www.politico.com/blogs/under-the-radar/2015/12/court-mulls-fbi-mosque-surveillance-216529

133. Stephenson E, Becker A. Trump backs surveillance of mosques despite criticism of rhetoric. Reuters, 15 Jun 2016. https://www.reuters.com/article/us-usa-election-idUSKCN0Z12AS

134. Crowley M. Trump's terror-fighting team yet to take shape. Politico, 20 Dec 2016. https://www.politico.com/story/2016/12/donald-trump-terrorism-232870

135. Wray CA. Hearing on the Nomination of Christopher Wray to be Director of the Federal Bureau of Investigation, Questions for the Record 16, 53 (2017), https://www.judiciary.senate.gov/imo/media/doc/Wray%20Responses%20to%20QFRs.pdf.

136. Posner RA. Privacy, surveillance, and law. Univ Chicago L Rev. 2008;75:245–247.

137. Bouie J. Facebook has been a disaster for the world. New York Times, 18 Sep 2020.

138. Barnes BD. Confronting the one-man wolf pack: Adapting law enforcement and prosecution responses to the threat of lone wolf terrorism. B U L Rev. 2012;92:1613–1660. .

139. Votava GJ, III. First Amendment concerns in governmental acquisition and analysis of mobile device location data. Univ Pitt J Tech L Pol'y. 2013;13:1–7.

140. See e.g., National Ass'n for Advancement of Colored People v. State of Ala. Ex rel. Patterson, 357 US 449 (1958).

141. See e.g., Griswold v. Connecticut, 381 US 479 (1965).

142. Richards NM. The dangers of surveillance. Harv L Rev. 2013;126(1934):1945–1946.

143. Waters S. The effects of mass surveillance on journalists' relations with confidential sources: A constant comparative study. Digital Journalism. 2017:1294–1313.

144. Strandburg KJ. Freedom of association in a networked world: First Amendment regulation of relational surveillance. B C L Rev. 2008;49:741–751.

145. Berman E. Regulating domestic intelligence collection. Wash & Lee L Rev. 2014;71:3, 22.

146. Moy KK. Monitoring "inspiration": First Amendment limitations on surveilling individuals who view terrorist propaganda. Stan L & Pol'y Rev. 2018;29:267, 285.

147. Berman, Regulating domestic intelligence collection, at 22.

148. Moy, Monitoring inspiration, at 285.

149. Berman, Regulating domestic intelligence collection, at 22

150. Ibid.

151. Toor A. "Our identity is often what's triggering surveillance": How government surveillance of #blacklivesmatter violates the first amendment freedom of association. Rutgers Computer & Tech L J. 2018;44:286, 311–312.

152. Judge Posner notes that "[t]o get a good job, to get health and life insurance, to get bank credit, to get a credit card, you need to reveal personal information. Every time you make a purchase other than with cash you convey information about your tastes, interests, and income that may well end up in some easily accessible database."

153. Teachout BR. Gotta collect it all!: Surveillance law lessons of Pokemon Go. Stan L Rev. 2016;69:83, 84.

154. "In general, content is that which a user intends to communicate (for instance, the body and subject of an e-mail), and noncontent is information about the means by which it is communicated (for instance, usage logs and header information other than the subject)."

155. Berman. Regulating domestic intelligence collection..

156. Solove DJ. Data mining and the security-liberty debate. Univ Chicago L Rev. 2008;75:343, 350.

157. The Third-Party Doctrine holds that "Any information that we have disclosed to a third-party individual or business entity, for example, lacks Fourth Amendment protection against unreasonable searches and seizures. Thus the Constitution places no limits on the collection of information contained in credit card transactions, bank records, Internet service provider (ISP) records, Amazon.com transaction histories, Facebook activities, electronic toll records, cell-tower location data (in some jurisdictions), and even statements made to undercover agents or government informants-regardless of whether

the agent or informant discloses his intention to share the contents of the conversation."

158. Hosein G, Wilson Palow C. Modern safeguards for modern surveillance: An analysis of innovations in communications surveillance techniques. *Ohio St L J.* 2013;74:1071, 1082–1090.

159. In re Warrant to Search a Target Computer at Premises Unknown, No. H-13-234M, 2013 WL 1729765, at *1 (S.D. Tex. Apr. 22, 2013).

160. Undercover policing in the age of social media. *Policing Project*, 17 Dec 2018. https://www.policingproject.org/news-main/undercover-policing-social-media

161. Rengel A. Privacy-invading technologies and recommendations for designing a better future for privacy rights. *Intercultural Hum Rts L Rev.* 2013;8:177–178.

162. *Zadvydas v. Davis*, 533 US 678 (2001).

163. *Rasul v. Bush*, 542 US 466 (2004).

164. Special Counsel Robert S. Mueller, III. Report on the Investigation into Russian Interference in the 2016 Presidential Election. 2019:1, 14. https://www.justice.gov/storage/report.pdf

165. Dennis ST, Brody B. Congress is likely to support new regulations on social media, senator says. Bloomberg, 13 Sep 2018. https://www.bloomberg.com/news/articles/2018-09-13/new-social-media-rules-can-get-majority-in-congress-warner-says

166. Chalfant M. Top intel dem says new Facebook finding "further evidence" of Russian meddling. *The Hill*, 31 Jul 2018. https://thehill.com/policy/cybersecurity/399711-top-democrat-says-new-facebook-findings-is-further-evidence-of-russian

167. Shane S, Goel V. Fake Russian Facebook accounts bought $100,000 in political ads. *New York Times*, 6 Sep 2017. https://www.nytimes.com/2017/09/06/technology/facebook-russian-political-ads.html

168. Steinmetz K. Lawmakers hint at regulating social media during hearing with Facebook and Twitter execs. *Time*, 3 Sep 2018. http://time.com/5387560/senate-intelligence-hearing-facebook-twitter/

169. Thompson BG. The National Counterterrorism Center: Foreign and domestic intelligence fusion and the potential threat to privacy. *Univ Pitt J Tech L Pol'y.* 2006;6:3.

170. Scott JD. Social media and government surveillance: The case for better privacy protections for our newest public space. *J Bus Tech L.* 2017;12:151, 157.

171. *Guest v. Leis*, 255 F.3d 325, 336 (6th Cir. 2001).

172. *United States v. Forrester*, 495 F.3d 1041, 1048 (9th Cir. 2007).

173. *United States v. Miller*, 425 US 435 (1976).

174. *United States v. Charbonneau*, 979 F. Supp. 1177, 1184 (S.D. Ohio 1997).

175. *United States v. Hambrick*, No. 99-4793, 2000 WL 1062039, at *4 (4th Cir. Aug. 3, 2000).

176. *State v. Reid*, 914 A.2d 310, 317 (N.J. Super. Ct. App. Div. 2007).

177. *United States v. Long*, 64 M.J. 57, 66-67 (C.A.A.F. 2006).

178. *United States v. Maxwell*, 45 M.J. 406, 418 (C.A.A.F. 1996).

179. R.S. ex rel. *S.S. v. Minnewaska Area Sch. Dist.* No. 2149, 894 F. Supp. 2d 1128, 1142 (D. Minn. 2012).

180. *People v. Harris*, 949 N.Y.S.2d 590, 594 (Crim. Ct. 2012).

181. *Romano v. Steelcase Inc.*, 907 N.Y.S.2d 650, 656 (Sup. Ct. 2010).

182. *United States v. Gines-Perez*, 214 F. Supp. 2d 205, 225 (D.P.R. 2002).

183. Mund B. Social media searches and the reasonable expectation of privacy. *Yale J L & Tech.* 2017;19:238, 248.

184. Semitsu JP. From Facebook to mug shot: How the dearth of social networking privacy rights revolutionized online government surveillance. *Pace L Rev.* 2011;31:291, 338 n.184.

185. *United States v. Gines-Perez*, 214 F. Supp. 2d 205, 225 (D.P.R. 2002)

186. *United States v. Meregildo*, 883 F. Supp. 2d 523, 526 (S.D.N.Y. 2012).

187. *Cheney v. Fayette Cty. Pub. Sch. Dist.*, 977 F. Supp. 2d 1308, 1315 (N.D. Ga. 2013)

188. *United States v. Ladeau*, No. CRIM 09-40021-FDS, 2010 WL 1427523, at *5 (D. Mass. Apr. 7, 2010)

189. *Hoffa v. United State*, 385 US 293 (1996).

190. *United States v. Gatson*, No. 13-705, 2014 WL 7182275, at *22 (D.N.J. Dec. 16, 2014).

191. *United States v. Sawyer*, 786 F. Supp. 2d 1352, 1355–56 (N.D. Ohio 2011).

192. Levinson-Waldman R. Government access to and manipulation of social media: Legal and policy challenges. *Howard L J.* 2018;61:523, 557.

193. *United States v. Warshak*, 631 F.3d 266, 288 (6th Cir. 2010).

194. Bedi M. Facebook and interpersonal privacy: Why the Third Party Doctrine should not apply. *B C L Rev.* 2013;54:1.

195. Kerr OS. The mosaic theory of the Fourth Amendment. *Mich L Rev.* Dec 2012;111:311, 313.

196. *United States v. Jones*, 565 US 400 (2012).

197. *Carpenter v. United States*, 138 S.Ct. 2206 (2018).

198. Kris D. Carpenter's implications for foreign intelligence surveillance. *Lawfare*, 24 Jun 2018. https://www.lawfareblog.com/carpenters-implications-foreign-intelligence-surveillance

199. Serrato JK, et al. US Supreme Court expands digital privacy rights in *Carpenter v. United States*. Data Protection Report, 27 Jun 2018. https://www.dataprotectionreport.com/2018/06/scotus-expands-digital-privacy-rights-carpenter/

200. Kerr O. When does a carpenter search start: And when does it stop? *Lawfare*, 6 Jul 2018. https://www.lawfareblog.com/when-does-carpenter-search-start-and-when-does-it-stop

201. Gallagher S. Barr says the US needs encryption backdoors to prevent "going dark." Um what? *Ars Technica*, 4 Aug 2019. https://arstechnica.com/tech-policy/2019/08/post-snowden-tech-became-more-secure-but-is-govt-really at-risk-of-going-dark/; Mylan Traylor J. Note: Shedding light on the "going dark" problem and the encryption debate. *Univ Mich J L Reform*. 2016;50:489, 491. https://repository.law.umich.edu/cgi/viewcontent.cgi?article=1175&context=mjlr

202. In The Matter of the Search of an Apple iPhone Seized During the Execution of a Search Warrant on a Black Lexus IS300, California License Plate 35KGD203, No. ED 15-0451M (C.D. Cal. Feb. 16, 2016) (Order Compelling Apple, Inc. to Assist Agents in Search) https://assets.documentcloud.org/documents/2714001/SB-Shooter-Order-Compelling-Apple-Asst-iPhone.pdf

203. Benner K, Lichtblau E. US says it has unlocked iPhone without Apple. *New York Times*, 28 Mar 2016. https://www.nytimes.com/2016/03/29/technology/apple-iphone-fbi-justice-department-case.html

204. Nicas J, Benner K. F.B.I. asks Apple to help unlock two iPhones. *New York Times*, 7 Jan 2020. https://www.nytimes.com/2020/01/07/technology/apple-fbi-iphone-encryption.html

205. Eadicicco L. For Months, Apple said it wouldn't break into an iPhone for the FBI. Attorney General Barr just said the FBI was able to do it without Apple's help. *Business Insider*, 28 May 2020. https://www.businessinsider.com/fbi-unlocks-pensacola-shooter-iphones-without-apple-2020-5

206. Dewan S, Winston A. In sea of hate, officials strain to spot threats. *New York Times*, 30 Apr 2019:A1. https://www.nytimes.com/2019/04/29/us/synagogue-shooting-fbi-warning.html

18

Pursuing Lone-Actor Terrorists

UK Counterterrorism Law and Policy

STUART MACDONALD

INTRODUCTION

The United Kingdom's strategy for countering international terrorism, CONTEST, consists of four strands.[1] Known as the four Ps, these strands are *Prepare*, which seeks to mitigate the impact of a terrorist incident by bringing any attack to an end rapidly and recovering from it; *Protect*, which is concerned with reducing the vulnerability of the United Kingdom and UK interests overseas; *Prevent*, which aims to safeguard and support those vulnerable to radicalization in order to stop them from becoming terrorists or supporting terrorism; and, *Pursue*, which seeks to stop terrorist attacks by disrupting terrorists and their operations. The focus of this chapter is the last of these, Pursue.

Given the potential severity of a successful terrorist attack, the need for special counterterrorism laws and powers to disrupt terrorists and their operations is widely accepted. Also widely accepted is the importance of these laws and powers being empirically grounded to ensure both their effectiveness and necessity. A challenge in this regard is the tendency toward security panics.[2] A stark example is the popularization of the term "lone wolf"—particularly since the attacks of July 22, 2011, in Norway, when Anders Behring Breivik killed 8 people in Oslo and a further 69 at the island of Utøya. In fact, "the term's connotations of a singular, stealthy, and deadly attacker poorly describe the reality."[3] Not only do so-called lone wolves often lack the implied levels of cunning and lethality, they also commonly "maintain plot-relevant social ties that render them vulnerable to detection."[4] Use of this sensationalist term may thus "perpetuate myths about these individuals' capabilities and modalities of attack planning and preparation that can hamper effective detection and interdiction efforts."[5]

Security panics can generate calls for further extension of special counterterrorism laws and policies, thus creating the possibility of legislative/executive overreach. It is essential to recognize, therefore, that another important component of an effective counterterrorism strategy is respect for human rights and rule of law values. In the years following the 9/11 attacks, for example, it was frequently suggested that the rights of suspected terrorists may justifiably be balanced away in return for an increase in security—a notion that was shown to be both flawed and counterproductive.[6] Today, counterterrorism strategies such as CONTEST emphasize the importance of respect for human rights and the rule of law.[7]

This chapter focuses on two requirements that flow from this respect for human rights and the rule of law. The first is that special counterterrorism laws and policies should be carefully circumscribed. They require principled justification, their scope should extend no further than necessary, and safeguards should be put in place to prevent their misuse. The second is that exceptional counterterrorism powers should not unquestioningly be transposed to other areas of criminal justice. The danger here is that, once enacted, laws and policies that were created in the name of counterterrorism become normalized and, in time, begin to permeate and contaminate other criminal law and justice areas.[8]

The chapter's examination of the Pursue strand of the UK CONTEST strategy focuses on three of the principal methods used to disrupt terrorist activity: prosecution, deportation, and Terrorism Prevention and Investigation Measures (TPIM). The chapter argues that, in certain respects, each of these methods fails to adhere to the two requirements outlined in the previous paragraph. The chapter begins by discussing prosecution, explaining that the definitions of a number of the United Kingdom's special terrorism offenses are overly broad, rely unduly on the responsible exercise of official discretion, and embody a relativistic approach to human rights. Turning next to deportation, the chapter details how the UK government's attempt to adopt a relativistic approach to the right not to suffer torture and other forms of ill-treatment was frustrated by the European Court of Human Rights. This led to the adoption of a policy of Deportation with Assurances (DWA), which places diplomatic relations, not universal legal prohibitions, at the forefront of efforts to prevent the ill-treatment of deportees. Finally, the chapter discusses TPIM. It explains that TPIM notices are imposed by the Home Secretary, with the court's role limited to a review jurisdiction, and review hearings may include closed sessions. Originally regarded as an exceptional measure, the TPIM regime now not only enjoys semi-permanent status but has also been transposed to other areas of criminal justice.

PROSECUTION

Of the methods of disrupting terrorist activity examined in this chapter, prosecution is the preferred option. This is for several reasons. From a due process perspective, prosecution requires the state to prove its case in open court beyond reasonable doubt and affords the suspect an opportunity to respond to the case against him. From a labeling perspective, a criminal conviction conveys the highest degree of censure. And, from a national security perspective, conviction for a serious criminal offense normally results in a lengthy period of imprisonment, which is more protective of the public than other forms of disruption such as deportation and TPIM.

In cases where a suspected terrorist has inflicted harm, a general application offense (such as murder, kidnap or hijack) will normally apply (with the terrorist connection operating as an aggravating factor that increases the seriousness of the offense, thus justifying a more severe sentence).[9] For cases in which a suspected terrorist has been prevented from inflicting harm, there are a number of general application inchoate offenses. While these offenses have a preventive rationale, efforts to deploy them in terrorism cases (particularly those involving lone actors) raise important practical issues. A defendant may only be convicted of attempting a crime if he engaged in activity that was more than merely preparatory to the commission of the full offense.[10] This has been interpreted by the courts as requiring

that the defendant "embark[ed] upon the crime proper."[11] Hence in *R v. Geddes* (1996) the conviction for attempted false imprisonment of a man found hiding in the boys' toilets of a school while in possession of a knife, rope, and masking tape was quashed on appeal on the basis that, since he had not yet come into contact with a pupil, he had not embarked upon the crime.[12] Similarly, in *R v. Campbell* (1990), the conviction for attempted robbery of a man stopped just outside a post office while in possession of an imitation firearm and a threatening note was quashed on appeal on the basis that, until he entered the post office, he had not embarked upon the crime.[13] This narrow scope of the law of criminal attempts means that it will only be relevant in terrorism cases in limited circumstances (as when someone planted a bomb unaware that it was faulty and incapable of exploding). Given the harm that a terrorist attack might inflict, it is infeasible to expect law enforcement to wait until the suspect has embarked upon the crime before intervening.

There are also practical issues with the general inchoate offenses of conspiracy[14] and encouraging/assisting crime.[15] For a start, these offenses are notoriously difficult to prove. It can be difficult to obtain evidence of an agreement or words of encouragement, especially if the suspects observe good communications security. Even if such evidence is obtained, it may not be admissible as a result of the United Kingdom's self-imposed ban on the use of intercepted materials as evidence in criminal trials.[16] And even if evidence is obtained and it is admissible, it may lack evidential value (perhaps because the suspects disguised the contents of the communication) and/or there may be public interest reasons not to disclose it in open court (perhaps because it would expose other ongoing investigations or reveal secret techniques or capabilities).[17] In addition, these offenses may not fit the facts of a case involving a lone actor. The offense of conspiracy requires proof of an agreement to commit an offense as a joint collaborative project, which is the very antithesis of acting alone.[18] The offense of encouraging/assisting crime, meanwhile, applies to those who seek to persuade or help others to commit an offense. So, while it might apply in some lone-actor cases, as when a suspect tries unsuccessfully to recruit others to join his terrorist plot, it will not apply where the suspect plans and prepares an attack alone.

These practical considerations—coupled with the conviction that, in terrorism cases, it is necessary to "defend further up the field"—have led to the creation of a raft of special, preventive, terrorism-related offenses.[19] Found predominantly in the UK Terrorism Acts of 2000 and 2006, these "precursor" offenses target a range of preparatory and facilitative activities, including: membership of a proscribed organization,[20] support for a proscribed organization,[21] fundraising for terrorist purposes,[22] failure to disclose information that might assist in preventing an act of terrorism,[23] collecting information or possessing a document likely to be useful to a terrorist,[24] encouraging terrorism,[25] dissemination of terrorist publications,[26] preparation of terrorist acts,[27] and training for terrorism.[28] Importantly, unlike the general offenses of conspiracy and encouraging/attempting crime, many of these offenses may straightforwardly apply in lone-actor cases. For example, those who download violent extremist propaganda might be charged with collecting information likely to be useful to a terrorist (maximum sentence 15 years imprisonment), while those who download bomb-making instructions or acquire a weapon might be charged with preparing a terrorist act (maximum sentence life imprisonment). Moreover, research has found that lone actors often interact and have social ties with other radical actors and are "alone largely and only with regard to the actual commission of the act of violence."[29] These wider interactions could potentially result in liability for being a member of or inviting support for a proscribed organization (maximum sentence: 10 years imprisonment), for disseminating terrorist publications (maximum sentence: 15 years imprisonment) or for another of the terrorism precursor offenses.

While the terrorism precursor offenses may avoid some of the practical difficulties with the general inchoate offenses and enable the disruption of terrorist activity, there is concern that, in an effort to facilitate early intervention, these offenses over-reach.[30] Some precursor offenses encompass activity that is quite far removed from the actual commission of a terrorist attack.[31] An example is the *membership of a proscribed organization offense* which, as noted earlier, is punishable by up to 10 years imprisonment. Section 11(1) of the Terrorism Act 2000 states that this offense applies not only to those who are in fact members of a proscribed organization but also to those who profess to be (but in fact are not). Moreover, proof of membership (or profession of membership) is all that is required to establish liability for the offense. The offense requires no proof of a terrorist purpose or intention, and, while the statute does provide a defense, this only applies

if the defendant adduces evidence that (a) the organization was not proscribed on the last (or only) occasion on which he became a member or began to profess to be a member and, (b) he has not taken part in the activities of the organization at any time while it was proscribed. In Attorney-General's Reference (No. 4 of 2002), the offense was described by Lord Bingham as a "provision of extraordinary breadth." He commented:

> It would cover a person who joined an organisation when it was not a terrorist organisation or when, if it was, he did not know that it was. It would cover a person who joined an organisation when it was not proscribed or, if it was, he did not know that it was. It would cover a person who joined such an organisation as an immature juvenile. It would cover someone who joined such an organisation abroad in a country where it was not proscribed and came to this country ignorant that it was proscribed here. . . . It would cover a person who wished to dissociate himself from an organisation he had earlier joined, perhaps in good faith, but had no means of doing so, or no means of doing so which did not expose him to the risk of serious injury or assassination.[32]

It would also apply to a fantasist who falsely claims to be a member of a proscribed group in a misguided attempt to show off.

There are also a number of precursor offenses that do not require proof of a sufficient degree of culpability. An example, also punishable by up to 15 years imprisonment, is the offense of collecting information or possessing a document likely to be useful to a terrorist. Such documents include bomb-making instructions, information on how to gain unauthorized entry to a military establishment, or any other material that "calls for an explanation,"[33] such as advice on how to conceal information from others.[34] Once it has been shown that the defendant collected or possessed such requisite information/documents, the only culpability requirements are that the defendant knew that he was in possession and had control of the information/document, knew the nature of its contents, and lacked a reasonable excuse. Notably, there is no requirement to prove a terrorist purpose or intention.[35]

This was a critical element in the outcome in *R v. G* (2009).[36] The defendant in this case had paranoid schizophrenia. He had been detained for a number of non-terrorism offenses. While in custody he collected information on explosives and bomb-making and also drew a map of the Territorial Army center in Chesterfield and wrote down plans to attack the center. The items were discovered during a search of his cell. His explanation for collecting the information was that he wanted to wind up the prison staff because he believed they had been whispering about him. The prosecution accepted expert evidence that he had collected the information as a direct consequence of his illness. The case reached the House of Lords.

In this case, since (a) the information on explosives that the defendant had collected called for an explanation and would be useful to a terrorist, (b) the defendant knew he was in possession and had control of the information and, (c) he knew the nature of the information, the key issue in the case was whether the defense of reasonable excuse was available to him. Here, the House of Lords held that proof of a non-terrorist purpose does not, in itself, constitute a reasonable excuse. The question is not whether the defendant had a terrorist purpose, but whether his excuse for collecting the information is objectively reasonable. Seeking to antagonize prison guards is not reasonable and could not be rendered *objectively* reasonable by the defendant's mental illness. G was therefore guilty of the offense, notwithstanding the absence of any terrorist purpose or connection. The effect is to "make a terrorist out of nothing," which raises important questions about fair labeling.[37]

The overreach of terrorism precursor offenses is an example of a wider contemporary legislative technique, in which deliberately broad powers are vested in the executive alongside an assurance that the powers will be exercised responsibly.[38] In the specific context of terrorism, the UK government has argued that widely drawn powers confer flexibility and that a "flexible statutory framework" is required to "ensure that our law enforcement and intelligence agencies can continue to disrupt and prosecute those who pose a threat to the public."[39] Yet such an approach is at odds with a human rights ethos that stresses the importance of tightly constraining state power in order to safeguard against potential abuse and has been criticized by the Supreme Court:

> The Crown's reliance on prosecutorial discretion is intrinsically unattractive, as it amounts to saying that the legislature, whose primary duty is to make the law, and to do so in public, has in effect delegated to an appointee of the executive, albeit a respected and independent lawyer, the decision whether an activity should be treated as criminal for the purposes of prosecution. Such a statutory device, unless deployed very rarely indeed and only when there is no alternative, risks undermining the rule of law. It involves Parliament abdicating a significant part of its legislative function to an unelected DPP, or to the Attorney General, who, though he is accountable to Parliament, does not make open, democratically accountable decisions in the same way as Parliament. Further, such a device leaves citizens unclear as to whether or not their actions or projected actions are liable to be treated by the prosecution authorities as effectively innocent or criminal—in this case seriously criminal.[40]

It is for this same reason that the terrorism precursor offenses have been dubbed "ouster offenses" because the effect of their over-inclusivity is to deprive the trial court of the opportunity to adjudicate on the underlying wrong that the offense is targeting.[41]

DEPORTATION

In some cases, prosecution is not an available option due to (a) insufficient admissible evidence to bring a prosecution, (b) sufficient admissible evidence but public interest reasons for not disclosing it, or (c) perhaps the individual was convicted of a crime and has served his sentence. One alternative tactic in such circumstances is to use nationality and immigration powers.[42] There are various powers aimed at British nationals who have traveled overseas to engage in terrorism, including Temporary Exclusion Orders and, in the case of dual nationals and naturalized citizens who have a reasonable prospect of attaining another nationality, removal of their British citizenship.[43] Meanwhile, foreign nationals who are suspected of involvement in terrorism-related activity may be deported from the United Kingdom.[44] Deportation of foreign suspected terrorists is intended to protect national security and send "a strong signal that foreign nationals who threaten our national security cannot expect to be allowed to remain in the UK."[45]

Deportation of a foreign national must comply with the European Convention on Human Rights. Of particular relevance here is Article 3, which states that "No one shall be subjected to torture or to inhuman or degrading treatment or punishment." Importantly, the scope of the Article 3 prohibition is not limited to cases in which the feared ill-treatment would be inflicted by a member state. According to the European Court of Human Rights in *Soering v. UK* (1989),[46] Article 3 also prohibits the extradition of a person to a non-member state in circumstances where there is a "real risk" that that person will suffer ill-treatment in the receiving country. The Court said that to hold otherwise would be "contrary to the spirit and intendment of the Article."[47]

In the subsequent case *Chahal v. UK* (1996), the UK government argued that the principle from *Soering v. UK* did not apply in cases involving the deportation of a suspected terrorist.[48] The UK wished to deport Mr. Chahal, allegedly a Sikh militant, to India on the grounds of national security. Mr. Chahal claimed that, if he were returned to India, he would suffer ill-treatment. Before the European Court of Human Rights, the UK government argued that, in spite of its absolute wording, Article 3 in fact contains an implied limitation that allows member states to deport an individual, even if there exists a real risk of ill-treatment, if the deportation is required on national security grounds. Alternatively, the UK government argued that in a case like *Chahal v. UK*, the gravity of the threat to national security should be balanced against the degree of risk of ill-treatment, so that deportation would be permissible where there is substantial doubt about the risk of ill-treatment and the threat to national security weighs heavily in the balance.

In its judgment, the Court acknowledged the challenges that states face in protecting their communities from terrorism but rejected both of the UK government's arguments, insisting that the Article 3 prohibition on ill-treatment is absolute. So, applying the principle from *Soering v. UK*, it followed from the Court's conclusion that there was a real risk he would suffer ill-treatment if deported to India, so Mr Chahal could not be returned there. Moreover, the Court stated that, according to Article 5(1)(f) of the Convention, a person may only be detained pending deportation while deportation proceedings are in progress. Since the Court's judgment marked the end of the process, there was therefore no possibility of continuing to detain Mr Chahal until it was safe to return him to India. To do so would have amounted to a violation of his Article 5 right to liberty.[49]

The judgment in *Chahal v. UK* was delivered in October 1996. Just over a decade later, in *Saadi v. Italy* (2008),[50] the United Kingdom sought to persuade the European Court to reconsider its

stance in *Chahal v. UK*, arguing that the threat posed by international terrorism had increased since the attacks of 9/11. It argued that the "rigidity" of the judgment in *Chahal v. UK* caused member states "many difficulties." In particular, it forced states to rely on other measures such as surveillance or restrictions on movement, which offer "only partial protection." In response, the Court acknowledged that member states "face immense difficulties in modern times in protecting their communities from terrorist violence." However, these difficulties do not, the Court insisted, "call into question the absolute nature of Article 3." The prohibition on torture and other forms of ill-treatment "enshrines one of the fundamental values of democratic societies" and applies to all people, irrespective of their conduct or the nature of any offense they have allegedly committed.[51]

While some criticized the decision in *Saadi v. Italy* for leaving "the UK a safe haven for some individuals whose determination is to damage the UK and its citizens,"[52] human rights commentators applauded the decision. As Moeckli has explained, any dilution of the principle from *Chahal v. UK* would have had the effect of creating a distinction between domestic and foreign suspected terrorists.[53] On the one hand, for domestic suspected terrorists the Article 3 right not to be ill-treated would have remained absolute. On the other hand, diluting the principle would have made it possible to expose foreign suspected terrorists to a real risk of ill-treatment. But to apply differing levels of protection on the basis of nationality would have been at odds with the ethos of *human* rights. As Judge Zupančič stated in his concurring opinion in *Saadi v. Italy*, the implication would have been that "such individuals do not deserve human rights . . . because they are less human."[54]

In an effort to facilitate the deportation of foreign suspected terrorists while also adhering to the judgments in *Chahal v. UK* and *Saadi v. Italy*, the UK government has pursued a policy of DWA. The idea behind DWA is a simple one: if the United Kingdom wishes to deport a foreign suspected terrorist to his country of origin, but there are concerns that he may suffer ill-treatment there, then the receiving country can be asked to provide a diplomatic assurance (or, in UK terminology, a *Memorandum of Understanding*) that no ill-treatment will be inflicted. This assurance will diminish any risk of ill-treatment that may have existed and so enable deportation to proceed consistently with the *Chahal v. UK* principle.

While DWA may sound straightforward, it in fact raises a number of difficult issues. Many of the states with which diplomatic assurances might be agreed are already parties to the UN Convention against Torture and/or the International Covenant on Civil and Political Rights and so have already committed not to resort to torture or other forms of ill-treatment under any circumstances.[55] It has therefore been argued that, by entering into such agreements, the UK government both undermines these universal legal prohibitions and implies that the ill-treatment of some detainees is more acceptable than the ill-treatment of others.[56] It has also been argued that diplomatic assurances are meaningless, especially as they are not legally binding and there are examples (such as Maher Arar) of individuals being ill-treated in breach of a diplomatic assurance.[57] The fact that it is felt necessary to seek an assurance is, in itself, an acknowledgment of the risk of ill-treatment, and there is little reason to regard as credible an assurance given by a state that disregards its obligations under international human rights law.

In addition, even if the assurance is given in good faith by the central government, in countries where there is a culture or subculture of ill-treatment the assurance may be "subverted by local officials who probably believe that their actions are necessary, condoned in practice, and certainly not the subject of potential sanction against them."[58] It is also difficult to monitor compliance since many forms of ill-treatment are deliberately difficult to detect and a detainee may well be reluctant to make an allegation of ill-treatment. Some have also argued that there is little incentive for either the United Kingdom or the receiving country to monitor the agreement: if the UK government were to allege ill-treatment this could upset the diplomatic relationship with the receiving country and damage the chances of deporting others there in the future, while if the foreign government were to discover ill-treatment has occurred, this would constitute a breach not only of internationally agreed standards but also the specific promise given to the UK government.[59]

Perhaps the most high-profile case involving DWA is that of Omar Othman (also known as Abu Qatada).[60] In this case, which was heard by the Fourth Section of the European Court of Human Rights, both Othman's counsel and the third-party interveners (Amnesty International, Human Rights Watch, and JUSTICE) expressed grave concern at the use of diplomatic assurances for the reasons just outlined. In its submissions

to the Court, the UK government responded to these concerns. It argued that to criticize a diplomatic assurance for not being legally binding is to "betray a lack of an appreciation as to how [they] worked in practice between states."[61] The fact that an agreement is a political, not a legal, one could mean that the receiving country has greater incentive to adhere to it. The obligation in a multilateral treaty is owed to many countries in general but none in particular. By contrast, a firm political commitment in a bilateral diplomatic assurance is owed to a specific country, so the implications of breaking it could be more acute. This is all the more so if, as in Othman's case, the assurance was agreed at the highest level of government.[62] Nor is it in the interests of the UK government for breaches of diplomatic assurances to remain undiscovered or hidden. Knowing how deportees have been treated helps the government assess the risk of ill-treatment in future cases.[63] Moreover, while some assurances had in the past proved to be unreliable, it does not follow from this that all assurances inevitably lack credibility. Each case must be assessed individually on its merits. Here, it is important to note that all decisions to deport are subject to appeal to the Special Immigration Appeals Commission (SIAC). SIAC is an independent, expert tribunal. It scrutinizes all diplomatic assurances carefully and has in the past stopped the deportation of some foreign suspected terrorists. Decisions of SIAC can in turn be appealed to the Court of Appeal, the UK Supreme Court, and, ultimately, the European Court of Human Rights. There are thus "extensive judicial safeguards to ensure that an individual will only be deported where compatible with, rather than in breach or avoidance of, the UK's [international] obligations."[64]

In its judgment in *Othman v. UK* (2012), the European Court stated that it is "not for this Court to rule upon the propriety of seeking assurances, or to assess the long term consequences of doing so." Rather, the Court's role is to assess whether the individual faces a real risk of ill-treatment in the receiving country. Any assurances that have been provided by the receiving country "constitute a further relevant factor" in making this assessment. The Court began by noting that, while torture is "widespread and routine" in Jordanian prisons, it did not necessarily follow that Jordan would not comply with a diplomatic assurance. The United Kingdom and Jordan had historically enjoyed a "very strong" bilateral relationship, and the assurance in Othman's case had the express support of the King of Jordan himself.

Othman's high profile also made it more likely that the Jordanian authorities would be careful to ensure that he was treated properly. Ill-treatment would have "serious consequences" for Jordan's relationship with the United Kingdom and also cause "international outrage."[65]

The text of the assurance was, the Court said, "superior in both its detail and its formality" to any assurance the Court had previously examined. Importantly, it included provision for an independent monitor: the Adaleh Centre. While the Court conceded that "the Adaleh Centre does not have the same expertise or resources as leading international NGOs such as Amnesty International, Human Rights Watch or the International Committee of the Red Cross," it concluded that "it was the very fact of monitoring visits which was important." It also noted that, thanks to funding from the UK government, the capacity of the Adaleh Centre had increased significantly and that given the government's "broader interest in ensuring that the assurances are respected, it can be expected that this funding will continue." So, according to the Court, if Othman was returned to Jordan there was no real risk that he would suffer ill-treatment and therefore deporting him would not violate his Article 3 right.[66]

In should be noted, however, that the European Court did hold that deporting Othman to Jordan would violate his Article 6 right to a fair trial.[67] On his return to Jordan, Othman faced being retried before the State Security Court on charges of conspiring to cause explosions. There was found to be a real risk that the prosecution case at his retrial would include evidence obtained by torture from his alleged co-conspirators. This evidence would be of considerable, perhaps decisive, importance against him. Admitting it at the retrial would, the European Court said, amount to a flagrant denial of justice: "a breach of the principles of fair trial guaranteed by Article 6 which is so fundamental as to amount to a nullification, or destruction of the very essence, of the right guaranteed by that Article."[68] Following the European Court's judgment, the United Kingdom and Jordan agreed to a treaty dealing with mutual assistance in tackling crime, one clause of which addressed the use of torture evidence in criminal trials.[69] Once both countries had ratified the treaty, Othman returned to Jordan voluntarily. At his retrial he was acquitted after the judges ruled that there was insufficient evidence against him.

The *Othman v. UK* judgment thus "gave its blessing to DWA in principle."[70] While the European Court did set conditions that require the sending country to "engage deeply with a receptive foreign partner,"[71] some unease remains that "the transfer of the issue into the diplomatic sphere means that human rights are no longer the sole or perhaps predominant issue."[72] At the same time, the engagement involved in agreeing a diplomatic assurance can have wider benefits. In his report on the topic, the United Kingdom's then Independent Reviewer of Terrorism Legislation, David Anderson, recounts a conversation with a Jordanian prison governor. Obliged by bilateral arrangements not to hood prisoners sent to him from the United Kingdom on their regular journeys from prison to court, the governor ordered the hoods to be removed from all his prisoners making that journey.[73] Yet this level of intensive engagement with a foreign partner is both costly and time-consuming. The litigation surrounding Othman, for example, lasted for 8 years and cost roughly £1.7 million.[74] In fact, since 2005, the total number of successful uses of the DWA policy currently stands at 12: 9 to Algeria; 2 (including Othman) to Jordan; and 1 to Morocco. Moreover, following the decision of SIAC in *BB & others v. Secretary of State for the Home Department* (unreported, 18 April 2016) that the lack of an effective system of verification meant that six men could not be deported to Algeria and the withdrawal of proceedings in the case of the Jordanian man N2 following Jordan's refusal to provide the requested assurances, there are no DWA proceedings currently in progress. Anderson and his special adviser, Clive Walker, thus conclude that "DWA can play a significant role in counter-terrorism, especially in prominent and otherwise intractable cases which are worth the cost and effort, but it will be delivered effectively and legitimately in international law only if laborious care is taken."[75]

TERRORISM PREVENTION AND INVESTIGATION MEASURES

There are a small number of people in the United Kingdom who pose a terrorist threat but who can be neither prosecuted (for the reasons explained earlier) nor deported (either because they are a British citizen or because of a real risk of ill-treatment in the receiving country).[76] In such cases, the United Kingdom has resorted to the use of executive measures. In 2001, in the aftermath of 9/11, the power to indefinitely detain foreign suspected terrorists was introduced.[77] After this power was held by the House of Lords to violate Articles 5 (right to liberty) and 14 (prohibition of discrimination) of the European Convention on Human Rights,[78] it was replaced in 2005 by a new system of Control Orders.[79] Control Orders were then themselves replaced in 2011 by TPIM.[80] TPIMs soon began to dwindle, and, by early 2014, there were no TPIM notices in force at all.[81] In early 2015, amendments created "TPIMs Mk II."[82]

Although TPIMs were intended to be "less intrusive" than the system of Control Orders, they may still impose significant restrictions on an individual's liberty.[83] There are a total of 14 types of possible measure listed in the legislation. These include an overnight residence measure (effectively a curfew of up to 10 hours duration[84]), travel and exclusion measures (requiring the individual not to leave, or to enter, a specified area), association measures (restrictions on the individual's association or communication with other persons), an electronic communication device measure (limiting the individual's use and possession of such devices—though, unlike the system of Control Orders, the individual must at a minimum be allowed to possess and use a landline telephone, a computer with internet access, and a mobile phone that does not have internet access, subject to any specified conditions on such use), a work or studies measure (restrictions on the individual's work or studies), financial services measures (imposing restrictions on the individual's use of, or access to, specified financial services), a reporting measure (a requirement to report to a particular police station at specified times), and a monitoring measure (such as a requirement to wear an electronic tag).[85]

In addition, a TPIM notice may impose forced relocation. This is particularly significant given that, when the Coalition Government introduced the TPIM legislation in 2011, it heralded the ending of forced relocation as one of the key liberalizing measures of the new TPIM regime.[86] Forced relocation requires the individual to reside in a place of the Home Secretary's choosing and away from their former associates. It was described by some as a form of "internal exile" and was "in some cases very strongly resented by those subject to it, and their families."[87] At the same time, forced relocation could be effective in disrupting terrorist networks that were concentrated in particular areas and was used regularly in practice (23 of the 52 men who received Control Orders from 2005 to 2011 were forced to relocate).[88] By removing an individual from their networks, forced relocation also made absconsion more difficult. So, following two high-profile instances of men subject to TPIM notices absconding (Ibrahim Magag in

December 2012 and Mohammed Mohamed in November 2013), the United Kingdom's then Independent Reviewer of Terrorism Legislation, David Anderson, recommended that the possibility of forced relocation be reintroduced.[89] This recommendation was reluctantly endorsed by Parliament's Joint Committee on Human Rights, which also urged the importance of "bringing forward ideas about how to mitigate the alienation and resentment likely to be caused in some minority communities."[90] It is the reintroduction of forced relocation in TPIM Mk II (albeit with a stipulation that an individual may not be relocated more than 200 miles from his home) that appears to have led to TPIM's renewed use. By the end of May 2018 there were a total of eight TPIM notices in force, and all eight imposed relocation.[91]

A TPIM notice lasts for a maximum of 2 years. Following this, a new TPIM notice may only be issued if there is evidence of fresh terrorism-related activity.[92] This is another respect in which TPIM differ from Control Orders. While Control Orders had a maximum duration of 1 year, there was no limit on how many times an Order could be renewed. In effect, therefore, Control Orders were of indefinite duration. Indeed, the longest period for which someone was subject to a Control Order was 55 months.[93] The Coalition Government explained that the 2-year maximum duration of TPIM was intended to "emphasise that they are a short term expedient not a long term solution."[94]

When TPIM were introduced, concern was expressed that this could result in the state being forced to rely on other methods of disruption, such as surveillance, that offer a lesser degree of protection. This concern was exacerbated by the fact that those subject to TPIM at the time included two men who, as members of the airline liquid bomb plot, were at the gravest end of the threat spectrum.[95] A 2-year maximum duration was, however, supported by the United Kingdom's former Independent Reviewer of Terrorism Legislation, Lord Carlile, who stated that, after 2 years, "at least the immediate utility of all but the most dedicated terrorist will seriously have been disrupted. The terrorist will know that the authorities retain an interest in his/her activities and contacts, and will be likely to scrutinise them in the future"[96]—and by his successor, David Anderson who, in 2014, reported that the 2-year maximum duration "is now generally perceived [by Home Office officials, MI5 and police] as part of the landscape."[97] Anderson did, however, say that more needed to be done to develop an exit strategy for each individual subject to a TPIM notice: "the question of how best to prevent [terrorism-related activity] in the longer term needs to be addressed not just in the final months, but from the start of a TPIM notice and in the light of the rare opportunity for dialogue that a TPIM notice provides."[98] In developing an exit strategy, consideration should be given to engagement, as well as coercive, strategies. While it might be naïve to suppose that all TPIM subjects could be diverted from further terrorism-related activity, Anderson stated

> All are however human beings; all are and will remain members of society; and some have first come under constraint while still quite young. If nothing else, an element of intervention could give them a point of reference distinct from those which are believed to have led them into [terrorism-related activity]. At best, it could help set them on a different path.[99]

Following Anderson's recommendation, TPIM Mk II now includes the possibility of *appointments measures*. These require the individual to attend appointments with specified persons, such as a specialist probation officer, with the aim of de-radicalization. However, Anderson's related recommendation that the legislation should state that information gathered in the course of such appointments may not be used in criminal or similar proceedings was not enacted.[100] Parliament's Joint Committee on Human Rights has expressed concern that the lack of such an assurance is at odds with the privilege against self-incrimination and may impede individuals' willingness to engage with de-radicalization programs.[101]

A TPIM notice is imposed by the Home Secretary.[102] Before issuing a TPIM notice, the Home Secretary must first seek permission from the courts (save in urgent cases, where permission may be obtained retrospectively). The permission hearing may take place without the individual concerned being present, without the individual having been notified of the application, and without the individual having been given an opportunity to make representations to the court. Once permission has been granted and the TPIM notice issued, a review hearing must be held. At the review hearing the role of the court is to review the Home Secretary's decision that the conditions for imposing a TPIM notice were met. The conditions are, first, that the Home Secretary is satisfied, on the balance of probabilities, that the

individual is or has been involved in terrorism-related activity. As stated earlier, this must be activity in respect of which no TPIM notice has previously been issued.

Second, the Home Secretary reasonably considers that it is necessary to impose TPIM on the individual to protect the public from a risk of terrorism. Each individual measure imposed on the individual must also satisfy this test. In respect of the first of these conditions, it is worth noting that the current standard of proof (balance of probabilities) is higher than it was both for TPIM Mk I (reasonable belief) and Control Orders (reasonable suspicion). However, David Anderson's recommendation that a TPIM notice should only be imposed if the reviewing court is itself satisfied, on the balance of probabilities, that the individual is or has been involved in terrorism-related activity was not accepted.[103] As such, the court's role is merely to review the decision of the Home Secretary that the conditions are met.

The review hearing may include closed sessions.[104] The purpose of closed sessions is to ensure that information is not disclosed contrary to the public interest, subject to the requirement that the individual must "be given sufficient information about the allegations against him to enable him to give effective instructions in relation to those allegations."[105] The individual and his lawyer are excluded from the closed sessions, with the interests of the individual instead represented by a Special Advocate (a practitioner with security clearance appointed by the Attorney General).[106] The Special Advocate may make submissions and cross-examine witnesses on behalf of the individual. Yet, while independent review has found the contribution of Special Advocates to be valuable in the protection of the individuals whose interests they represent, the Special Advocates themselves have expressed misgivings about their role.[107] Before the Special Advocate is shown the closed materials, he may communicate freely with the individual and the individual's lawyer. Once the Special Advocate has been served with the closed materials, the individual may still communicate with him (in writing and through his lawyer). But the Special Advocate may no longer communicate with the individual, except in two circumstances. First, to acknowledge receipt (in writing) of any communication received from the individual. Second, following a successful application to the court for authorization to communicate with the individual or his lawyer.

Before the court decides whether to grant authorization, however, the Home Secretary must be notified of the request and given the opportunity to object. In practice this means authorization to communicate with the individual or his lawyer is rarely sought. Not only is permission unlikely to be granted (since it is likely that parts of the closed materials could be inferred from any questions that the Special Advocate might wish to ask), it is also tactically undesirable because of the risk that "it might give away to the opposing party the parts of the closed evidence in relation to which the controlled person does not have an explanation."[108] This restriction on the ability to communicate with the individual (in addition to other concerns including lack of funding and access to justice, the lack of any practical ability to call evidence, and the practice of iterative disclosure) led a group of 57 Special Advocates to state that closed materials proceedings "are inherently unfair; they do not 'work effectively', nor do they deliver real procedural fairness."[109] Yet, following the Justice and Security Act of 2013, the availability of closed material proceedings has now been expanded to *all* civil proceedings.

Last, it is worth noting the requirement that Parliament review and renew the TPIM legislation every 5 years.[110] This is significantly longer than for Control Orders. which received Parliamentary scrutiny every 12 months. This means that, in contrast to Control Orders, TPIM enjoy a degree of semi-permanence.

CONCLUSION

The starting point of this chapter was that respect for individuals' rights and rule of law values is an essential component of an effective counterterrorism strategy. So, while special counterterrorism laws and policies are necessary, these require principled justification and should be carefully circumscribed. It is also important that laws and policies that are created in the name of counterterrorism are not readily and unquestioningly extended to other areas of criminal justice. Yet two recurring themes of the chapter's examination of the principal methods of disruption employed by the Pursue strand of the United Kingdom's CONTEST strategy have been the weakening of legal forms of protection of individuals' rights and the normalization of exceptional counterterrorism laws and powers.

The chapter expressed concern about the overreach of the terrorism precursor offenses, both in terms of the conduct they encompass and the level of culpability they require. As the Supreme Court has remarked, official assurances that the breadth of these offenses will in practice be tempered by the responsible exercise of the discretion to prosecute are not an appropriate substitute for the safeguard offered by more narrowly drawn offense definitions. A similar reliance on executive judgment was evident in the TPIM legislation. Notwithstanding the onerousness of the measures that can be imposed, a TPIM notice is imposed by the Home Secretary, with the courts' role limited to a review jurisdiction. The recommendation that a TPIM notice should only be imposed if the court, as well as the Home Secretary, is satisfied that the individual is or has been involved in terrorism-related activity was rejected. This was a missed opportunity to secure enhanced legal protection of individual liberty.[111] And the policy of DWA places diplomatic relations, not universal legal prohibitions, at the forefront of efforts to prevent torture and other forms of ill-treatment.

The chapter has also highlighted the potential for special counterterrorism laws and policies to become normalized. Closed sessions were originally only used in appeals in immigration and asylum cases for reasons of national security. They were then deployed in TPIM review hearings and certain other settings.[112] They may now be used in any civil proceedings where this is required in the interests of national security and the fair and effective administration of justice. The TPIM regime is also now a semi-permanent part of the United Kingdom's legal landscape and has permeated into other areas of criminal justice (e.g., in the form of Serious Crime Prevention Orders). Terrorism precursor offenses, meanwhile, may be understood as a form of "enemy criminal law"[113] in which "exceptional measures of the war on terror are legalized and incorporated into criminal law."[114] Enemy criminal law not only presents a danger of contamination of other parts of the criminal law. The underlying premise is that since the enemy can no longer minimally guarantee that he will conduct himself as a loyal citizen, sanctions should be imposed not as retrospective punishment for past wrongdoing but prospectively in order to prevent future harms. This premise presents human rights not as vested in the individual by virtue of their personhood, but as entitlements that have to be earned through loyalty to the law.[115] A similarly relativistic approach was evident in the United Kingdom's attempt to overturn the European Court of Human Rights judgment in *Chahal v. UK*. Had this attempt succeeded, the nationality of a suspected terrorist would have determined their level of protection against torture and other forms of ill-treatment.

Such conditionality is at odds with the universality of human rights.

The scale and severity of terrorist attacks, whether perpetrated by a lone actor or otherwise, warrant special counterterrorism laws and policies. As well as ensuring that these special powers are effective in disrupting terrorism-related activity, it is also important to ensure that they respect individuals' rights and rule of law values. This chapter has argued that this involves not just maximizing legal protection of these rights and values, but also guarding against the normalization of exceptional counterterrorism measures.

NOTES AND REFERENCES

1. HM Government. *CONTEST: The United Kingdom's Strategy for Countering Terrorism*. Cm 9608. London: Stationery Office; 2018
2. Sunstein CR. Fear and liberty. *Social Res*. 2004; 71:967–996
3. Schuurman B, Bakker E, Gill P, Bouhana N. Lone actor terrorist attack planning and preparation: A data-driven analysis. *J Forensic Sci*. 2018;63:1191–1200, 1191
4. Schuurman B, Lindekilde L, Malthaner S, O'Connor F, Gill P, Bouhana, N. End of the lone wolf: The typology that should not have been. *Stud Conflict Terrorism*. 2019;42:771–778, 772
5. Schuurman et al. Lone actor.
6. See, Macdonald S. The unbalanced imagery of anti-terrorism policy. *Corn J L Public Pol*. 2009;18:519–540;Macdonald S. Why we should abandon the balance metaphor: A new approach to counterterrorism policy. *ILSA J Intl Compar L*. 2009;15:95–146;Waldron J. Security and liberty: The image of balance. *J Political Phil*. 2003;11:191–210;Zedner L. Securing liberty in the face of terror: Reflections from criminal justice. *J L Soc*. 2005;32:507–533.
7. HM Government. CONTEST (e.g., "Successful disruption and prosecution of terrorists depends on effective international collaboration that is underpinned by the rule of law and human rights," para. 279).
8. Zedner L. Security, the state, and the citizen: The changing architecture of crime control. *New Crim L R*. 2010;13:379–403.
9. Criminal Justice Act 2003, schedule 21 (murder); Counter-Terrorism Act 2008, section 30 (other offenses).
10. Criminal Attempts Act 1981, section 1.
11. *R v. Gullefer* [1990] 1 WLR 1063.
12. [1996] Crim LR 894.
13. (1990) 93 Cr App R 350.
14. Criminal Law Act 1977, section 1.
15. Serious Crime Act 2007, sections 44–46.
16. Regulation of Investigatory Powers Act 2000, section 17. The ban has been reviewed a total of eight times since 1993. For the most recent review see HM Government. *Intercept as Evidence*. Cm 8989. London: Stationery Office; 2014.
17. *Privy Council Review of Intercept as Evidence*. Report to the Prime Minister and the Home Secretary. Cm 7324. London: Stationery Office; 2008.
18. *R v. Mehta* [2012] EWCA Crim 2824.
19. Anderson D. Shielding the compass: How to fight terrorism without defeating the law. *Eur Hum Rights L Rev*. 2013:233–246, 237
20. Terrorism Act 2000, section 11.
21. Terrorism Act 2000, section 12.
22. Terrorism Act 2000, section 15.
23. Terrorism Act 2000, section 38B.
24. Terrorism Act 2000, section 58.
25. Terrorism Act 2006, section 1.
26. Terrorism Act 2006, section 2.
27. Terrorism Act 2006, section 5.
28. Terrorism Act 2006, section 6.
29. Schuurman et al. End of the lone wolf.
30. Macdonald S, Carlile A. Disrupting terrorist activity: What are the limits to criminal methods of disruption? In Juss S, ed., *Beyond Human Rights and the War on Terror*. Abingdon: Routledge; 2018:125–142.
31. See, Macdonald S. Cyberterrorism and enemy criminal law. In Ohlin J, Govern K, Finkelstein C, eds., *Cyberwar: Law and Ethics for Virtual Conflicts*. Oxford: Oxford University Press; 2015:57–75; Macdonald S. Prosecuting suspected terrorists: Precursor crimes, intercept evidence and the priority of security. In Jarvis L, Lister M, eds., *Critical Perspectives on Counter-Terrorism*. Abingdon: Routledge; 2015:130–149.
32. 2004] UKHL 43, para. 47.
33. *R v. G* [2009] UKHL 13, para. 43.
34. *R v. Muhammed* [2010] EWCA Crim 227.
35. Carlile A, Macdonald S. The criminalisation of terrorists' online preparatory acts. In Chen T, Jarvis L, Macdonald S, eds., *Cyberterrorism: Understanding, Assessment and Response*. New York: Springer; 2014:155–173
36. [2009] UKHL 13.
37. Hodgson J, Tadros V. How to make a terrorist out of nothing. *Modern L Rev*. 2009;72:984–998.
38. Macdonald S. ASBOs and control orders: Two recurring themes, two apparent contradictions. *Parliamentary Affairs*. 2007;60:601–624.
39. HM Government. *The Government Response to the Annual Report on the Operation of the Terrorism Acts in 2013 by the Independent Reviewer of Terrorism Legislation*. Cm 9032. London: Stationery Office; 2015:8.
40. *R v. Gul* [2013] UKSC 64, para. 36.
41. Edwards J. Justice denied: The criminal law and the ouster of the courts. *Oxf J Legal Stud*. 2010;30:725–748.
42. HM Government. CONTEST.
43. Fenwick H. Terrorism threats and temporary exclusion orders: Counter-terror rhetoric or reality? *Eur Hum Rights L Rev*. 2017:247–271.

44. Immigration Act 1971, section 3.
45. HM Government. *Countering International Terrorism: The United Kingdom's Strategy.* Cm 6888. London: Stationery Office; 2006:18.
46. (1989) 11 EHRR 439.
47. (1989) 11 EHRR 439, para. 88.
48. (1997) 23 EHRR 413.
49. Ibid.
50. (2009) 49 EHRR 30.
51. (2009) 49 EHRR 30, paras. 127, 137.
52. Carlile A. *Sixth Report of the Independent Reviewer Pursuant to Section 14(3) of the Prevention of Terrorism Act 2005.* London: Stationery Office; 2011:31.
53. Moeckli D. *Saadi v. Italy*: The rules of the game have *not* changed. *Hum Rights L Rev.* 2008;8:534–548.
54. (2009) 49 EHRR 30, concurring opinion of Judge Zupančič, para. 2.
55. Nowak M. Diplomatic assurances not an adequate safeguard for deportees, UN Special Rapporteur Against Torture warns. United Nations Human Rights Office of the High Commissioner Press Release. 23 Aug 2005.
56. Joint Committee on Human Rights. *The UN Convention Against Torture (UNCAT).* 19th Report of 2005–06. London: Stationery Office; 2006.
57. Ibid.
58. Walker C. The treatment of foreign terror suspects. *Modern L Rev.* 2007;70:427–457, 446.
59. Human Rights Watch. "Diplomatic Assurances" against Torture: Questions and Answers. 10 Nov 2006. https://www.hrw.org/news/2006/11/10/diplomatic-assurances-against-torture
60. *Othman v. UK* (2012) 55 EHRR 1.
61. Ibid., para. 164.
62. Jones K. Deportations with assurances: Addressing key criticisms. *Intl Compar L Q.* 2008;57:183–194.
63. Ibid.
64. Ibid.
65. *Othman v. UK* (2012) 55 EHRR 1, paras. 186–196.
66. Ibid., paras. 194, 203.
67. Ibid.
68. Ibid., para. 260.
69. UK/Jordan. *Treaty on Mutual Legal Assistance in Criminal Matters between the United Kingdom of Great Britain and Northern Ireland and the Hashemite Kingdom of Jordan.* Cm 8612. London: Stationery Office; 2013.
70. Anderson D, Walker C. *Deportation with Assurances.* Cm 9462. London: Stationery Office; 2017:30.
71. Ibid.
72. Walker. The treatment of foreign terror suspects. See also Grozdanova R. The United Kingdom and diplomatic assurances: A minimalist approach towards the anti-torture norm. *Intl Crim L Rev.* 2015;15:369–395.
73. Anderson, Walker. *Deportation with Assurances.*
74. BBC News. Abu Qatada case has cost UK £1.7m, home secretary says. 14 Jun 2013. https://www.bbc.co.uk/news/uk-22909465
75. Anderson, Walker C. *Deportation with Assurances*, at 92.
76. HM Government. *Review of Counter-Terrorism and Security Powers: Review Findings and Recommendations.* Cm 8004. London: Stationery Office; 2011.
77. Anti-terrorism, Crime and Security Act 2001, Part IV.
78. *A (& others) v. Secretary of State for the Home Department* [2004] UKHL 56.
79. Prevention of Terrorism Act 2005.
80. Terrorism Prevention and Investigation Measures Act 2011.
81. Allen G, Dempsey N. Terrorism in Great Britain: The statistics. House of Commons Library briefing paper number CBP7613; 2018.
82. Anderson D. *Terrorism Prevention and Investigation Measures in 2014: Third Report of the Independent Reviewer on the Operation of the Terrorism Prevention and Investigation Measures Act 2011.* London: Stationery Office; 2015:20.
83. HM Government. *Review of Counter-Terrorism and Security Powers*, at 6.
84. *Secretary of State for the Home Department v. BM* [2012] EWHC 714 (Admin).
85. Terrorism Prevention and Investigation Measures Act 2011, Schedule 1.
86. HM Government. *Review of Counter-Terrorism and Security Powers.*
87. Anderson D. *Terrorism Prevention and Investigation Measures in 2012: First Report of the Independent Reviewer on the Operation of the Terrorism Prevention and Investigation Measures Act 2011.* London: Stationery Office; 2013:48, 50.
88. Ibid.
89. Anderson D. *Terrorism Prevention and Investigation Measures in 2013: Second Report of the Independent Reviewer on the Operation of the Terrorism Prevention and Investigation Measures Act 2011.* London: The Stationery Office; 2014 Ibid.
90. Joint Committee on Human Rights. *Legislative Scrutiny: Counter-Terrorism and Security Bill. Fifth Report of Session 2014–15.* London: Stationery Office; 2015:20.
91. Javid S. Terrorism prevention and investigation measures: March–May 2018. House of Commons Written Statement. HCWS851. 12 July 2018.
92. Terrorism Prevention and Investigation Measures Act 2011, s. 3.
93. Anderson D. *Control Orders in 2011. Final Report of the Independent Reviewer on the Prevention of Terrorism Act 2005.* London: Stationery Office; 2012.
94. HM Government. *Review of Counter-Terrorism and Security Powers*, at 41.

95. Anderson. *Terrorism Prevention and Investigation Measures in 2012.*

96. Carlile A. *Fifth Report of the Independent Reviewer Pursuant to Section 14(3) of the Prevention of Terrorism Act 2005.* London: Stationery Office; 2010:44.

97. Anderson. *Terrorism Prevention and Investigation Measures in 2013,* at 55.

98. Ibid., at 30.

99. Anderson. *Terrorism Prevention and Investigation Measures in 2012,* at 96.

100. Anderson. *Terrorism Prevention and Investigation Measures in 2014.*

101. Joint Committee on Human Rights. *Legislative Scrutiny: Counter-Terrorism and Security Bill. Fifth Report of Session 2014–15.* London: Stationery Office;2015

102. Terrorism Prevention and Investigation Measures Act 2011, s 2

103. Anderson. *Terrorism Prevention and Investigation Measures in 2014.*

104. Terrorism Prevention and Investigation Measures Act 2011, Schedule 4.

105. *Secretary of State for the Home Department v. AF* [2009] UKHL 28, para. 59.

106. Civil Procedure Rules, Part 80.

107. Macdonald S, Carlile A. Disrupting terrorist activity: What are the limits to criminal methods of disruption? In Juss S, ed. *Beyond Human Rights and the War on Terror.* Abingdon: Routledge; 2018:125–142.

108. Joint Committee on Human Rights. *Counter-Terrorism Policy and Human Rights: 28 Days, Intercept and Post-Charge Questioning.* Nineteenth Report of Session 2006-07. London: Stationery Office; 2007:53

109. McCullough A, Chamberlain M, Sadiq T, et al. Justice and Security Green Paper: Response to consultation from special advocates. 16 Dec 2011, para 15.

110. Terrorism Prevention and Investigation Measures Act 2011, s 21.

111. Macdonald S. The role of the courts in imposing terrorism prevention and investigation measures: Normative duality and legal realism. *Crim Law Philosophy.* 2015;9:265–283.

112. Ip J. The rise and spread of the special advocate. *Public Law.* 2008:717–741.

113. Macdonald S. Cyberterrorism and enemy criminal law. In Ohlin J, Govern K, Finkelstein C, eds., *Cyberwar: Law and Ethics for Virtual Conflicts.* Oxford: Oxford University Press; 2015:57–75.

114. de Goede M, de Graaf B. Sentencing risk: Temporality and precaution in terrorism trials. *Intl Pol Sociol.* 2013;7:313–331, at 328.

115. Macdonald. Cyberterrorism and enemy criminal law.

19

Lone-Actor Terrorism

Understanding Online Indoctrination

STEVEN HASSAN, JON CAVEN-ATACK, MANSI J. SHAH, AND
SIMRAN MALHOTRA

INTRODUCTION

Our concern is whether the psychological pressures experienced by members of destructive cults[1] also apply to fringe or lone-actor terrorists. In particular, we explore the influence of virtual societies and how they can groom and indoctrinate followers to take violent action. We contend that the "echo chamber" effect of the internet allows extremist and anti-social groups to promulgate messages that significantly increase the possibility of lone-terrorist acts. This chapter views such extremist and anti-social groups through the lens of destructive cults. We set out to judge them using cult mind control (or "brainwashing") models developed over the past seven decades. Destructive cult groups have an authoritarian structure. Cult dogma cannot be questioned. Once a "cultic" principle has been adopted, the believer becomes "impure" if it is not scrupulously followed.[2] We call such behavior "cult-like." We consider the cases of Elliot Rodger and Dylann Roof, assessing their behavior against Hassan's[3,4] Behavior, Information, Thought, Emotion (BITE) model of authoritarian control. This model analyzes a destructive cult's control of behavior, information, thought, and emotion in a destructive cult. We also consider insights from the work of psychiatrist Robert Jay Lifton[5] in his study of thought reform in China. Lifton's criteria include milieu control, loaded language, demand for purity, confession, mystical manipulation, doctrine over person (or ideology over experience), sacred science, and dispensing of existence.

ELLIOT RODGER

Elliot Rodger grew up in California in an affluent family. On May 23, 2014, he killed six people and injured numerous others in Isla Vista, California, before killing himself.[6] Rodger had a complicated past that involved a diagnosis of Asperger's syndrome, being bullied in school, and social isolation.[7] Isolation is a crucial factor of involvement in a destructive cult group: information control becomes self-motivated, with the rejection of other points of view and immersion in a separate world. Rodger escaped into the game World of Warcraft, and later into the *Song of Ice and Fire* books which are devoted to revenge and punishment. His relationship to the World of Warcraft became compulsive. Through his YouTube[8] vlog channel Rodger explained his refusal to take prescription risperidone, an anti-psychotic used to lessen irritability and aggression. Rodger posted videos on his channel in the weeks before the attack, explaining his murderous intent.[9] He had also worked on a manifesto that shows a familiarity with the *loaded language*[10] of "incel" or involuntary celibacy forums online, where participants speak of taking the "red pill"—from *The Matrix* (movie)—to wake up to the truth, or the "black pill," to achieve male dominance.

DYLANN ROOF

Dylann Storm Roof killed nine African Americans during a service at the Emanuel African Methodist Episcopal Church in Charleston, South Carolina, on June 17, 2015. Roof later confessed he had hoped to ignite a race war.[11] Roof's website, *The Last Rhodesian*, demonstrates his misguided view of history and his racist beliefs.[12] Like Rodger's, Roof's manifesto[13] was available online before he committed his crimes. In the manifesto, Roof insisted that he was not raised in a racist environment. He claims that he was "awakened" by the fatal shooting of Trayvon Martin,[14] in 2012, by George Zimmerman while on neighborhood watch. Zimmerman was a man of mixed race who described himself as "Hispanic," but Roof believed him to be white. Roof was 17, the same age as victim Trayvon Martin. In *The Last Rhodesian,* Roof made racist statements about Blacks, Hispanics, and Jews. His remarks ranged from referring to them as "enemies," to motivating others to "destroy" their identities, and claiming that segregation was necessary to protect whites. Roof also had an eccentric view of patriotism: "I hate the sight of the American flag. Modern American patriotism is an absolute joke. People pretending like they have something to be proud [sic] while White people are being murdered daily in the streets." While his internet research appears to have been the primary cause for Roof's "awakening," he was also motivated by the violent Japanese drama, *Himizu,* set after the Fukushima tsunami of 2011. He said the film was his "favorite" and cites a line spoken by the protagonist before he begins his violent rampage: "Even if my life is worth less than a speck of dirt, I want to use it for the good of society." He wrote, "this prompted me to type in 'black on White crime' into Google, and I have never been the same since that day."[15]

Roof ended his manifesto with, "I have no choice. I am not in the position to, alone, go into the ghetto and fight. . . . Well someone has to have the bravery to take it to the real world, and I guess that has to be me."[16]

NIDAL HASAN

In 2003, Nidal Hasan graduated from medical school and entered his internship and residency at Walter Reed National Military Medical Center. This timeframe, from 2003 to early 2009, can be seen as Hasan's "radicalization period."[17] During this time, patterns and indicators of radicalization develop in Hasan's beliefs and behavior. These include increasing isolation from family and colleagues, growing religious conservatism, and the adoption of views typically associated with jihadi-Salafism. These indicators are present in four different areas: his relationships with family members, his interactions with colleagues at Walter Reed, and two separate academic works focusing on Muslim soldiers and their potential religious conflicts with US military involvement in the Middle East. Hasan killed 13 and wounded 32 others at the Fort Hood military post in Killeen, Texas in November 2009. In August 2013 he was sentenced to death.[18]

MODELS FOR UNDERSTANDING MIND CONTROL, THOUGHT REFORM, AND UNDUE INFLUENCE

Elliott Rodger, Dylan Roof, and Nidal Hasan came from different worlds and adopted different dogmas that impelled them to take innocent lives through devotion to their causes. Let us now see how the models used to analyze cultic involvement can be applied to the virtual communities to which these three lone-actor terrorists belonged.

The Influence Continuum

The influence continuum, (see figure 19.1)[19] developed by one of the authors (SH) to explore the dynamics of involvement in destructive cult groups, shows the essential distinctions between ethical and unethical influence. Ethical influence is based on informed consent. No healthy person would join a group with the expectation of being exploited and abused, so no one readily joins a destructive cult. Members do not join with informed consent. They are systematically recruited, as these groups conceal their true nature from prospective recruits.[20] Destructive cults lure members. Information is hidden, distorted, and exaggerated, or outright lies are told. Usually, the recruit will not see the workings of the inner group. The core practices and beliefs are hidden unless and until the recruit has fully attached to the cult. The true nature of the cult is deliberately withheld. A promise of liberation, enlightenment, or a future paradise conceals the intent to enslave.

The World Wide Web has made it possible for hate speech to flourish and for the socially inept to believe misinformation and alluring propaganda, which is heavily weighted toward confirming any existing bias. The echo chamber of the virtual group restricts the believer's perception. An intervention with a cult specialist and a former member might well have averted the violent acts committed by online believers. With an accurate education in history, negative emotions are directed toward reform rather than mass murder. Neither Elliot Rodger nor Dylann Roof showed any devotion to a specific group or individual but rather to a set of beliefs, a dogma, which led to their interpretation of the world and the urge to dispense with the existence of perceived enemies (Lifton's "dispensing of existence").[5] Nidal Hasan had brief contact with al-Qaeda but was radicalized online.[21]

In their beliefs, Rodger and Roof found certainty—the *noetic* quality described by William

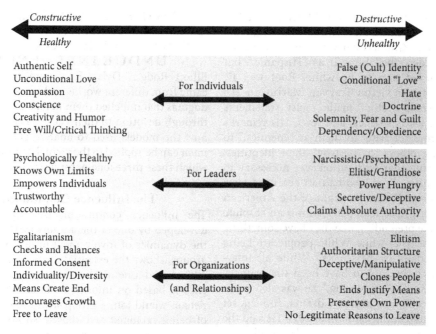

FIGURE 19.1 Influence Continuum

From The Bite Model: Behavior, Information, Thought And Emotional Control

From Combating Cult Mind Control (2015) by Steven Hassan

James[22] and neurologist Robert A. Burton[23]—and that certainty led them to exclude all alternatives to the dogma that came to control their actions. They were convinced of their beliefs because they were misinformed and incited by emotionally alarming discussions online. Noetic certainty is the "feeling of knowing," rather than a certainty based on evidence. On the World Wide Web, destructive cults have developed sophisticated recruiting processes. al-Qaeda and Daesh/Islamic State of Iraq and al-Sham (ISIS) make propaganda videos using themes and story lines from Hollywood movies and video games, including soundtracks, to lure new recruits.[24] They use long-established strategies to create phobia, guilt, and aversion to manipulate beliefs. Non-religious extremist groups also have a significant internet presence.[25] Through smartphones, people can potentially be unduly influenced 24 hours a day. These groups have long urged believers to commit acts of terror and violence without direction. The same is true in many hate communities, including some incel and white nationalist forums.[26]

Destructive Cults

Thousands of destructive cults exist, and these vary from huge international movements to single-member authoritarian relationships.[27] They may differ tremendously in their beliefs but share common features of control. The surrounding culture shapes the group to some extent, but it is always affected by the member's place in the hierarchy. The extent of control varies widely within larger cult groups. There are several significant variables. Those who live communally have a much more controlled experience than "public" members who attend periodic indoctrination sessions. Yet even a "public" member can become a "total convert" despite working outside the cult and being subjected to far less scrutiny than the "staff." Destructive cults often parade celebrity members, but their experience is usually very different and far more comfortable. Live-in members keep quiet about the privations of their often arduous daily lives so as not to discourage fee-paying "public" members.[28] Destructive cults have rules for information control—or "gatekeeping"—including punishing members if they criticize the group in any way, especially if they share negative information. Members are pressured to spy and inform on other members to avoid punishment and retain their own status. Some members will not be "total converts," and the interpretation of the belief system can be strikingly different from

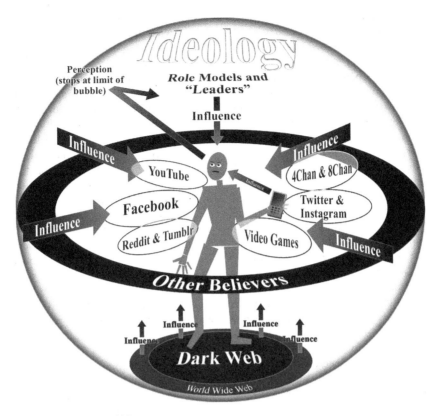

FIGURE 19.2 The Influence Bubble

Graphic by Karin Spike Robinson for Freedom of Mind

one member to another. Quite different interpretations of the world can exist side by side within members' minds in the same destructive cult. Information control usually becomes self-imposed (see figure 19.2).

Elliot Rodger's dogma came from the fantasy worlds of the *Song of Ice and Fire* (where revenge is a constant theme) and World of Warcraft (where punishment is meted out through a safe avatar), admixed with the virtual world created by incels (involuntary celibates) and bounded by his lack of social skills. His connection was to this dogma (Lifton calls this the "text as guru"): it seemed *just* for him to murder as many people as possible in "retribution." In his last video, Rodger acts a role as he punctuates his threats with histrionic laughter. "Day of Retribution" refers to the Judeo-Christian-Islamic idea of a Day of Reckoning, when the damned are punished.[29] Elliot Rodger had perhaps come to believe that this world would end with his own death. He became a solipsistic character in a malevolent fiction.

EVALUATING GROUPS AND SITUATIONS

In his ground-breaking *cognitive dissonance theory*, Festinger[30] showed that beliefs have cognitive, emotional, and behavioral components. The BITE model takes the three components of dissonance (cognitive, affective, and behavioral) and adds information as a fourth overlapping component.[31] Ethical influence always encourages the recipient to develop an internal locus of control within their authentic/autonomous personality. Subjected to undue influence or coercive control, the cult-identity dominates the authentic/autonomous personality, and the individual accepts direction from the outside, so the locus of control moves to the dogma of the cult. As Erich Fromm said, a "pseudo-identity" supplants the authentic self, and all actions are judged according to compliance with social expectations.[32] Elliot Rodger's videos make it clear that he had developed a dramatic persona—a pseudo-identity—for his videos.

BITE Model: Behavior Control

Obedience to the group and dependency on its dogma and leadership are the essential criteria of behavior control. Without explicit permission, a follower who acts independently will face criticism and even punishment. Freedom of movement may be restricted, and communication with nonbelievers may require permission. Individualism is frowned upon, and surrender to the group or its "God" (as interpreted by the leader) is demanded. Strict rules are enforced. Certain thoughts, feelings, and activities are censured and must be reported to superiors. The group may demand conformity in appearance, dress, or hairstyle. Behavior control often includes a restricted diet. Many live-in members will subsist on a high-carbohydrate diet. Some groups enforce a regime of fasting for days on end, which can lead to hallucinations and depersonalization or derealization.

Behavior is judged according to the cult's tenets: "good" behavior is praised and rewarded (especially bringing in new recruits, and even more so when bringing in wealthy new recruits), and "bad" behavior is criticized (often in front of other members) and punished. Virtual groups and online societies are often bound together by belief in a set of ideas rather than devotion to a charismatic leader. Members will tend to conform their behavior to group norms. Where groups propose violence, violent behavior becomes acceptable and even laudable. Both Elliot Rodger and Dylann Roof seemed to be immature and came to view their virtual groups as true family (a frequent notion in destructive cults: Sun Myung Moon, for instance, called himself "True Father").[33] They felt compelled to act out the inclinations fostered by their membership in extremist communities they found through the World Wide Web.

Information Control

An authoritarian group or individual uses information to exploit others. It is important to differentiate ethical and unethical use of information: an honest, ethical group is open about its beliefs, its history, and its expectations of a new member. Military recruits know that they may have to risk their lives. An ethical religion openly explains cultural restrictions—for instance, abstinence from pork or beef, or from any meat or animal products. An unethical group or individual will restrict, distort, or conceal important information, if not simply lie. Moonies use "heavenly deception," citing Jacob's deception of his father Isaac to receive a blessing.[34] Jehovah's Witnesses use the story of Rahab's protection of Israelite spies as a justification for deception.[35] The leaders decide what information members should have (also known as "gatekeeping"). Members are often persuaded to spy on other members and anyone critical of the group, including friends and family. In Scientology, "knowledge reports" are filed about any deviation from group "policy."[36] Any thought, feeling, or activity that deviates from the group's beliefs must be reported. Destructive cults are expert at propaganda. Web sites and videos are available every minute of the day; meetings are often livestreamed to followers. Large destructive cults have departments devoted to the production of every form of media, from traditional print to podcasts and apps. Many web-based groups influence their followers with such distorted material, and Rodger and Roof were clearly influenced in this way.

Independent thinking relies on access to reputable sources and the ability to determine which are credible and to make free choices. Both Rodger and Roof clearly lacked these skills. Destructive cults indoctrinate members to dismiss any negative report. Some groups forbid all public media sources. Aversion is aroused, so that members will not consider anything hostile to the group. Often, members are kept so busy that they simply have no time to read anything beyond the group's material or spend time with anyone who might question the group's beliefs. This creates an echo chamber where only material that reinforces group beliefs is ever studied. This "echo chamber" phenomenon is particularly important in studying people radicalized or recruited through the internet. Groups may control believers through frequent texting, calls, or even through their cell phones' GPS tracking. Scientology was criticized for sending out programs that included "net nannies" preventing access to critical web sites.[37,38] The echo chamber of the World Wide Web makes it possible for untrained minds to exclude or ignore differing opinions and evidence. Dylann Roof was profoundly misinformed but unwilling to check accepted historical sources. A review of Thomas Thistlewood's diaries[39] would have given him a far better idea of the horrific and inhuman punishments suffered by African slaves. Information control is often self-imposed: members of destructive cults may refuse to study any material that criticizes the group's dogma.

Thought Control

There are many thought control techniques. Hours of monotonous lectures can reduce critical, independent thinking. Cult lectures may be peppered with obscure or invented terms, and followers may have to memorize and regurgitate lists of information without any appeal to their understanding or practical application. Repetitive prayers, mantra chanting, speaking in tongues, rocking back and forth, or long periods of motionless silence can all induce altered states where analytical thinking and rational evaluation is inhibited. Repetition, fixation, and mimicry all tend to override critical skills. Destructive cults also use techniques that induce euphoria and elation. Visualization and "guided meditation" techniques tend to heighten suggestibility so that thoughts and beliefs can be implanted into followers.[40] Typically, destructive, authoritarian cults demand polarized thinking: everything is all-or-nothing, black or white, us versus them, and good versus evil: there are no shades of gray. The group's dogma is seen as the ultimate "Truth" and is considered both sacred and scientific (Lifton's "sacred science"[5]). Believers are armored against criticism through self-activated "thought-stopping" techniques. They are taught that this will keep them pure and safe from "evil" thoughts or influences. Krishna devotees are taught to chant the "Hare Krishna" mantra to drown out the world and any intellectual conflict.[41,42] Destructive cults close themselves off from the world with "loaded language,"[5] which can be incomprehensible to outsiders. Because our conceptual thinking is mediated by language, this can make it nearly impossible to think coherently or critically.

Elliot Rodger accepted the concepts of the blue, red, and black pills. Men who failed to share his belief in the inferiority of women were "betas."[43] Such "loaded language" is easily used to develop "thought-terminating cliches,"[5,44] to confine and restrict thought.

A destructive cult avoids or forbids any doubt or questioning about the leadership or group dogma. Any deviation from the teaching is viewed as a failure of faith. Followers are discouraged from critical thinking, and even constructive criticism is considered sinful or immoral. Other belief systems are dismissed as flawed, evil, or damaging. Empirical thinking and scientific analysis are rejected. Both Rodger and Roof developed rigid beliefs that were impervious to correction. They became certain that their information and their insights were beyond question. Having had social difficulties and been rejected by the few women he had approached, Rodger came to view women as enemies to men such as himself—the "incels." Dylann Roof accepted racist propaganda

as the truth—for instance, believing that black slaves wanted to be dependent on their white masters.[45]

As with information control, thought control is often self-imposed. Believers exclude thoughts that question the dogma they have come to accept. This closed-minded approach is to some extent a consequence of our educational institutions' obsession with memorizing data over developing critical thinking or intelligent disobedience. Roof accepted malign and false information about non-Caucasians because he believed in the authority of the websites he visited.[46] Rodger believed the rantings of misogynists without consulting better-informed sources.[47]

Emotional Control

Recruiters use flattery or "love-bombing" (a Moonie expression)[48] to create an emotional bond. The recruiter feels like a new best friend and offers an attractive vision of the group. As an al-Qaeda recruiting manual[49] says, "Don't criticize the candidate's behavior. Thank him for any help, even if it is just a little. Caution: don't disregard his opinion or his manner of thinking but let him express his opinion even if it opposes yours. . . . Be close to him in order to get to know more about his character."

Rodger and Roof both came to feel an emotional sense of belonging to their chosen online groups even though they did not meet their fellow believers in person or develop real-world relationships with them. In Rodger, this is a development of his isolated immersion in fantasy novels and the World of Warcraft. Both young men had dissociated from the world around them to take on roles in a fantasy world—a world that they could control.

Rodger was distressed when he left his online gaming, as he admits about a holiday in Morocco.[50] His emotional well-being depended on connection to that virtual world. This is comparable to the separation anxiety experienced by members of destructive cults when removed from their environments or teachings.

Membership of a destructive cult is maintained by creating frustration and dependency. Self-esteem is based on devotion to the leadership, the group, and the dogma rather than individual achievements. Guilt, fear (Hassan, 1988)[51] and aversion, or disgust (Atack, 2015, 2018)[52] are the three most frequently used emotional control techniques.

Phobia induction and indoctrination is found in all destructive cults (Hassan, 1988, 2000, 2012, 2018;[53,54,55,56] Lalich and Tobias 1994, 2006).[57,58]

Beset by phobias, followers find normal functioning impossible. They become dependent on the group and its teachings to protect them from the very fears that the group's dogma instills. These phobias create a pathway through which a destructive cult can introduce programed responses and create the overwhelming belief that life outside the group is impossible. Rodger and Roof took this sense of belonging to the extreme: they remained loyal to their beliefs by committing murder. Rodger took his own life, and Roof became a hero in the world of his followers, the Bowl Gang.[59] Both young men avoided anyone who might challenge their beliefs by isolating themselves in the virtual world of extremist communities online. They acted out the disgust nurtured in such forums. Rodger believed that through his actions he would show *all* women their error in rejecting him. Roof believed that he would incite a race war through his attack on innocent churchgoers. Guilt keeps the believer's attention inwardly focused. It changes the usual fundamental attribution error, whereby most people justify their own shortcomings through extenuating circumstances but believe others are deliberately falling short. In a destructive cult, this error justifies the group's excesses and magnifies the member's shortcomings. Many groups teach that we are entirely responsible for everything that happens to us, so even catching a cold can be seen as an implication of guilt.

The jargon of the incel movement can be considered a "loaded language,"[5] which interferes with rational thought and allows the ideas of incel media to limit and control thinking, so following the thought control aspect of the BITE model. The echo chamber limits access to helpful information and creates a dogma where differing ideas are scorned and rejected, also in line with the control of information.

CONCLUSION

Several works in recent years have explored the potentially harmful impact of social media on human behaviors. The documentary "The Social Dilemma" explores how the internet's most powerful companies track users' behavior in order to create targeted ads and induce addiction in a vicious cycle.[60,61] The film blends interviews with tech experts, including many former employees of Silicon Valley giants, and public service announcement-style dramatic scenarios illustrating the potential negative effects of social media on average Americans. Among the many issues the film touches on include how tech companies

have influenced elections, ethnic violence, and rates of depression and suicide. "The Great Hack" shows how strategic communications laboratories used data from 87 million Facebook users to influence the election of Donald Trump and the UK's Brexit campaign.[62]

The development of the World Wide Web has created both opportunities and challenges in this new century. The echo chamber of social media can perpetuate hatred: "Within the past two years, a number of zealous Roof fans and would-be copycats have emerged, including some who have crossed the line into criminal activity," Anti-Defamation League researchers say.[63] They list four individuals possibly inspired by Roof who were arrested before committing an attack. One of them said he wanted to "pull a Dylann Roof" and "make the news some more and shoot some Jews." Roof also inspired a following of adherents to his beliefs, who call themselves the "Bowl Gang": a reference to Roof's distinctive haircut.[64] Bowl Gang members spend time on social media sites like Gab,[65] spreading slogans like "Dylann Roof did nothing wrong" through memes with pictures of Roof's face set against a halo. Their posts encourage others to commit violent acts. One of those arrested for threats of violence used the online handle "DC Bowl Gang" (he lived in Washington, DC). He had praised the Pittsburgh synagogue shooter and gathered a stockpile of illegal weapons; he made threats to a journalist and had become progressively more extreme after his brother's suicide in October 2018. He was reported by his family, and the FBI arrested him.[66]

We need to be concerned about the relationships between online subcultures, extremism, and violent copycat incidents. Lone-actor terrorism is extraordinarily difficult to prevent. The cult-like influence of some online subcultures makes it highly likely that there will be more copycat attacks—just as Elliot Rodger followed in the footsteps of George Sodini.[67] Research by the counterextremism group Hope Not Hate found that children as young as 13 are becoming involved in a new wave of groups that are gathering support online: "The threat of far-right terrorism comes from both organised groups, like National Action, but increasingly from lone actors who get radicalised on the internet."[68]

Both Elliot Rodger and Dylann Roof would have benefited from critical thinking skills. It is vital that young people learn about methods of recruitment and the emotional manipulations common to destructive cults and other radical groups. Understanding cognitive dissonance and cognitive biases and our susceptibility to manipulation through heightened emotions could help to safeguard the next generation from involvement in antisocial groups and other toxic relationships.

Robert Jay Lifton's model of thought reform,[69] Robert Cialdini's[70] points of influence, the influence continuum, and the BITE model foster a more cautious—and sensible—approach to the many specious ideas that lead to antisocial behavior.

NOTES AND REFERENCES

1. We use the Shorter Oxford Dictionary definition of the term "cult": "Devotion to a particular person or thing, now especially as paid by a body of professed adherents." We do not consider the term pejorative, so are only concerned with "destructive" cults.
2. The demand for purity, one of Robert Jay Lifton's "eight deadly sins of thought reform" is discussed later in this chapter.
3. Hassan SA. *Combatting Cult Mind Control: The #1 Best-Selling Guide to Protection, Rescue, and Recovery from Destructive Cults.* Randolph, VT: Park Street Press; 1988.
4. Hassan SA. The BITE model of authoritarian control: Undue influence, thought reform, brainwashing, mind control, trafficking and the law. In press. 2020.
5. Lifton RJ. *Thought Reform and the Psychology of Totalism.* New York: Norton; 1961.
6. NBC News. California shooting suspect Elliot Rodgers life rage and resentment. 25 May 2014. https://www.nbcnews.com/storyline/isla-vista-rampage/california-shooting-suspect-elliot-rodgers-life-rage-resentment-n113996
7. Freedom of Mind. Asperger's/autism spectrum disorder and undue influence. https://freedomofmind.com/aspergers-autism-spectrum-disorder-and-undue-influence/
8. ABC News. Alleged gunman Elliot Rodger used his Youtube channel as a manifesto. 26 May 2014. https://www.youtube.com/watch?v=MQdAwSq9PiM&ab_channel=ABCNews
9. Rodger E. My twisted world: The story of Elliot Rodger. 2016.
10. Lifton. *Thought Reform.*
11. Block M. Dylann Roof said he wanted to start a race war, friends say. NPR, 19 Jun 2015. https://www.npr.org/2015/06/19/415809511/dylann-roof-said-he-wanted-to-start-a-race-war-friends-say
12. Neuman S. Photos of Dylann Roof, racist manifesto surface on website. NPR, 20 Jun 2015. https://www.npr.org/sections/thetwo-way/2015/06/20/416024920/photos-possible-manifesto-of-dylann-roof-surface-on-website
13. Robles F. Dylann Roof photos and a manifesto are posted on website. *New York Times,* 21 2015.
14. Hersher R. What happened when Dylann Roof asked google for information about race? NPR, 10 Jan 2017. https://www.npr.org/sections/thetwo-way/2017/01/10/508363607/what-happened-when-dylann-roof-asked-google-for-information-about-race
15. McWilliams J. Dylann Roof's fateful google search. *Pacific Standard,* 2 Jul 2018. https://psmag.com/news/dylann-roof-google-algorithms
16. Morgan D. Dylann Roof's Manifesto: "I have no choice." CBS News, 20 Jun 2015. https://www.cbsnews.com/news/dylann-roofs-manifesto-i-have-no-choice/
17. Poppe K. Nidal Hasan: A case study in lone-actor terrorism. 2018.
18. History.com Editors. Army major kills 13 people in Fort Hood shooting spree. History, 2 Jun 2011. https://www.history.com/this-day-in-history/army-major-kills-13-people-in-fort-hood-shooting-spree
19. Hassan. *Combatting Cult Mind Control.*
20. Atack J. *Scientology: The Cult of Greed.* Colchester, UK: Trentvalley Ltd.; 2014; Atack J. *Opening Minds: The Secret World of Manipulation, Undue Influence, and Brainwashing.* Colchester, UK: Trentvalley; 2013, 2016. 2018.
21. Poppe. Nidal Hasan.
22. James W. Varieties of Religious Experience.
23. Burton RA. *On Being Certain: Believing You Are Right Even When You're Not.* New York: St Martins; 2008
24. Hassan. *Combatting Cult Mind Control..*
25. Adam GK. *A Space for Hate: The White Power Movement's Adaptation into Cyberspace.* Duluth, MN: Litwin Books; 2009:217. ISBN 978-1-936117-07-9.
26. Waśniewska M. *The Red Pill, Unicorns and White Knights: Cultural Symbolism and Conceptual Metaphor in the Slang of Online Incel Communities*; 2020.
27. Singer MT, Lalich J. *Cults in Our Midst: The Hidden Menace in Our Everyday Lives.* San Francisco, CA: Jossey-Bass; 1995.
28. Hassan. *Combatting Cult Mind Control.*
29. Jeremiah 46:10, for instance.
30. Festinger L. *A Theory of Cognitive Dissonance.* Stanford, CA: Stanford University Press; 1957.
31. Hassan SA, Shah MJ. The anatomy of undue influence used by terrorist cults and traffickers to induce helplessness and trauma, so creating false identities. *Ethics Med Public Health.* 2019;8:97–107. https://doi.org/10.1016/j.jemep.2019.03.002
32. Fromm E. *Escape from Freedom.* New York: Ishi Press; 1941, 2011.
33. Hassan. *Combatting Cult Mind Control..*
34. Ibid.
35. Ibid.

36. Atack J. *Let's Sell These People a Piece of Blue Sky.* Colchester, UK: Lyle Stuart; 1990, 2018.

37. Xenu. Church of Scientology censors net access for members. https://www.xenu.net/archive/events/censorship/

38. Scientology Inc. Internet Nannies. Mark Rathbun, 2012/May 2019. https://markrathbun.blog/2012/05/29/scientology-inc-internet-nannies/.

39. World Heritage Encyclopedia. Thomas Thistlewood. Project Gutenberg. http://self.gutenberg.org/articles/thomas_thistlewood.

40. Hassan S. *Freedom of Mind: Helping Loved Ones Leave Controlling People, Cults, and Beliefs.* Newton, MA: Freedom of Mind Press: 2012.

41. Muster NJ. *Betrayal of the Spirit: My Life Behind the Headlines of the Hare Krishna Movement.* Foreword by Larry D. Shinn. Bloomington: University of Illinois Press; 2001. https://www-jstor-org.fgul.idm.oclc.org/stable/10.5406/j.ctt5hjjjv

42. Bryant E, Ekstrand M, eds. *The Hare Krishna Movement: The Postcharismatic Fate of a Religious Transplant.* New York: Columbia University Press; 2004.

43. Beauchamp Z. Our incel problem: How a support group for the dateless become one of the internet's dangerous subcultures. Zack Beauchamp. Vox, 23 Apr 2019. https://www.vox.com/the-highlight/2019/4/16/18287446/incel-definition-reddit

44. Lifton. *Thought Reform.*

45. Beauchamp Z. An online subculture celebrating the Charleston church shooter appears to be inspiring copycat plots: Inside the online group that treats a racist killer like a saint. *Vox,* Feb 2019. https://www.vox.com/policy-and-politics/2019/2/7/18215634/dylann-roof-charleston-church-shooter-bowl-gang

46. Hersher. What happened.

47. BBC News. Elliot Rodger: How misogynist killer became "incel hero." 25 Apr 2018. https://www.bbc.com/news/world-us-canada-43892189

48. Hassan. *Combatting Cult Mind Control.*

49. Al Qa'idy A. A course in the art of recruiting. No publisher; undated.

50. DailyMail.com. Nick Cravan. 24 May 2014. https://www.dailymail.co.uk/news/article-2638427/He-disturbed-boy-British-grandmother-Santa-Barbara-mass-killer-boy-grew-Hollywood-royalty-posted-chilling-blogs-vowing-revenge-against-women-rejected-him.html

51. Hassan. *Combatting Cult Mind Control..*

52. Atack. *Opening Minds.*

53. Hassan. *Combating Cult Mind Control .*

54. Hassan S. *Releasing the Bonds: Empowering People to Think for Themselves.* Newton, MA: Freedom of Mind Press; 2000.

55. Hassan. *Freedom of Mind.*

56. Hassan. *Combatting Cult Mind Control.*

57. Ibid.

58. Atack. *Opening Minds.*

59. Beauchamp Z. Dylann Roof Charleston church shooter Bowl Gang. Vox.com, 7 Feb 2019. https://www.vox.com/policy-and-politics/2019/2/7/18215634/dylann-roof-charleston-church-shooter-bowl-gang

60. https://www.cnbc.com/2020/09/21/netflix-movie-the-social-dilemma-slams-social-media-review.html

61. Orlowski J. (Director). *The Social Dilemma* [Film]. Exposure Labs; Argent Pictures; The Space Program; 2020.

62. Seadle M. *The Great Hack* [Documentary film]. Produced and directed by Karim Amer and Jehane Noujaim. Netflix. *J Assoc Information Sci Tech.* 2019.

63. Hardcore white supremacists elevate Dylann Roof to cult hero status. Anti-Defamation League. Feb 2019. https://www.adl.org/blog/hardcore-white-supremacists-elevate-dylann-roof-to-cult-hero-status.

64. Ibid.

65. Coaston J. Gab, the social media platform favored by the alleged Pittsburgh shooter, explained. *Vox,* Oct 2018. https://www.vox.com/policy-and-politics/2018/10/29/18033006/gab-social-media-anti-semitism-neo-nazis-twitter-facebook

66. FBI National Press Office. James Comey. 10 Jun 2015. https://www.fbi.gov/news/pressrel/press-releases/statement-by-fbi-director-james-comey-regarding-dylann-roof-gun-purchase

67. Langman P. Role models, contagions, and copycats: An exploration of the influence of prior killers on subsequent attacks. 2017. www.schoolshooters.info

68. Dearden L. How Facebook became one of the far-right's biggest recruitment tools. *Independent,* Apr 2019. https://www.independent.co.uk/news/uk/home-news/facebook-ban-edl-britain-first-tommy-robinson-farright-recruitment-a8876866.html

69. Lifton. *Thought Reform.*

70. Cialdini RB. *Pre-Suasion: A Revolutionary Way to Influence and Persuade.* New York: Simon & Schuster; 2016.

20

Hatred and Grievance as Constructs in Lone-Actor Terrorism

JACOB C. HOLZER, ARYA SHAH, ERIC Y. DROGIN, AND ROBERT P. GRANACHER, JR.

INTRODUCTION

In a broad review of academically based terrorism literature, the terms "hatred" and "grievance" are found but are not prevalent. As emphasized in this book, there are numerous variables that factor into the complex understanding of lone-actor terrorism, including developmental, environmental, ideological, social, criminological, etc. But, following a lone-actor terrorism incident, the concepts of hatred and acting on a grievance are front and center in news reports. This chapter reviews some aspects of hatred and grievance in relation to lone-actor terrorism.

DEFINITIONS AND CONCEPTS

The concepts of hatred and harboring a grievance may factor into many, if not all lone-actor terrorism incidents. "Hatred" can be defined as a strong aversion or dislike. It is fundamentally an emotional experience. There are numerous viewpoints by which to examine hatred. Hatred can be a generic experience at different levels— individually between people; between groups of people; based on geography, religion, or other entities; in the family, social, or occupational settings; between societies, regions, or countries, etc. It can be a fleeting emotion, as one would experience after a disagreement, or it can be chronic and pervasive. And it can vary in intensity, between a mild dislike and an extreme animosity. At times, hatred can evolve and move a relationship in a positive direction or become entrenched.

"Lone-actor terrorism," as defined in this volume, is the planning or commission of violence by one or two individuals outside of the command and control structure of an organized group.

Although a group may not be formally involved, the individual(s) may get informal direction or support through the use of social media. For purposes of this volume, the lone-actor is linked to a radicalized or extremist cause or ideology, which can vary across different political, extremist religious, geographic, single-issue, or other spectrums. A "hate crime" has a different definition. As described in the Hate Crimes section of the FBI website, a hate crime is defined as a "criminal offense against a person or property motivated in whole or in part by an offender's bias against a race, religion, disability, sexual orientation, ethnicity, gender, or gender identity." The FBI point out that hate itself is not criminal and that it is important to be mindful of the freedom of speech and other civil liberties in our society.[1]

Despite the divergence in these definitions, there is broad overlap. The complexity of understanding this relationship between lone-actor terrorism and hate/grievance is described in detail in a report by the National Consortium for the Study of Terrorism and Responses to Terrorism (START), where lone-actor terrorism and hate crimes have both overlapping and distinguishing features. Their report to the US Dept. of Homeland Security (DHS) describes several important findings: (a) lone-actor terrorism and violent hate crimes are not exactly the same, although they have similarities; (b) there is no correlation in occurrence between lone-actor terrorism events and violent hate crimes from year to year; (c) the amount of lone-actor terrorism in less populated states is greater than the amount of hate crimes; (d) at the county level, both lone-actor terrorism and hate crimes are more likely to occur in larger populations, where there is lower home ownership rates and higher percentages of non-Hispanic whites; (e) unlike violent hate crimes, lone-actor terrorism is not more likely in counties with higher percentages of residents in urban areas, higher percentages of teen/young adult male residents, or higher unemployment rates; and (f) where lone-actor terrorism occurs shares more demographically with locations of violent hate crimes, both in comparison to group-based terrorism.[2] The START report does stress common features: hate crime offenders are rarely part of an organized group and each type of behavior (lone-actor terrorism and violent hate crime) expresses a bias or intolerance against a target or what the target stands for. Some researchers have described hate crimes as strongly related to the extremist white supremacist movement, in which it is viewed that hate crimes are a type of leaderless resistance that shares a similarity with lone-actor terrorism.[2]

An important argument in considering how these two concepts merge is made by Daniel Byman in an article in *Foreign Policy*.[3] Byman points out that, after the 9/11 attacks, US focus was on foreign Islamist threats and that far less attention was given to far-right domestic groups, in part bolstered by First Amendment. In addition, there is no official US counterterrorism or legal response at the federal level to domestic threats or acts in the same context as the response to foreign terrorist threats, where the former may be handled at the local or state level. Byman makes a persuasive argument that, by considering far-right (and other) domestic violent groups as equivalent to foreign groups, several outcomes would be achieved: (1) more law enforcement budgetary resources at the federal level, (2) a faster and more robust law enforcement response if domestic individuals or groups were considered terrorists without the backdrop of First and Second Amendment protections, and (3) a clarity that could support technology companies in intervening in domestic group incitement in social media.

When one examines hatred and grievance in individual lone-actor cases, the pervasiveness of these concepts becomes clear. Byman points out in his *Foreign Policy* article that the Pittsburgh Tree of Life synagogue attacker posted hateful anti-Semitic content on social media.[3,4] Similarly, Cesar Sayoc, who was convicted of mailing pipe bombs to Democratic politicians and others he saw as "enemies" of President Trump, acted out of hatred.[5] In an examination of the case studies in chapter 2 volume, many had a prominent component of hatred or harboring a grievance that factored into the case incident. Anders Breivik harbored anti-Muslim and anti-feminist views, and his writings before the attacks were described as a "policy of hatred" for anything non-Nordic.[6,7] Ismaaiyl Brinsley harbored a hatred and grievance against the police, in retribution for the police killings of Michael Brown and Eric Garner.[8] James von Brunn, who was virulently anti-Jewish and anti-black,[9] had a history of hatred which he expressed on a website.[10] Baruch Goldstein had a manifest hatred of Arabs, and it was reported that, as a physician, he refused to treat Palestinians.[11] James Alex Fields Jr., who on August 12, 2017, drove his car into a crowd of people peacefully protesting the Unite the Right rally in Charlottesville, Virginia., killing one person and injuring more than two dozen, was reported as having committed a hate-inspired act of domestic terrorism by the US Attorney. Fields expressed and promoted white supremacy, the views of Nazism and Hitler, and advocated violence against members of racial, ethnic, and religious groups he perceived to be non-white.[12] Although on the surface holding a strong hatred or harboring a grievance may seem like the predominant motivation in lone-actor incidents, the underlying context may be more complex. An example of this complexity may be found in the Nidal Hasan case, where some reports indicated he held a personal grievance against the military for his potential deployment to fight a war he morally opposed. Katharine Poppe, in a case study of Nidal Hasan, described a confluence of three variables that may factor into the terrorism incident: the radicalization process, the primacy of religion and ideology in shaping his worldview and pushing him toward violence, and his relationship with Anwar al-Awlaki.[13] Hatred and harboring a grievance may be a necessary but insufficient variable in some lone-actor cases.

CLINICAL AND CONTEXTUAL BASIS

Hatred in the context of interpersonal violence has been a topic of great interest in forensic literature. Though there has been debate regarding how to legally categorize violence as hate crimes or as terrorism, and though current legal definitions may be biased in how they categorize violence based on the background and ideology of the perpetrator,[14] both forms of violence involve strong negative emotions and targeting of a negatively perceived "other." Individuals involved in acts of mass violence, hate crimes, and lone-actor terrorism have been categorized as engaging in "grievance-fueled violence."[15,16] Such forms of violence have continued to be at the forefront of public attention, with multiple recent examples of individual terrorism and targeted violence (e.g., the mass shooting at a Pittsburgh synagogue by a man named Robert Bowers and the mailing of 14 explosive devices by Cesar Sayoc, a supporter of President Trump, to multiple politicians of the opposition) continuing to drive research on the role of hate in motivating violence. Experts have posited that recognizing the role of hate in acts of terror and violence represents an urgent population health issue influencing the safety of all.[17]

The study of the psychological components of hate is relevant to understanding the actions of lone-actor terrorists for whom hatred in the form of personal grievance and moral outrage are felt to be major contributors to acts of violence. The Terrorist Radicalization Assessment Protocol (TRAP-18) represents a tool to assess risk of violence in individuals with extreme beliefs. This tool was developed to include 8 "warning behaviors" and 10 "distal characteristics" of lone terrorists, all of which were developed based on research and expert consensus. Among these distal characteristics is the category of "personal grievance and moral outrage" occurring in relation to life experience, loss, and difference of fundamental beliefs. In one analysis using the TRAP-18 to evaluate the actions of 111 lone terrorists in the United States and Europe,[18] this personal grievance and moral outrage category included feelings of being "degraded," "ignored or treated poorly," "lied to," and "disrespected," as well as being "the target of an act of prejudice/unfairness," "the victim of verbal or physical assault," "recently unemployed," or having recently "experienced financial problems." Of all analyzed individuals in this study, the prevalence of personal grievance and moral outrage in relation to act an of terror was found to be 78% overall. The concepts of "personal grievance" and "moral outrage" have continued to be studied in a literature aiming to better understand the actions of lone-actor terrorists.

Personal Grievance

In 2015, Hamm and Spaag analyzed 98 cases of lone-actor terror in the United States using the American Lone Wolf Terrorism Database; their findings led them to conclude that lone terrorists "feel deprived of what they perceive as values to which they are entitled, and form grievances against the government responsible for their unemployment, discrimination and injustices."[19]

Fox and colleagues describe common sources of interpersonal grievance as including loss of employment, financial difficulties, marital stress, and bullying; furthermore, sudden separation, loss, or termination can exacerbate existing feelings of victimization and ultimately precipitate acts of violence.[20-22] Levin and Madfis present the example of perpetrators of workplace massacres as feeling "entitled" to promotions they never received and of feeling that their contributions to their employer have gone unappreciated.[23]

Moral Outrage

Personal grievance has found to frequently be "framed by an ideology" that might serve to contribute to moral outrage and subsequently to violence; ideology has been described as beliefs that "justify the terrorist's intent to act."[18] Such ideologic beliefs might be based on political views, religious commitment, conflict associated with a discrete issue, or other reasoning. As Meloy describes, individual belief systems might be built using self-selected language that justifies the individual's actions and moral outrage.[18] One study highlighted the role of grievance and ideology in the case of Roshonora Choudhry who stabbed British politician Stephen Timms; while Choudhry stated that "millions of Iraqis are suffering" and that she had done "my Islamic duty to stand up for the people of Iraq," her choice of target in Timms was further influenced and motivated by a personal grievance she had. Prior to the attack, Choudhary had met Timms at his office and requested a grant to continue her education; the grant was not approved, and she subsequently withdrew from university.[24] In addition to personal grievance and moral outrage, the "hatred" in lone-actor terror and related violence might be understood as unique from other forms of general violence in added ways, such as from the perspectives of ideology, psychology, obsessional fixation, and group dynamics.

Ideological Framing

"Hate" as it relates to the occurrence of hate crimes is believed to be unique from other forms of interpersonal aggression in that it includes not only an intent to cause physical harm, but also to convey a symbolic message on behalf of those committing the acts of violence and to influence future actions of the community to which the victim belonged.[25] Ideologic beliefs might be based on political views, religious commitment, conflict associated with a discrete issue, or other reasoning. Such belief systems might be built using self-selected language that justifies the individuals actions, hatred, and moral outrage.[18] Aaron Beck identified a sense of "revulsion" as further being one of the common themes in personal or intergroup violence, with perpetrators perceiving the other as wrong, immoral, or threatening to a core ideology.[26]

Psychological Features

From a psychological standpoint, Aaron Beck described individuals who engage in acts in lone terror as exhibiting *dichotomous thinking, tunnel vision*, and *overgeneralization*, psychological characteristics that contribute to a deep conviction that an act of violence is justified.[26] Another cognitive feature that research has identified in individual perpetrators of mass violence includes externalization of blame.[21,22] Individuals might hold society or particular individuals responsible for their grievance and may view their societies and individuals in their communities as "persecutory" or as "malevolent objects."[27,28]

Pathological Fixation

From a psychiatric standpoint, hatred and grievance as they contribute to acts of lone terror can be understood to include unique aspects of fixation and obsession that have led many experts to posit that mental illness and lone-actor terrorism may be associated.[14,29-35] Pathological fixation, defined as intense preoccupations with an individual, place, or cause that are pursued to an excessive or irrational degree, has been associated with mental illness, as is abnormally intense focus placed on public figures.[36] Malkki described the "fixated individual" with the potential for grievance-fueled violence as follows:

> The so called fixated individuals combine grievances with socio-economic problems and psychiatric disorder, and project their anger on persons or institutions. Grievances and frustration are mostly connected with governmental actions, such as feelings that one is not being heard or respected by local authorities, loss of a court case, complaints not dealt with by the authorities, and so forth. Trigger events are believed to play an important role in an escalation of frustration and anger which may turn violent.[37]

McCauley and colleagues study assassins and school attackers, perpetrators that they posit are similar to lone-actor terrorists in terms of harboring grievances that eventually result in acts

of violence; they posit that mental illness might represent a risk factor for lone-actor violence.[16] Mental illness, including delusional disorders, major affective disorders, and psychotic disorders, is commonly associated with the presence of pathological fixations[38-40]; in the context of targets of potential violence, Walsh and colleagues propose fixation related to public figures might be the result of "grievances, real or otherwise, quests for 'justice' [or] of perceived rejection."[32] Rahman and colleagues posit that the "extreme overvalued belief," which has previously been associated with strong feelings of injustice and with individuals perceiving themselves as having been "slighted or judged unfairly," might be more likely to contribute to acts of terror because overvalued ideas might be more common and more ego-syntonic.[41]

In-Group Favoritism

Another unique feature of grievance-fueled violence in the context of lone-actor terror and hate-related crime might include the role of in-group and out-group formations.[42] Despite the moniker of "lone-actor terrorist" implying complete isolation of action, it has been found that a significant proportion of individuals responsible for acts of terror had some connection to an ideological group.[43] Moss went so far as to posit that, from a psychodynamic standpoint, that

> When we hate—racistly, homophobically, and misogynistically—we are hating not as isolated individuals but as part of a group; not in the first person singular but in the first person plural. Within the sphere of these hatreds, "I" hate not as "I" alone, but as a white person, a straight person, a man. Our hatred is directed, as it were, taxonomically downward. Disidentification downward, identification upward.[44]

Aaron Beck describes "the image of the enemy" and the "idealized collective self-image of members of the movement" as serving to "enhance the collective self-image as pure, righteous, and united." In the context of acts of terror by an individual, the image of the "enemy" becomes the target of violence. Beck further posits that individuals perceiving themselves or the groups that they identify with as threatened, often by a marginalized or stigmatized minority, will frequently view themselves as the representation of "goodness" that is in conflict with the "badness" of the other. Beck applies this phenomenon to understand the group psychology influencing the terrorist, stating that

> Like the terrorists, we are disposed at these times to see ourselves as the victims victimized by the others, who are vulnerable and innocent. Over time our view of the other person or group progresses from opponent to antagonist to Enemy. We see the Enemy as dangerous, needing to be isolated, punished, or eliminated. We may seek revenge for the damage that we believe we have sustained or we may make a pre-emptive strike to forestall damage.[26]

Neurobiological Aspects

Glaser,[45] in conversation with Kenneth Stern at a Holocaust conference in Scottsdale, Arizona, raised an important question: Had anyone considered studying the role of the brain to understand the neurobiological origins and mechanisms of hate? Stern advised Glaser that, to the best of his knowledge, little if any attention had been devoted to that question. Glaser was asked by Stern to review this topic. Glaser first experienced hate in a clinical fashion when he was functioning as a medical photographer for the US Army at the Nuremburg Medical Trials following World War II. Twenty-three defendant physicians were accused of experimenting on concentration camp victims and causing the deaths of untold numbers of them. We shall see later that there is nascent work on the neurobiology of hate under way for about 13 years. Glaser feels that most neuroscientists ignore hate because it is a too vague a term to work with: its existence is rarely acknowledged in brain research. He opines that hatred or hate signifies that the feeling being addressed is akin to odium.[45]

It is difficult to know when hate first entered the communication language of this planet. Early references to hate are found in the Old Testament at Leviticus 19:17, Numbers 10:35, and Deuteronomy 22:13. Specific references to hate are absent in the New Testament of the Christian Bibles.

There appears to be a changing face of terrorism in the twenty-first century according to some experts. Psychiatrist Jerrold Post worked for many years at the Central Intelligence Agency (CIA) where he began developing psychological profiles of world leaders. He left the CIA in 1986 and spent the rest of his career until 2015 developing a program of political psychology at George Washington University. Dr. Post's important work included "psychobiographies" of Begin and Sadat that helped achieve the successful Camp David Accords in September 1978, and the prescient work a year before the 2020 US election forecasting that if Trump lost the election, he would refuse to accept defeat and that his supporters would follow suit.[46] Dr. Post identified four ways in which terrorism can be categorized: (1) the "anarchist wave"; (2) the "anti-colonial wave" (nationalist-separatist), with minority groups seeking to be liberated from their colonial masters or from the majority in their country; (3) the "new left" wave (social-revolutionary); (4) and the "religious" wave.[47] With the communications and social media revolution, a new phenomenon is emerging that may presage a fifth wave: lone-actor terrorists who, through the internet, are radicalized and feel they belong to the virtual community of hatred. There seems to be a lone-actor terrorism typology developing however these appear devoid of insights from neurobiology [47] Unfortunately, the communications revolution does not get us any closer to the neurobiology of hate.

Most experts agree that the first neurobiological publication on hate was by Zeki and Romaya.[48] These researchers from Wellington, New Zealand studied 17 healthy subjects (10 male, 12 right-handed, mean age of 34.8 years) after informed consent was obtained. During a primary visit to the laboratory some 2 weeks prior to scanning, each subject provided picture portraits of the hated person and picture portraits of three other people of the same sex toward whom they had neutral feelings. All pictures were matched as far as possible for expression and general appearance. Each subject was exposed to either two or three identical stimulus sessions. Scanning was performed in a 1.5-T Siemens Magneton Sonata magnetic resonance imaging (MRI) scanner fitted with a head volume coil. An angled mirror was attached, allowing subjects to view a screen on which face stimuli were projected using an LCD projector. An echo-planar imaging sequence was applied for functional scans measuring blood-oxygen-level-dependent (BOLD) signals. Each brain image was acquired in a descending sequence comprising of 38 actual slices each, 2 mm thick with an interstitial gap of 1 mm. This covered nearly the whole brain. The stimulus for each subject was modeled as a set of aggressors in the SPM5 General Linear Model (GLM) analysis. The principal interest of the researchers was to learn whether any cortical areas were especially active in the contrast *Hated face > Neutral face*. Across all 17 subjects, there was voxel-level activation in the medial frontal gyrus. In addition, there were six activations significant at the cluster level.

To simplify this task in approaching so complex a sentiment, the researchers concentrated on the feeling of hate directed against an individual. These studies did indeed reveal a basic pattern unique to the sentiment of hate, even though individual sites within this pattern have been shown to be active in other conditions related to hate. The researchers identified components that had been important in (a) generating aggressive behavior and (b) translating this behavior into motor action through motor planning. The most intriguing finding was that this network involved regions of the putamen and insula that are almost identical to those activated by passionate, romantic love.[48] The authors opined that their results show that there is a unique pattern of activity in the brain in the context of hate ("hate circuit"): increased activity in the medial frontal gyrus, right putamen, and bilaterally in premotor cortex. This pattern, while being distinct from that obtained in the context of romantic love, nevertheless shares two areas with the latter, namely the putamen and the insula. This linkage may account for why love and hate are so intricately linked to each other in life.[48] Currently, the Zeki and Romaya research[48] has not been replicated. However, since their initial publication in 2008, other neurobiological research articles are signaling the rise of research into the neurobiology of hate. For instance, Tao et al.[49] have completed a functional MRI (fMRI) study on functional connectivity, and they argue that theirs is the first evidence for the involvement of the "hate circuit" in depression, and they suggest a potential reappraisal of the key neural circuitry involved. They hypothesize that their findings may reflect restricted cognitive control over negative feelings toward both self and others within the state of depression. The details of their research are beyond the scope of this chapter, and interested readers are encouraged to read the article. However, they note that their study differs from other methods, such as seed-based analysis and independent component analysis, and makes no assumptions about which circuits might be altered or that brain regions are independent of one another. Their approach identified the so-called "hate circuit" as showing the largest change in both first-episode major depressive disorder (FEMDD) patients and resistant major depressive disorder (RMDD) patients. These authors report uncoupling of the "hate circuit" in depressed patients. This circuit appears to be the same that Zeki and Romaya identified.[48] That

study noted that three areas comprised the "hate circuit." The insula region has been reported by others to be involved in feelings of disgust as well as other emotions.[50]

Also along these lines there is current evidence that numerous psychiatric illnesses are now being evaluated in terms of the "hate circuit." For instance, Fan et al.[51] have studied the bipolar mood state and its reflections in the functional connectivity of the "hate circuit." These researchers used fMRI studies to explore group differences of resting state functional connectivity within the "hate circuit" in controls and patients with bipolar mania, bipolar depression, and bipolar euthymia using seed-based functional connectivity analysis. Their findings revealed that there is significant variance among the "hate circuit" when it is analyzed in terms of distinctive mood phases of bipolar disorder. For instance, bipolar depressive patients revealed decreased "hate circuit" function compared with bipolar mania and bipolar euthymic patients. In addition, patients with bipolar euthymia had a similar connectivity pattern of the "hate circuit" to human controls. Exactly what these data mean for bipolar illness remains to be elucidated.

Only the surface has been scratched regarding the neurobiology of hate. However, if one reviews the literature of the "hate circuit," this research is broadening into many areas of psychiatric disorders, as is research on the differences and close kinship of love versus hate. This research will add to the neurobiological information available on terrorism where hate toward individuals is an issue.

Hate-Related Speech and Crimes

"Hatred" is not a psychiatric disorder; nor is it a recognized, free-standing symptom of such any such disorder. It does, however, have a featured role in the *Diagnostic and Statistical Manual of Mental Disorders* (DSM-5) "Glossary of Cultural Concepts of Distress" concerning the Haitian notion of *maladi moun* ("humanly sent illness"), which "may be caused by others' envy and hatred, provoked by the victim's economic success." In this scenario, "one person's gain is assumed to produce another person's loss, so visible success makes one vulnerable to attack."[52] Etiological and experiential parallels between *maladi moun* and lone-actor terrorism are readily apparent. Affording no coverage to *maladi moun*, *Campbell's Psychiatric Dictionary* refers those seeking definitions for "hate" and "hate propaganda" to entries on "aggression" and "propaganda," respectively.[53]

Must one hate in order to aggress? Does all hatred lead to aggression? Neurophysiological studies conducted with the use of fMRI have established, for example, that although "areas in the medial frontal gyrus, right putamen, premotor cortex, and medial insula" were activated for subjects who contemplated "images of a person they professed to hate" and that some of these areas are "also involved in initiating aggressive behavior," it is also true that an individual's "feelings of aggression itself—as well as anger, danger and fear—show different patterns in the brain than hatred does."[54] While "hate propaganda" seeks to instill and inflame hatred in its target audience,[55] there is technically no requirement that the authors of such material experience hatred themselves, and, more broadly, it is worth noting that there is also the medium of "positive propaganda."[56]

By contrast, from a legal perspective, *Black's Law Dictionary* defines a "hate crime" as an offense "motivated by the perpetrator's prejudice, usually an intense bigotry, on the basis of the victim's race, color, national origin, ancestry, gender, religion, religious practice, age, disability, or sexual orientation."[57] Here, the existence and particular cause of the perpetrator's personal malice are necessary prerequisites for criminal culpability. It would not be enough, for example, for prosecutors to establish beyond a reasonable doubt that the defendant was a notorious bigot, condemned out of his own mouth on the basis of countless video-recorded social media rants of an overtly racist nature. It would be necessary to establish that the offense in question was inspired by that racism, as opposed, say, to a robbery motivated by purely financial considerations. Similarly, the victims themselves would need to be—or would need to be believed by the perpetrator to be—members of a "suspect class,"[58] definable by one or more of the above-noted identities. The relevance of the designation of undesirable behavior as a hate crime has to do with much more than mere adverse categorization and public opprobrium. The primary reason, and in particular the driving legislative motivation for this characterization, is penalty enhancement.[59,60] Conviction of an illegal act committed with malign prejudicial intent can result in a longer prison sentence, incur stiffer financial penalties, and complicate options for post-conviction relief.[61] Currently, during an era notable for sharply drawn sociopolitical divisions, it is not surprising that hate crime designations have the potential to generate public controversy. Some will see pursuit of a hate crime conviction as more a reflection of the prosecutor's personal belief system than an attempt to bring about a just, objective proportionate legal outcome. Others will see failure to pursue a hate crime conviction as an act of victim abandonment and even outright discrimination. The very existence of hate crime legislation has become the subject of considerable legal and political debate.[62] Sometimes this reflects alleged difficulties in "deciding which identity groups are categorized as specific hate crime victim groups and which are not."[63] On occasion, resistance actually comes from representatives of some of these groups themselves, who, for example, "have repeatedly opposed the inclusion of sexual orientation and gender identity/expression in hate crime legislation."[64] Some approach inclusion from a markedly differently perspective, such as those who espouse the "Blue Lives Matter" movement [65,66] and advocate "for the expansion of hate crime statutes to include police and other first responders as protected victim categories."[67] Most of all, opposition to the notion of hate crime legislation springs from a conflation of the notion of hate crime with that of "hate speech," defined by *Black's Law Dictionary* as that "whose sole purpose is to demean people on the basis of race, ethnicity, gender, religion, age, disability, or some other similar ground," and particularly "when the communication is likely to provoke violence."[57] It should be acknowledged that there are indeed instances in which hate crime and hate speech are one and the same, and hate speech is often a prime source of inculpatory evidence for the commission of a hate crime.[68] In any event, the primary argument against hate speech restrictions—and, by extension, against any form of speech criminalization, in whole or in part—is based on the "free speech" guaranteed by the First Amendment.[69] In relation to the United States, such guarantees have never been viewed as absolute,[70] and those who wish to hide behind the First Amendment while issuing calls for violence by lone-actor terrorists will confront a well-established Constitutional jurisprudence that addresses such issues in considerable detail. In *Schenck v. United States*,[71] the Supreme Court of the United States opined that "[t]he question in every case is whether the words used are used in such circumstances and are of such a nature as to create a clear and present danger that they will bring about the substantive evils that Congress has a right to prevent." *Schenck* was followed half a century later by *Brandenburg v. Ohio*,72 in which the Court elaborated on this exception with reference to speech that is both "directed to inciting or producing imminent lawless action" and is "likely to incite or produce such action." In order to circumnavigate these standards, those attempting to pass off pro-terrorism harangues as "protected" speech would need to establish, concerning the consequences of such exhortations, that the "lawless action" in question would not be "imminent." Naturally, a higher level of security would follow from a legal test that "would no longer require imminence" but would instead require that "because of speech directing, advocating, or encouraging lawless action, there is a substantial likelihood of a high level of harm," with such speech representing "a fairly clear directive toward illegal action that could actually occur."[73]

CONCLUSION

Contemporary research stresses the multivariable context of lone-actor terrorism. Borum describes three dimensions—loneness, direction, and motivation—in analyzing lone-actor cases and the roles of mental illness and radicalization.[74] Corner and Gill describe the influence of several variables on mental illness, the latter having a significantly higher prevalence in lone-actor terrorists compared with those who join groups. These variables include a spouse or partner being a member of a larger group, preceding life changes, being a recent victim of bias, and experiencing acute and chronic stress.[30] Schuurman and colleagues report on a number of common lone-actor terrorist characteristics, including poor operational security maintenance, leaking motivations and capabilities to others in advance of an attack, and maintaining social connections.[75] In his behavioral analysis of lone-actor terrorism, Gill discusses the inaccuracy of attempting to place an individual lone-actor in a "master narrative" (such as school shooter, terrorist, mentally ill, politically driven, acting on a grievance, etc.) and emphasizes that offenders may span a number of these categories.[76] These findings, along with other lone-actor terrorism research, support the principle that an array of variables and experiences crystallize within the offender and that no one variable should be considered "pivotal: in the planning and implementation of lone-actor events. A review of lone-actor terrorism literature underscores the constructs of hatred and grievance as factors in some, if not most cases, but hatred/grievance alone cannot explain the complexity of lone-actor terrorism (i.e., there are plenty of people who hate but do not commit terrorism).

NOTES AND REFERENCES

1. https://www.fbi.gov/investigate/civil-rights/hate crimes
2. Asal V, Deloughery K, King RD. Understanding lone-actor terrorism: A comparative analysis with violent hate crimes and group-based terrorism. National Consortium for the Study of Terrorism and Responses to Terrorism, Department of Homeland Security Science and Technology Center of Excellence, University of Maryland. Sep 2013. https://www.dhs.gov/sites/default/files/publications/OPSR_TP_TEVUS_Comparing-Lone-Actor-Terrorism_Hate crimes_Group-Terrorism_2013-508.pdf
3. Byman D. When to call a terrorist a terrorist. *Foreign Policy*, 27 Oct 2018. https://foreignpolicy.com/2018/10/27/when-to-call-a-terrorist-a-terrorist/
4. Turkewitz J, Roose K. Who is Robert Bowers, the suspect in the Pittsburgh synagogue shooting? *New York Times*, 27 Oct 2018. https://www.nytimes.com/2018/10/27/us/robert-bowers-pittsburgh-synagogue-shooter.html
5. Weiser B, Watkins A. Cesar Sayoc, who mailed pipe bombs to Trump critics, is sentenced to 20 years. *New York Times*, 5 Aug 2019. https://www.nytimes.com/2019/08/05/nyregion/cesar-sayoc-sentencing-pipe-bombing.html
6. Jones JC. Anders Breivik's chilling anti-feminism. The Guardian, 27 Jul 2011. https://www.theguardian.com/commentisfree/2011/jul/27/breivik-anti-feminism
7. BBC News. Profile: Anders Behring Breivik. 12 Apr 2012. https://www.bbc.com/news/world-europe-14259989
8. Holley P. Two New York City police officers are shot and killed in a brazen ambush in Brooklyn. *Washington Post*, 20 Dec 2014. https://www.washingtonpost.com/national/two-new-york-city-police-officers-are-shot-and-killed-in-a-brazen-ambush-in-brooklyn/2014/12/20/2a73f7ae-8898-11e4-9534-f79a23c40e6c_story.html
9. Beirich H. Holocaust Museum shooter had close ties to prominent neo-Nazis. SPLC, 10 Jun 2009. https://www.Splcenter.Org/Hatewatch/2009/06/10/Holocaust-Museum-Shooter-Had-Close-Ties-Prominent-Neo-Nazis
10. Emery T, Robbins L. Holocaust Museum shooter James von Brunn had history of hate. Seattle Times, 12 Jun 2009. https://www.seattletimes.com/nation-world/holocaust-museum-shooter-james-von-brunn-had-history-of-hate/
11. Pringle P. Hebron massacre: Brooklyn doctor with a prescription for hatred. Independent, 27 Feb 1994. https://www.independent.co.uk/news/world/hebron-massacre-brooklyn-doctor-with-a-prescription-for-hatred-1396680.html

12. Office of Public Affairs, US Department of Justice. Ohio man sentenced to life in prison for federal hate crimes related to August 2017 car attack at rally in Charlottesville, Virginia. Department of Justice, 28 Jun 2019. https://www.justice.gov/opa/pr/ohio-man-sentenced-life-prison-federal-hate-crimes-related-august-2017-car-attack-rally

13. Poppe K. Nidal Hasan: A case study in lone-actor terrorism. Program on Extremism. George Washington University, Oct 2018. https://extremism.gwu.edu/sites/g/files/zaxdzs2191/f/Nidal%20Hasan.pdf

14. Erlandsson Å., Reid Meloy J. The Swedish school attack in Trollhättan. *J Forensic Sci.* 2018;63(6):1917–1927.

15. James D. *The Fixated, Lone Actors and Grievance Fuelled Violence.* Bangkok: Asia Pacific Association of Threat Assessment Professionals; 2015.

16. McCauley C, Moskalenko S, Van Son B. Characteristics of lone-wolf violent offenders: A comparison of assassins and school attackers. *Perspect Terrorism* 2013;7(1):4–24.

17. Shultz JM, Zakrison TL, Galea S. Hate and the health of populations. *Milbank Q.* 2018;97(1):11–15.

18. Meloy JR, Gill P. The lone-actor terrorist and the TRAP-18. *J Threat Assess Manage.* 2016;3(1):37.

19. Hamm, M, Spaaij, R. Lone wolf terrorism in America: Using knowledge of radicalization pathways to forge prevention strategies. 2015. https://www.ncjrs.gov/pdffiles1/nij/grants/248691.pdf

20. Aitken L, Oosthuizen P, Emsley R, Seedat S. Mass murders: Implications for mental health professionals. Int J Psychiatry Med 2008;38(3):261–269.

21. Fox JA, Levin J. Mass murder: An analysis of extreme violence. J Appl Psychoanal Stud. 2003;5:47–64.

22. Duwe G. The patterns and prevalence of mass murder in twentieth century America. Justice Q 2004;21(4):729–761.

23. Levin J, Madfis E. Mass murder at school and cumulative strain: A sequential model. Am Behav Sci. 2009;52(9):1227–1245.

24. Gill P, Corner E. Lone-actor terrorist target choice. *Behav Sci Law.* 2016;34(5):693–705.

25. Craig KM. Examining hate-motivated aggression: A review of the social psychological literature on hate crimes as a distinct form of aggression. *Aggression Violent Behav.* 2002;7(1):85–101.

26. Beck AT. Prisoners of hate. *Behav Res Therapy.* 2002;40(3):209–216.

27. Mullen PE. The autogenic (self-generated) massacre. *Behavioral Sciences & the Law* 2004; 22(3):311–323.

28. Hempel A, Melroy J, Richards T. Offender and offense characteristics of a nonrandom sample of mass murderers. J Am Acad Psychiatry Law. 1999;27:213–225.

29. Liem M, van Buuren J, de Roy van Zuijdewijn J, Schönberger H, Bakker E. European lone actor terrorists versus "common" homicide offenders: An empirical analysis. *Homicide Stud.* 2018;22(1):45–69.

30. Corner E, Gill P. A false dichotomy? Mental illness and lone-actor terrorism. *Law Hum Behav.* 2015;39(1):23.

31. Gill P, Corner E. There and back again: The study of mental disorder and terrorist involvement. *Am Psychologist.* 2017;72(3):231.

32. Barry-Walsh J, James DV, Mullen PE. Fixated Threat Assessment Centers: Preventing harm and facilitating care in public figure threat cases and those thought to be at risk of lone-actor grievance-fueled violence. *CNS Spectrums.* 2020;25(5):630–637.

33. van der Meer BB, Bootsma L, Meloy R. Disturbing communications and problematic approaches to the Dutch Royal Family. J Forensic Psychiatry Psychol. 2012;23:571–589.

34. Hoffmann J, Meloy JR, Guldimann A, Ermer A. Attacks on German public figures, 1968–2004: Warning behaviors, potentially lethal and nonlethal acts, psychiatric status, and motivations. Behav Sci Law. 2011;29:155–179. doi:10.1002/bsl.979.

35. James DV, Mullen P, Meloy JR, Pathé M, Farnham F, Preston L, Darnley B. The role of mental disorder in attacks on European politicians, 1990–2004. Acta Psychiatrica Scand. 2007;116:334–344. doi:10.1111/j.1600-0447.2007.01077.x. J.

36. Mullen PE, James DV, Meloy JR, Pathé MT, Farnham FR, Preston L, et al. The fixated and the pursuit of public figures. *J Forensic Psychiatry Psychol.* 2009;20(1):33–47.

37. Malkki L. School shootings and lone actor terrorism. In Michael F, ed. *Understanding Lone Actor Terrorism: Past Experience, Future Outlook, and Response Strategies.* Abingdon: Routledge; 2016:198–221.

38. Every-Palmer S, Barry-Walsh J, Pathé M. Harassment, stalking, threats and attacks targeting New Zealand politicians: A mental health issue. Aust N Z J Psychiatry. 2015 Jul;49(7):634–641.

39. Pathé MT, Lowry TJ, Haworth DJ, Winterbourne P, Day L. Public figure fixation: Cautionary findings for mental health practitioners. *Behav Sci Law.* 2016;34(5):681–692.

40. James D, Kerrington TR, Forfar R, Farnham FR, Preston L. The fixated threat assessment center: Preventing harm and facilitating care. J Forensic Psychiatry Psychol. 2010;21:521–536. doi:10.1080/14789941003596981.

41. Rahman T, Meloy JR, Bauer R. Extreme overvalued belief and the legacy of Carl Wernicke. *J Am Acad Psychiatry Law.* 2019;47(2):180–187.

42. Greenwald AG, Pettigrew TF. With malice toward none and charity for some: Ingroup

favoritism enables discrimination. *Am Psychologist.* 2014;69(7):669.

43. Horgan J, Shortland N, Abbasciano S, Walsh S. Actions speak louder than words: A behavioral analysis of 183 individuals convicted for terrorist offenses in the United States from 1995 to 2012. *J Forensic Sci.* 2016;61(5):1228–1237.

44. Moss D. On hating in the first person plural: Thinking psychoanalytically about racism, homophobia, and misogyny. J Am Psychoanalyt Assoc. 2001;49(4):1315–1334. https://doi.org/10.1177/00030651010490041801

45. Glaser EM. Is there a neurobiology of hate? *J Hate Stud.* 2009;7:7–20.

46. Risen C. Jerrold M. Post, specialist in political psychology, dies at 86. New York Times, 12 Dec 2020. https://www.nytimes.com/2020/12/12/us/jerrold-m-post-dead.html

47. Post JM, McGinnis C, Moody K. The changing face of terrorism in the twenty-first century: The communications revolution and the virtual community of hatred. *Behav Sci Law.* 2014;32(3):306–334.

48. Zeki S, Romaya JP. Neural correlates of hate. *PLoS ONE.* 2008;3(10):e3556. https://doi.org/10.1371/journal.pone.0003556

49. Tao H, Guo S, Ge T, et al. Depression uncouples brain hate circuit. *Mol Psychiatry.* 2013;18:101–111.

50. Chen YH, Dammers J, Boers F, et al. The temporal dynamics of insula activity to disgust and happy facial expressions: A magnetoencephalography study. *Neuroimage.* 2009;47:1921–1928.

51. Fan Z, Yang J, Zeng C, et al. Bipolar mood state reflected in functional connectivity of the hate circuit: A resting-state functional magnetic resonance imaging study. *Front Psychiatry.* 2020;11:1–10.

52. American Psychiatric Association. *Diagnostic and Statistical Manual of Mental Disorders.* 5th ed. Arlington, VA: American Psychiatric Association; 2013.

53. Campbell R. *Campbell's Psychiatric Dictionary.* 9th ed. New York: Oxford University Press; 2009:445.

54. Harmon K. The origin of hatred. *Sci Am*, 19 Aug 2009. https://www.scientificamerican.com/ article/the-origin-of-hatred

55. Lanning R. Irrationalism: The foundation of hate propaganda. *J Hate Stud.* 2012;10(1):49–71.

56. Rusu M, Herman R. The implications of propaganda as a social influence strategy. *Sci Bull.* 2018;23(2):118–125.

57. Gardner B, ed. *Black's Law Dictionary.* 11th ed. St. Paul, MN: Thomson Reuters; 2019:467.

58. Ross B, Li S. Measuring political power: Suspect class determinations and the poor. *Calif Law Rev.* 2016;104:232–291.

59. Iganski P. Hate crimes hurt more. *Am Beh Sci.* 2001;45(4):626–638.

60. Iganski P, Lagou S. Hate crimes hurt some more than others: Implications for the just sentencing of offenders. *J Interpers Violence.* 2015;30(10):1696–1718.

61. Sherry M. *Disability Hate Crimes: Does Anyone Really Hate Disabled People?* New York: Routledge; 2016.

62. Mathis J. Motive, actions, and confusions in the debate over hate crime legislation. *Crim Justice Ethics.* 2018;37(1):1–20.

63. Garland J. Difficulties in defining hate crime victimization. *Int'l Rev Victimology.* 2012;18(1):25–37:25.

64. Swiffen A. New resistance to hate crime legislation and the concept of law. *Law Cult Humanit.* 2018;14(1):121–139, at 121.

65. Solomon J, Martin A. Competitive victimhood as a lens to reconciliation: An analysis of the black lives matter and blue lives matter movements. *Conflict Resolut Q.* 2019;37(1):7–31.

66. Thomas M, Tufts S. Blue solidarity: Police unions, race and authoritarian populism in North America. *Work Employ Soc.* 2020;34(1):126–144.

67. Mason G. Blue lives matter and hate crime law. *Race Justice*, 16 Jun 2020. https://journals.sagepub.com/doi/abs/10.1177/2153368720933665

68. Gould R. Is the "hate" in hate speech the "hate" in hate crime? Waldon and Dworkin on political legitimacy. *Jurisprudence.* 2019;10(2):71–87.

69. Beausoleil L. Free, hateful, and posted: Rethinking First Amendment protection of hate speech in a social media world. *BC L Rev.* 2019;60(7):2101–2144.

70. Kendrick L. Use your words: On the "speech" in "freedom of speech. *Mich L Rev.* 2018;116:667–704.

71. *Schenck v. United States*, 249 US 47 (1919).

72. *Brandenburg v. Ohio*, 395 US 444 (1969).

73. Leibowitz Z. Criminalizing terrorist incitement on social media through doctrinal shift. *Fordham Law Rev.* 2017;86:795–824.

74. Borum R. Informing lone-offender investigations, policy essay: Loner attacks and domestic extremism. *Criminol Public Pol.* Feb 2013;12(1):103–112.

75. Schuurman B, Bakker E, Gill P, Bouhana N. Lone actor terrorist attack planning and preparation: A data-driven analysis. *J Forensic Sci Oct.* 2017;63(1).

76. Gill P. *Lone-Actor Terrorism: A Behavioural Analysis.* New York: Routledge; 2015.

21

Comparing Lone-Actor Terrorism to Other High-Threat Groups

*JACOB C. HOLZER, EMILY THRELKELD, WILLIAM COSTANZA, PATRICIA R. RECUPERO, AND SAMARA E. RAINEY**

INTRODUCTION

Preliminary research examining lone-actor terrorists with others involved in mass violence and threats to national security have shown overlapping and divergent findings. This area of study is important because it may add to a better understanding of both the complex landscape of lone-actor terrorism and how better to combat it and reduce the risk it poses to society. Three comparison groups reviewed in this chapter are (a) individuals who have breached national security and committed treason, (b) individuals who have committed mass violence without a clear associated ideology, and (c) school shooters.

TREASON AND ESPIONAGE: NATIONAL SECURITY RISKS

US history is replete with examples of individuals who have, for varied reasons, breached national security and committed espionage. *Espionage* in this context is defined broadly as a criminal act by a US citizen which may result in damage to national security. In some cases, the US Espionage Act was violated.[1] In other cases, the Espionage Act has been applied in controversial contexts where an individual acted as or claimed to be a whistleblower acting for altruistic reasons.[2] Examples reviewed in this preliminary study were drawn from open non-classified news and media sources and were divided into categories based on motivation. Reasons for security breaches include (1) greed, (2) acting on behalf of another country,

or (3) altruism. These and other motives may overlap in some cases and are not mutually exclusive. Based on a review by the authors, the altruistic group were noted to be outliers in a number of characteristics and were excluded from this preliminary analysis. The other two groups (those acting for money and those acting for another country) appeared similar and were combined. An individual's decision to "cross the line" and act as an agent of a foreign country is driven by a complex constellation of motivational factors that come together at a particular point in time that is unique to that individual. This crystallization of variables may parallel the lone-actor terrorism group. The goal of case officers is to carefully assess the potential recruitment target for susceptibilities that would make the individual vulnerable to a recruitment pitch. In this chapter, several high-profile espionage cases are reviewed, followed by a discussion about their relationship to lone-actor terrorism cases.
Espionage Case Reviews

Robert Philip Hanssen

Hanssen[3–10] is a former FBI agent who was arrested in February 2001 for selling US secret information to the former Soviet Union and Russian Federation for cash and diamonds. He pled guilty and is serving life imprisonment in Florence, Colorado. Hanssen, like Aldrich Ames, offered his services rather than being recruited. Two factors may have driven Hanssen's behavior— financial stress and the excitement of engaging

---

* The opinions expressed in this chapter are the chapter author's and not that of the Central Intelligence Agency.

in illegal behavior involving classified material. It appears the primary reason for his actions was to make money, with reports indicating he made more than a half-million dollars in cash and diamonds. Although Hanssen perceived the need for money, he was underpaid for the information that he was providing to the Soviets. He assumed that he would be caught someday, stating on arrest "What took you so long?" A sense of excitement was clearly part of his motivation, fueled by resentment. A psychological evaluation on Hanssen showed the presence of clinical issues such as psychopathic, narcissistic, and dependency features. References indicate he was intelligent and one of the FBI's top counterintelligence officers before engaging in espionage. A review of material indicated a mix of psychological issues— early physical and emotional abuse, unhealthy sexual practices, personality traits—within the context of his fundamentalist religious views and practices. These internal and external factors fed into his decision-making process to varying degrees. Hanssen was exceedingly complex, driven by a series of motivations that tended to change over time given the length of years he spied for the Soviets.

Aldrich Ames

Ames[11-15] was a CIA career officer convicted of espionage in 1994 after spying for the Soviet Union and Russia; he is now serving a life sentence without the possibility of parole. His early career was marked by conflicts—he was enthusiastic and performance ratings were excellent, but he also had security violations, affairs, drank heavily, and got into a drunken argument with a foreign official. Unlike Hanssen, Ames received approximately $2.5 million for the information he provided, and he lived extravagantly. Events leading to his arrest included a change in his appearance—his wearing of tailored suits, having cosmetic dental procedures, and buying an expensive house and car inconsistent with his salary.

Ames's early years provide a context to understand the evolution of the behavioral patterns later in life that would make him vulnerable to espionage. His father, a CIA analyst, was an alcoholic with poor job performance. Ames's alcoholism no doubt impacted on his decision-making when he decided to volunteer to work with the Russians. (It should be noted that a volunteer or "walk-in" is not the same as a defector. A volunteer becomes a defector if the individual does not agree to go back to his or her original position to report classified information. If the person agrees to go back to their position, as Ames did, he is referred to as a *penetration* of that foreign service and is viewed as a volunteer; i.e., a spy). Ames appeared better suited for a staff position that drew on his knowledge of Soviet matters rather than for operations. The prevalence of alcohol use and alcohol-related incidents followed him during his career, and, within the setting of marital conflict and the start of his relationship with Rosario Casas Dupuy during his Mexico tour, added financial pressure ensued. He reported that his indebtedness had grown during that relationship. In that context, he rationalized (enabled by alcoholism) crossing the line to volunteer to work with the Russians, whom he had plausible reason to contact given his operational duties.

Jonathan Pollard

Pollard,[16-25] an intelligence analyst for the US Navy, pleaded guilty in 1987 to providing classified information to Israel. He was sentenced to life imprisonment and released on parole in 2015; he completed his sentence in November 2020. He arrived in Israel in Dec. 2020. Although in part Pollard was driven to spy due to his allegiance to Israel and belief that Israel needed US classified information for its own defense, he was also paid for providing that information. It was alleged that Pollard may also have passed classified information to other countries. During the vetting process for his classified work in the Navy, it was (later) discovered that Pollard had withheld or lied about personal information, including his history of drug use, and claims about his father, his language abilities, and education. Reports indicate a history of heavy marijuana use and that he had at times told fantastical stories about his life, such as being an agent for the Mossad and a Colonel in the Israeli Army. A CIA analysis indicated that Pollard's lack of awareness into his misjudgments and his modifying of events to fit his self-image were consistent with narcissistic personality traits. Before committing espionage, Pollard experienced financial and psychological stressors which may have contributed to his decision. After a transfer to a more sensitive job, he expressed ideas thought to be aberrant to the Naval Intelligence Command staff, which raised concerns about him, leading to an eventual investigation. A lie detector test was equivocal, and Pollard admitted to giving false information, resulting in a temporary reduction in his security clearance. He eventually regained a higher level security clearance and worked as an analyst for Naval Intelligence.

John Anthony Walker

Walker[26-31] was a US Navy Warrant Officer convicted of spying for the Soviet Union from the 1960s through the 1980s, as part of the Walker spy ring. He made a plea arrangement to testify against a co-conspirator in exchange for a lesser sentence for his son. He died in 2014 in prison. His early life was unstable—his father was an alcoholic and the family moved around a lot. He was involved in petty crime as a youth and was given the option of going to jail or enlisting in the military. While stationed in South Carolina, he opened a bar which failed and resulted in his being in debt. It was around this time that he experienced conflicts in his marriage and engaged in affairs. Walker subsequently was motivated to spy for financial gain, and, around 1967, he offered to spy for the Soviet Union. Walker's callousness, need for excitement, and exploitative behavior were consistent with psychopathic traits. In the mid-1970s, after retiring from the Navy, he became a private investigator, traveling the world, passing classified information on to the Soviet Union. It was believed that his psychopathic and maladaptive traits coupled with alcoholism allowed him to leverage his access to classified information to provide to an adversary for money.

David Sheldon Boone

Boone[32-38] is a former US Army analyst who worked for the National Security Agency (NSA) and was convicted of espionage in 1999 relating to selling classified information to the Soviet Union a decade earlier. He received training in cryptographic analysis and took two Russian-language training courses at the Defense Language Institute. In the Army, Boone served in Signals Intelligence, and, toward the latter part of his career in the late 1980s, in the context of worsening debt, marital problems, and anger problems, it was reported that he separated and turned over his income and children to his wife prior to initiating a relationship with the Soviet Union. Boone was paid for the classified information he turned over to the Soviets. Reports indicate that a cause of his anger was that so much of his money was being turned over to his ex-wife. Based on a report of his sentence, he is scheduled for release in June 2023.

Harold James Nicholson

Nicholson[39-46] is a former CIA officer convicted of spying for Russia. He joined the CIA after serving in the US Army, and he was assigned to CIA stations around the world, in part working on intelligence operations against foreign intelligence services. While stationed in Malaysia in the early 1990s, he volunteered to the Russian intelligence service and began providing national defense information until his arrest in the mid-1990s. Reports indicated that, as his career developed, his home life suffered, in part related to his assignments. His marriage ended in divorce and financial stress when he gained custody of his children and paid alimony. His son Nathaniel was later arrested for acting as a courier between his father in prison and Russia intelligence during the mid-2000s. In one magazine article, a number of variables were identified as triggers for his selling national defense information to the Russians, including financial stress, greed, ego, desperation, and anger at his CIA superiors.

Jeffrey Carney

Carney, [47-50] a former US Air Force airman who worked as a linguist, was convicted of spying for East German state security (Stasi) while stationed in Berlin in the early 1980s. News reports indicate a number of variables which could have factored into his spying, including challenges to his sexual orientation while in the military and discouragement and resentment with the Air Force. Reports indicate that family problems, drinking, and isolation may have been added variables. While spying for the Stasi, he was recognized with awards from East Germany. In the mid-1980s, he was transferred from Germany back to the United States, where his spying continued until he sought refuge and escaped to East Germany in 1985. With the fall of the Berlin Wall and reunification of Germany, Carney was eventually apprehended and convicted; he spent 12 years in prison for espionage, desertion, and conspiracy. Reports indicate that ideology was not a factor in his attempt to defect to and assist East Germany.

Literature Review

An individual's susceptibility to engage in espionage is a psychologically complex process unique to the individual's psychosocial development. There are limited number of reviews and reports describing characteristics and patterns related to espionage and security risks. One comprehensive review by Dr. Ursula M. Wilder described behavioral patterns and personality traits associated with espionage: psychopathy and personality disorders, narcissism and grandiosity, impulsiveness and immaturity, impaired relationships, vindictiveness, paranoia, and risk-seeking, among other traits and patterns,[51] and defined three key elements which set the conditions for someone to engage in espionage: personality dysfunction, crisis state, and ease of opportunity. In a project involving interviews with people convicted of espionage, most initially were found trustworthy and loyal but later changed. Three variables were identified as critical: (a) a character weakness; (b) a personal, financial, or career crisis; and (c) friends and co-workers had not recognized the signs of a serious problem.[52] In a CIA review of defectors titled "Psychology of Treason," severe mental illness was not considered a major factor, and some difficulties were felt to have a late or insidious onset.[53] In this review, characteristics such as immaturity, impulsivity, sociopathy, and narcissism were described as a pattern in some defections. The literature describes a number of characteristics as factoring in at least some espionage cases—such as disgruntlement, seeking revenge, the practice of ingratiation, and self-importance. In an article titled "Treason on Their Minds," the author indicates that ideology and financial motives alone cannot fully explain why some turn to espionage. In discussing the importance of underlying psychological issues, the author states that treason "is usually the last act of an employee's long simmering emotional crisis."[54]

Espionage Typology

Based on a review of the literature and case examples, individuals committing espionage can be divided into two broad categories (a) *recruited*, or those individuals who have been taken through the recruitment cycle (spotting, assessing developing, recruiting) and are handled by a case officer; and (b) volunteers (walk-ins) who make independent decisions to contact the adversarial service and who become assets if they are "turned" and agree to go back to their jobs to work in place to provide classified information. If the individuals cannot be "turned" to work in place they are known as *defectors*, are debriefed by the service they defect to, and are sometimes later called on to consult. In each circumstance, the individual is driven by their perceived need to offer their services (i.e., providing access to classified information) to an adversarial service as a means of addressing their psychological and material needs and potentially longer term goals.

As discussed, individuals are motivated by a constellation of factors (psychological, emotional, survival, financial, etc.) that peak at a specific point in time under the right conditions (i.e., access to classified, protected information of interest to foreign intelligence services). Some individuals are more resilient than others; that is, they have some personality traits that may counter those that make an individual susceptible to a recruitment pitch or that lead them to make a faulty cost-benefit analysis and choose to volunteer to a foreign intelligence service. The bottom line is that it is difficult to generalize motivations to an individual case. An individual's self-assessment of their motivations as a reliable indicator can be highly suspect. It is also difficult to make assumptions about educational level. Many educated people do appalling things; academic achievement doesn't necessarily equate to acting rationally across all of life's challenges. High academic achievement may have assisted in positioning them to obtain a sensitive job in the national security bureaucracy but that seems to have more to do with them acquiring access to classified information. It is only after they have been in the career that circumstances changed or the conditions were just right and the individual made the decision to spy.

Based on one author's preliminary research (JH), high-profile cases reviewed described a broad array of individuals with varying backgrounds, education, and motivators related to their behaviors. Motivators were seen as fitting into subcategories—volunteer, money, foreign allegiance, resentful/vengeance, or altruism, with some overlap. As a group, most of the sample reviewed were educated and intelligent. For example, Hanssen received his master's degree in accounting and information systems from Northwestern University, and Pollard completed his undergraduate degree at Stanford. Although no major mental illness was described, reports indicated many of the individuals had some underlying psychiatric or psychological difficulties, including paraphilias, alcohol/substance abuse, temper dyscontrol, and antisocial traits. Ames struggled with alcohol abuse, and the behaviors of Hanssen and Pollard indicated narcissistic personality traits. Early life trauma was a factor in some of the cases. Hanssen endured emotional abuse as a child from his father, and Walker also suffered abuse and abandonment from his alcoholic father. Many individuals in the espionage group achieved success in their careers (in contrast to a finding of disruption in the military or civilian careers in many individuals in the lone-actor terrorism group). Another finding was that some individuals initially "flirted" with the idea of committing espionage as a stimulation, to gain excitement.

The authors drew a distinction between those acting for motivations of money, foreign allegiance, or resentment/vengeance, and the concept of altruism. As opposed to other motivations, those motivated by altruism appeared to have less of a burden related to mental health factors, conflicts, or problems in goals or careers; they appeared as "outliers" and were dropped from this preliminary study. The case example in this preliminary study that fit with the altruistic group (and was therefore not included) was Daniel Ellsberg.

The role of a foreign intelligence case officer or "handler" was important to consider in some cases of individuals at risk to commit espionage; the handler may offer the right amount of incentive to drive that individual to then commit espionage. The foreign case officer is a critical element in a recruitment and handling operation in all espionage cases. Whether a foreign case officer takes an individual through the recruitment cycle—spotting, assessing, developing, recruiting, handling—or handles and guides a volunteer, there is no sustained operation without the handling case officer. The foreign case officer continues to assess the production of the case and will terminate continued contact of the case if it is no longer productive, if there is a threat to the asset's security, or if deception is discovered. To recruit an asset a foreign case officer will determine whether an individual has access to classified information of interest and carefully cultivate and assess the individual to determine vulnerabilities that could lead to recruitment. Another important consideration is that the cases cited in this section are representative of those who were apprehended and who committed penetrations of US intelligence organizations. The findings based on the espionage cases may not generalize to those who were never detected or those who committed penetrations of foreign governments. It is important to note that intelligence cultures around the world differ and may lead to a variety of motivations that are unique to their own intelligence culture.

An important assessment using a "critical-path method" for evaluation of insider threats (in both espionage and lone-actor terrorism cases) outlines the key variables of personal predisposition, stressors, concerning behaviors, and problematic organizational responses as leading to the adverse event.[55]

Commonalities
Pilot research comparing high-profile espionage to lone-actor terrorism groups found some common variables, although there was also substantial

individual variability. As outlined in earlier chapters in this volume, some key variables found in the lone-actor terrorism group included some type of clinical mental health symptoms or difficulties; that individuals had changed and acted differently or unusually to peers; that although people acted individually or with one other there were in some cases encouragement and guidance from others; rhetoric and social media played a role; individuals were impressionable and may have had a history of violence; some had maladjustments at work or in the military; and some had contradictory beliefs and behaviors in their backgrounds.[56] In the comparison study, an important finding in many cases was a history of some form of conflictual or contradictory views or behaviors, which was strikingly similar to findings in the lone-actor terrorism group of individuals studied. For example, Hanssen was very active in the church and held strong religious beliefs, yet he engaged in contradictory behaviors, such as public displays of he and his wife being intimate without her knowledge, frequenting strip clubs, and befriending a stripper.[57] He expressed a hatred of communism despite betraying his country. Hanssen was a complex character who was able to compartmentalize aspects of his life. Other findings in some of the cases that overlapped with the lone-actor terrorism group, included (a) presence of clinical mental health symptoms or difficulties, (b) unfulfilled goals in the military or career, and (c) usually acting in isolation or with few others.[58,59]

Distinctions
An analysis of the preceding projects reveal a number of key differences between the two groups. An important distinction between those who commit espionage and lone-actor terrorism (in most cases) is that the former had background investigations, received adjudicated clearances, and consequently were not perceived as a security threat at the time of entry on duty (one obvious example in the lone-actor group would be Nidal Hasan). While both lone-actor terrorists and those who commit espionage typically act alone or with few others, those who commit espionage are part of structured organizations and, as such, were initially vetted and accepted into the organization. In contrast, lone-actor terrorists are not members of organized terrorist groups, and organized terrorist groups may weed out those who seem incompetent or pose a security threat to the group, although recently organized groups may encourage followers to act alone.[60] Membership in

a group (occupation/career) for those who commit espionage points to a fundamental difference when compared to lone-actor terrorists.

Another key difference is motivation. The motives of individuals who commit espionage may fall into one or more of several general categories: money (may not be the sole motivating factor), foreign allegiance, resentment/revengeful, and altruism. In many cases, motivation may be more complex. Those who breach national security typically do so in response to a personal crisis. As outlined earlier, recruitment almost always relies on a constellation of factors coming together at a particular point in time that is exploited by the case officer in contact with the target or when an individual reaches a crisis point that leads them to volunteer to a foreign intelligence service. A spy is assessed to see if there is a financial need and payments are made to address that specific need—this may or may not be based on greed (i.e., the individual "target" may have a selfless need, such as a sick relative in need of expensive treatment, which the case officer may then identify and exploit). There are of course basically venal people who are greedy and want money for the sake of accumulating possessions, but case officers are always assessing them to see if assets are living beyond their means. If so, they have a higher probability of getting caught. Money is basically a means to an end; it may be a proximate cause to spy but not the underlying motivation. In contrast, lone-actor terrorists are motivated by a specific context or ideology, and there may be a triggering event inspiring the terrorist activity.[56] Based on the preliminary studies under discussion, monetary payment was not a variable in lone-actor terrorism behavior (although monetary payment could be a factor in individuals acting on behalf of an organized group). For example, prior to providing classified information to the Soviet Union for money, Boone experienced marital problems, lost custody of his children, and was forced to pay part of his income to his ex-wife. In contrast, Timothy McVeigh, the lone-actor terrorist who committed the Oklahoma City bombing, was motivated by anti-government sentiment and the Waco and Ruby Ridge incidents.[56] There is some potential overlap, however, in motivation, in that harboring resentment and seeking revenge could be common to both. Additionally, in both groups— lone-actor terrorists and those committing treason/espionage—the "common pathway" involves a constellation of variables coming together at the right time, rather than simply one predominant factor or element. In summary, there are a range of potential motivations that combine uniquely in each individual based on their distinctive psychological issues, life experiences, and personal relationships. These converge in a way that allows an individual to violate the norms of society (in the case of a terrorist) and an individual's legal secrecy agreement (in the case of a spy).

Another difference is the way that each group's behavior is perceived by others. In some of the espionage cases, supervisors and colleagues failed to recognize the signs of a serious change in behavior prior to the espionage. For instance, those at the FBI did not detect any suspicious behavior in Hanssen's day-to-day life, and even after committing several security breaches, Hanssen's behavior was ignored.[3] Despite his security violations, affairs, and relationships with foreign nationals that violated CIA regulations, Ames's behavior was not considered suspicious and was apparently disregarded.[11-15] In the Walker case study, multiple sailors who worked with Walker noted unethical behavior and large financial transactions; however, he was not suspected of espionage.[61] In contrast, those in the lone-actor terrorist group may be characterized as presenting as odd or changed to others, and research has shown that, in at least some cases, there are preexisting suspicion or warning signs.[56] Dylann Roof, the terrorist who committed the Charleston church shooting, displayed a noticeable change in behavior, becoming quieter and "emotionless."[58,59] The broader histories of those in the lone-actor group are distinct to those in the espionage group. The rate of prior criminal behavior in the lone-actor group is high, with almost half having previous criminal convictions.[62] However, those in the espionage group did not display criminal behavior prior to breaching national security (prior criminal behavior would have been inconsistent with their employment in a national security setting).

Interpretation

Although individuals committing acts of espionage and acts of violence in the context of an ideology would seem to comprise disparate groups, there is an eventual confluence in that both espionage and terrorism result in damage to US national security and society as a whole. As discussed earlier, preliminary research shows some overlap in these groups in behavioral and clinical variables and, in some cases, motivation. As a group, those who commit espionage or treason are well-educated and have, to some degree, a successful career, although somewhere in the course of their career something failed. Numerous psychological variables have been identified which may play a role or influence an individual to commit espionage, including money, ideology, compromise, ego, disgruntlement, ingratiation, and thrill seeking.[63] In overlap with the lone-actor terrorism group, there will always be a constellation of factors (internal/psychological, external/group influences) that come together at a particular point in time to make an individual susceptible. Very few are driven by allegiance to a foreign government (particularly given the vetting process to get a clearance). The decision to betray one's country for money can be viewed as a means to satisfy a more complex need. Case officers look at financial vulnerabilities to measure a person's motivational need for money as one dimension in a vulnerability assessment (i.e., gambling, mistress, pay a debt, etc.). The multiple and integrated motivational factors unique to an individual's personal situation reflect a closer approximation of the drivers that lead an individual to commit espionage, at least in the context of threats to US national security. Future research into the underpinnings of individuals acting to commit espionage may also provide information to better understand and counter those individuals who would act violently on behalf of a belief.

MASS VIOLENCE WITHOUT AN IDEOLOGY

There is a limited literature reviewing the comparison of lone-actor terrorists with those committing mass violence and mass murder without a clear ideology. This section reviews case examples of the latter and discusses some research findings in this area. As stressed throughout this volume, case examples tend to be complex and multilayered, and, in some instances, individuals included in the lone-actor group may have had non-ideological motivations alongside ideological. An example of the latter would include Omar Mateen, the 2016 Orlando nightclub shooter, who identified himself as an Islamist soldier, yet, after the shooting, reports indicated that his sexual orientation may have been a separate variable,[64,65] although the relevance of this latter issue was debatable. Although on the surface these groups overlap to a significant degree, the literature points to some distinguishing features. Three case examples are briefly reviewed as an introduction to this topic, although these cases are not meant to be a comprehensive review.

Non-Ideology Case Examples

James Holmes

Holmes committed a mass shooting at an Aurora, Colorado, movie theater in July 2012, killing 12 and injuring 70 (from gunfire and other injuries). He confessed to the shooting, pleaded not guilty by reason of insanity, was found guilty, and was sentenced to life without parole.[66] Reports of his early life indicate his being a gifted student during childhood, but becoming withdrawn and having difficulty making friends when, at age 12, he and his family moved. He did well academically as an undergraduate but was described later as "rudderless"; he had difficulty getting into top graduate programs until he was accepted at the University of Colorado's Medical Campus in Aurora.[67] In the months before the shooting, Holmes met with psychiatrists on the campus and discussed homicidal thoughts, and one psychiatrist he worked with became concerned enough to alert the university threat assessment team, although reports indicate that authorities felt he did not reach the threshold of involuntary hospitalization.[68] He was evaluated by a forensic psychiatrist during the trial who indicated Holmes was "genetically loaded" for mental illness.[67] Another court-appointed psychiatrist who interviewed Holmes indicated that what led Holmes to open fire in the movie theater was a combination of mental illness, personality, his circumstances, and other unknown factors that may not be uncovered.[69] Although reports indicate mental illness was clearly established, prosecutors were able to persuade the jury that Holmes was criminally responsible at the time of the shooting.[70]

Andreas Lubitz

In March 2015, Lubitz, a co-pilot on a Germanwings airline flight from Barcelona to Düsseldorf, intentionally crashed the plane in the Alps, killing all passengers and crew on board.[71,72] Lubitz had a history of depression, at one point taking a leave from flight training in 2009 for several months.[73] Reports indicate Lubitz had reoccurrences of his depression; in December 2014 he developed depression with psychosis and was prescribed psychotropic medication.[74] In February and March 2015, reports indicate he had been reevaluated psychiatrically and diagnosed with several conditions, including psychosomatic disorder, anxiety, and a possible psychotic disorder, for which medications were prescribed and an inpatient psychiatric hospitalization was recommended.[75] The accident report by the French Civil Aviation Safety Investigation Authority indicated that no action could have been taken by the authorities or employer to prevent him from flying on the day of the crash because they were not informed by Lubitz or other parties of Lubitz's clinical picture.[74]

Following the crash, investigators found evidence that Lubitz was searching ways to commit suicide, that he feared he was going blind, and he was not sleeping.[76] Reports indicate no evidence was found that the co-pilot's actions were politically or religiously motivated.[77]

Stephen Paddock

In October 2017, Paddock opened fire from an elevated position in a hotel onto a crowd attending a concert in Las Vegas Nevada, killing 60 and wounding several hundred.[78] After the shooting, an array of weapons and ammunition was found in his hotel room, including assault weapons and "bump stocks" that allow for rapid fire simulating fully automatic fire.[79,80] Paddock killed himself before police could apprehend him.[81] A post-incident analysis by the FBI Behavioral Analysis Unit Las Vegas Review Panel (LVRP),[82] a group of experts from within and outside of the FBI, culminated in several important findings regarding Paddock's motivation and pre-attack behaviors:

- There was no ideology-motivated group or individual related to the attack; Paddock acted alone, and there was no clear single motivation.
- An apparent important factor was Paddock's desire to commit suicide.
- He had a desire to attain infamy through a mass casualty attack.
- His decision to murder people while they were being entertained was consistent with his personality.
- There was no indication that the attack was motivated by a grievance or revenge against a casino, Las Vegas institution, the festival, or an individual who was killed or injured in the attack.
- Once he decided to attack, he devoted time, attention, and energy to the attack, and he took multiple calculated steps to ensure his suicide would be under his control.
- He maintained interpersonal relationships and was not completely isolated.
- He was, in many ways, similar to other active shooters the FBI has studied.

The police and FBI found no motive in the attack and closed the investigation.[83] Knoll and Meloy developed a thoughtful analysis of the underlying psychology and dynamics related to Paddock,[84] describing his initial functioning in a more "internalized" mode with his earlier financial success and success in developing interpersonal relationships and that psychosis did not appear to be a factor. They note he was intelligent and methodical. The FBI noted he had minimal empathy throughout his life. Knoll and Meloy describe factors, including his alcohol use, gambling, despondency, financial stress, and alleged affair, along with the influence of his biological father (who had achieved notoriety on the FBI's Ten Most Wanted list), that led to a regression from an internalizing to an externalizing domain and that, within a context of psychopathy and with a destructive conviction, ultimately led to murder-suicide.[84] An unusual finding is that, in addition to the influence of his biological father, it was found that a distantly related gunman named Paddock (a fourth cousin to Stephen Paddock), a retired dentist-anesthetist, committed murder-suicide in 1888.[85]

Analysis and Literature Review

At first glance, it would appear that these two groups—individuals committing mass violence with an identified ideological drive and those committing mass violence without one—would overlap considerably. In some respects, they do, in that many lone-actor terrorism cases involve a complex mix of beliefs, variables, drives, etc., and not one pure ideology, and that many of the individuals not identified with an ideology (such as the examples just cited) are not apolitical and immune from stressors (interpersonal, biases, prejudices, beliefs, etc.) that may factor into their thinking and planning. To some extent, rather than distinct groups, individuals in both groups may fall along a continuum, with extremes being those with a clear ideology driving the behavior at one end, and, at the opposite end, those in whom no ideological drive can be identified. Although some of the cases cited in this volume may fall at the extremes, many would be somewhere in between. Despite this, research has shown some distinctions between these groups.

In a recent research study,[86] co-editor Paul Gill and colleagues compared lone-actor terrorists and those committing public mass murder on a number of variables. Results indicate a number of important findings: (a) there was little distinction in sociodemographics; (b) lone-actor terrorists were more likely to have military experience, criminal records convictions, engage in dry-runs and reconnaissance preparation, and verbalize their intent to commit violence; whereas (c) mass murderers were more likely to have a history of substance abuse and experience recent and chronic stress. Gill and his team found both groups shared similar background states including the prevalence of mental illness and financial problems in the 2-year period before the attack. In a comprehensive analysis by Horgan et al. comparing lone-actor terrorism with mass murderers, several findings were noted. Although there was little distinction between offender types with regard to sociodemographic profiles, there were distinctions involving the degree of interaction with co-conspirators, antecedent behaviors, and antecedent leakage of information.[87]

In a separate European study examining differences between lone-actor terrorists and a broader sample of homicide offenders, a number of distinguishing characteristics were found.[88] Lone-actor terrorists were found to be younger, more often single, and more often educated; they tended to attack strangers in public settings and use fire-arms. Homicide offenders were more likely to attack their victims in private settings using more "hands-on" methods.[88] In an interesting essay examining lone-actor terrorists, a case is made that, rather than individuals being cast as religious fanatics influenced by organized groups, many lone-actors are confused; they tend to fuse political and personal agendas, an argument that may support the continuum model of ideological drive in lone actors.[89] In a study by Clemmow et al. examining lone-actor terrorists and mass murderers, their research supported merging these groups into the concept of *lone-actor grievance-fueled violence* (LAGFV) *offenders*, rather than as distinct types, with results showing that, although differences exist, there is a "noteworthy shared space" between them.[90] This research parallels earlier work by Hallgarth into the complexities of motivation in offenders, indicating that lone-actor terrorism is a subset of other grievance-fueled violence, such as mass murders and workplace violence.[91] Several important observations were noted from this research, including motivational complexity and the difficulty in making distinctions between motivational factors in lone-actor terrorism when compared with other forms of grievance-fueled violence. This research noted the "interwoven grievances" of some lone-actor terrorists in whom strong ideological adherence may not be as prevalent compared with others who have no clear group guidance or direction but who may have high ideological motivation based on an internalized interpretation of an ideology.[91]

In keeping with the model of a broader overlap between lone offenders with and without a clear identified ideology, it may be time to reconsider the terms "lone-actor" or "lone-wolf" terrorism based on two points: (a) relationships with online and offline radical environments are often critical as related to motivation and capability, and (b) pre-attack behaviors in the majority of lone-actor terrorism cases are not as stealthy and highly capable as the lone-wolf title would suggest.[92]

SCHOOL SHOOTERS

Perpetrators of mass shootings at educational institutions ("school shooters") may possess characteristics that differentiate them from lone-actor terrorists although the two terms are not mutually exclusive. For the purposes of this review, "school shooters" will be understood to mean individuals not motivated primarily by political ideology. School shooters have been studied and described extensively elsewhere in the literature. This necessarily brief review serves only to outline some frequent characteristics among this subset of mass violence offenders. Some research suggests that the differences between lone-actor terrorists and school shooters are superficial.[93]

Empirical research and anecdotal reports support the existence of a contagion effect for all mass killings that is especially pronounced for school shootings.[94] This effect is believed to be due, at least in part, to the extensive and sensationalistic media coverage which such events typically receive.[95] Although school shootings date back at least as far as the nineteenth century, the mass public shooting from a bell tower at the University of Texas at Austin in 1966 is significant for having received an "unprecedented" level of news media coverage at the time.[95] This event claimed 14 lives and wounded another 32 individuals and inspired several subsequent mass shootings.[96, 97]

Like lone-actor terrorism, school shootings are statistically very rare,[98,99] which makes quantitative research into them challenging. Just as with research on lone-actor terrorism, research on school shootings is limited by the lack of a uniform definition of the phenomenon.[98] The frequency of school shootings appears to have been increasing recently,[99] and school shootings account for a significant proportion of casualties from active shooter events.[100] As is the case for lone-actor terrorists, there is no single unified "profile" for the school shooter.[101–103] For the purposes of this discussion and comparison to lone-actor terrorism, school shooters can be grouped according to four characteristics. These driving factors sometimes overlap, and an individual perpetrator's motives may be mixed or unclear.[104]

Revenge and Grievance-Fueled Shootings

Most school shootings occur in the context of a grievance of some kind, such as gang disputes.[105] Accidental shootings are more common than the targeted attacks or mass shootings that are often associated with the phrase "school shooting."[105] Because this analysis is focused on differences and similarities between lone-actor terrorists and other high-threat groups, "school shooters" in this chapter will be understood to mean perpetrators of targeted mass violence. More than half of all fatalities from shootings in K–12 schools are from such incidents.[105] Consistent with the finding that most school shootings are grievance-fueled incidents, a desire for revenge is a common motive.[104,106] Most school shootings in the United States have involved perpetrators who had experienced social isolation and rejection or persecution by their peers,[103,104,106] including prolonged bullying victimization observed by others[101] or stressors in relationships with romantic partners.[101] The experience of "aggrieved entitlement" has been proposed as a mechanism in the pathway toward violent action among school shooters.[107]

Some violence researchers[106,108] have described common "'cultural scripts"—prescriptions for behavior—that implicitly suggest firearm violence as an acceptable means of responding to interpersonal grievances, "particularly for altering the shooter's reputation from that of a loser to that of a notorious antihero."[108 (p. 1294)] Many school shooters have sought to recast themselves in such a light as a way of reclaiming power after subjective experiences of disempowerment and humiliation through bullying, rejection, or other forms of social exclusion. In many recent school attacks, perpetrators have distributed multimedia manifestos or suicide notes through the internet and social media as a way of explaining their reasons for the shooting. Public dissemination of such messages may perpetuate harmful cultural scripts and reinforce the notion that revenge through violent means is an acceptable or logical response to grievances.[106]

One of the most extensively studied school shootings to date is the massacre at Columbine High School in Littleton, Colorado, on April 20, 1999.[109] This incident has become so imprinted on the public consciousness that the mere mention of the word "Columbine" is likely to conjure up images of a school shooting rather than flowers, and the term "pulling a Columbine" has become shorthand for mass shootings, particularly in school settings.[97,107,110] The Columbine attack resulted in 15 dead (including the two shooters) and 23 wounded, garnered extensive and sensationalistic media coverage, and later served as the inspiration (and, in some cases, the template) for numerous subsequent school shootings and other acts of mass violence.[109,111] The shooting also appears to have had a snowball-type effect in that it inspired future shootings which themselves inspired subsequent attacks, many of which were committed by perpetrators also fascinated by the Columbine shooters.[96,109] Many of these perpetrators, such as the student who committed the mass shooting at Virginia Tech in 2007, were also motivated in part by grievances and a desire for revenge.[112,113]

Mental Health and Emotional and Developmental Difficulties

A history of some form of mental health condition or other emotional or developmental difficulties is common among school shooters.[108,114] The US Secret Service has reported that nearly all perpetrators of targeted school attacks had experienced some form of negative experiences in their homes, such as parental divorce or family members facing criminal charges.[101] Fernandez and colleagues found that the majority of mass shootings (including school shootings) have been committed by individuals experiencing significant levels of anger in response to psychological or psychosocial triggers (as opposed to physical stressors).[115]

Media reports of school shootings often initially present speculative information about the perpetrator's mental health (e.g., suspected schizophrenia or Asperger's disorder in the Sandy Hook shooter, suspected paranoid schizophrenia in the Virginia Tech shooter, or sociopathy in one of the Columbine shooters).[111] These reports are often made with minimal evidence to support the use of such diagnostic terminology, and they are believed to be a factor in perpetuating stigma toward persons with mental illness, potentially having a chilling effect on treatment-seeking.[102,116-118] Inaccurate statements that most school shooters were taking psychotropic prescription medicines prior to their attacks have also proliferated through social media, potentially contributing to public fears that such medications may increase the risk of violence.[102]

The Safe Schools Initiative of the US Secret Service found that 78% of school shooters had attempted or seriously considered suicide prior to their attacks.[103] Other research has confirmed the prevalence of suicidal ideation among school shooters.[101,106,107,114] Lankford has noted that school shooters and other perpetrators of mass violence, including lone-actor terrorists, typically exhibit many of the known risk factors for suicide.[93] Several school shooters, including the perpetrators of the Columbine shooting and the Red Lake High School shooting in 2005, shared their suicidal thoughts online prior to their attacks.[98,108]

Many school shooters had experienced significant personal losses or failures and had difficulty coping.[103] It bears noting that nearly 50% of the population in the US will meet criteria for some mental health diagnosis during their lifetimes.[119] In the Safe Schools Initiative sample, despite the high prevalence (61%) of a documented history of feeling extremely depressed or desperate, most school shooters had not received a mental health evaluation or diagnosis prior to their attacks.[103] However, research suggests that a history of mental health treatment may be growing more common, as roughly half of school attackers in a more recent sample had received some form of mental health services before the attack.[101] Whether school shooters are more likely to have been referred for mental health treatment than their peers who do not go on to commit mass violence is currently unknown because referral for psychological treatment or counseling has become more common among youth in general.

Fascination with and Admiration of Previous Perpetrators

Many school shooters have idolized and admired the perpetrators of previous school shootings, often viewing them as role models[96-98,108] and participating in subcultures online that glorify them.[97,109] This tendency to revere persons responsible for previous attacks is common among mass violence offenders in general, including lone-actor terrorists.[94,97] However, the phenomenon appears to be most pronounced among younger perpetrators, particularly those in their teenage and young adult years.[96] Some killers have expressed the desire to outdo the death counts of previous attacks.[96,111,114,120] Admiration of the Columbine school shooters has been apparent in internet-based subcultures around school shootings and numerous subsequent school shootings, with fans and perpetrators imitating their clothing[97,108,109] and musical tastes[109]; characterizing them as "gods,"[96] "saints,"[96] and "martyrs"[96,111] planning attacks on anniversaries of the Columbine shooting[96,98,108]; and even traveling to Littleton prior to the commission of an offense.[96] The Columbine attack was found to have had a strong copycat effect in the months following the incident,[106] and the incident has continued to inspire numerous school shooters and other perpetrators of mass violence (both thwarted and successful) in subsequent years.[96,108,109]

The perpetrator of the school shooting at Virginia Polytechnic Institute and State University ("Virginia Tech") on April 16, 2007 that claimed 32 lives idolized the Columbine shooters.[96,108,111] At age 15, not long after the Columbine incident, he wrote a disturbing essay involving themes of homicide and suicide (Murray 2017), stating that he "wanted to repeat Columbine."[96 (p. 221)] Despite evidence that the media frenzy following the tragedy in Littleton inspired the Virginia Tech shooter, news media coverage of the massacre at Virginia Tech also contained extensive and sensationalistic commentary about the perpetrator, including large photographs of him, some of which he had staged and taken himself, anticipating such coverage and publicity.[111,121] As had occurred in the wake of the Columbine attack, individuals responsible for planning and executing numerous subsequent mass shootings identified with and admired the Virginia Tech shooter, who has also become the subject of considerable commentary on the internet and social media.[96]

One of these individuals was a teenager who later killed 27 and wounded 2 at Sandy Hook Elementary School in Newtown, Connecticutt, in December 2012.[100] The Sandy Hook shooter was fascinated with mass killers in general and kept an extensive spreadsheet listing details from more than 500 attacks, including the perpetrators' names, weapons used, number of victims, and circumstances of the attack.[111] He especially admired the Columbine and Virginia Tech shooters[111] and participated regularly in internet forums wherein previous school shooters were idolized and analyzed.[109,114] As was the case for the Virginia Tech shooter, the fascination with earlier school shooters had begun at an early age and continued up until the commission of an attack in early adulthood. At the time of their crimes, the Virginia Tech and Sandy Hook shooters were 23 and 20 years of age, respectively.[100] Again, news coverage following the event contained detailed and extensive information about the perpetrator,[122] and subsequent school shooters have exhibited fascination with the Sandy Hook shooter.[109,123]

Desire for Fame and Notoriety

Some school shooters are motivated, at least in part, by a desire for fame and notoriety.[96,97,108,109,114,123,124] This motive appears to be more common among younger perpetrators (i.e., teenagers and young adults).[96,97,114] Although a desire for fame and notoriety was identified in only 10% of targeted school attackers in a recent Secret Service analysis,[101] this motive has figured prominently in some of the deadliest school shootings in US history,[97] attacks which have inspired copycat plots and a desire to "outdo" previous perpetrators in terms of death counts.[97,120] The Columbine high school shooters foresaw the lasting fame and notoriety that their attack would have and speculated about which Hollywood director would produce a movie about them.[97,114] The shooting did subsequently appear in various media, including feature films known by later school shooters.[98] The Virginia Tech shooter sent videos of himself directly to news outlets.[114] Compared to non–fame-seeking perpetrators of mass killings, attacks by persons seeking notoriety tend to have higher numbers of victims.[114]

For the perpetrator of the mass shooting at Sandy Hook Elementary School, the desire for fame was significant. He was "obsessed with movies about mass shooters, . . . participated in online debates about which was the 'the most famous school shooting,' and posted 'just look at how many fans you can find for all different types of mass murderers.'"[123 (p. 262)] Lankford has suggested that the Sandy Hook shooter's decision to target young children for his attack may have been motivated by this desire for fame and notoriety.[114]

Among those inspired by the Sandy Hook shooting was the fame-seeking perpetrator of the shooting at Marjorie Stoneman Douglas High School in Parkland, Florida, whose attack in February 2018 claimed the lives of 17 people.[125] He had expressed the desire to be known as a "professional school shooter,"[97,125] and in several videos recorded before the shooting, he stated a desire for his name to be remembered.[125] He also appears to have had mixed motives for the shooting in that he expressed racist, homophobic, xenophobic, and anti-Semitic views on social media[126] as well as feelings of loneliness and worthlessness.[125] Several months after the Parkland shooting, another fame-seeking school shooter killed 10 and wounded 13 at a high school in Santa Fe, Texas, wearing clothes evocative of the Columbine shooters and later telling investigators that he let some classmates live so that his story could be told.[97]

Characteristics Shared with Lone-Actor Terrorists

Several factors that school shooters frequently share with lone-actor terrorists and other mass violence perpetrators include male gender,[93,95,101] a fascination with violence and weapons (particularly firearms),[98,112,113,127] a fascination or obsession with previous incidents of mass violence,[125] the tendency to construct detailed plans for their attacks long before acting on them (i.e., their acts are not impulsive, unlike most other forms of homicide),[101,104,127,128] the presence of depression or other mental health difficulties before the attack,[101,128] the experience of significant personal crisis (e.g., failure in school or military training, recent major loss),[127,128] a lack of motivation for material profit,[128] a tendency to act alone,[128] and the existence of a perceived grievance.[101,112–115,128] As is the case among lone-actor terrorists, the presence of multiple and mixed motives is common in school shooters.[101] School shootings and lone-actor terrorist attacks receive a disproportionate percentage of media coverage of mass violence.[95]

Common Characteristics of School Shooters

Most school shooters exhibit some pre-attack behavior that arouses concern among others, such as classmates, family, or school personnel.[101,104,106,111,120,129] The majority display weapons or threaten others with weapons before the attack,[120] most (81%) use handguns in their attacks,[99] and most possess a fascination with other school shooters and other mass-violence perpetrators.[120] Many express a desire to influence others and inspire future attacks.[96] School shooters are often outsiders who are isolated from the social world of their peers at school, but not necessarily "loners"; most are subjected to bullying and ostracism.[101,111] As noted earlier, many school shooters experience suicidal ideation prior to their attacks,[101,103] and most had experienced a recent personal crisis such as significant loss or failure.[128] Most are male,[101,107,128] white,[115,128] and between the ages of 12 and 18.[101,105,128] A history of disciplinary actions in school is also common.[101] The majority of school shooters in K–12 settings are themselves students at the school which they target,[100] while the perpetrators of shootings at college and university settings tend to be older and more socially isolated.[108] School shooters, on average, tend to be significantly younger than other perpetrators of mass violence, such as lone-actor terrorists.[93] In school settings, as the offender's age increases, so, too, does the likely severity of the attack,[99] and the use of rifles or shotguns increases the likely number of fatalities.[99] These characteristics and comparisons, however, must be interpreted with caution; mass shootings at higher education settings like colleges were very rare prior to 2002,[108] and school shootings in general remain statistically rare events.

CONCLUSION

Research involving groups posing higher risk of violence to society have shown a fairly large overlap in characteristics and patterns although, as outlined in this chapter, each of these groups— lone-actor terrorists, those committing treason, individuals committing mass violence without an identified ideology, and school shooters—have distinguishing characteristics. This unique area of study can inform law enforcement, security, intelligence, clinicians, policymakers, and society as a whole on the associated risks and the potential for future mitigation of these risks.

NOTES AND REFERENCES

1. Espionage Act of 1917 ("An Act to punish acts of interference with the foreign relations, the neutrality, and the foreign commerce of the United States, to punish espionage, and better to enforce the criminal laws of the United States, and for other purposes"). 18 USC. Ch. 37 (18 USC. § 792 et seq.), Pub. L. 65-24, 40 Stat. 217 (1917).

2. Myre G. Once reserved for spies, Espionage Act now used against suspected leakers. NPR.org, 28 Jun 2017. https://www.npr.org/sections/parallels/2017/06/28/534682231/once-reserved-for-spies-espionage-act-now-used-against-suspected-leakers

3. United States Department of Justice, Office of the Inspector General. *A Review of the FBI's Performance in Deterring, Detecting, and Investigating the Espionage Activities of Robert Philip Hanssen.* Washington, DC: United States Department of Justice, Office of the Inspector General; August 2003. https://www.hsdl.org/?abstract&did=442330

4. United States Federal Bureau of Investigation. *History: Robert Hanssen.* Washington, DC: US FBI National Press Office, 20 Feb 2001. https://www.fbi.gov/history/famous-cases/robert-hanssen.

5. Robert Philip Hanssen. Times Topics. *New York Times.* 2020. https://www.nytimes.com/topic/person/robert-philip-hanssen

6. Wise D. *Spy: The Inside Story of How the FBI's Robert Hanssen Betrayed America.* New York: Random House; 2003.

7. Mangold T. When betrayal and paranoia are part of the job. New York Times, 2 Jan 2002. https://www.nytimes.com/2002/01/02/opinion/when-betrayal-and-paranoia-are-part-of-the-job.html

8. ABC News. Spycatcher: Bringing down Robert Hanssen. ABC News, 6 Jan 2006. https://abcnews.go.com/2020/story?id=123776

9. Nix E. Robert Hanssen: American traitor. History.com, 10 May 2017; updated 10 Apr 2019. https://www.history.com/news/robert-hanssen-american-traitor

10. Sanford JS, Arrigo BA. Policing and psychopathy: The case of Robert Philip Hanssen. *J Forensic Psychol Pract.* 2007;7(3):1–31.

11. DeConcini D, Warner JW, Metzenbaum HM, et al. *An Assessment of the Aldrich H. Ames Espionage Case and Its Implications for US Intelligence.* Washington, DC: US Senate Select Committee on Intelligence, November 1, 1994. https://www.intelligence.senate.gov/sites/default/files/publications/10390.pdf

12. Weiner T, Johnston D, Lewis NA. *Betrayal: The Story of Aldrich Ames, An American Spy.* New York: Random House; 1995.

13. United States Federal Bureau of Investigation. History: Aldrich Ames. https://www.fbi.gov/history/famous-cases/aldrich-ames

14. Weiner T. Why I spied: Aldrich Ames. *New York Times Magazine*, 31 Jul 1994:sect 6, p. 16. https://www.nytimes.com/1994/07/31/magazine/why-i-spied-aldrich-ames.html

15. Shapira I. "Rick is a goddamn Russian spy": Does the CIA have a new Aldrich Ames on its hands? Washington Post, 26 Jan 2018. https://www.washingtonpost.com/news/retropolis/wp/2018/01/26/rick-is-a-goddamn-russian-spy-does-the-cia-have-a-new-aldrich-ames-on-its-hands/

16. Blitzer W. *Territory of Lies.* New York: Harper & Row; 1989.

17. Hersh S. The traitor. *The New Yorker.* 18 Jan18, 1999:26–33.

18. Olive RJ. *Capturing Jonathan Pollard: How One of the Most Notorious Spies in American History Was Brought to Justice.* Annapolis, MD: Naval Institute Press; 2006.

19. Best RA Jr, Mark C. *Jonathan Pollard: Background and Considerations for Presidential Clemency.* Washington, DC: Congressional Research Service, US Library of Congress, 31 Jan 2001.

20. Bernstein A. Sumner Shapiro, long-serving director of Naval Intelligence (obituary).

Washington Post, 16 Nov 2006. https://www.washingtonpost.com/wp-dyn/content/article/2006/11/16/AR2006111600153.html

21. Lauer E, Semmelman J. Don't be fooled by Ronald Olive (op-ed). *Jerusalem Post*, 28 Nov 2006. https://www.jpost.com/Opinion/Op-Ed-Contributors/Dont-be-fooled-by-Ronald-Olive

22. Barnes JE. Jonathan Pollard, convicted spy, completes parole and may move to Israel. *New York Times*, 20 Nov 2020. https://www.nytimes.com/2020/11/20/us/politics/jonathan-pollard-parole-ends.html

23. Halbfinger DM, Kershner I. Jonathan Pollard, spy for Israel, gets hero's welcome from Netanyahu: 'You're home.' *New York Times*, 30 Dec 2020. https://www.nytimes.com/2020/12/30/world/middleeast/jonathan-pollard-israel-us-spy.html

24 Jonathan Pollard: American civilian defense analyst and spy. *Encyclopedia Britannica*, 25 Mar 2020. https://www.britannica.com/biography/Jonathan-Pollard

25. Associated Press. Convicted US spy Pollard is greeted by Netanyahu as he arrives in Israel. *Politico*, 30 Dec 2020. https://www.politico.com/news/2020/12/29/jonathan-pollard-spy-israel-452235

26 Herbig KL, Wiskoff MF. *Espionage Against the United States by American Citizens, 1947–2001* (Technical Report 02-5). Monterey, CA: Defense Personnel Security Research Center; July 2002.

27. Earley P. *Family of Spies: Inside the John Walker Spy Ring*. New York: Bantam; 1989.

28. Cornwell R. John Walker: American naval officer who formed a family spy ring that passed highly damaging secrets to the Soviet Union (obituary). *The Independent*, 1 Sep 2014. https://www.independent.co.uk/news/obituaries/john-walker-american-naval-officer-who-formed-family-spy-ring-passed-highly-damaging-secrets-soviet-union-9704890.html

29. Prados J. The John Walker spy ring and the US Navy's biggest betrayal. *US Naval Institute (USNI) News*, 2 Sep 2014. https://news.usni.org/2014/09/02/john-walker-spy-ring-u-s-navys-biggest-betrayal

30. Well M. John A. Walker Jr., who led family spy ring, dies at 77. *Washington Post*, 30 Aug 2014. https://www.washingtonpost.com/national/john-a-walker-who-led-family-spy-ring-dies/2014/08/30/dbc41a56-2f9d-11e4-bb9b-997ae96fad33_story.html

31. United States Federal Bureau of Investigation. History: Year of the spy (1985). n.d. https://www.fbi.gov/history/famous-cases/year-of-the-spy-1985

32. Rafalko FJ. Russia. In Rafalko FJ, ed. *A Counterintelligence Reader, Vol. 4: American Revolution into the New Millennium*. Washington, DC: Federation of American Scientists / National Counterintelligence Center (US); 2004:79–186.

33. Affidavit in support of criminal complaint, arrest warrant, and search warrants against David Sheldon Boone. Alexandria, VA: United States Attorney's Office, Eastern District of Virginia, US Department of Justice, 15 Oct 1998.

34. Thompson N. Bitter NSA worker allegedly turns spy: A former Army sergeant with life in tatters stands accused of selling secrets. *Baltimore Sun*, 9 Nov 1998. https://www.baltimoresun.com/news/bs-xpm-1998-11-09-1998313039-story.html

35. Kilian M. Ex-soldier accused of spying for Soviets caught in FBI sting. *Chicago Tribune*, 14 Oct 1998. https://www.chicagotribune.com/news/ct-xpm-1998-10-14-9810140108-story.html

36. *Espionage cases, 1975–2004: Summaries and sources*. Monterey, CA: Defense Personnel Security Research Center (PERSEREC), United States Department of Defense / Homeland Security Digital Library, Naval Postgraduate School; November 2004. https://www.hsdl.org/?view&did=482512

37. Risen J. Spy agencies' ex-analyst charged with selling secrets to Soviets. *New York Times*, 14 Oct 1998. https://www.nytimes.com/1998/10/14/world/spy-agencies-ex-analyst-charged-with-selling-secrets-to-soviets.html

38. *Espionage cases: National Security Agency*. Monterey, CA: Defense Personnel and Security Research Center (PERSEREC). United States Department of Defense, n.d. https://www.dhra.mil/PERSEREC/Espionage-Cases/nsa/

39. Bhattacharjee Y. My father and me: A spy story. GQ.com, 15 Jun 2012. https://www.gq.com/story/my-father-and-me-spy-story-russia

40. Grier P. Ex-wife's view of life with an accused CIA spy. *Christian Science Monitor*, 27 Jan 1997. https://www.csmonitor.com/1997/0127/012797.us.us.1.html

41. Lichtblau E. Jailed C.I.A. mole kept spying for Russia, via son, US says. *New York Times*, 29 Jan 2009. https://www.nytimes.com/2009/01/30/us/30spy.html

42. Joint CIA-FBI press release on arrest of Harold James Nicholson. United States Central Intelligence Agency and Federal Bureau of Investigation, 18 Nov 1996. Washington, DC: Federation of American Scientists; 1996. https://fas.org/irp/cia/news/pr111896.html

43. United States Federal Bureau of Investigation. All in the family: Spy and his son indicted. FBI, 2 Feb 2009. https://archives.fbi.gov/archives/news/stories/2009/february/familyspies_020209

44. Weiner T. C.I.A. traitor severely hurt US security, judge is told. *New York Times*, 4 Jun 1997. https://www.nytimes.com/1997/06/04/us/cia-traitor-severely-hurt-us-security-judge-is-told.html

45. Chamberlain G. Harold Nicholson. *History of Spies*. https://historyofspies.com/harold-nicholson/

46. United States Department of Justice, Office of Public Affairs. Imprisoned spy pleads guilty to conspiracy to act as an agent of the Russian government and money laundering (Press Release No. 10-1261). US Department of Justice, 8 Nov 2010; updated 15 Sep 2014. https://www.justice.gov/opa/pr/imprisoned-spy-pleads-guilty-conspiracy-act-agent-russian-government-and-money-laundering

47. Gee A. Jeff Carney: The lonely US airman turned Stasi spy. *BBC World Service*, 19 Sep 2013. https://www.bbc.com/news/magazine-23978501

48. Dahlkamp J. No country more beautiful. *Spiegel International*, 14 Jul 2003. https://www.spiegel.de/international/spiegel/agents-no-country-more-beautiful-a-257041.html

49. Catching an Air Force spy. Wright-Patterson AFB, OH: National Museum of the US Air Force; 1 Jun 2015. https://www.nationalmuseum.af.mil/Visit/Museum-Exhibits/Fact-Sheets/Display/Article/197642/catching-an-air-force-spy/

50. Kidwell D. Jeffrey Martin Carney: An AF deserter turned spy. Quantico, VA: United States Air Force, Office of Special Investigations; 23 Apr 2020. https://www.osi.af.mil/News/Features/Display/Article/2161575/jeffrey-martin-carney-an-af-deserter-turned-spy/

51. Wilder UM. Why spy now? The psychology of espionage and leaking in the digital age. *Stud Intelligence*. 2017;61(2):1–36. https://www.cia.gov/static/db3b29681fc4ba71b0220d16bb979ddd/Psych-of-Leaking-Espionage.pdf

52. Gelles M. Exploring the mind of the spy. NOAA Western Regional Center: Treason 101. United States Department of Commerce Office of Security, Western Region Security Office; 28 Nov 2001. https://www.wrc.noaa.gov/wrso/security_guide/mind.htm

53. Marbes W. Psychology of treason. *Stud Intelligence*. 1986;30(2):1–11. https://www.cia.gov/readingroom/docs/DOC_0006183135.pdf

54. Stein J. Treason on their minds. *Washington Post*, 12 Jan 1997. https://www.washingtonpost.com/archive/opinions/1997/01/12/treason-on-their-minds/2d7d89a5-f101-4bee-af80-2942cee59000/

55. Shaw E, Sellers L. Application of the critical-path method to evaluate insider risks. *Stud Intelligence*. 2015;59(2):1–8.

56. Holzer JC, Trosch ZS, Bursztajn H, Giella P. Anti-government rhetoric, violence, and psychiatric vulnerability. Poster presented at: American Academy of Psychiatry and the Law 43rd Annual Meeting; 26 Oct 2012, Montreal, Quebec, Canada.

57. Zahn P, Shannon E. Look at FBI spy Robert Hanssen. *American Morning with Paula Zahn* (show transcript). CNN.com, 8 Jan 2002. http://archives.cnn.com/TRANSCRIPTS/0201/08/ltm.08.html

58. Holzer JC. Lone-actor terrorism: Clinical and behavioral patterns. Presentation to the US Federal Bureau of Investigation, Boston, MA. April 2019.

59. Holzer JC. Lone-actor terrorism: Clinical and behavioral patterns. Presentation to START. July 2020.

60. Connor J, Flynn CR. Report: Lone wolf terrorism. Security Studies Program, National Security Critical Issue Task Force, Georgetown University, 27 Jun 2015. https://georgetownsecuritystudiesreview.org/wp-content/uploads/2015/08/NCITF-Final-Paper.pdf.

61. Heath LJ. *An Analysis of the Systemic Security Weaknesses of the US Navy Fleet Broadcasting System, 1967–1974, as Exploited by CWO John Walker*. Masters thesis. Leavenworth, KS: US Army Command and General Staff College; 2005. https://fas.org/irp/eprint/heath.pdf

62. Gill P. *Lone-Actor Terrorists: A Behavioural Analysis*. New York: Routledge; 2016.

63. Charney DL, Irvin JA. The psychology of espionage. Guide to the study of intelligence, the psychology of espionage. *Intelligencer*. 2016;22(1):71–77. https://www.afio.com/publications/CHARNEY_The_Psychology_of_Espionage_DRAFT_2014Aug28.pdf

64. Robles F, Turkewitz J. Was the Orlando gunman gay? The answer continues to elude the F.B.I. *New York Times*, 25 Jun 2016. https://www.nytimes.com/2016/06/26/us/was-the-orlando-gunman-gay-the-answer-continues-to-elude-the-fbi.html

65. Mitchell J, Bauerlein V, Paletta D. Before Orlando shooter's routine last days, hints of instability. *Wall Street Journal*, 14 Jun 2016. https://www.wsj.com/articles/before-orlando-shooters-routine-last-days-hints-of-instability-1465858489

66. O'Neill A. Theater shooter Holmes gets 12 life sentences, plus 3,318 years. *CNN*, 27 Aug 2015. https://www.cnn.com/2015/08/26/us/james-holmes-aurora-massacre-sentencing/index.html.

67. O'Neill A. James Holmes' life story didn't sway jury. *CNN*, 11 Aug 2015. https://www.cnn.com/2015/08/02/us/13th-juror-james-holmes-aurora-shooting/

68. Goode E, Kovaleski SF, Healy J, Frosch D. Before gunfire, hints of "bad news." *New York Times*, 26 Aug 2012. https://www.nytimes.com/2012/08/27/us/before-gunfire-in-colorado-theater-hints-of-bad-news-about-james-holmes.html

69. Elliott D. Psychiatrist: Much is still hidden in theater shooter's mind. *Washington Times*, 5 Aug 2018. https://www.washingtontimes.com/news/2018/aug/5/psychiatrist-much-is-still-hidden-in-theater-shoot/

70. Koppel N. James Holmes found guilty of murder in Colorado theater shooting trial. *Wall Street Journal*, 16 Jul 2015. https://www.wsj.com/articles/james-holmes-found-guilty-in-colorado-theater-shooting-trial-1437085199

71. What happened on the Germanwings flight. *New York Times*, 27 Mar 2015. https://www.nytimes.com/interactive/2015/03/24/world/europe/germanwings-plane-crash-map.html

72. Bilefsky D, Clark N. Fatal descent of Germanwings plane was "deliberate," French authorities say. *New York Times*, 26 Mar 2015. https://www.nytimes.com/2015/03/27/world/europe/germanwings-crash.html

73. Bryan V. Lufthansa flight school knew of crash pilot's depression. *Reuters*, 31 Mar 2015. https://www.reuters.com/article/us-france-crash-pilot-idUSKBN0MR1EJ20150401

74. Bureau d'Enquêtes et d'Analyses pour la sécurité de l'aviation civile. Final Report: Accident on 24 March 2015 at Prads-Haute-Bléone (Alpes-de-Haute-Provence, France) to the Airbus A320-211 registered D-AIPX operated by Germanwings (courtesy translation). Le Bourget Cedex, France: Bureau d'Enquêtes et d'Analyses (BEA); March 2016. https://www.bea.aero/uploads/tx_elyextendttnews/BEA2015-0125.en-LR_04.pdf

75. Germanwings crash: Co-pilot Lubitz 'researched suicide.' *BBC News*, 2 Apr 2015. https://www.bbc.com/news/world-europe-32159602

76. Germanwings crash: French prosecutors open new probe. *BBC News*, 11 Jun 2015. https://www.bbc.com/news/world-europe-33098797

77. What we know about A320 co-pilot Andreas Lubitz. News.com.au, 28 Mar 2015. https://www.news.com.au/travel/travel-updates/incidents/what-we-know-about-a320-copilot-andreas-lubitz/news-story/ce1230b88c2742f5abcfa-41768f9afeb

78. Newburg K. Sisolak: "We will never, never forget" those killed in Oct. 1 shooting. *Las Vegas Review-Journal*, 1 Oct 2020. https://www.reviewjournal.com/local/local-las-vegas/sisolak-we-will-never-never-forget-those-killed-in-oct-1-shooting-2134042/

79. Multiple weapons found in Las Vegas gunman's hotel room. *New York Times*, 2 Oct 2017. https://www.nytimes.com/2017/10/02/us/las-vegas-shooting.html

80. Pane LM. Once an obscure device, "bump stocks" are in the spotlight. *AP News*, 4 Oct 2017. https://apnews.com/article/north-america-us-news-ap-top-news-las-vegas-shootings-ff26110203da4a28bfd1d99022fb401c

81. Moore J. Vegas shooter Stephen Paddock planned to escape but shot himself as SWAT team moved in. *Newsweek*, 5 Oct 2017. https://www.newsweek.com/vegas-shooter-stephen-paddock-planned-escape-left-note-shooting-himself-678572

82. United States Federal Bureau of Investigation. Key findings of the Behavioral Analysis Unit's Las Vegas review panel. US Department of Justice, 2019. https://www.hsdl.org/?abstract&did=820782

83. Romo V. FBI finds no motive in Las Vegas shooting, closes investigation. *NPR*, 29 Jan 2019. https://www.npr.org/2019/01/29/689821599/fbi-finds-no-motive-in-las-vegas-shooting-closes-investigation

84. Knoll JL IV, Meloy JR. The mass shooter and his mental functioning. *Psychiatric Times*, 17 Feb 2020. https://www.psychiatrictimes.com/view/mass-shooter-and-his-mental-functioning

85. Kumar BJ, Bause GS. Related gunmen Paddock committed murder-suicide in 1888 and in 2017. *J Anesth Hist*. 2018;4(3):193–195.

86. Gill P, Silver J, Horgan J, Corner E, Bouhana N. Similar crimes, similar behaviors? Comparing lone-actor terrorists and public mass murderers. *J Forensic Sci*. 2021;66(5):1797–1804.

87. Horgan JG, Gill P, Bouhana N, Silver J, Corner E. Across the universe? A comparative analysis of violent behavior and radicalization across three offender types with implications for criminal justice training and education. Final Report to the United States Department of Justice, June 2016. Washington, DC: US Department of Justice, Office of Justice Programs; 2016. https://www.ojp.gov/pdffiles1/nij/grants/249937.pdf

88. Liem M, van Buuren J, Schönberger H. *Cut from the Same Cloth? Lone Actor Terrorists Versus Common Homicide Offenders*. The Hague: International Centre for Counter-Terrorism; 2018. https://icct.nl/app/uploads/2018/04/ICCT-Liem-et-al-Cut-from-the-Same-Cloth-April2018.pdf

89. Pascarelli P. Ideology à la carte: Why lone actor terrorists choose and fuse ideologies. *Lawfare*, 2 Oct 2016. https://www.lawfareblog.com/ideology-à-la-carte-why-lone-actor-terrorists-choose-and-fuse-ideologies

90. Clemmow C, Gill P, Bouhana N, Silver J, Horgan J. Disaggregating lone-actor grievance-fuelled violence: Comparing lone-actor terrorists and mass murderers [published online ahead of print February 19, 2020]. *Terrorism and Political Violence*. doi:10.1080/09546553.2020.1718661.

91. Hallgarth JG. *A Framework for Violence: Clarifying the Role of Motivation in Lone-Actor Terrorism*. [Masters thesis]. Monterey, CA: Naval Postgraduate School; 2017. https://www.hsdl.org/?view&did=800859

92. Schuurman B, Lindekilde L, Malthaner S, O'Connor F, Gill P, Bouhana N. End of the lone wolf: The typology that should not have been. *Stud Conflict Terrorism*. 2019;42(8):771–778.

93. Lankford A. A comparative analysis of suicide terrorists and rampage, workplace, and school shooters in the United States from 1990 to 2010. *Homicide Stud*. 2013;17(3):255–274.

94. Towers S, Gomez-Lievano A, Khan M, Mubayi A, Castillo-Chavez C. Contagion in mass killings and

school shootings. *PLoS One*. 2015;10(7):e0117259. doi:10.1371/journal.pone.0117259.

95. Silva JR, Capellan JA. A comparative analysis of media coverage of mass public shootings: Examining rampage, disgruntled employee, school, and lone-wolf terrorist shootings in the United States. *Crim Justice Policy Rev*. 2019;30(9):1312–1341.

96. Langman P. Different types of role model influence and fame seeking among mass killers and copycat offenders. *Am Behav Sci*. 2018;62(2):210–228.

97. Silva JR, Greene-Colozzi EA. Fame-seeking mass shooters in America: Severity, characteristics, and media coverage. *Aggress Violent Behav*. 2019;48:24–35.

98. Abel MN, Chermak S, Freilich JD. Pre-attack warning behaviors of 20 adolescent school shooters: A case study analysis [published online ahead of print April 17, 2021]. *Crime Delinquency*. doi:10.1177/0011128721999338.

99. Livingston MD, Rossheim ME, Hall KS. A descriptive analysis of school and school shooter characteristics and the severity of school shootings in the United States, 1999–2018. *J Adol Health*. 2019;64:797–799.

100. Blair JP, Schweit KW. *A Study of Active Shooter Incidents, 2000–2013*. Washington, DC: Texas State University and Federal Bureau of Investigation, US Department of Justice; 2014.

101. Alathari L, Drysdale D, Driscoll S, et al. *Protecting America's Schools: A US Secret Service Analysis of Targeted School Violence*. Washington, DC: National Threat Assessment Center, US Secret Service, Department of Homeland Security; 2019.

102. Hall RCW, Friedman SH, Sorrentino R, Lapchenko M, Marcus A, Ellis R. The myth of school shooters and psychotropic medications. *Behav Sci Law*. 2019;37:540–558.

103. Vossekuil B, Fein RA, Reddy M, Borum R, Modzeleski W. *The Final Report and Findings of the Safe School Initiative: Implications for the Prevention of School Attacks in the United States*. Washington, D.C.: United States Secret Service and United States Department of Education, July 2004.

104. United States Department of Justice, Federal Bureau of Investigation, Behavioral Analysis Unit. *The School Shooter: A Quick Reference Guide*. Quantico, VA: National Center for the Analysis of Violent Crime; March 2018.

105. United States Government Accountability Office. *K-12 Education: Characteristics of School Shootings*, GAO-20-455. Washington, DC: US GAO; June 2020.

106. Preti A. School shooting as a culturally enforced way of expressing suicidal hostile intentions. *J Am Acad Psychiatry Law*. 2008;36(4):544–550.

107. Kalish R, Kimmel M. Suicide by mass murder: Masculinity, aggrieved entitlement, and rampage school shootings. *Health Sociol Rev*. 2010;19(4):451–464.

108. Newman K, Fox C. Repeat tragedy: Rampage shootings in American high school and college settings, 2002–2008. *Am Behav Sci*. 2009;52(9):1286–1308.

109. Raitanen J, Oksanen A. Global online subculture surrounding school shootings. *Am Behav Sci*. 2018;62(2):195–209.

110. Muschert GW. The Columbine effect on culture, policy, and me. *J Contemp Crim Justice*. 2019;35(3):357–372.

111. Murray JL. Mass media reporting and enabling of mass shootings. *Cult Stud Crit Methodol*. 2017;17(2):114–124.

112. Knoll IV JL. The "pseudocommando" mass murderer: Part I, the psychology of revenge and obliteration. *J Am Acad Psychiatry Law*. 2010a;38(1):87–94.

113. Knoll IV JL. The "pseudocommando" mass murderer: Part II, the language of revenge. *J Am Acad Psychiatry Law*. 2010b;38(2):263–272.

114. Lankford A. Fame-seeking rampage shooters: Initial findings and empirical predictions. *Aggress Violent Behav*. 2016;27:122–129.

115. Fernandez E, Callen A, Johnson SL, Gaspar C, Kulhanek C, Jose-Bueno C. Prevalence, elicitors, and expression of anger in 21st century mass shootings. *Aggress Violent Behav*. 2020;55:101483. doi:10.1016/j.avb.2020.101483.

116. Appelbaum PS. Public safety, mental disorders, and guns. *JAMA Psychiatry*. 2013;70(6):565–566.

117. *Final Report of the Sandy Hook Advisory Commission*. Presented to Governor Dannel P. Malloy, State of Connecticut, 6 Mar 2015.

118. McGinty EE, Webster DW, Barry CL. Effects of news media messages about mass shootings on attitudes toward persons with serious mental illness and public support for gun control policies. *Am J Psychiatry*. 2013;170(5):494–501.

119. Kessler RC, Angermeyer M, Anthony JC, et al. Lifetime prevalence of and age-of-onset distributions of mental disorders in the World Health Organization's World Mental Health Survey Initiative. *World Psychiatry*. 2007;6(3):168–176.

120. Meloy JR, Hoffmann J, Guldimann A, James D. The role of warning behaviors in threat assessment: An exploration and suggested typology. *Behav Sci Law*. 2012;30(3):256–279.

121. Dahmen NS. Visually reporting mass shootings: US newspaper photographic coverage of three mass school shootings. *Am Behav Sci*. 2018;62(2):163–180.

122. Kovner J, Altimari D. More than 1,000 pages of documents reveal Sandy Hook shooter Adam Lanza's dark descent into depravity. *Hartford*

Courant, 9 Dec 2018. http://www.courant.com/news/connecticut/hc-news-sandy-hook-lanza-new-documents-20181204-story.html

123. Lankford A, Madfis E. Don't name them, don't show them, but report everything else: A pragmatic proposal for denying mass killers the attention they seek and deterring future offenders. *Am Behav Sci*. 2018;62(2):260–279.

124. Larkin RW. The Columbine legacy: Rampage shootings as political acts. *Am Behav Sci*. 2009;52(9):1309–1326.

125. Robles F. 'You'll all know who I am,' Parkland suspect said in video. *New York Times*, 30 May 2018. https://www.nytimes.com/2018/05/30/us/nikolas-cruz-parkland-video.html

126. Shortell D, Flores R, Perez E, Liptak K. Exclusive: Group chat messages show school shooter obsessed with race, violence and guns. *CNN*, 17 Feb 2018. https://www.cnn.com/2018/02/16/us/exclusive-school-shooter-instagram-group/index.html

127. Meloy JR, Hempel AG, Gray BT, Mohandie K, Shiva A, Richards TC. A comparative analysis of North American adolescent and adult mass murderers. *Behav Sci Law*. 2004;22(3):291–309.

128. McCauley C, Moskalenko S, Van Son B. Characteristics of lone-wolf violent offenders: A comparison of assassins and school attackers. *Perspect Terrorism*. 2013;7(1):4–24.

129. Lankford A, Adkins KG, Madfis E. Are the deadliest mass shootings preventable? An assessment of leakage, information reported to law enforcement, and firearms acquisition prior to attacks in the United States. *J Contemp Crim Justice*. 2019;35:315–341.

22

A Risk Analysis Framework of Lone-Actor Terrorism

NOÉMIE BOUHANA, EMILY CORNER, AND PAUL GILL

INTRODUCTION

Syntheses of the violent extremism research literature highlight the diversity of factors, indicators, mechanisms, processes, and overall concepts that have been associated, analytically or empirically, with the search for an explanation of (lone-actor) radicalization and behavior.[1] Empirical efforts to unify this knowledge into general frameworks have been largely aimed at producing typologies of lone actors.[2] This taxonomic approach, while a necessary step toward progress in any scientific field,[3] has some important limitations. While well-designed and validated typologies can provide useful definition and organization in a new area of research, their purpose remain essentially to organize observations: a typology *describes what it is*, but it does little to *explain why it is so*. It may be tempting to think that understanding has been improved by slotting a particular event under a labeled category, but an explanation requires more than a taxonomic exercise: it requires conceptual statements about the causes and causal processes which account for the outcome under study. The ability to tell apart (even deep) description from explanation and to move from the one to the other is crucial when the ultimate goal is to do away with the outcome: to prevent a problem from (re)occurring we need to remove or disrupt its causes.

Because empirical findings do not speak for themselves (e.g., statistics tell us about the presence and strength of a relation, not what it means), a knowledge base capable of supporting policy must be made up of more than a catalogue of statistically significant relationships between a set of factors (i.e., descriptive results). It must include theories which advance explanations about the role these factors play in producing the outcome of interest (e.g., radicalization) and the conditions under which they may come to interact.[4] This necessitates going beyond empirical generalizations to conjecture inherently unobservable but plausible causal mechanisms.[5] Progress is contingent on the emergence of theories which can not only make sense of accumulated observations and are compatible with established scientific knowledge in major disciplines, but which can also bridge disciplinary silos to integrate levels of analysis and, crucially, produce general rather than strictly local explanations.[6]

While observations about lone actors and their behavior have multiplied in recent years, few, if any, meta-models or theories of lone actor radicalization and lone actor extremist behavior have been put forward that articulate systematically how the kinds of factors discussed in the prior literature review interact to produce one or the other and that are able to differentiate between those factors which may act as indicators (needed for the design of detection and mitigation measures) of lone-actor extremist events and those which may be considered causes (needed for the design of prevention and disruption measures). To arrive at this point, a number of key problems remain to be tackled, namely:

- integrating the levels of explanation (i.e., establishing through which concrete mechanisms the different macro and micro levels interact) in order to tackle the problem of specificity (why some individuals radicalize when most others do not);
- transcending the problem of locality (i.e., getting beyond local explanations to general theories), and;
- achieving conceptual clarity, in the absence of which neither of the other problems are solvable.

In spite of a noticeable uptake in data-driven research,[7] the study of the causes of terrorism and radicalization remains theoretically fragmented, leading at least one prominent scholar to express concern about the so-called stagnation of scientific research in this field.[8] In a review of research on Islamic-inspired home-grown radicalization in Europe, Anja Dalgaard-Nielsen[9] identified three main categories of accounts of radicalization, each concerned with a different level of analysis: French sociological accounts, which focus on the role of the macro cultural and socioeconomic context in the radicalization process, with a particular emphasis on the factors that could explain the appeal of radical Islam for seemingly well-integrated Muslims; social movement and network theories, which privilege the individual's immediate psychosocial environment to explain how they become exposed to and eventually adopt radicalizing ideologies to the point of involvement in terrorism; and largely atheoretical accounts, which mine the background characteristics of terrorists in search of empirically grounded indicators and typologies of radicals, their motivations, or their "pathways" into radicalization.

Nielsen concludes that, while each category of account addresses salient elements of the radicalization process, all of them come short of a full theory that could tackle the "problem of specificity"[10] and explain why a majority of individuals experiencing these particular conditions (e.g., an inimical socioeconomic context, membership in a social network containing radicalized individuals, sociopolitical grievances) do not undergo a process of radicalization. Nielsen goes on to suggest that these accounts should be seen as complementary, rather than competing.

Similarly, Schmid[11] contends that radicalization studies have privileged the *micro* level of analysis, but that full explanations should integrate the *meso* (community) and *macro* (structural) levels as well, although the strategy to adopt to effect this integration is not outlined. Taylor and Horgan[12] (p. 587) recommend that the study of terrorism should be brought "within a broader ecological framework," but again their process model of terrorism involvement falls short of articulating those processes through which factors at different levels of analysis are theorized to interact (see, likewise, Hafez and Mullins[13] for a more recent synthesis that leaves out interaction mechanisms). The choice to draw from the criminological notion of "individual pathway" leads to the inevitable conclusion that routes into

terrorism are discrete, which would seem to preclude the statement of a general developmental model. Meanwhile, the psychological perspective adopted, while legitimate in itself, means that an examination of the emergence of ecological conditions which support radicalization or terrorist involvement is largely out of bounds. Veldhuis and Staun[14] have put forward a "root cause model" of radicalization in response to the weaknesses of "phase models"—which offer, at best, chronological deep descriptions of the radicalization process in a particular context[15] and as such do not provide a framework to differentiate between indicators (symptoms or markers) and genuine causal factors. Veldhuis and Staun[16] contribute a valuable synthesis of factors associated with radicalization at several levels of analysis, but their "model" relies on enumeration more than integration. How one should determine the exact role and assess the relative importance, of each category of factors is unspecified; the lack of an explicit integrative framework manifests in the omission of an intermediate level linking the macro and micro levels of explanation. Kruglanski and colleagues'[17] significance quest theory does take care to articulate the interaction between situational and individual factors but leaves out a full appraisal of the social ecology of radicalization (e.g., selection and emergence processes; see later discussion), which is likely necessary to explain variation in incidence between countries and communities at any given time.

This kind of theoretical fragmentation will be familiar to criminologists. In an ambitious paper published in *Crime and Justice*, Weisburd and Piquero[18] set out to test the respective "explanatory power" of theories of crime located at different levels of analysis. They conclude that all theories leave the bulk of the variance unexplained and advise that each theoretical framework should look to "what is not explained,"[18] (p. 453) if scientific progress is to continue. One might be tempted to address this difficulty by throwing any and all "risk factors"—individual, situational, social, ecological, macro-social—into the pot and hunt for statistical covariates of the outcome of interest (here: terrorism), but the limitations of this approach are recognized even by its proponents[19] and have been discussed at length elsewhere.[20] In the search for risk factors or so-called indicators, one quickly finds themselves overwhelmed by ever-expanding lists of significant correlates, with no way to discriminate between symptoms, markers, cause, or mere statistical accidents.

Alternatively, one might take the more difficult road, stop "segregat[ing] the "ingredients"" of crime or terrorism, or, conversely, "including everything" willy nilly, but instead seek to articulate the "rules of interaction" between levels of analysis[21]; between the individual and her (developmental or behavioral) environment: in other words, abandon a factor-based approach in favor of mechanism-based accounts, where *mechanism* is defined, in the scientific realist tradition, as the causal process that links the cause to its effect (i.e., that explains *how* the cause brings about the effect).

Beyond theories of terrorism, the logic and value of such an approach to explanation was deftly illustrated in a seminal paper by analytical sociologists Lieberson and Lynn,[22] in which the authors argue that, rather than emulate the deterministic and deductivist model of the physical sciences, a successful and relevant social science should learn from the example of the natural sciences. Like sociology (and criminology), evolutionary science seeks to understand the trajectory of complex organisms embedded in complex ecological systems. Yet evolutionary theory, arguably one of the most successful theoretical frameworks in scientific history, did not emerge out of attempts to isolate statistically the (potentially infinite number of) possible conditions that could impact the evolution of species and attribute to them some fixed amount of variance, net of other influence. Rather, early evidence in evolutionary theory was gathered from observation of natural experiments, and the powerful frame of the theory is not made up of a long list of statistically significant factors, but of a small set of interlocking general mechanisms (e.g., natural selection, migration, and genetic drift), resulting in a meta-model or framework that is adaptable and universally generalizable.

It is true that the general character of a meta-model can come at the cost of predictive power: evolutionary science does not set out to *predict* the evolution of specific species. To do so would require information about local ecological conditions in the very distant future, and it would require ignoring that evolutionary events (as social events) are also the product of chance.[23] Yet one would be hard-pressed to say that this lack of predictive power means evolution by natural selection is a failed theoretical framework. Nor does the ontological status of natural selection as more of a functional metaphor than a concrete causal mechanism in a physical system diminish the value of the explanation. Natural selection (as,

e.g., "exposure" in the model discussed in the next section) operates as a fertile synthetic construct which has guided, and continues to guide, the search for the lower-level processes and context-specific factors involved in bringing it about.

Developing a general, analytical meta-framework capable of explaining, organizing, and reconciling a knowledge base as patchy and disparate as the one synthesized later in this chapter, however, is not easily achieved from scratch. To the extent that crime and terrorism research can be considered cognate domains (see Bouhana and Wikström[24], for a development of this argument), criminologists have increasingly argued that there is much to learn from research on crime and criminality that could advance our understanding of the causes of non-state political violence, be it in terms of transferable research methodologies, analytical concepts, approaches to prevention, or theoretical frameworks.[25]

Owing perhaps to the availability of large open datasets which aggregate event-level information, such as the Global Terrorism Database,[26] this criminological enterprise has added chiefly to our knowledge of the characteristics, distribution, and predictors of terrorist events thanks to a number of studies guided by opportunity-focused approaches, such as rational choice, routine activities, crime pattern, and repeat victimization,[27] or by deterrence perspectives.[28] By comparison, efforts to apply general criminological theories to the development of terrorist criminality and individual involvement in terrorist action have been less conspicuous, with some notable exceptions.[29] Yet, to the extent that blocking opportunities for terrorist activity and deterring terrorists have not proved (to date) enough to control the threat of terrorism, and to the extent that governments continue to promote prevention efforts aimed at suppressing the disposition to commit acts of terrorism in the population,[30] then robust theories are needed which can organize and articulate our knowledge-base of how individuals come to perceive acts of terrorism as an alternative for action—the process commonly known as *radicalization*.

As previously stated, when dealing with a field which faces as many analytical and methodological hurdles as the study of terrorism in general and lone actor extremism in particular, it is arguably worth drawing on existing theories from areas where understanding (e.g., the ability to validate constructs and test hypotheses) is somewhat advanced.

To provide a robust foundation for its risk analysis framework (RAF), this chapter draws on a well-developed general theory of crime causation known as *situational action theory* (SAT). Previously, SAT was used to organize a systematic review of empirical observations associated with al-Qaeda–influenced radicalization.[31] The resulting meta-model clearly hypothesized the general processes (exposure and emergence) which connect categories of causal factors (individual, social ecological, and systemic) in the process of radicalization while at the same time relating them to the discrete markers (predictors or indicators) that flag the presence of those processes in specific (e.g., geographical) contexts.

SAT has been fruitfully applied *both* to the explanation of terrorism acts and to the process of individual radicalization,[32] thereby demonstrating that it can provide a unifying framework for the whole of the process including radicalization, attack preparation, and attack. SAT has the advantage of being an empirically well validated, general framework that articulates both developmental and action processes—a necessity for our RAF which aims to model all stages of the lone actor event, from radicalization to attack. Specific aspects or stages of the RAF may, however, benefit from insights from other accounts.

The analysis of attack processes (e.g., target selection; modus operandi) will indubitably draw from the extensive literature on opportunity theories (i.e., rational choice theory, routine activities theory, crime pattern theory) and situational crime prevention, while the analysis of the roles of selection processes and social emergence in radicalization will benefit from accumulated research in social movements, social networks, and other relational approaches, as has been made amply clear in the first section of this report. One of the many advantages of a RAF supported by an integrative general theory such as SAT is that it allows, by definition, the organized integration of different analytical approaches that may not have been brought together previously.

THE RISK ANALYSIS FRAMEWORK

As a general theory, SAT sets out the key mechanisms and processes involved in the acquisition of individual action propensities and in individual action. In this section, these general mechanisms are put in the context of our knowledge of radicalization and terrorism, with particular reference to lone actors. Given evidence of the growing role of exposure to online settings in the radicalization and actions of lone actors, examples of social ecological processes and systemic factors relevant to the online environment are provided. These mechanisms are summarized in a risk analysis matrix.

RADICALIZATION

In light of the analytical background provided by SAT, the categories of factors and mechanisms which are key to explaining how lone actors acquire the propensity to commit acts of terrorism—in other words, *radicalize*—can be summarized in terms of processes that play a role in the emergence of their *individual vulnerability* to moral change, their *exposure* to settings with terrorism-supportive moral contexts, and the *emergence* and maintenance of such settings in these people's activity fields. For convenience, this analytical model or meta-framework of radicalization is referred to as IVEE.

Cognitive Susceptibility

At the individual level of explanation, SAT suggests how certain experiences that contribute to moral education and cognitive nurturing play a part in the emergence of personal propensities for action. This process of personal emergence is, of course, continuous throughout the life course, meaning that, in effect, the person is continually *emerging*. It is the outcome of *antecedent* experiences of moral education and cognitive nurturing which determine an individual's level of vulnerability at the onset of the radicalization process. This outcome we may call *cognitive susceptibility* to moral change. The research observations summarized in a later section suggest that vulnerability to radicalization is partly a factor of an individual's prior commitment, or lack thereof, to a moral framework, their capacity for response regulation and executive functioning (EF; self-control, adaptability, and flexibility), and their lifestyle exposure to situations which deplete their (neuro)-cognitive resources.

EF is made up of the discrete but interacting higher-order neurocognitive processes which are involved in people's ability to engage in goal-oriented behavior, maintain motivation and attention, and adapt flexibly to contingencies that require new plans and decisions.[33] EF develops early in life and is responsible for such key tasks as inhibiting responses, updating working memory, and shifting mental sets (switching back and forth between tasks).[34] These processes are cognitively costly, and resources can become depleted after use. Because automatic or routine responses demand less energy and guide behavior much of the time, EF is only solicited when new and/or complex situations arise.[35] Rules of conduct, acquired through socialization and maintained through habit, moderate EF. As long as it is appropriate to the behavioral context, commitment to well-established rule-guidance allows for automatism, therefore less call for effortful deliberation and self-control, *ergo* lower energy expenditure and less drain on limited resources.[36]

People vary in their capacity for self-regulation and executive control.[37] Some are known for their impulsivity; others for being efficient decision-makers under stressful conditions.[38] A number of observations support the hypothesis that this variability could account, in part, for individual differences in susceptibility to radicalizing moral change. Many individuals undergo radicalization as adolescents or young adults. Age, as a marker of biological development, may be indicative of differences in executive capability. The prefrontal cortex, the seat of EF, is one of the last brain areas to develop, all the way through young adulthood,[39] with implications for young people's continuing openness to socialization. Low self-control is one of the factors most consistently associated with crime and substance abuse.[40] A delinquent past or a history of addiction (a notable subgroup among the radicalized population) could be evidence of weaknesses in executive control. This might, in turn, provide an explanation about why individuals who cling to a legalistic rule system cannot help but stray from it: they lack the capacity to inhibit responses to day-to-day situations, such as prescriptions about what to eat, drink, or wear, even if these situations challenge their new moral guidance. It might also contribute to the explanation about why newly radicalized persons or people in the process of radicalizing seem to systematically cut ties with friends and family who (may) disapprove of their new value system: those individuals may be trying to protect themselves from further stress on their neurocognitive resources (an experience generally accompanied by negative affect and therefore to be avoided) by ensuring they will not be exposed to competing moral rule guidance that might challenge their newly acquired morality and force them to reconcile contradictions and make choices.

Lifestyle changes (brought on, e.g., by life events such as migration, incarceration, or going to university) create opportunities for individuals to be confronted with new and challenging situations which require effortful control, flexibility, and adaption. Not all people may be equally able to handle such circumstances, especially if social support (attachments to relatives, networks of friends, supportive social institutions) has been lost. For individuals whose early socialization did not equip them ideally for the demands of life away from home and community of origin—as may be the case of second-generation immigrants caught between parental values and the diverging expectations of the host society—growing up and gaining independence may bring on its own plethora of taxing situations. Those less able to handle cognitive demands or facing circumstances that unrelentingly drain their psychological reserves (situations which generate intense and sustained anxiety, negative affect, and so on) may find relief in categorical rule guidance that alleviates the burden of decision-making.

A stable religious upbringing or a prior commitment to a non-violent value system is reportedly a protective factor in young people: this ties in well with the notion that commitment to context-relevant rules of conduct entails less reliance on costly decision-making processes, therefore less energy depletion, with its attendant negative effects of stress and exhaustion.[41]

While much work remains to be done to establish the specific (lower-level) mechanisms and processes responsible for individual differences in cognitive susceptibility to radicalization (see, however, Kruglanski et al.[42] for valuable work in this domain), the growing literature in cultural neuroscience (see, e.g., Kitayama and Park's model of brain-culture influence[43]), social cognitive neuroscience (see, e.g., McGregor et al.[44] for an application of goal regulation theory to violent religious radicalization) and molecular genetics (see, e.g., Bakermans-Kranenburg and van Ijzendoorn[45] for a discussion of differential susceptibility to rearing environments) suggests fruitful avenues. This literature, and research in other problem domains, also suggests that susceptibility to moral change is a general feature of human populations (which doesn't invalidate variation within and between individuals) and is not radicalization-specific.[46]

Susceptibility to Selection

Another kind of susceptibility is implied in the SAT framework, which bridges the individual (person), situational (setting), and social ecological (environment) levels of analysis.

Cognitive susceptibility alone cannot account for vulnerability to radicalization in the sense that, while an individual may be more or less susceptible to the influence of radicalizing teachings, it does not fully make sense to say that they are vulnerable to radicalization if nothing puts them at risk of ever being exposed to such teachings. To the extent that radicalizing practices are found in particular settings at particular times, people will vary in the level to which they possess characteristics which make it more likely that they will find themselves in these settings.

Research findings point to a number of personal characteristics which could be linked to susceptibility to selection, notably social selection. Place of residence is one: people who have undergone radicalization live in communities where radicalizing moral contexts are found. Age is another. Most people undergo radicalization as young adults or teenagers, a time associated with lifestyle changes. Monitoring from parents and teachers decreases. Personal agency increases. More time is spent outside the house, in a greater variety of places. More control is gained over whom to spend time with. In short, the activity field of young people changes and expands, bringing with it opportunities for exposure to new settings, some of which may have radicalizing moral contexts. Youth, then, may be an (admittedly general) factor of selection. Other factors may play a similar role. Some of the older men implicated in home-grown radicalization, like the expatriates discussed by Sageman,[47] are immigrants. Migration is an instance of a life event that will drastically impact an individual's activity field, not unlike moving out of the family home to attend a distant university. Many events have the potential to bring about changes in the types of environments people experience, which is why the discrete nature of life events matters less to the explanation of radicalization than the process they trigger: a lasting change in a person's activity field and, consequently, in her exposure to certain kinds of moral contexts.

Beyond its impact on activity fields, life experience may also be implicated in *preference formation* (acquisition of personal likes and dislikes). Over the course of their lives, people acquire preferences for particular kinds of setting—settings where they believe they will be able to fulfil their desires (pubs, dance clubs, libraries, malls, and so on). In the context of home-grown radicalization, these preferences impact susceptibility to selection if they result in people being exposed to radicalizing environments. For instance, repeated experiences of ethnic discrimination and associated negative feelings may, quite reasonably, lead individuals to develop a preference for settings where discrimination is less likely to occur, such as ethnically homogeneous settings. Experiences of victimization in prison might result in a preference for settings that offer physical protection. The experience of "moral shock" said to accompany the viewing of disturbing videos may spur a need to share one's reaction or to seek advice on how to cope with disruptive moral emotions.

In the first case, the person who feels discriminated against begins to spend more time in places frequented only by members of her own ethnic group. In doing so, she exposes herself to opportunities for contact with radicalizing agents who belong to the same group. In the second, the inmate in search of protection starts to hang out with members of a prison gang, some of whom may hold radical views. In the third, the young man morally outraged by images of suffering searches for a sympathetic ear and ends up in an internet forum, where users happen to hold both conventional and radicalizing views. Through these examples, one can see how personal characteristics and experiences—through their impact on activity fields and the formation of personal preferences—can interact with ecological features to lead to the exposure of certain individuals to radicalizing moral contexts.

Exposure

Radicalizing Settings

Building on the SAT concept of criminogenic settings, radicalizing settings can be understood as places whose features support the acquisition of personal morals supportive of terrorism. They enable terrorism-promoting socialization—the internalization of terrorism-supportive moral rules of conduct, values, and emotions. All radicalizing settings share key features.

First, these settings host radicalizing moral norms that are either transmitted person-to-person or through media. They convey terrorism-supportive ideas and associated emotions that promote the legitimate use of terrorism and may be delivered through "narrative" devices. Anecdotal evidence suggests that effective radicalizing teachings tend to be couched in a narrative form, which is communicated by perceived sources of moral authority and is characterized as transcendental (about "meaning-of-life stuff"), categorical (good/evil), and prescriptive (action-oriented) in a way that appeals particularly to the young, given their cognitive needs.[48] Settings differ in the extent to which these teachings coexist with others.

Second, these settings are further characterized by ineffective supervision. The level of formal and/or informal behavioral monitoring in these settings is ineffective or in some other way inadequate. Generally, crime-promoting settings are those where people spend time with like-minded peers and where they can express or enact rule violations without interference from formal or informal authorities.[49]

Third, the research synthesis suggests that, like other crime-promoting settings, radicalizing settings suffer from *ineffective monitoring*. Terrorism-promoting socialization activity is allowed to take place and go on without effective challenge. Lack of trust can mean that people with responsibility over the setting are reluctant to involve outside authorities in sanctioning and deterring unconventional activity. Generational and cultural divides can lead to spaces where young people associate unsupervised and isolated from counter-influence (so-called *enclaves*). Surveillance may displace activity to more private spaces. In sum, lack of awareness, willingness, and/or resources to intervene creates spaces where radicalizing practices go on unchallenged.

Finally, these settings provide opportunities for individuals to form *attachments* to radicalizing agents. Socialization is an interpersonal process. For the majority of people, the agents of socialization with the greatest influence over their lives are their parents or guardians. Within families, the main mechanisms of socialization are the teaching of rules of conduct and the supervision of behavior (i.e., moral education). How effective family socialization practices turn out to be depends in large part on the strength of the child's attachment to his guardians. That attachment, in turn, is a function of the caring (caregiving) relationship between child and guardians. Humans tend to get attached to the people who provide for their physical and emotional well-being.[50] Eventually, people form attachments beyond the circle of family—with friends, teachers, and spouses who care for them and come to have their own influence (e.g., in terms of moral education) over them. Attachment, as a mechanism, is closely associated with criminality and delinquency.[51]

The research on radicalization previously reviewed supports the notion that, like any other instance of socialization or criminal behavior,[52] effective radicalization entails attachment to the sources of radicalizing teachings. Radicalizing settings are those which facilitate, promote, or otherwise support the conditions necessary for radicalizing agents (kin, peers, activists, so-called spiritual sanctioners) to form lasting attachments to (susceptible) others—notably through caring or caregiving. This requires that the setting allows for genuine and lasting associations between individuals. When radicalizing agents approach individuals in positions of susceptibility, such as recent migrants or prison inmates facing a new and unknown moral context, and offer food, shelter, and spiritual comfort, they are trying to encourage a relation of *attachment* between themselves and the individual; in some sense, they may be said to emulate the parent–offspring relationship, which is the basis of human socialization. Once attachment is created, the process of socialization (propensity change) can proceed apace. Of course, a single setting is unlikely to offer opportunity for lasting exposure; instead, the constellation of settings in the individual's activity field may allow for repeated association.

Selection

As stated in the discussion of SAT, selection processes are the main social ecological processes that explain why individuals with particular characteristics (e.g., cognitive susceptibility) are more likely to find themselves in certain places at particular times and engaged in particular activities.

The operation of *self-selection* in the radicalization process is illustrated, for example, by Olsen,[53] who recounts how a preference for political engagement led one young individual to take part in a demonstration where he was given to observe a group of young rioters. The youth thought that this "was really exciting . . . this group, they were all my age, I could identify with them and they made something of themselves."[53] [(p.14)] He later approached them. The example shows how the non-radicalizing features of a setting can act as a personal draw, incidentally exposing people to terrorism-promoting influences. Self-selection being an ongoing process, preferences acquired during the earlier stages of radicalization can result in more intense and sustained exposure, such that some individuals may eventually graduate from sporting grounds in Birmingham and internet cafes in London to training camps in Afghanistan.

When supporters of terrorist movements upload videos purporting to depict scenes of Western soldiers harming civilians in Muslim lands, they may also lead people to expose themselves to radicalizing settings though self-selection. Viewing such videos may spark anger and eventually crystallize into grievance. These emotions, in turn, may give rise for a preference for settings where negative feelings can be aired and alleviated by sharing the experience with like-minded individuals.

More positive preferences may also lead to self-selection. For example, an article published in *Foreign Affairs* entitled "The World of Holy Warcraft" discusses how the "gamified" features of some online forums entice young people to involve (i.e., expose) themselves to these forums, some of which have radicalizing features, with ever greater intensity as they develop a (personal) taste for competition.[54] Hence self-selection can take someone from YouTube, Facebook, and discussion forums to, eventually, Syria.

Social selection sets the stage for *self-selection* by constraining the kinds of settings people are likely to find themselves in. Observations have suggested, for example, that individuals who belong to certain groups—young people, residents in Muslim communities, students, immigrants, people with a criminal history—are overrepresented among home-grown terrorists (for a full review, see Bouhana and Wikström[55]). Nor are radicalizing settings distributed randomly: they appear more likely to be found in some kinds of environments, which in turn are more likely to be frequented by members of particular groups. Social selection means that group membership is likely to affect the chance of exposure to radicalizing contexts, something echoed by the research on social movements and radical milieus already reviewed. For instance, individuals from an Islamic ethno-religious background are significantly more likely to find themselves in a setting where Muslims routinely congregate (mosque, Islamic study group, halal restaurant) compared with individuals from a non-Muslim background. Students are more likely to have the opportunity to spend several hours a day surfing the internet than most working adults. Unemployed individuals are more likely to have the freedom to spend time in cafes during working hours than most office workers. People with a criminal history are more likely than non-offenders to be exposed to a prison environment, and asylum seekers are more likely to spend time in immigration centers—two examples of so-called hotbeds associated with radicalization. Given the organization of social life and the location of radicalizing settings, some categories of people are more likely to be exposed compared to the rest of the population as a result of social selection.[56]

In sum, selection means that *who* ends up being radicalized is influenced as much by the characteristics of the settings in which radicalization takes place as it is by the characteristics of the individuals who undergo the process. Social selection is likely to be the key process which explains why members of particular terrorist cells, groups, or particular campaigns may share some sociodemographic characteristics—they met in places which draw people with these characteristics—yet the search for general terrorist "profiles" remains futile: radicalizing settings are found in new environments over time—if only as a result of counterterrorist activity—therefore, the kinds of people socially selected for exposure changes.

To explain why some (susceptible) individuals rather than others radicalize (*the problem of specificity*) is to explain why some people rather than others are exposed to the radicalizing settings in their environment through processes of selection.

Emergence

As discussed earlier, observations suggest that settings that promote terrorism are not equally distributed in space and time. Some streets, neighborhoods, communities, prisons, societies, even some countries have more of these kinds of settings compared to others at any given time. Processes of emergence link systemic factors (community-level factors and up) with social ecological processes of exposure, such as selection. At the systemic level are those factors and mechanisms which explain why radicalizing settings appear and remain in some environments rather than others. To explain *why radicalization occurs in particular places at particular times* is to explain why radicalizing settings emerge where and when they do and are sustained.

A given systemic factor is likely to matter to the extent that it facilitates (or constrains) the emergence and maintenance of (1) ineffectively monitored settings, in which (2) susceptible individuals come into lasting or repeated contact with radicalizing agents who (3) promote terrorism-supportive moral norms. Hence, in any given context, those systemic factors relevant to radicalization are likely to be those which allow for radicalizing moral norms to spread, for certain places to experience low levels of formal and informal social control, for radicalizing agents to move around freely among the rest of the population, and for susceptible individuals to be selected for exposure into particular settings.

Hence, at the systemic level, many factors are likely to matter, yet not just any factor. When confronted with analytical or statistical claims about the impact of meso- or macro-level characteristics on radicalization, one way to assess their (potential) relevance is to ask how they might be implicated in a causal chain which ends in the emergence of radicalizing environments or the exposure of susceptible individuals.

Scholarship on systemic factors and crime would suggest that levels of residential segregation and social disorganization; the collective efficacy of communities, schools, and families; and formal mechanisms of social control will affect the emergence of radicalizing settings inasmuch as these factors impact the organization of daily routines, the establishment of cohesive rules of conduct, and the availability of resources (the willingness and the means) to enforce these rules. One can also conceive of how macro-level political processes such as civil war could, given their ultimate effect on community rules and resources, affect emergence. Historical and political processes involved in the formation of groups like al-Qaeda, processes of norms promotion which contribute to the formation of competing moral contexts at the international level, factors which affect the movement of persons—all can be reasonably linked to radicalization in this way. Inasmuch as they facilitate contact between radicalizing agents, allow their activity to escape surveillance, and are a vector for the introduction of terrorism-supportive norms in activity fields, media outlets and the rules that govern them are also plausible contributors.

Research on radicalization at the systemic level of analysis is the least developed to date, which is understandable because investigating causes of causes (or, in this case, causes of causes of causes) is much more challenging that investigating proximate conditions, especially when studying low-incidence phenomena.

THE EMERGENCE OF RADICALIZING ENVIRONMENTS ONLINE

As just stated, empirical research on the topic of emergence is underdeveloped in radicalization and terrorism studies, all the more so regarding the emergence of virtual radicalizing settings, a relatively recent phenomenon. Nevertheless, to illustrate the analytical uses of the RAF, some factors are discussed and their role in the emergence of radicalizing settings online hypothesized:

- *The diffusion of internet access and mobile communication technologies.* The obvious first: without the internet and associated technologies, there would be no online radicalizing spaces. The diffusion of these technologies beyond public (e.g., universities and libraries) toward private and semi-private spaces (e.g., private accommodations and personal mobile devices) is one of those systemic trends which has affected internet use, reshaped people's routines and activity fields to include increasingly more virtual environments, and, therefore, created new opportunities for exposure to a variety of moral contexts. The democratization of broadband access and peer-to-peer technology has made the sharing of large files possible, enabling, for example, the transmission of videos with radicalizing content.[57] Any future technological development that would impact cyber access and content diffusion has the potential to play a part in online radicalization as a systemic factor.

- *The diffusion of "dark technologies."* Likewise, the democratization of technologies which provide access to the so-called *dark internet*, such as Tor, and the availability of encryption software are likely to impact the emergence of unsupervised and unmonitored settings, some of which may host radicalizing activity.

- *The diffusion of social networking platforms.* Social networking platforms are reported to play a number of roles in online radicalization. Notably, they are a vector of selection in the sense that they put individuals in (witting or unwitting) contact with radicalizing agents by creating connections between networks; they create a mechanism through which moral narratives can be propagated and amplified, and, because some of them enable anonymous and/or restricted interaction (e.g., friends-only spaces), they interfere with social monitoring of socializing activity.

- *The regulatory environment.* Governments, international agencies, internet service providers, platform owners, all are subject to rules and regulations which limit or enable their ability to regulate internet content[58] and therefore monitor and interfere with activity taking place in online settings or stem the propagation of radicalizing messages. The regulatory environment may be one of the single most important factors impacting the emergence of online radicalizing settings.

• *The deficit of digital media literacy.* Several factors come under this heading: notably, an intergenerational gap, which means that parents are not always equipped with an understanding of the technology sufficient to be able to monitor the online behavior of their children and that agents of law enforcement and other authorities may not always be *au fait* of the latest developments in terms of cyber-technology and risk being always one step behind. *Literacy* also refers to the skills, or lack thereof, one can call upon to interpret, evaluate, and interact with media content in a mature way. Though the concern about a lack of literacy is often aimed at children and young people, adults, too, may experience psychological distortions when interacting in the new media environment. All of these factors will have an impact of the level of formal and informal supervision of various online settings.

• *The collective efficacy (or lack thereof) of online communities.* "Collective efficacy" is defined as "social cohesion among neighbors combined with their willingness to intervene on behalf of the common good"[59] and is consistently associated with lower crime and violence in neighborhoods. Likewise, the capacity and willingness (or unwillingness) of online communities to intervene to counter radicalizing activity (e.g., by challenging radicalizing moral norms) which occurs within their corner of cyberspace is likely to have a major influence on the moral context of online settings and, therefore, on their effectiveness as radicalization-supportive environments. Witness grassroots initiatives to lobby Facebook or Twitter to take down various kinds of offensive content. Neumann,[60] however, observes that there appears to be an "enthusiasm gap" between online extremists and other internet citizens, with the former hogging some fora while the majority, who undoubtedly disagree with much of their discourse, remains silent.

• *The availability of radicalizing and other moral narratives.* Radicalizing, and counter-radicalizing, moral norms are often effectively conveyed in the form of narratives. The availability of such narratives (and counter-narratives), which can be readily transmitted by socializing agents, is also likely to be a factor that influences the emergence (or the suppression, in the case of counter-narratives) of radicalizing settings.

ANALYTICAL MODELS AS GUIDE FOR ACTION

Such analytical frameworks may also have value as cross-contextual guides for action. Whether one is faced with a resurgence of ethno-nationalist terrorism in a foreign country or with sporadic cases of homegrown radicalization, the first set of questions to ask before intervention can be designed are the same. Chiefly

• Where is the radicalizing activity taking place?
• On what basis (sociodemographic characteristics and personal preferences) are individuals selected for exposure to settings where this activity is taking place?
• What are the factors which have allowed (or failed to suppress) the emergence of these settings in this particular environment?
  o What stands in the way of these settings being effectively supervised, either by state authorities or by community members?
  o What makes it possible for radicalizing agents to gain access to these settings?
  o What makes it possible for radicalizing moral norms to be introduced into these settings and what forms do these norms take?
• Why are some of the individuals who are exposed to these settings susceptible to moral change?

The point has already been made that it is analytically crucial to distinguish the process of development of propensities for action (e.g., radicalization) from processes of action (e.g., terrorist act), if only because a person can engage in an action without having acquired the propensity to do so. Like radicalization, the situational model of terrorist action articulates how processes at different levels of analysis interact in the explanation of terrorist action.

A terrorist propensity results from the internalization of terrorism-supportive personal morals (terrorism-supportive moral beliefs, values, and commitments to terrorism-promoting rules of conduct and associated moral emotions), as well as the level of capacity to exercise self-control. As expounded earlier, terrorist propensity is the outcome of the process commonly called radicalization.

However, as previously stated, a terrorist propensity is not necessary for someone commit an act of terrorism: sufficient external pressures (e.g., peer pressure, a setting where terrorism is enforced as a social norm, acute stress or emotion, presence of drugs or alcohol) can override personal morals and internal controls in the face of the motivation to offend (e.g., being blackmailed into taking part in a terrorist plot). While such a configuration may be unlikely to arise in cases of lone actors, it should nevertheless be mentioned.

The same mechanisms of social and self-selection which place (or not) particular people in radicalizing settings operate to place them (or not) in particular criminogenic settings. Place of residence, group membership, personal preferences and routines—here again these factors will play a part in explaining how a person came to be exposed to a setting in which she eventually committed an act of terrorism (or from which she acquired the capability to do so).

Criminological research has shown that people with a high criminal propensity will select themselves into settings which present opportunities for offending, while individuals with a low criminal propensity will not spend time in criminogenic environments.[6] Though the same kind of longitudinal data are not available, there is every reason to believe that the relationship holds for terrorism. This means that radicalized individuals are more likely to place themselves in situations which present opportunities for involvement in terrorism than the non-radicalized.

The *situation* in which the terrorist action takes place arises from the interaction between the person and their propensity and a setting with particular characteristics that encourage and enable acts of terrorism (or not, as the case may be).[61] The notion of setting overlaps with that of place in the sense that the setting is the part of a place that the actor can perceive through his or her senses at any given time. A number of characteristics of settings, recapitulated here, are hypothesized to play a pivotal role in the terrorist action process.

Criminogenic settings are characterized by the presence of features that can be perceived by actors as temptations, provocations, or frictions that may result in the emergence of the motivation to act. When a jihadist group uploads videos depicting scenes of Western soldiers harming civilians in Muslim lands, they are trying to expose people, some of whom may already have a propensity for terrorism, to situational frictions and provocations from which the motivation to act can emerge. In other words, they are trying to get terrorism-prone individuals, most of whom would not feel inclined to move, "off the couch."

Closely associated with the motivational features of a setting are opportunities and affordances,[62] which are understood as more or less immediate properties of situations which enable the commission of crime (without compelling it). The concept of opportunity is discussed at length in the situational crime prevention literature.[63] In short, settings afford opportunities for the planning and commission of terrorist acts to the extent that they present attractive targets, allow access to convenient and effective weapons, or make available other tools that support the commission of terrorist acts (e.g., finances).

As per Wikström,[64] *motivation* is defined as "goal-directed attention." It is a situational process; in other words, *it is not a stable individual characteristic*, but the outcome of the interaction between the person and her environment. Motivation triggers the action process. It is necessary to move people to action (colloquially again, to "get them off the couch") and must be sustained through time for the action process to carry on. It can direct (motivations tend to entail a set of actions), but does not *determine* the type of action which will be taken in response to the motivation (the same motivation can be served by many kinds of actions).

Because motivation is a situational process, any change in the environment can lead to a change in the situation perceived by the actor and therefore a change in their motivation to carry out a particular act. This is a fact that terrorist groups are well aware of. When a handler accompanies a suicide bomber to the scene of the attack, they are arguably trying to ensure the continuity of a situation that may have started long before the attack process was under way and are therefore trying to maintain the bomber's *motivation* up until the last moment. Any change in the action-relevant features of the situation (e.g., a child or pregnant woman spotted in the crowd; unexpected security measures) has the potential to disrupt the motivation to act.

This underlines again an important point of difference between propensity and motivation—their respective "lastingness." On the one hand, propensity is the outcome of a developmental process, which, as previously noted, results in "a lasting change in the way a person perceives and deals with her environment."[65] On the other hand, motivation is the outcome of a situational process, which results in a short-term change of behavior. In sum, propensity change is slow but lasting, while the kind of behavioral change that is brought about by a change in situation (and therefore motivation) is fast but may only last as long as the source of motivation (the situation) remains. This has clear implications for prevention, as those interventions which target propensity and those which target motivation are likely to require very different kinds of efforts and will have effects of different longevity.

The RAF includes the hypothesis that one of the main conditional elements that affects the maintenance (or not) of motivation is the *perception of capability*. For motivation to be sustained beyond the initial perception of a temptation or provocation, a person has to perceive (a subjective process) that they have the capability to carry out the action successfully. Without some sense that something is *doable*, most people will not "stay off the couch," assuming they stood up in the first place.

During the attack process, the situation faced by the assailant may change and a chosen course of action will appear to outstrip their capability; as suggested earlier, motivation will then wane and is likely to fade. Capability explains why the majority of predisposed individuals who consider involvement in terrorism end up doing nothing, while a good number of those who do something end up getting caught. When an article like "Make a Bomb in the Kitchen of Your Mom" is published in *Inspire Magazine*,[66] the author's intent is likely to shore up the *perception of capability* of individuals who are already terrorism-prone and already moved to act but whose motivation may flag in the face of the challenges that have to be overcome before they can carry out a terrorist attack.

While capability entails physical, material, but also neuropsychological (cognitive) and spiritual resources, people can, of course, misjudge their abilities and *perceive* that they own capabilities which they have not, in fact, acquired (e.g., the ability to remain calm and determined under pressure, a sufficient knowledge of explosives, a reliable group of co-conspirators), which is why a distinction must be made between subjective and objective capability (resources). Banding together with co-conspirators is arguably another way to shore up one's perception of capability and address the potential problem of flagging motivation as well as pull together material resources. This may offer a hypothesis to explain the relatively low incidence of lone- compared to group-actor terrorism.

Among the features most relevant to the criminogeneity of a setting are the moral norms which are in force in the setting and how strongly (or weakly) these norms are enforced, formally (e.g., by police) or informally (e.g., passers-by)—what is traditionally called *deterrence*. Some settings may enable the preparation and commission of terrorist acts because the norms which are socially promoted and enforced encourage terrorism and other acts of crime (e.g., neighborhoods controlled by terrorist organizations and their sympathizers).

When the ideologues of a terrorist movement formulate lengthy moral and legal arguments that promote the view that terrorists are soldiers in a time of war and therefore that the usual rules of conduct prohibiting killing do not apply, they are aiming to change the moral context to influence individuals' perception of action alternatives in favor of terrorism. In this sense, much of the same observations made about radicalizing settings apply to some of the settings where acts of terrorism are planned and prepared.

Arguably, terrorism occupies a special place in most societies' legal and moral discourses specifically because, unlike most other crimes, the offenders do not limit themselves to breaking moral norms. The declared aim of their criminal activity is to usher in new rules of conduct altogether, which threatens the social order. This would entail that their (public) efforts to influence the moral context are more likely to be deterred (trigger a stronger reaction from authorities and citizens) than would the promotion of milder, less system-threatening forms of deviance.

Someone who perceives terrorism as a possible action alternative in a particular situation still has to choose to carry it out. Importantly, that choice does not have to be rational (e.g., weighing different options); it can be habitual. Habits tend to arise when people are exposed to the same settings again and again, where they perform the same actions. It may seem counterintuitive to think that habit could play any part in terrorism acts, but one may think of the training that soldiers undergo: the purpose of some of these exercises (e.g., endless repetition of bodily gestures) is to ensure that when faced with the decision to kill the enemy, the soldier does not stop to think about it but proceeds from automatism. The same kind of process may be implicated in the commission of terrorist acts; in fact, they may be part and parcel of the planning and preparation phase and address what a would-be attacker perceives as a weakness in their capability to act.

When not acting out of habit, people have to make the choice whether or not to get involved in terrorist action and, most likely, renew that choice each time they encounter new situations, which each time creates an opportunity for other agents to influence their decision-making. Agents can interfere in the deliberation process by making the actor perceive an action alternative he or she was not aware of. This works both ways, in that this applies to supporters and preventers alike. An agent can make the actor see terrorism as an alternative (as a co-conspirator), or they can provide them with an *alternative to terrorism*, which would still allow them to act upon their motivation. External agents can also interfere in the deliberation process by weakening the person's self-control (e.g., applying stressful social pressure, supplying drink or drugs), but also by strengthening it (e.g., sobering them up).

Much as was the case with the analysis of radicalization, social ecological and systemic factors are relevant to the analysis of acts of terrorism and their preparation to the extent that they support or suppress the emergence of any of the situational features involved in exposure. Taken together, these features can be thought of as the "opportunity structure" that enables (or suppresses) the terrorist activity of lone actors. Examples of such factors are what Clarke and Newman (2006) term "facilitating conditions," such as the general availability of access to firearms in a given jurisdiction, the proliferation of anonymous communication technologies, the resources granted intelligence services, or any factors that affect the level of trust between authorities and communities, whose members are natural guardians and potentials witnesses to an lone-actor's preparatory behaviors.

RISK ANALYSIS MATRIX

The RAF is synthesized in a matrix (Table 22.1). Each column of the matrix represents an analytical phase of the lone-actor extremist event (radicalization, attack preparation, attack), each row represents a level of analysis (individual, situational, social ecological, systemic), and each cell is populated with the key categories of causal factors and mechanisms involved. Theoretically, disrupting any causal factor or mechanism should prevent, interdict, or mitigate the lone-actor extremist event process.

As with any representation of multilevel processes and events, analytical distinctions are to some extent arbitrary and conventional. For example, as explained earlier, to the extent that motivation is a property emerging out of the interaction of the characteristics of individual (actor) and situational (setting) entities,

TABLE 22.1 RISK ANALYSIS MATRIX

		Phase of event		
		Radicalization	Attack preparation	Attack
Level of Analysis	Individual	Susceptibility to moral change Susceptibility to social selection Susceptibility to self-selection	Social, physical, and cognitive resources Susceptibility to social and self-selection	Social, physical, and cognitive resources
	Situational	Exposure to radicalizing settings Radicalizing agents Radicalizing teachings Social monitoring context	Opportunity structure Moral context Perception of action alternative Perception of capability (risk) Emergence of motivation	Opportunity structure Moral context Perception of action alternative Perception of capability (risk) Maintenance of motivation
	Social ecological	Emergence and maintenance of radicalizing settings	Emergence and maintenance of opportunity structure	Emergence and maintenance of opportunity structure
	Systemic	Emergence and maintenance of radicalization-supportive social ecologies Emergence of social selection processes	Emergence and maintenance of opportunity-supportive social ecologies Emergence of social selection processes	Emergence and maintenance of opportunity-supportive social ecologies

it does not belong *strictly* to any one analytical level. Furthermore, the RAF draws from SAT in theorizing individual susceptibilities, propensities, and relevant features of situational settings as direct influences on the development of lone-actor extremists (i.e., radicalization) and their behavior (i.e., attack preparation and attack), while ecological and systemic factors and processes are theorized as indirect influences (i.e., "causes of causes") of propensity development or behavior.

This has implication for data collection because relevant information is much more likely to be recorded and accessible regarding direct influences, rather than indirect ones. The cells of the matrix are differently shaded for this purpose. The darker the shading of the cell, the more likely it is estimated that it will be possible to capture data relevant to the factors and processes it contains. The lighter the shading, the less likely.

CONCLUSION

To conclude, the categories contained in the matrix, organized by level, can be described as follows. For the individual level, we need to account for

- *Susceptibility to moral change.* Evidence of cognitive susceptibility to moral change (or lack thereof) and of the historical factors involved in the personal emergence of this susceptibility (or lack thereof).
- *Susceptibility to social selection.* Evidence of factors of social selection that dispose the lone-actor extremist to exposure to radicalizing settings in their environment (or lack thereof).
- *Susceptibility to self-selection.* Evidence of factors of self-selection (personal preferences) that dispose the lone-actor extremist to exposure to radicalizing settings in their environment (or lack thereof).
- *Social, physical, and cognitive resources.* Evidence of resources relevant to the commission of the terrorist act (e.g., skills, intelligence, money, military experience; i.e., objective capability; see Ekblom and Tilley[67]) present at the outset of the action process.

For the situational level, it is important to consider:

- *Exposure to radicalizing settings.* Characteristics of the settings (real or virtual) in which exposure to radicalizing teachings took place and factors that explain the

presence of the actor in the setting (e.g., type of personal preference).
- *Radicalizing agents.* Characteristics of the actors (including virtually present) who transmit the radicalizing teachings and evidence of relationship between the lone actor and the actors (or lack thereof).
- *Radicalizing teachings.* Content and format of radicalizing teachings present in the setting (e.g., specific narrative).
- *Social monitoring context.* Evidence of willingness and capacity of formal and informal guardians to monitor and control the socializing activities taking place in the setting (or lack thereof).
- *Opportunity structure.* Characteristics of opportunities and affordances for preparation and commission of a terrorist act afforded by the environment (or lack thereof).
- *Moral context.* Characteristics of agents and measures of formal (e.g., police) and informal (e.g., neighbors) deterrence against the preparation of a terrorist act present in the environment (or lack thereof); characteristics of moral norms enforced in the environment (e.g., terrorism-supportive community values).
- *Perception of action alternative.* Characteristics of the situation in which the lone-actor extremist came to perceive terrorism (as opposed to another course of action) as a viable action alternative.
- *Perception of capability (risk).* Evidence of lone-actor extremist's self-assessment of their own capability to carry out preparation and attack (i.e., subjective capability).
- *Emergence of motivation.* Characteristics of the situation in which the lone-actor extremist acquired the motivation to engage in an act of terrorism and evidence of the nature and maintenance of this motivation (or lack thereof).
- *Maintenance of motivation.* Evidence that the motivation to engage in an act of terrorism was affected by changes in perception of capability at any point of the preparation and attack process (or not) (e.g., downgrades ambitious attack as a result of perception that capability is insufficient; evades site of attack when faced with police).

For the social ecological level, the following warrant consideration:

- *Emergence and maintenance of radicalizing settings.* Proximate factors which influence the emergence and maintenance (or lack thereof) of radicalizing settings in the lone-actor extremist's environment and which influence selection processes into these settings (e.g., neighborhood segregation).

- *Emergence and maintenance of opportunity structure.* Proximate factors which influence the emergence and maintenance (or lack thereof) of opportunities for terrorist attacks in the lone-actor extremist's environment (e.g., immediate facilitating conditions[68]).

And finally, the systemic level entails examining:

- *Emergence and maintenance of radicalization-supportive social ecologies.* Distal factors which influenced the emergence and maintenance (or lack thereof) of environments that produce radicalizing settings and which influenced selection processes into these settings (e.g., foreign policy).
- *Emergence and maintenance of opportunity-supportive social ecologies.* Distal factors which influenced the emergence and maintenance (or lack thereof) of opportunities for terrorist attacks in the lone-actor extremist's environment (e.g., gun laws).
- *Emergence of social selection processes.* Distal factors that influence social selection in society (e.g., residential segregation between social groups).

NOTES AND REFERENCES

1. Desmarais S, Simons-Rudolph J, Brugh CS, Schilling E, Hoggan C. The state of scientific knowledge regarding factors associated with terrorism. *J Threat Assess Manage.* 2017;4(4):180–209.
2. Borum R, Fein R, Vossekuil B. A dimensional approach to analyzing lone actor terrorism. *Aggression Violent Behav.* 2012;17;389–396; Pantucci R. *A Typology of Lone Wolves: Preliminary Analysis of Lone Islamist Terrorists.* London: International Centre for the Study of Radicalisation and Political Violence; 2011.
3. Bailey K D. *Typologies and Taxonomies: An Introduction to Classification Techniques.* Thousand Oaks, CA: Sage; 1994.
4. Wikström PO. Does everything matter? Addressing the problem of causation and explanation in the study of crime. In McGloin JM, Sullivan CJ, Kennedy LW, eds. *When Crime Appears: The Role of Emergence.* New York: Routledge; 2011:53–72.
5. Bunge M. How does it work? The search for explanatory mechanisms. *Philosophy of the Social Sciences.* 2004;34(2):182–210. doi:10.1177/0048393103262550.
6. Bouhana N, Wikström PO. *Theorising Terrorism: Terrorism as Moral Action. Report to the Ministry of Defence, Science and Technology Counter-Terrorism Centre.* London: UCL Jill Dando Institute; 2008.
7. LaFree G, Ackerman G. The empirical study of terrorism: Social and legal research. *Ann Rev Law Soc Sci.* 2009;5:347–374. doi:10.1146/annurev.lawsocsci.093008.131517.
8. Sageman M. The stagnation in terrorism research. *Terrorism Political Violence.* 2014;26:565–580. doi:10.1080/09546553.2014.895649.
9. Dalgaard-Nielsen A. Violent radicalisation in Europe: What we know and what we do not know. *Stud Conflict Terrorism.* 2010;33(9):797–814.
10. Sageman M. *Understanding Terror Networks.* Philadelphia: University of Pennsylvania Press; 2004.
11. Schmid AP. Comments on Marc Sageman's polemic "The stagnation in terrorism research." *Terrorism Political Violence.* 2014;26(4):587–595. doi:10.1080/09546553.2014.895651.
12. Taylor M, Horgan J. A conceptual framework for understanding psychological process in the development of the terrorist. *Terrorism Political Violence.* 2006;18(4): 585–601.
13. Hafez M, Mullins C. The radicalization puzzle: A theoretical synthesis of empirical approaches to homegrown extremism. *Stud Conflict Terrorism.* 2015;38(11):958–975. doi:10.1080/1057610X.2015.1051375.
14. Veldhuis T, Staun J. *Islamist Radicalization: A Root Cause Model.* Clingendael. The Hague: Netherlands Institute of International Relations; 2009.
15. Moghaddam A. The staircase to terrorism: A psychological exploration. *American Psychologist.* 2005;60:161–169; Silber MD, Bhatt A. *Radicalization in the West: The Homegrown Threat.* New York: The New York Police Department; 2007.
16. Veldhuis, Staun. *Islamist Radicalization.*
17. Kruglanski AW, Gelfand MJ, Bélanger JJ, Sheveland A, Hetiarachchi M, Gunaratna R. The psychology of radicalization and deradicalization: How significance quest impacts violent extremism. *Political Psychology.* 2014;35:69–93. doi:10.1111/pops.12163.
18. Weisburd D, Piquero A. How well do criminologists explain crime? Statistical modeling in published studies. *Crime Justice.* 2008;37(1): 453–502.
19. Farrington DP. Explaining and preventing crime: The globalization of knowledge. The American Society of Criminology 1999 Presidential Address. *Criminology.* 2000;38(1):1–24.
20. Wikström. Does everything matter?.
21. Sullivan CJ, McGloin JM, Kennedy LW. Moving past the person or context: Thinking about crime as an emergent phenomenon. In McGloin JM, Sullivan CJ, Kennedy LW, eds., *When Crime*

Appears: The Role of Emergence. New York: Routledge; 2011:17–30.

22. Lieberson S, Lynn FB. Barking up the wrong branch: Scientific alternatives to the current model of sociological science. *Ann Rev Sociol.* 2002;28(1):1–19.

23. Bunge M. *Chasing Reality: Strife Over Realism.* Toronto: University of Toronto Press; 2006.

24. Bouhana N, Wikström PO. *Al Qai'da-Influenced Radicalisation: A Rapid Evidence Assessment Guided by Situational Action Theory, RDS Occasional Paper 97.* London: Home Office Research, Development and Statistics Directorate; 2011.

25. Deflem M. Introduction: Towards a criminological sociology of terrorism and counter-terrorism. In Deflem M, ed., *Terrorism and Counter-Terrorism: Criminological Perspectives.* Amsterdam: Elsevier; 2004:1–8; Forst B, Greene JR, Lynch JP. *Criminologists on Terrorism and Homeland Security.* New York: Cambridge University Press; 2011; Freilich JD, Chermak SM, Gruenewald J. The future of terrorism research: A review essay. *Intl J Compar Applied Crim Justice.* 2015;39(4):353–369; LaFree G, Freilich JD. Editor's introduction: Quantitative approaches to the study of terrorism. *J Quant Criminol.* 2011;28(1):1–5; LaFree G, Dugan L. Introducing the Global Terrorism Database. *Terrorism Political Violence.* 2007;19(2):181–204. doi:10.1080/09546550701246817; Rosenfeld R. Why criminologists should study terrorism. *Criminologist.* 2002;27(6):1–4.

26. LaFree, Dugan. Introducing the Global Terrorism Database.

27. Braithwaite A, Johnson SD. Space–time modeling of insurgency and counterinsurgency in Iraq. *J Quant Criminol.* 2011;28(1):31–48. doi:10.1007/s10940-011-9152-8; Canetti-Nisim D, Mesch G, Pedahzur A. Victimization from terrorist attacks: Randomness or routine activities? *Terrorism Political Violence.* 2006;18(4):485–501. doi:10.1080/09546550600880237; Clarke RV, Newman GR, *Outsmarting the Terrorists.* New York: Praeger; 2006; Dugan L, LaFree G, Piquero AR. Testing a rational choice model of airline hijackings. *Criminology.* 2005;43(4):1031–1066; Hamm MS, van de Voorde C. Crimes committed by terrorist groups: Theory, research, and prevention. *Trends Organized Crime.* 2005;9:18–50. doi:10.1007/s12117-005-1023-y; Parkin WS, Freilich JD. Routine activities and right-wing extremists: An empirical comparison of the victims of ideologically-and non-ideologically-motivated homicides committed by American far-rightists. *Terrorism and Political Violence.* 2015;27(1):182–203.

27. Argomaniz J, Vidal-Diez A. Examining deterrence and backlash effects in counter-terrorism: The case of ETA. *Terrorism Political Violence.* 2015;27(1):160–181. doi:10.1080/

09546553.2014.975648; Dugan L, Chenoweth E. Moving beyond deterrence: The effectiveness of raising the expected utility of abstaining from terrorism in Israel. *Am Sociol Rev.* 2012;77(4):597–624. doi:10.1177/0003122412450573; Faria JR. Terrorist innovations and anti-terrorist policies. *Terrorism Political Violence.* 2006;18(1):47–56. doi:10.1080/095465591009377; Hafez MM, Hatfield JM. Do targeted assassinations work? A multivariate analysis of Israel's controversial tactic during al-Aqsa uprising. *Stud Conflict Terrorism.* 2006;29(4):359–382. doi:10.1080/1057610060641972; Lafree G, Dugan L, Korte R. The impact of British counterterrorist strategies on political violence in Northern Ireland: Comparing deterrence and backlash models. *Criminology.* 2009;47(1):17–45. doi:10.1111/j.1745-9125.2009.00138.x; Parkin WS, Freilich JD. Routine activities and right-wing extremists: An empirical comparison of the victims of ideologically-and non-ideologically-motivated homicides committed by American far-rightists. *Terrorism Political Violence.* 2015;27(1):182–203.

29. Agnew R. A general strain theory of terrorism. *Theoretical Criminol.* 2010;14(2):131–153. doi:10.1177/1362480609350163; Fahey S, Lafree G. Does country-level social disorganization increase terrorist attacks? *Terrorism Political Violence.* 2015;27(1):81–111. doi:10.1080/09546553.2014.972156; Pauwels L, Schils N. Differential online exposure to extremist content and political violence: Testing the relative strength of social learning and competing perspectives. *Terrorism Political Violence.* 2016;28(1):1–29. doi:10.1080/09546553.2013.876414.

30. HM Government. *Prevent Strategy.* 2011. https://www.gov.uk

31. Bouhana, Wikström. *Al Qai'da-Influenced Radicalisation.*

32. Bouhana, Wikström. *Theorising. Terrorism*; Bouhana N, Wikström PO. Theorizing terrorism: Terrorism as moral action. *Contemp Readings Law Soc Justice.* 2010;2(2):9–79; Schils N, Pauwels L. Explaining violent extremism for subgroups by gender and immigrant background using SAT as a framework. *J Strategic Security.* 2014;7(3):27–47; Wikström PO, Bouhana N. Analysing radicalisation and terrorism: A Situational Action Theory. In LaFree G, Freilich J, eds., *The Handbook of the Criminology of Terrorism.* New York: Wiley; 2017:175–186.

33. Suchy Y. Executive functioning: Overview, assessment, and research issues for non-neuropsychologists. *Ann Behav Med.* 2009;37:106–116.

34. Friedan NP, Miyake A, Corley RP, Young SE, DeFries JC, Hewitt JK. Not all executive functions are related to intelligence. *Psychol Sci.* 2006;17:172–179.

35. Suchy. Executive functioning.

36. Gino F, Schweitzer ME, Mead NL, Ariely D. Unable to resist temptation: How self-control depletion promotes unethical behavior. *Organizational Behav Hum Decision Processes*. 2011;115:191–203.
37. Williams PG, Suchy Y, Rau HK. Individual differences in executive functioning: Implications for stress regulation. *Ann Behav Med*. 2009;37(2):126–140.
38. Baumeister RF, Vohs KD. Self-regulation and the executive function of the self. In Leary MR, Tangney JP, eds., *Handbook of Self and Identity*. New York: Guilford Press; 2003:197–217.
39. Beaver KM, Wright JP, Delisi M. Self-control as an executive function: Reformulating Gottfredson's and Hirschi's parental socialization thesis. *Crim Justice Behav*. 2007;34:1345–1361.
40. Pratt TC, Cullen FT. The empirical status of Gottefredson and Hirschi's General Theory of Crime: A meta-analysis. *Criminology*. 2000;38(3):931–964.
41. Baumeister, Vohs. Self-regulation and the executive function of the self; Mick DG, Broniarczik SM, Haidt J. Choose, choose, choose: Emerging and prospective research on the deleterious effects of living in consumer hyperchoice. *J Business Ethics*. 2004;52:207–211.
42. Kruglanski et al. The psychology of radicalization and deradicalization.
43. Kitayama S, Park J. Cultural neuroscience of the self: Understanding the social grounding of the brain. *Soc Cogn Affect Neurosci*. 2010;5(2–3):111–129. doi:10.1093/scan/nsq052.
44. McGregor I, Hayes J, Prentice M. Motivation for aggressive religious radicalization: Goal regulation theory and a personality × threat × affordance hypothesis. *Front Psychol*. 2015;6:1–18. doi:10.3389/fpsyg.2015.01325.
45. Bakermans-Kranenburg MJ, van Ijzendoorn MH. Differential susceptibility to rearing environment depending on dopamine-related genes: New evidence and a meta-analysis. *Develop Psychopathol*. 2011;23(1):39–52. doi:10.1017/S0954579410000635
46. Bouhana, Wikström. *Al Qai'da-Influenced Radicalisation*.
47. Sageman. *Understanding Terror Networks*.
48. Bouhana, Wikström. *Al Qai'da-Influenced Radicalisation*.
49. Wikström PO, Sampson RJ. Social mechanisms of community influences on crime and pathways in criminality, In Lahey BB, Moffit TE, Caspi A, eds., *Causes of Conduct Disorder and Juvenile Delinquency*. New York: Guilford Press; 2003:118–148.
50. Wikström PO. Individuals, settings, and acts of crime: Situational mechanisms and the explanation of crime. In Wikström PO, Sampson RJ, eds., *The Explanation of Crime: Context, Mechanisms and Development*. Cambridge: Cambridge University Press; 2006:61–107.
51. Yuksek DA, Solakoglu O. The relative influence of parental attachment, peer attachment, school attachment, and school alienation on delinquency among high school students in Turkey. *Deviant Behav*. 2016;9625:1–25. doi:10.1080/01639625.2015.1062683.
52. Sampson RJ, Laub JH. Life-course desisters? Trajectories of crime among delinquent boys followed to age 70. *Criminology*. 2003;41(3):555–592.
53. Olsen JA. *Roads to Militant Radicalization: Interviews with Five Former Perpetrators of Politically Motivated Organized Violence*. Copenhagen: Danish Institute for International Studies; 2009.
54. Brachman JM, Levine AN. You too can be Awlaki! *Foreign Affairs*. 2011;35(1):25–46.
55. Bouhana, Wikström. *Al Qai'da-Influenced Radicalisation*.
56. Wikström, Bouhana. Analysing radicalisation and terrorism.
57. Edwards C, Gribbon L. Pathways to violent extremism in the digital era. *RUSI J*. 2013;158(5):40–47.
58. Neumann PR. Options and strategies for countering online radicalization in the United States. *Stud Conflict Terrorism*. 2013;36(6):431–459.
59. Sampson RJ, Raudenbush SW, Earls F. Neighborhoods and violent crime: A multilevel study of collective efficacy. *Science*. 1997;277(5328):918–924.
60. Neumann. Options and strategies.
61. Although we speak of *a* setting and *a* situation, this is for analytical clarity only; it is evident that an action can be an extended process that carries across a series of settings.
62. Pease K. No through road: Closing pathways to crime. In Moss K, Stephens M, eds., *Crime Reduction and the Law*. London: Routledge; 2006:50–66.
63. Clarke, Newman. *Outsmarting the Terrorists*.
64. Wikström. Individuals, settings, and acts of crime.
65. Bronfenbrenner U. *The Ecology of Human Development*. Cambridge, MA: Harvard University Press; 1979.
66. Lemieux AF, Brachman JM, Levitt J, Wood J. Inspire magazine: A critical analysis of its significance and potential impact through the lens of the information, motivation, and behavioral skills model. *Terrorism Political Violence*. 2014;26(2):354–371. doi:10.1080/09546553.2013.828604.
67. Ekblom P, Tilley N. Going equipped: Criminology, situational crime prevention and the resourceful offender. *Br J Criminol*. 2000;40:376–398.
68. Clarke, Newman. *Outsmarting the Terrorists*.

23

A Framework for Preempting Lone-Actor Terrorists During the Pre-Incident Phases

JOSHUA SINAI

INTRODUCTION

For counterterrorism agencies, violent attacks by lone-actor terrorist perpetrators are a relatively frequent occurrence in the United States because they are easier to carry out than are attacks by organized groups: it is easier for counterterrorism agencies to identify the presence of a larger group for effective preemption. As a result, a minority of terrorist incidents in the United States have been committed by combat cells of organized terrorist groups, such as al-Qaeda's 9/11 attacks, or by their loosely affiliated networks, such as the Taliban-directed plot by Najibullah Zazi and his associates to attack the New York City subway system in September 2009 and al-Qaeda in the Arabian Peninsula's directed the plot by its operative Mohammed Saeed Alshamrani to conduct a shooting rampage on December 6, 2019, at the Naval Air Station in Pensacola, Florida, killing three people and wounding eight others. These and other factors have resulted in a majority of plots and attacks to be conducted by lone actors without a direct link to a terrorist group, although they may be influenced by them in extremist social media sites to carry out their attacks, which are self-funded.

For counterterrorism agencies, preempting lone-actor terrorists is thus more difficult and differs from thwarting organized terrorist groups or their loosely networked affiliates. This chapter primarily focuses on how such lone actors can be identified and preempted during the pre-incident phases of their planning and execution activities, if possible. To illustrate the importance of such early preemption, out of this study's sample of 56 lone-actor terrorists who had plotted to conduct a terrorist attack in the United States during the period of 2001 to

early 2020, 42 (75.0%) had succeeded in carrying out their attacks, inflicting varying numbers of casualties or, at the very least, placing or detonating explosives at their targeted locations. Of these "successful" plotters, however, many were already known to those associated with them as susceptible to violent extremism, with a few even interviewed by law enforcement officers for warning purposes prior to their attacks. However, only 14 potential attackers (25.0%) in this study's sample of cases were successfully preempted by law enforcement agencies prior to their attempted attacks. For legal reasons, several additional cases were not included in which the perpetrators were in a state of pre-trial/not convicted as of August 2020, so the cases included should be considered as a representative sample rather than as an inclusive list.

To increase the level of successful preemption of such attacker types, this study presents a framework to enable analysts in the counterterrorism and public policy/academic communities to identify such perpetrators' mindset and behavioral characteristics for effective preemption during the crucial pre-incident warning phases when their suspicious intentions and activities can be identified and thwarted.

To analyze these issues, this chapter begins by presenting a definition of lone-actor terrorists, which is followed by an analysis of an eight-phase trajectory into violence that such individuals progress through prior to their attacks. Drawing on this trajectory into violence, the final section presents a framework for preventing such potential lone-actor terrorists during the formative pre-incident phases. This is followed by an appendix that provides a database of the study's sample of 56 cases, with separate columns indicating whether the attacks were completed or prevented by law enforcement.

CRITERIA FOR IDENTIFY-ING LONE-ACTOR TER-RORISTS FOR INCLUSION IN STUDY'S CASES

For the purpose of this study, seven criteria are employed to identify lone-actor terrorists in the United States for inclusion in the study's cases. These include their role as domestic (US) actors; how their domestic and/or foreign-based extremist ideologies apply; that, if two attackers are involved in an attack, one of the attackers must be the attack's primary architect and actor; and certain gray areas in distinguishing between lone actors and those who are loosely affiliated with a terrorist group. Understanding these criteria is crucial because it enables counterterrorist agencies to distinguish lone-actor terrorists from other types of terrorist actors (i.e., those who have a more formal affiliation with a terrorist group), especially the suspicious characteristics and activities that might need to be monitored for pre-incident preemption. Also, by educating community leaders where such susceptible individuals might exist, they will be able report their suspicious mindsets and behaviors to appropriate authorities to identify the potential terrorist actors who might be operating in their midst for follow-up, including mental health or professional counseling, if necessary.

In the first criteria for inclusion, the selected violent lone actors must plot, attempt to, or complete a terrorism-motivated attack in the United States. Although numerous violent lone actors in the US commit mass fatality attacks, such as psychologically driven active shooters, in this study only ideologically driven terrorists are selected, with their attacks having a political dimension. This is not intended to imply that some ideologically driven terrorists are not considered psychologically disordered individuals as well, but that being driven by extremist ideologies is the primary distinguishing characteristic of such violent perpetrators. For this reason, Aaron Alexis's shooting rampage at the Washington, DC, Navy Yard (September 16, 2013) or Stephen Paddock's mass shooting in Las Vegas, Nevada (October 1, 2017) are not included because a terrorism motivation had not been proved as a motivating factor in their mass shooting attacks. In the case of Alexis, in particular, although he had attacked a US Navy facility, his motivation was reportedly workplace-focused, as he was seeking revenge for his imminent firing from his employment as a contractor to the Navy.[1]

In the second selection criteria, the lone actors included in this sample are categorized as domestic terrorists. Although this is not an official US government definition, but the author's own formulation, domestic terrorism is defined broadly to include persons who attack other Americans in the United States for political objectives, which may be domestic or foreign (e.g., global jihad). To be considered for inclusion under the third criteria, such lone actors decide to conduct their attacks while in the United States, as opposed to foreigners planning their operations prior to arrival in America. Residing in the United States at the time of their attack is a crucial component in the definition, whether they are US citizens or foreigners on a student or work visa. Thus, not falling under this criteria are "one-person" foreign-based terrorists who are deployed by a foreign terrorist organization to conduct an attack in the United States. For this reason, foreign-deployed "single terrorists" are not included, such as British national Richard Reid ("Transatlantic Shoe Bomber"; December 22, 2001) or Nigerian national Umar Farouk Abdulmutallab ("Transatlantic Christmas Bomber"; December 25, 2009). On the other hand, this study's cases include Khalid Aldawsari, a Saudi Arabian national who was studying in the United States on an expired student visa and who was arrested for plotting an attack in Dallas, Texas, in February 2011.

Moreover, not included in the listed cases are several high-profile US homegrown terrorist operatives such as Adam Gadahn, Anwar al-Awlaki, Samir Khan, and Omar Shafik Hammami (aka Abu Mansoor al-Amriki) because they had traveled overseas to join foreign terrorist groups as opposed to attempting to carry out terrorist attacks in America.

In the fourth criteria, to qualify as domestic terrorists, the extremist ideologies motivating them either are US- or foreign-based (or a combination of the two). This is my own definition: this definition does not represent any government definition because the United States, at least as of mid-2020, has not legislated an official definition of domestic terrorism that addresses both domestic- and foreign-based ideologies as motivating domestic terrorists.

Generally, the extremist ideologies motivating domestic terrorists are primarily far right-wing, far left-wing, or Islamist. The far right-wing groups that inspire them include white supremacists, neo-Nazis, Christian Identity, the Sovereign Citizens Movement, anti-abortionists, and others. The far left-wing ideologies that motivate them include extremist environmentalists (including anti-modern technology), anti-law enforcement, anti-globalists, and others. In a few cases, the extremist ideologies driving such lone actors are a blend of conspiratorial anti-government libertarianism that cannot be characterized either as far right-wing or far left-wing, including a recent phenomenon, "incel," an online movement of mostly men who view themselves as "involuntarily celibate" and promote violence against women.

Fifth, the status of "loner" makes such perpetrators unique, as opposed to being members of organized terrorist groups or loosely affiliated networks.[2] This is particularly the case due to their lack of training, provision of weapons, and other forms of logistical support by organized terrorist groups at the time of their plots or attacks, although several such perpetrators underwent military training during their military service in the United States (such as Timothy McVeigh, the perpetrator of the Oklahoma City bombing on April 19, 1995). This category includes certain gray areas, such as informal links between lone actors (e.g., Nidal Hasan's November 2009 correspondence with his ideological "mentor" Anwar al-Awlaki, who was based in Yemen, or Zachary Chesser [July 2010] and his fellow extremist American jihadi bloggers, who were not formal members of jihadi groups).

Sixth, their status as "loners," however, does not imply that they must be single actors, although it is the case that most lone actors are single perpetrators. As explained by the FBI's study, to qualify as lone actors, if two perpetrators are involved, one of them must be the primary architect and actor in the attack.[3] Thus, in the case of the Tsarnaev brothers who carried out the April 2013 Boston Marathon bombing, it was Tamerlan, the elder brother, who allegedly was the plot's primary architect, with Dzhokhar, the younger brother, acting in a supporting role.

As demonstrated by this discussion, formulating the criteria for inclusion as lone actors is the subject of controversy in the academic literature. To resolve this controversy, Hamm and Spaaij write that "Some experts use an expansive definition of lone wolf terrorism in terms of both motives and the number of perpetrators involved."

They cite Jeffrey Simon's definition as "the use or threat of violence or nonviolent sabotage, including cyber-attacks, against government, society, business, the military . . . or any other target, by an individual acting alone or with minimal support from one or two other people . . . to further a political, social, religious, financial, or other related goal,"[4] to create fear and disruption that provokes heightened government reaction.

Building on these expanded selection criteria for inclusion, as part of the sixth criteria, this chapter accepts the definitions by Simon and the FBI that lone actors can cooperate with one or two other individuals as long as one of them is the primary attack perpetrator. I add that their operations are not directed by an organized terrorist group and that they self-fund and self-weaponize their operations during the pre-incident preparatory phases. Examples for inclusion are the cases of the Beltway Snipers (October 2002); the Tsarnaev brothers (Boston Marathon, April 13, 2013); Jerad Miller and Amanda Miller (June 2014), the husband-and-wife mass shooters (San Bernardino, California, December 2, 2015); and David N. Anderson and Francine Graham (Newark, New Jersey, December 2019). These acted as "joint" actors: one of them was the primary attacker, they had no direct affiliation with a terrorist group, and their plots were self-funded and self-weaponized.

In a final selection criteria, this chapter terms these "lone actors" as opposed to "lone wolves" (the most commonly used term) because, as Bart Schuurman et al. point out, the "latter implies a high level of cunning and lethality that is often not present among" such perpetrators.[5]

TRAJECTORY INTO VIOLENCE

The lone-actor terrorists (like psychologically driven violent lone actors, such as active shooters) transition through a *pathway to violence* trajectory. As lone actors, this trajectory does not involve individuals who are members in a terrorist group, whose recruitment differs markedly because it generally takes place within a hierarchical organizational structure, including provision of a training facility (of varying degrees of sophistication) as opposed to the self-recruitment that characterizes lone actors and with their attacks organized and financed largely on their own.

This lone-actors' trajectory into violence is composed of a series of eight progressively escalating phases, with each phase characterized by corresponding risk factors exhibited by such attackers that can be thwarted once they are pre-emptively identified and reported to appropriate authorities. It begins with the three preparatory phases of (1) cognitive opening, (2) a traumatic triggering event (or events), which is followed by an (3) ideation/fantasy (or homicidal ideation) phase. A fourth phase, (4) threshold, is crucial in determining whether such susceptible individuals respond in a violent way to the previous two phases and embark on the pre-violence phases of (5) planning, (6) preparation, and (7) approaching the target. The final phase is (8) the execution of an attack.

The transition along the pathway to violence trajectory is not necessarily linear, with some individuals progressing along such a trajectory potentially deciding on their own to backtrack and turn away from embarking on the final three pre-attack phases. This might be due to what are called "risk-reducing factors," which include constructive and healthy personal coping mechanisms, the persuasive influence of friends and family, the support of professional mental health counselors, and intervention by law enforcement.

Phase 1: Triggers

Terrorist attacks by lone actors either are conducted impulsively or evolve over time. Although like other lone actor attacks, such as those by psychologically driven active shooters, assessing such perpetrators' precise motivation for conducting a terrorist attack may not "be known with complete certainty,"[6] the pre-incident preparatory phases often produce early warning signals that can be identified to prevent them. The first grouping of early warning signals is usually the result of triggers, such as a spectrum of traumatic events. These usually include traumatic personal, professional, or ideological crises that lead to the formation of strong grievances that influence susceptible individuals to decide to engage in some sort of retributive violence to redress them. In the case of ideologically driven terrorists, these crises—whether actual or self-perceived—might include a sense that they are members of a religious or civil community that is being unjustly victimized, oppressed, or under illegitimate foreign subjugation. For right-wing white supremacists, for example, politicians' demagoguery about threats to their survival posed by the pervasiveness of non-white populations in society through illegal immigration and its impact on their own economic hardship, can spur grievances that need to be redressed through violence. Thus, when traumatic events such as failed personal relationships,

lack of employment, and an ideology that promises to redress their various problems converge, such triggers will cumulatively drive susceptible individuals to transition into a violent phase.

Examples of how such triggers might motivate lone actors to engage in terrorist-type attacks include the case of Nidal Hasan. The trigger for his violent shooting rampage at the Ft. Hood military base may have been a combination of his Islamist jihadist anger against US military intervention in Afghanistan and Iraq, with his fellow soldiers viewed as the agents of such injustice. In the case of Paul Anthony Ciancia's targeting of the passenger terminal at the Los Angeles International Airport, his attack was reportedly triggered by his perceived grievance against the US government in general and the Transportation Security Agency (TSA) in particular.[7]

In evaluating such triggers for their role in formulating a threat assessment, it is important to consider them in a wider context involving other risk factors, such as those listed in phases 2–4, since only a tiny proportion of individuals motivated by such triggers are likely to "go operational" and conduct a terrorist attack against their perceived targets, whether they are intentional or random. To transition into the violent phases, susceptible individuals need to be "cognitively open" to consider engaging in retributive violence in the first place.

Phase 2: Cognitive Opening

Based on this chapter's sample of incidents, all 73 of its extremist, ideologically driven lone-actor terrorists (with seven of the cases involving two actors), like their psychologically driven active shooter counterparts, appeared to be troubled individuals whose "collection of grievances" (whether legitimate or not) drove them to engage in targeted violence against their perceived adversaries. The notion of "troubled individuals" is employed as a general category, as opposed to the American Psychological Association's *Diagnostic and Statistical Manual of Mental Disorders* (DSM-5) categorization of psychological disorders because access to these perpetrators' case files is not available to make such mental health determinations. The notion of "troubled individuals" should be sufficient to characterize some sort of psychological problem because "normally" disposed individuals are likely to find constructive and non-violent ways to redress their various grievances as opposed to the lone-actor terrorists who are determined to be arrested or killed while carrying out their vengeful, targeted violence.

In a second component of this phase, individuals become lone actors (as opposed to members of a group) because, according to the literature, on the one hand, they prefer not to be "formally involved with terrorist networks that would have happily given guidance and material support,"[8] while, on the other hand, many are social misfits who would not be accepted by such groups due to their "social ineptitude" and other psychological factors.[9] This was the case with Timothy McVeigh and Terry Nichols, the perpetrators of the bombing of the Alfred P. Murrah Federal Building in Oklahoma City (April 19, 1995) who were "ostracized by the Michigan Militia because they advocated for violence."[10]

With regard to the several lone-actor terrorists who were married, while each appeared to be motivated by different psychological drivers, they shared certain commonalities. In the case of husband-and-wife Syed Rizwan Farook and Tashfeen Malik (December 2015) both had self-radicalized themselves into violent extremism to such an extent that, even though they had an infant child, they had become desensitized to the consequences of their violent attacks on the fate of their children and families.[11] Although Faisal Shahzad (May 2010), Tamerlan Tsarnaev (April 2013_), and Omar Mateen (June 2016) were married, their wives were not directly involved in their attacks (although Mateen's wife was later arrested as an accessory), but, like Farook and Malik, despite having young children, they persisted in conducting their attacks with no concern for the negative consequences of their attacks on the future lives of their wives and children.

In a third component, several of the lone-actor terrorists had a history of engaging in domestic violence. With men constituting all the primary architects of the 49 "successful" attacks (and only three of their co-attackers being women), as Joan Smith explains, such perpetrators share a sense of perverse entitlement that causes them to "seek to control every aspect of the lives of their wives and children" without any interest in "considering their long-term welfare" or "protecting them from the consequences of [their] horrific public acts of violence. It is a chilling view of family relationships in which becoming a husband and father appears to have more to do with confirming a man's status . . . than forming close attachments."[12] The literature describes numerous examples of lone-actor terrorists who had reportedly abused their wives or girlfriends.

Phase 3: Violent Ideation/Fantasy

Even for troubled individuals who experience traumatic triggers and who possess a cognitive opening to violence may not actually transition into the third phase's violent ideation/fantasy. This psychological state, also known as *homicidal ideation*, refers to the adoption of thoughts about pursuing homicide to avenge a grievance. This may range from vague ideas of taking revenge while not committing homicide, to deciding to cross into phase 4's threshold into engaging in violence to redress the grievances against their perceived adversaries.

While for most "normal" individuals phase 1's triggering events will be sufficiently traumatic to cause some sort of ideation/fantasy involving anger and even fury, it will not necessarily lead to the build-up of violent thoughts against their alleged victimizers that will drive them to cross phase 4's threshold into violence.

In the latter component of this phase, those fantasizing about embarking on vengeful violence will begin to dehumanize their intended victims (whether they have any direct relation to them or not) and imagine the event in which their revenge takes place. They might also begin to romanticize the media coverage, headlines, and notoriety produced by their vengeful event.

Phase 4: Threshold into Violence

Once the susceptible individuals' sense of grievance is strong enough, they cross phase 4's threshold into violence. This phase has two components. In the first component, to pass through this phase, it will be necessary for them to bypass any psychological internal or external constraints that might stop them from following their homicidal ideation to its violent endpoint.

In the second component, once such individuals are prepared to follow through on their violent vengeance, there are two possible responses for them to transition into the next phase of planning an attack: reactive or predatory. In a *reactive response*, also referred to as "in the heat of the moment," the decision to launch an attack is relatively quick, usually immediately in the aftermath of the infliction of a perceived grievance. A *predatory response* could still take place within a short period in response to a perceived grievance, but it generally involves a lengthier degree of preparation and planning that for some perpetrators can last days, weeks, or even a year or two. Some of these individuals might appear outwardly "calm" and "silently determined" in order not to let others be aware of their violent intentions.

Phase 5: Planning

Orchestrating a violent attack is something that the lone actor fantasizes about, plans for, prepares for (e.g., by purchasing the weapon[s] for the attack), and then rehearses in advance. It is during the planning phase that decisions will be made on the tactics to be used, weaponry, the intended targeting, date, and location for the attack. Adhering to these components in the planning phase thus enables the potential attacker to control "the day, time, location and the weapon he's going to use."[13]

Phase 6: Preparation

During the preparation phase, the attacker will seek to obtain the weapon(s) necessary to carry out the incident. The attempt to obtain the weapon(s) will be made legally or by theft. The weapons will likely be hidden in a designated place. The attacker will attempt to become proficient in employing the weapon(s), rehearse the attack, and surveil the target.

Phase 7: Approach

At this phase—the closest and most lethal period prior to the planned event—the attacker will likely develop the attack plan, deploy the weapon(s), and begin to execute the plan for the attack. The attacker will travel to the target location while armed.

As an example of such cold-blooded attackers, on the morning of November 5, 2009, when Nidal Hasan drove through the checkpoint at Fort Hood and proceeded to the Soldier Readiness Processing Center, he is reported to have exhibited no outward behavior to arouse suspicion about his imminent intentions to open fire within minutes of his arrival.[14]

This was also the case with Jared Lee Loughner on the morning of his planned attack in Tucson, Arizona, on January 8, 2011. At 7:04 AM, he went to a Walmart store in the area to purchase ammunition. At 7:34 AM he was stopped by an Arizona police officer for running a red light; once the officer determined there were no outstanding warrants for him, he was allowed to proceed to his destination with a warning to drive carefully. That morning, he took a taxi to the Safeway supermarket location in Casas Adobes, where he proceeded to carry out his shooting rampage at Representative Gifford's outdoor constituents meeting.[15]

Similarly, on December 2, 2015, Syed Rizwan Farook arrived at his office's holiday party at the Inland Regional Center in San Bernardino, California, at around 8:30 AM. Throughout the party, he posed for photos with his other co-workers. He left the party's midpoint at around 10:30 AM. It is reported that he left a backpack containing explosives on top of a table. At around 10:59 AM, he returned with his wife to carry out their joint shooting attack.[16]

In another example, Omar Mateen (June 2016) is reported to have visited the Pulse nightclub on several occasions prior to his attack, so he was likely recognizable to some of the staff when he entered the club to carry out his attack.[17]

Phase 8: Attack

At this phase, the attacker begins to execute his attack. Because he is tightly focused on attacking his targets, the event will generally evolve quickly, and the attacker will not stop until he runs out of ammunition, the bomb explodes, all the victims die, he takes his own life, or he decides that sufficient fatalities were inflicted that he can escape from the scene. The attack may take place in an indoor or outdoor environment. Finally, the attack may involve single or multiple locations or be mobile, with the attacker moving along multiple locations until he is stopped and neutralized.

PREVENTING LONE-ACTOR TERRORIST ATTACKS

Based on the warning signs generated by this trajectory into violence's eight phases, six measures are proposed to preempt and prevent perpetrators during their pre-incident preparatory phases. These consist of, first, identifying expressions of violent extremism, including leakages of such views and intentions; second, identifying those who are "trusted insiders" within an organization who express extremist views that might point to a possible attack; third, identifying pre-incident planning and preparation activities; fourth, identifying potential perpetrators on their approach to their intended target; and, fifth, identifying released prisoners with a proclivity to re-engage in violent extremism. Once a sufficient number of these (as well as other) suspicious indicators are identified by law enforcement and those associated with such individuals, a sixth measure is for law enforcement to covertly engage potential perpetrators into thinking they are involved in a potential attack and then arrest them for successful preemption when they attempt to follow-up with their intentions.

Identifying "Troubled" Personalities and Trajectory into Violent Extremism

As highlighted in phase 2 "cognitive opening," as part of their "troubled" personalities, many of these perpetrators tend to be frustrated with their personal lives, are mostly unmarried (although a few who are married or in a relationship will engage in such violence), and are frustrated with the pace of their professional lives (with no known lone-actor terrorists being well-to-do financially). In the case of those lone-actor terrorists who had a history of engaging in domestic violence, when they become radicalized into extremism, correlating their proclivity to domestic violence and adopting an extremist ideology may point to a potential for them to engage in terrorist violence as well. It is for these reasons that it is crucial to be aware of the risky mindsets that might point to such susceptible individuals potentially engaging in a lone actor-type terrorist attack.

Following the first phase's triggering events, throughout the trajectory into violence's subsequent six pre-incident phases, lone-actor perpetrators tend to leak their attack intentions to others, whether in person or on internet social media sites, making it possible for others to notice suspicious signs that could be reported to appropriate authorities for preemption. Because lone actors are not bound by the secrecy that is usually demanded by a terrorist cell, they are freer to express their vengeful grievances and rage prior to their attacks. One of the reasons such individuals express their grievances, rages, and, in the most extreme cases, their violent intentions to strike back at their self-perceived adversaries, is that some exhibit the characteristics of psychopaths (and, in this analysis, this should be understood as a thesis that must be examined within each investigatory case). As explained by Dave Cullen, the author of a book on the April 1999 Columbine High School shootings, "they love giving us clues."[18] As further explained by Mary Ellen O'Toole, a retired FBI behavioral profiler, this phenomenon can be explained by the term "leakage," with internet social media sites supplanting diaries and videos as the vehicle for such individuals to "hint or even announce their plans far in advance of carrying them out."[19] Since it is difficult for outsiders to know about a potential suspect's private diaries and notes, monitoring such social media sites, "where most young people have a presence and share much of their lives," therefore can "pinpoint potential problems before they start."[20]

Monitoring social media sites where extremist sentiments are expressed, therefore, has become an important tool for law enforcement and others charged with tracking such individuals because, whether prior to their attacks or as postmortems, their social media "footprints" are becoming a sort of Rorschach test that can produce a profile of individuals who might demonstrate an inclination to conduct violent attacks.[21]

Once these early warning indicators are identified, their trajectory into violent extremism can be preempted through various preventative community-level approaches. In addition to mental health counseling, if this is possible, other programs would promote peaceful alternatives to the pursuit of violence to fulfill their ideological objectives by providing them a sense of belonging and meaning in life.[22] This is important "because the best way to stop terrorism is by preventing its causes."[23]

Identifying Radicalized "Trusted" Insiders

The previous response measures focused on the need to identify suspicious mindsets and behaviors by individuals who were largely unknown to their attackers. With 6 out of the 49 (12.24%) lone-actor terrorists who had carried out "successful" attacks known to their intended victims, whether as fellow employees or students, a crucial preventative measure is to identify the characteristics of such radicalized "insider" threats. As employees in an organization or as students at an educational institution, "trusted" insiders have legitimate access to their targeted facilities, where they frequently interact with their fellow employees or students. As employees who are assigned trust once they are hired or as students trusted to observe a school's general rules, there is a tacit assumption that they are trustworthy. In the case of such "trusted" insiders who become ideologically motivated terrorists, there are often changes in their behavioral patterns over time that can indicate a change in their trustworthiness. Often, changes that affect their personal circumstances impact on the quality of their work as well. This was most evident in Nidal Hasan, whose fellow medical students and workers had frequently complained about his extremist views and inadequate work performance. Similarly, although G4S, the security corporation that employed Omar Mateen as a security guard did not appropriately follow-up with him after he was interviewed by the FBI in 2013 for possible radicalization and association with other extremists.

This enabled him to proceed with his further radicalization, ultimately leading to his shooting rampage at the Pulse nightclub, in Orlando, Florida, on June 12, 2016.[24]

As these six cases of "trusted" insiders demonstrate, their radicalization into violent extremism while working at their jobs was missed by their respective organizations, thus thwarting effective preemption. They all exhibited the early warning indicators of a radicalized insider threat. These included expressing hatred of American society, expressing sympathy for foreign organizations that promote anti-American violence, associating with or expressing loyalty to foreign terrorists, browsing websites that promote violence against the United States, expressing outrage against US military operations abroad, adopting an extremist ideology that advocates violence, purchasing a large amount of firearms and ammunition that was reflective of violent intentions, and keeping a social distance from their co-workers. While in isolation, these concerning activities might not indicate potential terrorist activity, once correlated with each other, they indicated a high risk of becoming a violent insider threat to fellow workers.

The question then becomes how such suspicious radicalized mindset and behavioral manifestations can be identified by supervisors, fellow employees, or school colleagues and reported to the appropriate authorities to mitigate and minimize the risk of their potential turn to violence.

Identifying Pre-Incident Planning and Preparation

Beginning in the trajectory's fifth and sixth phases of planning and preparation, potential perpetrators will attempt to acquire the weapon(s) to be used in the attack. Their weapon(s) are likely to be low-tech firearms, followed by bombs, although one should also anticipate other weapons to be employed, such as vehicles, weaponized letters/packages, knives, and drones. As demonstrated by the anthrax letter attacks, however, even some lone actors may be capable of developing certain types of high-tech weapons, so these types of sophisticated approaches need to be considered in formulating threat assessments of the types of weapons likely to be employed. When individuals of concern attempt to acquire weapon(s), this also presents an opportunity to identify suspicious activities and report them to appropriate authorities.

This is crucial because in several high-profile mass casualty attacks such suspicious attempts to acquire weapons, including pre-cursor explosives, were not identified for pre-emptive alert to the appropriate authorities. These included the lethal handgun purchase by Nidal Hasan (November 2009) at the Guns Galore store in Killeen, Texas; the purchase by Tamerlan Tsarnaev (April 2013) of pre-cursor bomb-making materials of fertilizer and fireworks; and the purchase of a handgun by Mohammed Saeed Alshamrani (December 2019). These all would have raised suspicion in those who sold them the items if they had been properly briefed beforehand about identifying suspicious purchases. In fact, following Hasan's attack and after the salespeople at Guns Galore were briefed by law enforcement, when Nasser Jason Abdo (July 2011) attempted a suspicious gun purchase, the store's salesmen immediately contacted local law enforcement who arrested Abdo.

Elliot Rodgers presents an example of unsuccessful preemption, in which law enforcement officers interviewed him, but did not properly follow-up. Rodger carried out a shooting rampage on May 23, 2014, in Isla Vista, California, near the campus of the University of California, Santa Barbara, killing 6 people and wounding 14 others. Several weeks prior to his shooting rampage, his parents contacted their local police over their concern about his threatening online postings. When police officers interviewed him at his apartment on April 30, they found him to be "reasonable" and did not follow-up by searching his apartment, where he had stockpiled four guns and hundreds of rounds of ammunition, all legally purchased.[25]

Identifying Approaching the Target

In the trajectory's fourth phase, approaching the target, there will still be sufficient opportunities to identify warning signs, although they may be more difficulty to notice than those exhibited in previous phases. As in the cases of Hasan (November 2009) and Jared Loughner (January 2011), street patrol officers might encounter a potential attacker through encounters ranging from a traffic stop to routine screening when they enter a military facility's guarded entrance. It might be difficult for law enforcement to identify risky behaviors during such pre-incident encounters because the attacker has the upper hand: he knows exactly what he intends to do, so he might adopt an innocent demeanor. Nevertheless, such deception might still be possible to detect. Contact with the attacker at this point might also be dangerous because he might act as though he knows he is under surveillance;

if he feels threatened, he might attack. In the case of a co-worker who might be plotting an attack, as was the case with Syed Rizwan Farook (December 2, 2015), a trained observer might have been able to detect suspicious behavior at the holiday party that might have pointed to an imminent attack.

Identifying Violent Extremism by Released Prisoners

In this sample database, at least three of the "successful" perpetrators—John Allen Mohammad (October 2002), Cesar Sayoc Jr. (October 2018), and David Anderson (December 2019)—had been previously incarcerated for criminal activity, were radicalized into extremism while in prison, and subsequently turned to terrorism following their release. This was confirmed by an FBI study of some 50 cases of lone-actor terrorists over a 40-year period in the United States, where 35 offenders (70% of their sample) were arrested at least once as an adult before their terrorist attack. In such cases, it is the responsibility of parole bodies to continue watching them during their post-release phase to ensure they do not engage in terrorist violence. With such lone actors likely to self-fund their terrorist attacks through criminal activities, law enforcement authorities need to be aware of possible precursor crimes. Most of these crimes when viewed singly may not necessarily indicate a link to terrorism, but when operatives are identified as motivated by an extremist ideology, possible correlations will likely point to a nexus to a potential terrorist attack. It is at this point that these warning indicators represent the probable establishment of a seed-bed for lone-actor or cell activity in that locality, thus warranting the activation of a counterterrorism target zone investigation.

Covert Preemption

Once lone actors move from the third phase of violent ideation to cross the fourth phase's threshold, suspicious behaviors and preparatory activities that might point to an imminent attack will be present. These situations present law enforcement authorities with an opportunity to intervene and preempt a potential lone-actor attacker, whether overtly or covertly. Overt intervention, as in the form of an immediate arrest, is possible if a suspect is open about his attack intentions (e.g., in social media postings or in attempting to purchase a weapon under suspicious circumstances).

In other cases, however, covert intervention may be necessary. To gain accurate and timely intelligence about intentions to commit a future attack, information needs to be collected from a variety of sources ranging from government intelligence agencies to a suspect's family and friends who express concern to law enforcement about a possible trajectory into violence. When sufficient suspicious indicators are correlated to initiate an investigation accompanied by continuous monitoring and surveillance, at this point covert engagement with the suspect will be established. An agent will attempt to befriend the suspect, claiming to be associated with other terrorist operatives who are interested in helping the suspect accomplish his intended attack. The agent may provide the suspect with a weapon (usually one that is non-functioning) in order to arrest him once he attempts to execute the attack.

This covert measure is not a form of entrapment because the law enforcement agency is not promoting an attack by a suspect who lacks a predisposition to engage in such an attack. As explained by Oroszi and Ellis, the FBI is the lead agency in investigating acts of terrorism in the United States. Once it receive a tip from a bystander who notices a susceptible individual's expression of extremist beliefs (whether in social media or in person) or suspicious activities, the FBI deploys an undercover agent or informant to "befriend" the suspect. In such cases, the FBI arranges a sting operation in which the potential terrorist has the opportunity discuss an operation, attempt to acquire a weapon (with a "defective" weapon usually provided by an undercover agent), and then attempt to carry out the attack, such as detonating the "bomb" supplied to them. This covert practice is justified, Oroszi and Ellis argue, because "if the person shows a predisposition toward perpetrating the crime, ultimately chooses the crime and the target, and takes steps toward accomplishing the infraction, then they were not entrapped, they were caught."[26] In this study's 17 cases of successful preemption efforts, all involved such law enforcement covert preemptive operations.

CONCLUSION

As this chapter has demonstrated, for effective preemption, suspicious early warning signs exhibited by potential lone-actor terrorists need to be identified and correlated by close others throughout the suspect's trajectory into violence seven pre-incident phases. No single warning indicator may be sufficient on its own to anticipate a trajectory to violence; fantasizing about taking revenge for extremist ideological reasons without acquiring a weapon may not indicate that a potential attack is under way. However, when a susceptible individual does acquire a weapon, whether legally or illegally, and begins to engage in selecting a target to attack, it is at this point that pre-incident preemption is required. Even if an attack fails to result in casualties, such as Faisal Shahzad's unsuccessful vehicular bombing attack in Times Square in May 2010, the fact that such a lone-actor perpetrator had succeeded in reaching this final phase in the trajectory into violence represents a preventative failure because the early warning signs could have been observed by close others. To successfully preempt such lone-actor terrorists during the pre-incident phases, this chapter proposed six preventative measures, with the 14 cases of successful preemption compiled by the study examples of best practices in prevention. They also validate

the effectiveness of the Department of Homeland Security's motto that "when you see something, say something." Hopefully the widespread implementation of such best practices in prevention will increase the success rate in preventing lone-actor terrorists from approximately 25% of overall cases in this study's sample to a much higher rate of effectiveness.

APPENDIX A

This appendix presents a table of significant attacks and thwarted plots by lone-actor terrorists in the United States, from 2001 to 2020, in which the perpetrators were convicted in a trial or were killed in the attacks. Note that in a few recent cases the alleged perpetrators' scheduled trials were delayed due to the outbreak of the COVID-19 pandemic. The table's fifth and sixth columns indicate whether the attacks were completed or preempted during the pre-incident phases. The sources for the cases are provided below the table.

Lone-actor terrorist attacks/ plots, 2001–2020	Date	Plot/Attack	Outcome	Completed	Preempted
1	September 2001	Bruce Ivins, 55, alleged to have sent a series of poisonous anthrax letters; 22 infected, with 5 killed.	He committed suicide on July 28, 2008. On August 6, 2008, the FBI and Department of Justice formally announced that the government had concluded that Ivins was solely responsible for carrying out the attacks.[27]	X	
2	July 2, 2002	Hesham Mohamed Hadayet, 41, carried out a shooting rampage at airline ticket counter of El Al, Israel's national airline, at Los Angeles International Airport. Two people were killed and 4 others were wounded.	Hadayet was fatally shot by an El Al security guard after being wounded by him.[28]	X	

Lone-actor terrorist attacks/ plots, 2001–2020	Date	Plot/Attack	Outcome	Completed	Preempted
3	October 2002	John Allen Muhammad, 41, and Lee Boyd Malvo, 17, carried out drive-by sniper attacks in Maryland and Virginia. Ten people were killed and 3 others were wounded.	Muhammad was convicted on November 17, 2003, and executed on November 10, 2019. Malvo was convicted on December 18, 2003, and on November 8, 2006 was sentenced to life with parole.[29]	X	
4	July 28, 2006	**Naveed Afzal Haq, 30, carried out a shooting attack at the Jewish Federation of Greater Seattle building, in Washington; 1 person killed and 5 others wounded.**	On December 15, 2009 Haq was convicted for the crime. In January 2010, he was sentenced to life in prison without parole.[30]	X	
5	June 1, 2009	**Carlos Bledsoe (aka Abdulhakim Mujahid Muhammad), 23, carried out a drive-by shooting attack on US Army soldiers in front of a US military recruiting office in Little Rock, Arkansas, killing 1 soldier and wounding another.**	On July 25, 2011 Bledsoe was sentenced to life in prison.[31]	X	
6	June 10, 2009	James Wenneker von Brunn, 89, carried out a shooting attack at the US Holocaust Museum, in Washington, DC, killing a Museum Special Police Officer.	On January 6, 2010, Brunn died in prison while awaiting trial.[32]	X	

Lone-actor terrorist attacks/ plots, 2001–2020	Date	Plot/Attack	Outcome	Completed	Preempted
7	September 24, 2009	Michael C. Finton (Talib Islam), 39–40, was arrested for attempting to bomb the Paul Findley Federal Building and the adjacent offices of Congressman Aaron Schock in downtown Springfield, Illinois.	Finton pleaded guilty in federal court on May 9, 2011, and was sentenced to 28 years in prison.[33]		X
8	September 24, 2009	Hosam Maher Husein Smadi, 19, was arrested for planning a terrorist bombing of Fountain Place, a building in Dallas, Texas.	Following his conviction, in October 20, 2010, Smadi was sentenced to 24 years imprisonment.[34]		X
9	November 5, 2009	Nidal Hasan, 39, carried out a shooting rampage at the Fort Hood Army base near Killeen, Texas; 13 people killed; more than 30 others wounded.	On August 23, 2013, he was convicted by a military jury for all charges against him and sentenced to death.[35]	X	
10	February 18, 2010	Andrew Joseph Stack III, 53, allegedly intentionally crashed his light aircraft into an office building that housed an Internal Revenue Service (IRS) field office in Austin, Texas. An IRS manager was killed; 13 other people were wounded.	Stack died in the attack.[36]	X	
11	March 4, 2010	John Patrick Bedel, 36, used a handgun to attack Pentagon police officers at a security checkpoint at the Pentagon's metro station, in Arlington, Virginia, wounding 2 of them.	Bedel was killed in the exchange of fire.[37]	X	

Lone-actor terrorist attacks/ plots, 2001–2020	Date	Plot/Attack	Outcome	Completed	Preempted
12	May 1, 2010	Faisal Shahzad, 30, attempted to detonate a bomb inside his Nissan Pathfinder car in Times Square, New York; no casualties.	On June 21, 2010, Shahzad confessed to the attempted bombing and was convicted on October 5, 2010.[38]	X	
13	October 27, 2010	Farooque Ahmed, 43–44, was arrested for plotting to bomb Washington DC Metro stations at Arlington Cemetery, Pentagon City, Crystal City, and the Court House.	After pleading guilty, on April 11, 2011, Ahmed was sentenced to 23 years in prison, followed by 50 years of supervised release.[39]		X
14	October–November 2010	Yonathan Melaku, 22, used a rifle to carry out a series of drive-by shootings at several military facilities in Northern Virginia; no casualties.	Following his conviction, on January 11, 2013, Melaku was sentenced to 25 years in prison.[40]	X	
15	November 26, 2010	Mohamed Osman Mohamud, 19, was arrested after attempting to set off a vehicle bomb at an annual Christmas tree lighting ceremony in Portland, Oregon. The FBI had provided him the dud bomb.	On January 31, Mohamud was convicted, and, in October 2014, he was sentenced to 30 years in federal prison with credit for time served.[41]		X
16	December 8, 2010	Antonio Martinez (aka Muhammad Hussain), 20, was arrested and charged with plotting to bomb a military recruiting station in Catonsville, Maryland.	After pleading guilty in January 2011, he was sentenced on April 6, 2012, to 25 years in federal prison.[42]		X

Lone-actor terrorist attacks/ plots, 2001–2020	Date	Plot/Attack	Outcome	Completed	Preempted
17	January 8, 2011	Jared Lee Loughner, 22, carried out a shooting attack at an outdoor rally for US Representative Gabrielle Giffords in Tucson, Arizona; 6 people were killed, with 13 others wounded, including Representative Giffords.	Following his conviction, on November 8, 2012, Loughner was sentenced to life in prison.[43]	X	
18	January 17, 2011	Kevin William Harpham, 36, placed a remote-controlled bomb-laden backpack on a bench along the route of a Martin Luther King, Jr. Day parade in Spokane, Washington. The backpack containing the bomb was discovered and defused, with no casualties.	Following his conviction, on December 20, 2011, Harpham was sentenced to 32 years in prison for the attempted bombing.[44]	X	
19	February 2011	Khalid Aldawsari, 20, was arrested for plotting a bombing attack against the home of former President George W. Bush in Dallas, Texas.	On June 27, 2012 Aldawsari was convicted for plotting his attack.[45]		X
20	June 22, 2011	Abu Khalid Abdul-Latif (aka Joseph Anthony Davis), 33, and Walli Mujahidh (aka Frederick Domingue, Jr.), 32, were arrested for possession of machine guns that they planned to use in an attack on the Military Entrance Processing Station (MEPS) located on East Marginal Way, Seattle.	Abdul-Latif pleaded guilty in December 2012,[46] while Mujahidh pleaded guilty in December 2011.[47]		X

Lone-actor terrorist attacks/ plots, 2001–2020	Date	Plot/Attack	Outcome	Completed	Preempted
21	July 28, 2011	Nasser Jason Abdo, 21, was arrested near Fort Hood, Texas, for possession of an unregistered firearm and allegedly planning to attack a restaurant frequented by soldiers from the military base.	On May 24, 2012, he was convicted in federal court for his plot and on August 10, 2012, he was sentenced to two consecutive sentences of life in prison, plus 60 years.[48]		X
22	September 28, 2011	Rezwan Ferdaus, 27–28, was arrested for plotting to attack the Pentagon and the US Capitol using large remote-controlled aircraft filled with C-4 plastic explosives.	On July 10, 2012, Ferdaus pleaded guilty to federal charges of attempting to damage and destroy a federal building by means of an explosive and attempting to provide material support to terrorists and a terrorist organization.[49]		X
23	November 2011	Jose Pimentel, 27, was charged with plotting to build and use a bomb to assassinate members of the US military returning from active duty in Afghanistan in New York City.	On February 19, 2014, Pimentel pleaded guilty to a state terrorism charge.[50]		X
24	August 5, 2012	Wade Michael Page, 40, carried out a shooting attack at the *gurdwara* (Sikh temple), in Oak Creek, Wisconsin; 6 people were killed, 4 others were wounded.	After being shot in the hip by a responding officer, Page committed suicide.[51]	X	

Lone-actor terrorist attacks/ plots, 2001–2020	Date	Plot/Attack	Outcome	Completed	Preempted
25	February 3–12, 2013	Christopher Jordan Dorner, 33, carried out a series of shooting in Orange County, Los Angeles, and Riverside County, California; 4 people were killed and 3 others were wounded.	On February 12, 2013, Dorner died in a shootout with the San Bernardino Sheriff's deputies.[52]	X	
26	April 15, 2013; April 19, 2013	Tamerlan Tsarnaev, 26, and Dzhokhar Tsarnaev, 19 detonated two pressure cooker bombs near the finish line of the Boston Marathon, killing 3 persons and wounding an estimated 264 others. This was followed by a related shooting in nearby Watertown, Massachusetts, on April 19, in which they fatally shot an MIT policeman.	At the shootout in Watertown, Massachusetts, Tamerlan was killed by the responding police. On April 8, 2015, Dzhokhar was convicted for his role in the bombing.[53]	X	
27	November 1, 2013	Paul Anthony Giancia, 23, carried out a shooting rampage with a rifle in Terminal 3 of the Los Angeles International Airport, killing a US government Transportation Security Administration (TSA) officer and wounding 7 other persons.	On September 6, 2016, Ciancia pleaded guilty in exchange for a life sentence.[54]	X	

Lone-actor terrorist attacks/ plots, 2001–2020	Date	Plot/Attack	Outcome	Completed	Preempted
28	April 13, 2014	Frazier Glenn Miller, Jr., 73, carried out a pair of shootings at the Jewish Community Center of Greater Kansas City and Village Shalom, a Jewish retirement community, both located in Overland Park, Kansas. Three people were killed, 2 at the community center and 1 who was fatally shot at the retirement community.	On August 31, 2015, Miller was convicted and was sentenced to death on November 10, 2015.[55]	X	
29	May 23, 2014	Elliot Rodger, 22, carried out a shooting rampage in Isla Vista, near the campus of University of California, Santa Barbara, killing 6 and wounding 14 others.	Rodger committed suicide following his attack.[56]	X	
30	June 9, 2014	Jerad Miller, 31, and Amanda Miller, 22, husband and wife, ambushed two Las Vegas policemen at a restaurant and then killed a civilian in a nearby Walmart store.	The couple died in a shootout with the responding officers.[57]	X	
31	July 18, 2014	Ali Muhammad Brown, 29–30, was arrested for four terrorism-related killings in Washington state. He told investigators that the slayings were motivated by his Muslim faith.	After being charged with terrorism offenses in July 2015, he was convicted in Essex County Court on numerous charges, including terrorism, on March 6, 2018.[58]	X	

Lone-actor terrorist attacks/ plots, 2001–2020	Date	Plot/Attack	Outcome	Completed	Preempted
32	April 10, 2015	Mohammed Abdullah Hassan (previously known as John T. Booker), 20, was arrested for plotting to plant a bomb outside an Army post in northeast Kansas.	On February 3, 2016, Hassan pleaded guilty in federal court to two counts for plotting to plant a bomb outside the Army post.[59]		X
33	June 17, 2015	Dylann Roof, 21, shot and killed 9 people, wounding 1 other person, during a prayer service at the Emanuel African Methodist Episcopal Church in downtown Charleston, South Carolina.	After formally pleading guilty to state murder charges, on April 10, 2017, Roof was sentenced to nine consecutive sentences of life without parole.[60]	X	
34	July 16, 2015	Mohammad Youssef Abdulazeez, 34, carried out a drive-by shooting rampage at a recruiting station and a naval reserve center in Chattanooga, Tennessee; 4 Marines and a Navy petty officer were killed.	Abdulazeez was eventually fatally shot by the responding police officers in a shootout outside the facility.[61]	X	
35	October 1, 2015	Chris Harper-Mercer, 26, carried out a shooting rampage at Umpqua Community College, near Roseburg, Oregon; an assistant professor and 8 students in a classroom were killed, 8 others were wounded.	After being wounded by the responding police, Harper-Mercer killed himself with his gun.[62]	X	

Lone-actor terrorist attacks/ plots, 2001–2020	Date	Plot/Attack	Outcome	Completed	Preempted
36	November 27, 2015	Robert Lewis Dear Jr., 57; carried out a shooting attack at a Planned Parenthood clinic in Colorado Springs, Colorado; 3 were killed and 9 others were wounded.	After being charged in state court with first-degree murder, in May 2016 it was determined that Dear was incompetent to stand trial, and was ordered to be indefinitely confined to a Colorado state mental hospital.[63]	X	
37	December 2, 2015	Syed Rizwan Farook, 28, and Tashfeen Malik, 29, husband and wife, conducted a shooting rampage at the husband's office's holiday party at the Inland Regional Center, in San Bernardino, California; 14 people were killed and 22 others were wounded.	During their escape by car, Farook and Malik were subsequently killed by the responding police in a shootout.[64]	X	
38	June 12, 2016	Omar Mateen, 29, carried out a shooting rampage at the Pulse Nightclub, in Orlando, Florida; 49 persons were killed and 58 others were wounded.	Mateen was killed in a shootout with the responding police at the scene of his rampage.[65]	X	
39	September 17-19, 2016	Ahmad Khan Rahimi, 28, planted several bombs in the New York City metropolitan area, including at a seaside marathon in New Jersey. Three of the bombs exploded and several did not explode. The three bombings wounded 31 people.	After a shootout with the responding police, Rahimi was arrested, and on October 16, 2017, he was convicted in US federal court of eight federal crimes arising from the attack.[66]	X	

Lone-actor terrorist attacks/ plots, 2001–2020	Date	Plot/Attack	Outcome	Completed	Preempted
40	November 28, 2016	Abdul Razak Ali Artan, 18 (?), carried out a car ramming and stabbing attack at Ohio State University, in Columbus; 11 persons were wounded.	Artan was killed by a responding campus policeman.[67]	X	
41	June 14, 2017	James Hodgkinson, 66, carried out a shooting rampage at a Republican baseball practice session in Alexandria, Virginia, wounding 6 people.	Hodgkinson was killed by the responding police.[68]	X	
42	August 12, 2017	Jerry Drake Varnell, 23, was arrested after he attempted to detonate a van full of what he believed were explosives in an alley beside the downtown branch of BancFirst, Oklahoma's largest state-chartered bank. The site of the Alfred P. Murrah Federal Building was a few blocks away.	On February 25, 2019, Varnell was convicted of trying to detonate the supposedly explosives-laden van.[69]		X
43	August 12, 2017	James Alex Fields Jr., 20, intentionally drove his car into a crowd of people in Charlottesville, Virginia, who were demonstrating against a white supremacist rally. One person was killed and 28 others were wounded.	After pleading guilty, on June 28, 2019, Fields was sentenced to life in prison on federal hate crime charges.[70]	X	

Lone-actor terrorist attacks/ plots, 2001–2020	Date	Plot/Attack	Outcome	Completed	Preempted
44	December 11, 2017	Akayed Ullah, 27, attempted to detonate an improvised, low-tech explosive device, which was attached to his body in a crowded underground corridor of the subway system that connects Times Square to the Port Authority Bus Terminal, in mid-town Manhattan. The bomb only partially exploded, injuring the bomber and 3 bystanders, who sustained minor injuries.	On November 6, 2018, Ullah was convicted of offenses related to his attack.[71]	X	
45	March 23, 2018	Hafiz Kazi, 51, drove a minivan through the main gate of Travis Air Force Base, near Fairfield, California. His minivan was filled with five propane tanks, three plastic 1-gallon gas cans, several lighters, three phones, and a gym bag with personal items, which were deliberately ignited.	Kazi was fatally burned in his attack.[72]	X	
46	Mid-to-late October 2018	Cesar Sayoc, Jr., 56, embarked from Aventura, Florida, on a several weeks-long mailing of 16 explosive-laden packages against two former presidents, public figures, and media organizations such as CNN. He had a long criminal history. On October 26, he was arrested.	After being convicted on March 21, 2019, on August 5 that year he was sentenced to 20 years in prison.[73]	X	

Lone-actor terrorist attacks/ plots, 2001–2020	Date	Plot/Attack	Outcome	Completed	Preempted
47	November 2, 2018	Scott Paul Beierle, 40, shot 6 women, 2 fatally, as well as wounding a male, at a yoga studio in Tallahassee, Florida. He was allegedly an adherent of the "involuntary celibate" community.	Following his rampage, Beierle fatally shot himself.[74]	X	
48	January 16, 2019	Hasher Jallal Taheb, 22, was arrested for plotting to use a firearm or explosive to attack the White House and the Statue of Liberty.	On April 1, 2020, Taheb pleaded guilty for planning his attack.[75]		X
49	February 15, 2019	Christopher Paul Hasson, 50, was arrested for allegedly plotting to kill journalists, Democratic politicians, professors, Supreme Court Judges, and "leftists."	In October 2019, Hasson pleaded guilty and was sentenced to 160 months in federal prison.[76]		X
50	March 28, 2019	Rondell Henry, 28, was arrested by the FBI in Germantown, Maryland, for driving a stolen van, allegedly plotting to ram it into pedestrians at National Harbor, Maryland, as part of his provision of material support ISIS.	Following his arrest and indictment, in early July 2020, a federal judge extended Henry's court-ordered hospitalization, deeming him mentally unfit for trial.[77]	X	
51	July 28, 2019	Santino William Legan, 19, carried out a shooting rampage at the annual Gilroy Garlic Festival, Gilroy, California; 3 people were killed and 12 others wounded.	Legan committed suicide following a shootout with the responding police officers.[78]	X	

Lone-actor terrorist attacks/ plots, 2001–2020	Date	Plot/Attack	Outcome	Completed	Preempted
52	August 4, 2019	Connor Stephen Betts, 24, carried out a shooting rampage outside a bar in Dayton, Ohio; 9 people were killed and 17 others wounded.	Betts was fatally shot by the responding police officers.[79]	X	
53	December 10, 2019	David N. Anderson, 47, and Francine Graham, 50, a couple, carried out two shooting attacks in Jersey City, New Jersey, that killed 4 people. After killing a police officer at a park, the pair drove their van to a kosher supermarket in Jersey City, where they killed 2 employees and a shopper inside the store.	Anderson and Graham were killed in a shootout with the responding police officers.[80]	X	
54	December 12, 2019	Grafton E. Thomas, 37, carried out a stabbing rampage at a Hanukkah party in Monsey, New York. At the time, 5 people were injured, with 1 later dying of his injuries.	After being arraigned and indicted on December 29, 2019, on April 20, 2020, a federal judge ruled that Thomas was incompetent to stand trial and ordered him to be hospitalized in a mental facility.[81]	X	
55	April 15, 2020	John Michael Rathbun, 36, placed a homemade incendiary device at the entrance of Ruth's House, a Jewish-sponsored assisted living residential facility for seniors of all faiths, located on Converse Street in Longmeadow, Massachusetts. The device did not detonate.	On June 23, 2020 Rathbun was indicted for his attempted attack, with a pre-trial hearing held in mid-June 2020.[82]	X	

Lone-actor terrorist attacks/ plots, 2001–2020	Date	Plot/Attack	Outcome	Completed	Preempted
56	May 21, 2020	Adam Salim Alsahli, 20, drove to the entrance of Naval Air Station (NAS), Corpus Christi, Texas, and after failing to drive over the barrier, exited his vehicle and drew a handgun, firing at a military policewoman, striking her ballistic vest and injuring her.	Alsahli was shot and killed by the responding military police.[83]	X	

NOTES AND REFERENCES

1. Independent review of the Washington navy yard shooting. *Security from Within*, Nov 2013:4. https://fas.org/sgp/library/within.pdf.
2. Hamm M, Spaaij R. *The Age of Lone Wolf Terrorism*. New York: Columbia University Press; 2017:7.
3. FBI. *Lone Offender: A Study of Lone Offender Terrorism in the United States, 1972–2015*. Quantico, VA: FBI National Center for the Analysis of Violent Crime, Behavioral Threat Assessment Center; Nov 2019:7. https://www.fbi.gov/file-repository/lone-offender-terrorism-report-111319.pdf/view
4. Simon JD. *Lone Wolf Terrorism: Understanding the Growing Threat*. Amherst, NY: Prometheus Books, 2013:266.
5. Schuurman B, Lindekilde L, Malthaner M, O'Connor F, Gill P, Bouhana N. End of the lone wolf: The typology that should not have been. *Stud Conflict Terrorism*. 2019;42(8):771–778.
6. O'Toole ME. *The School Shooter: A Threat Assessment Perspective*. Quantico, VA: Critical Incident Response Group, National Center for the Analysis of Violent Crime, FBI Academy; 2000:6.
7. Simpson S. LAX shooting: Latest on suspect, victims and warning that may have come too late. *CNN*, 5 Nov 2013.
8. Capellan JA. Killing alone: Can the work performance literature help us solve the enigma of lone wolf terrorism? In Valeri RM, Borgeson, K, eds., *Terrorism in America* New York: Routledge; 2018:76.
9. Ibid.
10. Ibid.
11. Smith J. *Home Grown: How Domestic Violence Turns Men Into Terrorists*. London: Riverrun; 2019:152–153.
12. Ibid., 5.
13. Thornsley S. Cited in Philips A. Psychology 101: The mind of a shooter. *Officer.Com*, 15 Jun 2007. http://www.officer.com/article/10249728/psychology-101-the-mind-of-a-shooter
14. US Department of Defense. Fort Hood: Army Internal Review Team: Final report. 4 Aug 2010: 52–62. file:///C:/Users/Owner/Desktop/Prevent%20LA%20OUP%20(Apr%2020)/ft-hood_airt_final-report.pdf
15. Wagner D. FBI files: Jared Loughner apparently wrote poem for 2011 killing spree. *The Republic, azcentral.com*, 6 Apr 2018. https://www.wgrz.com/article/news/nation-now/fbi-files-jared-loughner-apparently wrote-poem-for-2011-killing-spree/465-5a696f3e-dce6-491d-a0d1-4149911d49db
16. Nagourney A, Lovett I, Pérez-Peña R. San Bernardino shooting kills at least 14: Two suspects are dead. *New York Times*, 2 Dec 2015. https://www.nytimes.com/2015/12/03/us/san-bernardino-shooting.html
17. Pilkington E, Elgot J. Orlando gunman Omar Mateen "was a regular" at Pulse nightclub. *The Guardian*, 14 Jun 2016. https://www.theguardian.com/us-news/2016/jun/14/orlando-shooter-omar-mateen-was-a-regular-at-nightclub
18. Cited in Walker M. Social media helps experts understand, prevent school shooters. *USA Today*, 29 Jan 2014.
19. Ibid.
20. Ibid.

21. Ibid.
22. Valeri RM, Borgeson K, eds. *Terrorism in America*. New York: Routledge; 2018:234.
23. Ibid.
24. Mazetti M, Lichtblau E, Blinder A. Omar Mateen, twice scrutinized by F.B.I., shows threat of lone terrorists. *New York Times*, 13 Jun 2016. https://www.nytimes.com/2016/06/14/us/politics/orlando-shooting-omar-mateen.html
25. Sandell C. Officers visited suspected gunman in the weeks before deadly attack. *ABCNews.com*, 26 May 2014. https://abcnews.go.com/US/police-miss-chance-stop-santa-barbara-rampage/story?id=23867478
26. Oroszi T, Ellis D. *The American Terrorist: Everything You Need to Know to be a Subject Matter Expert*. Dayton, OH: Greylander Press; 2019:179.
27. https://www.fredericknewspost.com/news/continuing_coverage/hindsight/hindsight-2020-bruce-ivins-takes-his-own-life-in-2008-days-before-fbi-charges-him/article_99a86997-12df-5a7b-80b1-df7d6bb56cd4.html
28. https://abcnews.go.com/US/story?id=91485&page=1
29. https://www.cnn.com/2013/11/04/us/dc-area-sniper-fast-facts/index.html
30. https://www.latimes.com/archives/la-xpm-2010-jan-15-la-na-seattle-jewish-center15-2010jan15-story.html
31. file:///C:/Users/Owner/Downloads/788760.pdf.
32. https://www.adl.org/sites/default/files/documents/assets/pdf/combating-hate/James-Von-Brunn-An-Adl-Backgrounder.pdf
33. https://herald-review.com/news/state-and-regional/michael-c-finton-formerly-of-decatur-begins-sentence-for-attempted-courthouse-bombing-in-springfield/article_f33d38d3-8267-5180-b194-40f399cb7beb.html
34. https://www.justice.gov/opa/pr/man-sentenced-24-years-prison-attempting-use-weapon-mass-destruction-bomb-skyscraper-downtown
35. https://www.washingtonpost.com/world/national-security/nidal-hasan-sentenced-to-death-for-fort-hood-shooting-rampage/2013/08/28/aad28de2-0ffa-11e3-bdf6-e4fc677d94a1_story.html
36. https://www.kvue.com/article/news/local/echelon-austin-plane-crash-10th-anniversary/269-278585ad-f221-499d-b3d9-cade96218b74
37. https://archives.fbi.gov/archives/washingtondc/press-releases/2010/wfo030510.htm
38. https://archives.fbi.gov/archives/newyork/press-releases/2010/nyfo100510.htm
39. https://www.bbc.com/news/world-us-canada-13044187
40. https://archives.fbi.gov/archives/washingtondc/press-releases/2013/alexandria-man-sentenced-to-25-years-for-shooting-military-buildings-in-northern-virginia
41. https://www.nytimes.com/2013/02/01/us/man-21-convicted-in-oregon-bomb-plot.html?searchResultPosition=5
42. https://archives.fbi.gov/archives/baltimore/press-releases/2012/maryland-man-pleads-guilty-to-attempted-use-of-a-weapon-of-mass-destruction-in-plot-to-attack-armed-forces-recruiting-center
43. https://archives.fbi.gov/archives/phoenix/press-releases/2012/jared-lee-loughner-sentenced-in-arizona-on-federal-charges-in-tucson-shooting
44. https://archives.fbi.gov/archives/seattle/press-releases/2011/washington-man-sentenced-to-32-years-for-attempted-bombing-of-martin-luther-king-unity-march
45. https://www.justice.gov/opa/pr/saudi-student-sentenced-life-prison-attempted-use-weapon-mass-destruction
46. https://archives.fbi.gov/archives/seattle/press-releases/2013/seattle-man-sentenced-to-18-years-in-prison-for-plot-to-attack-seattle-military-processing-center
47. https://archives.fbi.gov/archives/seattle/press-releases/2013/former-los-angeles-man-sentenced-to-17-years-in-prison-for-role-in-plot-to-attack-seattle-military-processing-center
48. https://archives.fbi.gov/archives/sanantonio/press-releases/2012/naser-jason-abdo-sentenced-to-life-in-federal-prison-in-connection-with-killeen-bomb-plot
49. https://archives.fbi.gov/archives/boston/press-releases/2012/man-sentenced-in-boston-for-plotting-attack-on-pentagon-and-u.s.-capitol-and-attempting-to-provide-detonation-devices-to-terrorists
50. https://www.nytimes.com/2014/03/26/nyregion/judge-imposes-16-year-term-for-manhattan-man-in-pipe-bomb-case.html
51. https://www.splcenter.org/fighting-hate/intelligence-report/2012/sikh-temple-killer-wade-michael-page-radicalized-army
52. https://www.bbc.com/news/magazine-21476904
53. https://www.bostonherald.com/2020/10/07/boston-marathon-bomber-case-u-s-justice-department-asks-supreme-court-to-reinstate-death-penalty-for-dzhokhar-tsarnaev/
54. https://www.justice.gov/opa/pr/california-man-sentenced-life-plus-60-years-2013-shooting-spree-los-angeles-international
55. https://www.splcenter.org/fighting-hate/extremist-files/individual/frazier-glenn-miller.
56. https://www.nytimes.com/2014/06/02/us/elliot-rodger-killings-in-california-followed-years-of-withdrawal.html
57. https://www.washingtonpost.com/news/morning-mix/wp/2014/06/24/las-vegas-cop-killers-packed-ammo-and-wore-adult-diapers-as-they-prepared-for-their-revolution/

58. https://www.counterextremism.com/extremists/ali-muhammad-brown

59. https://www.justice.gov/usao-ks/pr/topeka-man-sentenced-conspiracy-fort-riley-bomb-plot

60. https://www.nytimes.com/2017/01/10/us/dylann-roof-trial-charleston.html

61. https://time.com/3962344/chattanooga-muhammad-youssef-abdulazeez/

62. https://www.nytimes.com/2015/10/03/us/chris-harper-mercer-umpqua-community-college-shooting.html

63. https://www.denverpost.com/2018/10/26/colorado-springs-planned-parenthood-shooter-incompetent/

64. https://www.cnn.com/2015/12/03/us/syed-farook-tashfeen-malik-mass-shooting-profile/index.html

65. https://www.nytimes.com/2016/06/19/us/omar-mateen-gunman-orlando-shooting.html

66. https://www.nbcnewyork.com/news/local/crime-and-courts/convicted-chelsea-bomber-ahmad-khan-rahimi-gets-2nd-life-sentence-in-attempted-cop-killings/2266059/

67. https://www.nytimes.com/2016/11/30/us/ohio-state-university-attack-abdul-razak-ali-artan.html

68. https://www.washingtonpost.com/local/public-safety/law-enforcement-officials-identify-shooter-at-congressional-ballgame-as-illinois-man/2017/06/14/ba6439f4-510f-11e7-91eb-9611861a988f_story.html

69. https://www.justice.gov/usao-wdok/pr/man-who-attempted-bomb-downtown-oklahoma-city-bank-sentenced-25-years

70. https://www.nbcnews.com/news/us-news/james-alex-fields-driver-deadly car-attack-charlottesville-rally sentenced-n1024436

71. https://www.justice.gov/opa/pr/akayed-ullah-convicted-detonation-bomb-new-york-city.

72. https://www.dailyrepublic.com/all-dr-news/solano-news/fairfield/travis-air-force-base/one-year-later-motive-for-sausalito-mans-death-at-travis-main-gate-still-a-mystery/

73. https://www.nbcnews.com/news/us-news/pipe-bomb-mailer-cesar-sayoc-who-targeted-trump-critics-sentenced-n1039261

74. https://www.nbcnews.com/news/us-news/fbi-received-warning-about-gunman-yoga-studio-shooting-police-say-n971006

75. https://www.justice.gov/opa/pr/forsyth-man-sentenced-attempted-attack-white-house

76. https://www.justice.gov/usao-md/pr/christopher-hasson-sentenced-more-13-years-federal-prison-federal-charges-illegal

77. https://baltimore.cbslocal.com/2020/07/04/rondell-henry-court-case-maryland-latest/

78. https://www.usatoday.com/story/news/nation/2019/07/29/santino-willian-legan-lagan-picture-rifle-might-makes-right/1860828001/

79. https://www.daytondailynews.com/news/dayton-shooter-left-decade-red-flags/E5UoTI-8To1CJDaWUndXBlO/

80. https://www.fox29.com/news/officials-nj-kosher-deli-shooters-planned-attack-for-months

81. https://www.nbcnews.com/news/us-news/suspect-hanukkah-machete-attack-rabbi-s-ny-home-not-fit-n1188426

82. https://www.wwlp.com/news/crime/mistrial-declared-in-case-of-attempted-arson-at-longmeadow-assisted-living-facility/

83 https://dfw.cbslocal.com/2020/05/27/fbi-confirms-only 1-gunman-texas-naval-base-shooting/

24

Threat Assessment

The TRAP-18 and Application to a Lone-Actor Terrorism Incident

J. REID MELOY AND JACOB C. HOLZER

INTRODUCTION

Terrorists do not snap. The notion that terrorist violence is an impulsive and irrational act—at least in the mind of the terrorist—is a misguided belief. In the larger context of violence risk assessment in general, it is partially a conceptual failure to distinguish between two modes of violence, affective and predatory, which has dogged the violence risk literature for at least four decades. *Affective violence* is emotional, impulsive, a reaction to an imminent perceived threat, and it is a common mode of violence we see in our species— its evolutionary genesis was to defend against a sudden threat to survival. *Predatory violence* is emotionless, planned, purposeful, and without a discernable and imminent threat—its evolutionary genesis was to hunt for food. These modes of violence have been studied for the past 80 years,[1–3] are biologically distinctive in mammals,[4] yet have generally failed to be integrated into existing instruments for assessing the risk of violence.[5] Synonyms in the research for affective violence include reactive, emotional, impulsive, defensive, and hot-blooded or heat of passion violence; synonyms for predatory violence include targeted, instrumental, premeditated, and cold-blooded violence. The legal corollaries are manslaughter and murder, respectively.

Acts of terrorism are ideologically motivated incidents of predatory violence which rarely occur, whether perpetrated by a terrorist organization or a lone actor.[6] This fact has posed a number of problems for those who have attempted to forecast violence in terrorists in the same manner as violence risk assessment has been traditionally practiced: terrorist acts cannot be accurately predicted because of their very low base rates in any population of concern[7]; traditional variables associated with general violence risk (e.g., drug use, history of violence) are usually absent among lone-actor terrorists[8,9]; violence risk assessment is often a static enterprise that results in a one-time opinion of general risk and largely focuses on characteristics of the individual being assessed in a contained setting (hospital, jail, or prison), and violence risk assessment usually does not account for the variability of the situational/environmental context nor the target that is being contemplated by the terrorist.

The scientific and operational discipline of *threat assessment and management* (TAM) has attempted to rectify this problem in the larger context of risk assessment by focusing on behaviors of concern which precede acts of targeted, or predatory violence.[10–12] Originating toward the end of the twentieth century, the TAM model is now utilized in colleges, universities, corporations, and other private and governmental entities in North America, Europe, Asia, and the Middle East where threats of targeted violence are most apparent. The research on TAM is now substantial and has focused on behaviors of concern which have preceded acts of targeted violence by public figure attackers, stalkers, adolescent and adult mass murderers, targeted attackers in public venues, domestic violence perpetrators, and lone-actor terrorists.[13,14] The point of these efforts, however, is not to predict but to prevent. The paradox of such work is that one can never know—with the exception of a last-minute tactical intervention by law enforcement—whether the efforts of threat assessment and management, if *not* done, would have resulted in an act of targeted violence. The good news is that prevention does not *require* prediction.

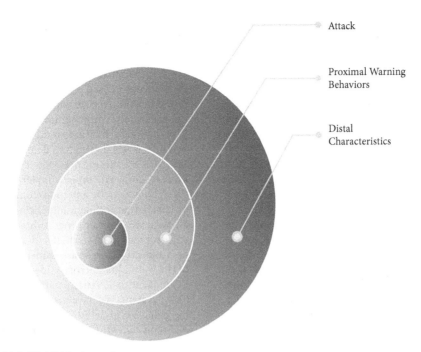

Attack

Proximal Warning
Behaviors

Distal
Characteristics

FIGURE 24.1 TRAP-18 schematic

The application of TAM to lone-actor terror-ism has resulted in exceptional advances in the understanding of the pathways to violence of such individuals.[15,16] It has also produced a threat assessment method, developed by the first author (Dr. Meloy derives income from the marketing of both the TRAP-18 manual and code sheets and any training associated with the instru-ment), which is showing promise as a structured professional judgment instrument to help law enforcement and counterterrorism investiga-tors prioritize cases and actively risk-manage the most acute situations. It is called the Terrorist Radicalization Assessment Protocol (TRAP-18).[17] There are several other instruments used to assess risk of terrorist violence, including the Extremism Risk Guidelines (ERG 22+)[18] and the Violent Extremism Risk Assessment (VERA),[19] which are also structured professional judgment tools: they help investigators identify charac-teristics of a person of concern for carrying out an act of terrorist violence. Other scales and instruments are addressed in a separate chapters in this book. Multimethod approaches are best for the assessment of terrorism risk, and other instruments for general risk of violence, such as the HCR-20 V3,[5] are also very useful as well-validated and complementary sources of impor-tant data collection. This chapter focuses on the TRAP-18.

THE TRAP-18

The TRAP-18 is composed of 8 proximal warn-ing behaviors and 10 distal characteristics which were theoretically and rationally derived from the extant research on terrorism.[17,20-22] The model assumes that the proximal warning behaviors are more closely related in time to the violent act of the terrorist than are the distal characteristics (see Figure 24.1). Monahan and Steadman pro-posed a very helpful weather analogy for violence prediction.[23] They opined that the meteorologi-cal terms "watch" and "warn" are useful in both specificity and imminence when thinking about and communicating violence risk.[23] This analogy is very useful in the juxtaposition of the proxi-mal warning behaviors and the distal character-istics for the TRAP-18. Any presence of a cluster of distal characteristics would suggest a "watch" strategy: there are storm clouds forming on the horizon, but one does not know if or when they will coalesce into a fierce weather event. The presence of one proximal warning behavior sug-gests that the storm is in one's backyard. In other words, monitoring of a potential event—in this case mobilization for terrorist violence—shifts to active management of a more imminent event (see Figure 24.1). There are no empirically derived cutoffs for the TRAP-18 since it is a structured professional judgment instrument and not a psy-chological test. Nevertheless, the model advances the hypothesis that one proximal warning behavior is necessary for active risk management, and data indicate that all targeted violence subjects to date have exhibited multiple warning behaviors prior to their attacks.

These 18 indicators are considered *patterns* of risk to correct for the assessor's tendency to focus on a discrete variable and to facilitate a more wide-angle view by capitalizing on our natural ability to see patterns and organize stimuli. Pattern analysis has its roots in gestalt psychology[24-26] and capitalizes on our normal cognitive-perception to organize bits of detail into meaningful patterns.

The focus of these 18 indicators are present behaviors of concern, the core of threat assessment, and not the traditional mental health approach of an initial diagnostic formulation through the development of psychological inferences, often based on fairly remote historical data,[13] to determine general violence risk. Each indicator is coded as present, absent, or insufficient data. The typology consists of the following 8 proximal warning behaviors:

1. *Pathway Warning Behavior* is research, planning, preparation for, or implementation of an attack. This first warning behavior combines the concept of a *pathway* for targeted violence[10] with the late-stage markers formulated by Calhoun and Weston.[12] When there is evidence of these behaviors, it indicates that the person of concern has moved into operational space and there is intent to be violent. A recent problem in counterterrorism work is the increased brevity of pathway behavior and the weaponizing of common household and family items, such as knives and cars. In some cases, "the pathway has become a runway."[27]

2. *Fixation Warning Behavior* is an increasingly pathological preoccupation with a person or a cause, accompanied by a deterioration in social and/or occupational life. The work on fixation evolved from the Fixated Research Group, funded by the Home Office in London, to investigate threats to the British Royal Family and other political figures. This project spanned 5 years and resulted in a number of scientific publications between 2004 and 2010 (available in PDF at drreidmeloy.com). Fixation is a preoccupation of thought, usually on a person or a cause. A simple key to the presence of a pathological fixation—beside the deterioration in work and love—is the disjuncture between the social setting in which it is voiced and the fixation itself. In virtual reality, the more intense the fixation, the greater the number of constant social media postings for others to see. For instance, when they accelerate, there is usually increased perseveration, stridency, negative characterization of those who oppose the cause, or an angry emotional undertone.[20] A pathological fixation could be cognitively and affectively driven by a delusion, an obsession, or an "extreme overvalued belief."[28,29]

3. *Identification Warning Behavior* is a psychological desire to be a pseudo-commando[30] or have a warrior mentality[31]; closely associate with weapons or other military or law enforcement paraphernalia; identify with previous attackers or assassins; or, in the case of the individual terrorist, identify oneself as an agent to advance a particular cause or belief system. We have discussed this warning behavior in detail,[32] including its roots in A. Freud's *identification with the aggressor*[33] and the concept of identity in the history of psychoanalytic thought.[34] Simply put, fixation is what one constantly thinks about; identification is what one becomes. In the context of terrorism, the key is a shift from fixation to identification[6] as the pathological preoccupation metamorphosizes into a self-identity (e.g., a soldier for ISIS).

4. *Novel Aggression Warning Behavior* is an act of violence that appears unrelated to the intended act of concern and is committed for the first time; it is typically done to test the subject's ability to carry out his or her act of violence. This warning behavior is difficult to discern and easy to miss. However, the testing of one's ability to be violent may be critical to the subject moving into operational space. MacCulloch, Snowden, Wood, and Mills referred to this as a *behavioral tryout* in the context of the sexually sadistic offender, and Hull would likely define the term as a measure of motivation to act on the environment.[35,36]

5. *Energy Burst Warning Behavior* is an increase in the frequency or variety of any noted activities related to the target, even if the activities themselves appear relatively innocuous, usually in the weeks, days, or hours before the attack. Social media activity will usually decrease during this period of time. This warning behavior cannot be assessed unless a baseline of general activity for the person of concern has been established by the threat assessor. Energy burst is a notable increase

from baseline and is likely due to the person of interest running out of time to complete all necessary tasks before implementing his attack, rather than a psychiatric disturbance such as manic acceleration. Virtual reality presence (social media) during this brief period before an attack will likely decrease due to encryption to enhance secrecy (two of the currently most common applications are Telegram and WhatsApp) or an actual time limitation due to final preparations in terrestrial reality.

6. *Leakage Warning Behavior* is communication to a third party of an intent to do harm to a target through an attack.[37] The third party may be an internet audience and/or any social media audience. In the context of psychotherapy, this could prompt a legal obligation on the part of the mental health professional to warn the third party and/or law enforcement. This warning behavior is the Achilles heel of the lone-actor terrorist and others intending to engage in targeted violence. A majority of such individuals will leak their intent to third parties, lone-actor terrorists more frequently than non-ideologically motivated mass murderers.[38] Motivations vary greatly and tend to evolve around vulnerabilities created by a narcissistic sense of impunity or various anxieties. The paradox is that most attackers will leak their intent, while most persons of concern with no intent will also engage in leakage. This is exacerbated by the subsequent reluctance of third parties to report following knowledge of a leak, a likely derivative of the "bystander effect," a validated phenomenon from social psychology that individuals are less likely to help in an emergency when others are present—or perceived as being so.[39] The threat assessment risk with leakage is that the professional assessor becomes complacent due to the frequency of false positives he or she encounters.

7. *Last Resort Warning Behavior* is evidence of a "violent action and/or time imperative."[40] It may be a signal of desperation or distress. Often it is the result of an unexpected triggering event or one which is anticipated, which involves a loss in love or work. The subject believes he has no other choice and must act now. Sometimes there is no external triggering event, yet the subject imposes on himself the necessity of action through various psychological defense maneuvers, often narcissistically colored, such as characterizing

himself as the last man standing or the only one with the courage to act. This is a pattern of behavior which may contain within it "final acts"[11,12]: the subject will complete tasks that suggest he believes his life is about to end, such as giving away possessions, settling debts, or closing bank accounts. It has also been referred to as "end of tether" behavior.[41]

8. *Directly Communicated Threat Warning Behavior* is the communication of a direct threat through any means to the target or law enforcement beforehand. Although directly communicated threats are quite infrequent among those who engage in targeted violence of any kind, including terrorism,[13] they always warrant active investigation because they may turn out to be true positives: in a few cases they are actually signaling an intent to act. We found this to be the case in one out of five lone-actor terrorists.[22] The paradox is that research among approachers and attackers of public figures, for example, indicates that a directly communicated threat may actually *reduce* the likelihood of an attack when analyzed as group data.[13] The operational issue, however, is that one cannot afford to be wrong when conducting a threat assessment, and therefore the default position should always be that all direct threats are taken seriously.

The 10 distal characteristics are as follows:

1. *Personal grievance and moral outrage* is the joining of both personal life experience and particular historical, religious, or political events. Personal grievance is often defined by a major loss in love or work, feelings of anger and humiliation, and the blaming of others. Moral outrage is typically a vicarious identification with a group which has suffered, even though the lone-actor terrorist usually has not experienced the same suffering.

2. *Framed by an ideology* is the presence of beliefs that justify the subject's intent to act. It can be a religious belief system, a political philosophy, a secular commitment, a one-issue conflict, or an idiosyncratic justification. Beliefs are usually superficial and selected to justify violence.

3. *Failure to affiliate with an extremist or other group* is the experience of rejecting or being rejected by a radical, extremist, or other group with which the subject initially wanted to affiliate.

4. *Dependence on the virtual community* is the

use of the internet through social media, chat rooms, emails, listservs, texting, tweeting, posting, searches, etc., for virtual interaction (e.g., reinforcement of beliefs) or virtual learning (e.g., planning and preparation).

5. *Thwarting of occupational goals* is a major setback or failure in a planned academic and/or occupational life course.

6. *Changes in thinking and emotion* is a pattern over time wherein thoughts and their expression become more strident, simplistic, and absolute. Argument ceases and preaching begins. Persuasion yields to imposition of one's beliefs on others. There is no critical analysis of theory or opinion, and the mantra, "don't think, just believe," is adopted. Emotions typically move from anger and argument to contempt and disdain for others' beliefs, to disgust for the out-group and a willingness to homicidally aggress against them.[42] Violence is cloaked in self-righteousness and the pretense of superior belief. Humor is lost. Engagement with others in virtual and/or terrestrial reality may greatly diminish or cease once the subject has moved into operational space.

7. *Failure of sexually intimate pair bonding* is the historic failure to form lasting sexually intimate relationships. The sexualization of violence is a secondary component. It refers to the finding of a sexual attitude or behavior in the subject which appears to substitute for the absence of a sexual pair bond, such as the sexualization of weapons, the anticipation of unlimited sexual gratification in the afterlife, the exclusive use of prostitutes and other unbonded sources of sexual gratification, or compulsive use of pornography: all of these behaviors may be rationalized by the ideology.[43]

8. *Mental disorder* is evidence of a major mental disorder by history or in the present. The ideology may help to reduce anxiety surrounding the mental disorder or utilize the symptoms to advance the attack (e.g., suicidal thoughts and depression become motivations for martyrdom; delusions of grandeur solidify commitment).

9. *Creativity and innovation* is evidence of tactical thinking "outside the box." The planned terrorist act is creative (a major aspect has not been done before in contemporary times) and/or innovative (may be imitated by others).

10. *Criminal violence* is evidence of instrumental criminal violence in the subject's past, demonstrating a capacity and willingness to engage in predation for a variety of reasons, such as a history of armed robberies or planned assaults on others for material gain.

The proximal warning behaviors were assumed to be both sensitive and specific to lone-actor terrorist acts, while the distal characteristics were assumed to be sensitive to acts of terrorism, and not necessarily specific (e.g., criminal violence). However, these assumptions needed to be empirically tested.

EMPIRICAL VALIDATION OF THE TRAP-18

The first published study of the TRAP-18 coded a sample of 22 individuals who carried out acts of terrorism in Europe between 1980 and 2015.[44] Fifteen subjects acted alone and 7 formed autonomous cells of two or more individuals whose actions were not commanded or controlled by a terrorist organization, which included the *Charlie Hebdo* attackers in Paris, in January 2015. The mean interrater reliability (Cohen's kappa) was 0.895 and ranged from 0.69 to 1.0 for the warning behaviors and 0.75 to 1.0 for the distal characteristics. The terrorists who acted alone and the autonomous cell members showed no significantly different frequencies across the eight warning behaviors, with a majority positive for 72% of the indicators. There were more differences when comparing the distal characteristics between the lone actors and the cell members, but both groups showed a frequency of greater than 70% on personal grievance and moral outrage, framed by an ideology, thwarting of occupational goals, and changes in thinking and emotion. The only significant difference ($p = .0048$, phi = 0.70) was a much greater frequency of criminal violence (100%) by history among the autonomous cell members than the lone actors.

There are some important take-aways from this study. Gill, Horgan, Corner, and Silver noted the risk of a "time cohort effect" when a sample covered a lengthy time period, but in our study 64% of the cases occurred during the past decade, thus lowering the likelihood of such an effect.[45] This study also provided some basic evidence of criterion validity for the TRAP-18 when applied to these small samples and also the generalizability (the real-world fit) of the instrument when applied to both lone actors and autonomous cell subjects. There was not, however, a comparison group of those of concern but without intent, as we had in a previous school shooting study[46] with just the warning behaviors; therefore, evidence for the TRAP-18's discriminant validity was not demonstrated.

The second study[22] used an open source sample of 111 lone-actor terrorists from the United States and Europe as criteria to further validate the TRAP-18. Terrorism was defined as "the use or threat of action where the use or threat is designed to influence the government or to intimidate the public or a section of the public, and/or the use or threat is made for the purpose of advancing a political, religious, or ideological cause."[47] The sample, however, was composed of only those who planned and carried out an attack (in some cases thwarted) between 1990 and 2014. Seventy percent of the terrorists were positive for at least half or more of the indicators; 77% or more evidenced four proximal warning behaviors: pathway, fixation, identification, and leakage. When the sample was divided into Islamic terrorists ($n = 38$), extreme right-wing terrorists ($n = 43$), and single-issue terrorists, mostly anti-abortionists ($n = 30$), there were no significant differences across the 18 indicators except for four: personal grievance and moral outrage, dependence on the virtual community, thwarting of occupational goals, and fixation. Islamic extremist lone actors were significantly more likely to display dependence on the virtual community than were the single-issue terrorists. Extreme right-wing lone actors were significantly less likely to display personal grievance and moral outrage, thwarting of occupational goals, and fixation warning behaviors than either the Islamic extremists or the single-issue terrorists. Single-issue lone actors were significantly less likely to display dependence on virtual communities than were the Islamic extremists.

We then divided the sample according to successful ($n = 67$) versus thwarted ($n = 44$) attackers. The successful attackers actually carried out their violent act, while a thwarted attack covered plots which were developed by lone-actor terrorists but were interrupted, uncovered, or stopped by some form of police, intelligence, or security organization *and* subsequently led to a conviction. Individuals caught up in FBI sting operations or "material support" cases were not included. These are cases in which a person knowingly and intentionally provides training, expert advice, service, or personnel for terrorist endeavors.[48] The successful attackers were significantly more fixated, creative, and innovative and failed to have

a sexually intimate pair bond. They were significantly less likely to have displayed pathway warning behavior to others and be dependent on a virtual community of like-minded true believers. Effect sizes for these comparative differences were small to medium (phi = 0.19–0.32).

These differences make operational sense. Less evidence of pathway behavior would suggest less observation by others, whether through luck or stealth. Fixation, the second warning behavior more frequent among the successful attackers, suggests an intensity of pursuit in a larger stalking context.[13] A history of failed sexual pair bonding lowers the risk of an intimate becoming familiar with one's activities and disrupting the operation. Creativity and innovation, another distal characteristic more frequent among the successful attackers, helps outwit the counterterrorism investigator, and less dependence on the virtual community means a lessened chance of having one's postings or social media communication picked up by a third party and communicated to authorities.

Meloy and Gill advanced the construct validation of the TRAP-18, with important within-group comparisons from an ideological and operational perspective.[22] However, a comparison group of subjects of concern but without intent (false positives) was not available, and therefore discriminant validity was not demonstrated.

In a postdictive study of US domestic terrorists (Sovereign Citizens), Challacombe and Lucas compared 58 individuals, 30 who had committed violent or dangerous actions and 28 who committed nonviolent criminal actions.[49] Interrater reliability was excellent (kappa = .76). All incidents occurred between 2004 and 2014. Ten TRAP-18 indicators significantly correlated with violence with medium to large effect sizes (phi = 0.33–0.70): the warning behaviors of pathway, identification, leakage, and last resort, and the distal characteristics of personal grievance and moral outrage, framed by ideology, thwarting of occupational goals, and criminal violence, were all more frequent among the violent right-wing extremists. Two warning behaviors negatively correlated with violence: novel aggression and energy burst. A binary logistic regression was then performed using the summed TRAP-18 score and correctly explained 44–59% of the variance. The TRAP-18 correctly classified 75.9% of the cases as either violent or non-violent. Odds ratio was 2.10 (p = .000).

Another comparative study of North American terrorist attackers ($n = 33$) and persons of national security concern who were successfully risk managed (n = 23) found significant differences with medium to large effect sizes (phi = .35–.70) across half of the TRAP-18 indicators.[6] The subjects in this study were an ideological mix of violent jihadists, extreme right-wing nationalists, and single-issue terrorists, usually anti-abortionists. Findings indicated that the proximal warning behaviors which differentiated the attackers from those of concern where there had been successful intervention and risk management were pathway, identification, energy burst, last resort, and the absence of a directly communicated threat. The distal characteristics which were more frequent in the attackers were ideological framing, changes in thinking and emotion, and creativity and innovation. Mental disorder was significantly less frequent. Odds ratios and 95% confidence intervals were also computed in this study. Goodwill and Meloy, using the same sample, demonstrated through multidimensional scaling that the proximal warning behaviors clustered together (co-occurrence) among the attackers and not among the non-attackers and that there was less clustering among the distal characteristics, which were apparent in both groups.[50] What has emerged across all the targeted violence studies to date is the ubiquity of the proximal warning behaviors of pathway, fixation, identification, leakage, energy burst, and last resort, and, within the lone-actor terrorist domain, the evolution from fixation to identification—what one thinks about all the time to what one becomes—may be a critical marker for imminent risk. Two studies[6,50] also empirically supported the theoretical model of the TRAP-18: proximal warning behaviors were virtually absent among the non-attackers, while both groups showed a plethora of distal characteristics. One of the ironies in these studies was the significantly *greater frequency* of directly communicated threats among the non-attackers when compared to the attackers, a finding which supports the conventional belief across threat assessors in general that direct threats often lower the risk for targeted violence.[12,13]

The march of science is the interplay of nomothetic and idiographic research. Several studies have also been published to advance a fuller understanding of the TRAP-18 in the context of the individual terrorist. Meloy, Habermeyer, and Guldimann studied the proximal warning behaviors of a 2011 extreme right-wing Norwegian mass murderer.[51] Bockler et al. wrote a detailed study of the violent jihadist Frankfurt Airport attacker utilizing the TRAP-18 and identified 15 out of 18 indicators.[52] Meloy and Genzman studied the case of the violent jihadist Ft. Hood mass murderer with a particular focus on threat assessment using the TRAP-18 by mental health clinicians; he evidenced 13 out of 18 indicators.[53] Bockler et al. scrutinized the violent jihadist Berlin Christmas market attacker's proximal warning behaviors, which included pathway, fixation, identification, leakage, and last resort.[54] Erlandsson and Meloy studied an extreme right-wing Swedish school attacker and found 15 out of 18 TRAP indicators.[55] The only proximal warning behavior that was not in evidence was a directly communicated threat. Case studies do not provide predictive data but allow for a more nuanced and deeper contemplation of each fact pattern and how it correlates with the TRAP-18 indicators.

THE APPLICATION OF THE TRAP-18 TO THE OKLAHOMA CITY BOMBER

On April 19, 1995, Timothy McVeigh detonated a 5,000-pound ammonium nitrate and fertilizer bomb in front of the Alfred P. Murrah Federal Building in downtown Oklahoma City, Oklahoma: 168 adults and children died, and hundreds more were injured. Although it was initially thought by the popular media to be a jihadist attack, McVeigh was a right-wing ethnic nationalist, a member of the Patriot Movement at the time, who believed that his attack would usher in the Second American Revolution. He was subsequently tried and eventually executed 2 months before the 9/11 attacks on the World Trade Center and the Pentagon. McVeigh's history and behaviors are viewed through the lens of the TRAP-18 to illustrate the application of the instrument, in retrospect, to a lone-actor terrorist. The data for this study are drawn from the author's case files while retained as an expert witness for the US Attorney in *United States v. Timothy James McVeigh* and *United States v. Terry Nichols*, and other sources as referenced. Such an analysis, however, is inherently unfair to those responsible for counterterrorism at the time since all evidence is now aggregated and known to the public and the extreme difficulties of threat management at the time, such as separating the signal from the noise, are lost. Such an analysis is also subject to hindsight bias: the "knew-it-all-along" effect; that is, the inclination, after an event has occurred, to see the event as having been predictable despite there having been little known data for predicting it.

Nevertheless, individual cases allow for a more granular look at the indicators which may be useful to contemporary threat assessors. Here are the eight proximal warning behaviors which were present or absent:

1. *Pathway warning behavior.* McVeigh planned and prepared for the attack at least 18 months earlier. He formed a three-man cell with Michael Fortier and Terry Nichols, and target selection eventually settled on the Murrah building due to its easy access and the presence of the federal law enforcement offices (ATF) which had been involved in the Branch Davidian siege in Waco, Texas, 2 years earlier. During the course of the preparation, McVeigh and Nichols engaged in a burglary from a quarry in Marion, Kansas (September 1994) and a robbery of gun dealer Roger Moore's home for money (November 1994) near Hot Springs, Arkansas. The bomb was eventually constructed using 55-gallon drums in a shaped charge in a Ryder Truck.

2. *Fixation warning behavior.* McVeigh was pre-occupied with the siege and eventual destruction of the Branch Davidian compound by FBI and ATF agents on April 19, 1993. He was convinced that all members who died, including women and children, had been deliberately murdered by the federal government. Prior to this event, he was incensed by the Ruby Ridge incident in August 1992, when Randy Weaver and his family had an armed confrontation with the FBI in Idaho; Weaver's wife, son, and a federal agent were killed. His anger and perseveration on these topics were noted by others and cemented his belief that the federal government and its employees were his enemy. His social and occupation functioning was in isolated limbo.

   His fixation also met the definition of an *extreme overvalued belief.* An extreme over-valued belief is one that is shared by others in a person's cultural, religious, or subcultural group. The belief is often relished, amplified, and defended by the possessor of the belief and should be differentiated from an obsession or a delusion. The belief grows more dominant over time, more refined, and more resistant to challenge. The individual has an intense emotional commitment to the belief and may carry out violent behavior in its service.[28]

3. *Identification warning behavior.* McVeigh saw himself as "the first hero of the second American revolution" and believed that the bombing would begin a national uprising against the federal government (in letters to sister Jennifer reviewed by author). He closely identified with the US founding forefathers, especially Thomas Jefferson, and wore a t-shirt during his bombing imprinted on the back with Jefferson's words: "the tree of liberty must from time to time be replenished with the blood of patriots and tyrants." On the front was a depiction of President Abraham Lincoln and the phrase, "sic semper tyrannis" (thus always to tyrants), purportedly yelled by John Wilkes Booth immediately after the Lincoln assassination. He had become a soldier for the Patriot Movement.

4. *Novel aggression warning behavior.* McVeigh showed no evidence of this warning behavior. He didn't need to test his capability for violence since he had a history of sanctioned violence during "Desert Storm," as a Bradley vehicle machine gunner (August 1990–February 1991). He allegedly killed several Iraqis and was considered by some of his US Army colleagues at his trial as a "soldier's soldier."

5. *Energy burst warning behavior.* The bomb was constructed in the back of a Ryder truck at Geary State Lake in Kansas—an enormous physical task involving the mixing of nitro-methane, ammonium nitrate, diesel fuel, and fertilizer in thirteen 55-gallon drums. It is unclear who helped him. One witness reported seeing a total of five people at the truck site; others saw no trucks. McVeigh stated it was only Nichols and him.[56–58] McVeigh then drove 250 miles on back roads to Oklahoma City and slept in the truck the night of April 18, 1995. Just after 9 AM, he parked the truck under the overhang of the Murrah building, having lit two fuses as he approached. He then jogged away from the truck, the bomb detonated, and he accessed his 1977 yellow Mercury Marquis several blocks from the site where he had parked it a week earlier. He began driving north at exactly the speed limit to avoid attention.

6. *Leakage warning behavior.* McVeigh discussed his intent with his two cell members, Nichols and Fortier. Fortier withdrew from the conspiracy, testified at trial, was given a reduced sentence, and released to witness protection (WITSEC) in 2006. Nichols pulled back, but then helped McVeigh construct the bomb. Neither one contacted authorities prior to the

bombing. Nichols was eventually sentenced to 161 consecutive life sentences in federal prison without possibility of parole. McVeigh also showed Lori Fortier, the wife of Michael, how he would construct a bomb in the back of a truck by stacking soup cans on the floor in Lori's kitchen in Kingman, Arizona. She was granted immunity at trial to testify against McVeigh and appeared to have full knowledge of the attack. In the months prior to the bombing, he also told his sister Jennifer his plans that something big would happen in Spring 1995, "there's going to be a revolution," but did not tell her the weapon or the specific target. She then communicated this to several other people. Her friends reported that she became boastful at a Christmas party. "You'll see in either April or May something big is going to happen with my brother. I don't know what it is, but it's going to be big. There's going to be a revolution and you're either going to be with us or against us. I know I'm going to be ready."[57] Later McVeigh sent her a letter, "something is going to happen in the month of the bull" and then told his sister to burn the letter.[57]

7. *Last resort warning behavior.* McVeigh believed that violence was the only answer to destroy the federal government, and his mission was to begin the second American Revolution. In February1992, he wrote an op-ed piece for his hometown newspaper saying, in part, "Is civil war imminent? Do we have to shed blood to reform the current system? I hope it doesn't come to that, but it might."[59] In the months prior to the bombing, he gave his personal belongings to his sister, Jennifer. He wrote to her, "Who else would come to the rescue of those innocent women and children at Waco?!? Surely not the Sheriff or the state police! Nor the Army—whom are used overseas to 'restore democracy,' while at home are used to destroy it (in full violation of the Posse Comitatus Act), at places like Waco. I'm no longer in the propaganda stage. . . . Now I'm in the action stage."[57]

8. *Directly communicated threat warning behavior.* There is no evidence that McVeigh communicated his intent to law enforcement or the target beforehand, consistent with other research on targeted violence.[13]

Here are the 10 distal characteristics which were either present or absent:

1. *Personal grievance and moral outrage.* McVeigh's personal grievance was his failure to pass the selection process at Ft. Bragg, North Carolina, to become a US Army Green Beret in 1991. He was invited to return again once he was back in shape, but declined to do so. He finished his enlistment at Ft. Riley and left the Army later that year. His dream of becoming the "ultimate warrior" was shattered. His moral outrage was his identification with both Randy Weaver, a retired special forces soldier, and Weaver's family, whom he saw as victims of the federal government at Ruby Ridge in August 1992; and his identification with members of the Branch Davidians, whom he saw as the murder victims of the federal government in Waco, Texas, on April 19, 1993. This was the spark on the oil slick of Timothy McVeigh's mind. He changed his birthday to April 19.

2. *Framed by Ideology.* Following his US Army service, McVeigh drifted further to the right and embraced the ideology of the Patriot Movement: the US Constitution was being violated, the federal government was the enemy, and power should only reside at the county level (posse comitatus). Within the Patriot Movement was a strong defense of the Second Amendment, as well as white ethnic Christian superiority and dominance, the latter often manifest through anti-Semitic and racist literature. His ideological framing supported two aspects of his terrorist planning and preparation: the bombing should occur on Patriot's Day (April 19), a celebration of the date in 1775 when the colonialists fired their first shot against the occupying British at Lexington-Concord and began the American Revolution, and the use of William Pierce's book, *The Turner Diaries*, as a partial template for bombing a federal building. Pierce, a trained physicist, was the founder and head of the National Alliance, a very large, extreme right-wing ethnic nationalist organization. He was an anti-Semite and neo-Nazi. McVeigh attempted to contact Pierce by telephone in the days prior to the bombing.

3. *Failure to affiliate with an extremist or other group.* Although McVeigh and Nichols attended some meetings of the Michigan militia, a local paramilitary group, after the bombing, members of the group insisted that they leave due to their advocacy of violence. One other source reports that McVeigh

served as a bodyguard to its leader, Mark Koernke, on a trip to Florida following the Branch Davidian compound conflagration.[56]

4. *Dependence on the virtual community.* There was no public internet or social media at the time of the Oklahoma City bombing, so this characteristic is absent.

5. *Thwarting of occupational goals.* McVeigh's rejection from special selection for the Green Berets, his personal grievance, thwarted his larger goal of being the "ultimate warrior" and a career soldier, although he could have continued to pursue this occupation but for his humiliation when he failed one endurance run. He tried other related paths—armed security guard, application to become a US Marshal—but was met with either boredom or failure.

6. *Changes in thinking and emotion.* McVeigh became more isolative after leaving the US Army, living as a drifter, selling paraphernalia at gun shows, and traveling between Decker, Michigan, the home of the Nichols family, and Kingman, Arizona, the home of the Fortiers. He became more angry, strident, and absolutist in his beliefs following the Waco conflagration. His writings to his sister Jennifer reflected an increasing paranoia and grandiosity as the date of the bombing approached. He became more brooding and humorless. He left a note for the ATF on his sister's word processor: "ATF Read: ATF, all you tyrannical motherfuckers will swing in the wind one day for your treasonous actions against the Constitution and the United States. Remember the Nuremburg War Trials. But . . . but . . . but . . . I was only following orders. Die, you spineless cowardice bastards!"[57,58] There was no longer any small talk. On February 10, 1995, he wrote Gwenn Strider, an older friend in Caro, Michigan, who had written to him about a local problem. He wrote at length about his commitment to militancy and ended with the following statement: "Sorry I can't be of more help, but most of the people sent my way these days are of the direct-action type, and my whole mindset has shifted from intellectual to animal (rip the bastards heads off and shit down their necks! And I'll show you how with a simple pocket knife . . . etc.)." He signed it, "Seeya, The Desert Rat."[57,58] He could no longer stand to be around children. He was stressed and edgy. The primitivity of this latter comment may reflect his

emotional shift from anger to contempt and disgust for his enemy. Such emotional change has been shown to correlate with politically violent action.[42]

His internal fantasies were also apparently becoming more violent and grandiose. He communicated to his sister that he would become the first hero of the second American Revolution and was intent on becoming the "ultimate warrior."[58] As is often the case, he wore clothing and carried amulets consistent with these fantasies on the day of the bombing. Along with the t-shirt noted earlier, McVeigh carried in his pocket a gold commemorative coin inscribed on one side, "Battle of Lexington/Concord, April 19, 1775" and on the other side, "shot heard round the world," a reference to the famous poem by Ralph Waldo Emerson.

7. *Failure of sexually intimate pair bonding.* There is no evidence that McVeigh had any experience with sexually intimate bonding from puberty until his death. There is suggestive evidence that he engaged in sexual relations with women on occasion, but no enduring sexually intimate attachments whatsoever. He bemoaned the fact that he had not reproduced prior to his execution.[43,59]

8. *Mental disorder.* McVeigh had no known diagnosable mental disorder, and no mental condition was introduced by his defense team during trial to mitigate responsibility for his crimes. He may have been clinically depressed following his discharge from the US Army. Standardized IQ testing in the military found him to have an IQ in the superior range (FSIQ 120–129). He was an introvert by temperament, but could be intentionally friendly and talkative. He did not trust others and did not form close relationships easily. His personality suggested a poised, overcontrolled individual, self-sufficient and self-reliant, who believed he was superior to others. He was usually serious and gravitated toward esoteric political and philosophical beliefs. He nurtured a lifelong anger toward authority figures whom he believed were arbitrary and unreasonable. McVeigh was abandoned by his mother in mid-adolescence, and his father was chronically emotionally withdrawn from the children.[60] There was no evidence of any diagnosable psychiatric condition as a child nor any antisocial behavior. Others viewed

him as quiet and ruminative. His adult personality was similar to the "hypervigilant narcissist" described by Gabbard.[58,60,61]

9. *Creativity and innovation*. The bombing was innovative in size and consequences since it was at that time the largest terrorist attack in the history of the United States. However, the modus operandi was taken from Pierce's novel, *The Turner Diaries*, and an ammonium nitrate/fuel oil bomb and Ryder Truck were utilized by al-Qaeda in the first World Trade Center bombing in February 1993. The Oklahoma bombing, however, was imitated, most recently by Anders Breivik on July 22, 2011, in Oslo, Norway. Breivik also idolized McVeigh and closely identified with him as a warrior for a nationalist cause.[62]

10. *Criminal violence*. McVeigh did have one act of criminal violence by history prior to the bombing: the robbery of Roger Moore in November 1994, in Hot Springs, Arkansas.

McVeigh was positive on 14 out of 18 indicators (78%). If one extrapolates the 43 extreme right-wing terrorists from the Meloy and Gill lone-actor terrorist sample,[22] McVeigh was positive on the four most prominent warning behaviors in that subgroup: pathway (81%), fixation (65%), identification (86%), and leakage (88%). The McVeigh findings, in retrospect, have no predictive value, but do demonstrate the goodness of fit—the ecological validity—when the TRAP-18 is applied to an individual terrorist. It also provides an organized template for understanding both proximal and distal risk indicators in a person of concern and for planning appropriate and timely intervention strategies. Group-based comparative studies are necessary to draw conclusions concerning the predictive and discriminant validity of the TRAP-18, as reviewed earlier. McVeigh was a soldier for the extreme right, the white power movement, a political and social problem of underestimated magnitude that continues to haunt both North American and European countries.[56]

CONCLUSION

Prevention does not require prediction. In other words, one does not require specific prediction of a terrorist act in order to engage in countermeasures to thwart those who may pose a threat and divert those who present early-stage concerns into more prosocial and nonviolent pathways. With this principle in mind, the TRAP-18 was designed to document both proximal and distal indicators of risk. When only distal indicators are present, research suggests that the case need only be monitored. When one or more proximal warning behaviors are present, the case should be actively managed. Such an approach to threat assessment of lone-actor terrorism allows for the *prioritization* of cases, a problem endemic in counterterrorism efforts since the base rate for actual violence is very low even within a population of general concern, the intelligence noise is very high, and the civil rights of individuals must be protected.

In this chapter the TRAP-18 was introduced as a threat assessment tool, and its 18 indicators defined. The extant empirical research on the TRAP-18 was presented, which is beginning to demonstrate interrater reliability, content validity, construct validity, discriminant validity, and postdictive validity across multiple studies. The instrument was also applied to one case of domestic terrorism in the United States, the bombing of the federal building in Oklahoma City in 1995. The TRAP-18 demonstrated both directionality and depth of understanding in assessing retrospectively the threat presented by Timothy McVeigh.

Eric Hoffer wrote in his book, *The True Believer*, a passage utilized by the author in one of his reports to the federal trial judge concerning McVeigh and his co-conspirator, Terry Nichols[63]:

> For there is often a monstrous incongruity
> between the hopes,
>   however noble and tender, and the actions
> which follows them.
>   It is as if ivied maidens and garlanded
> youths were to herald
>   the four horsemen of the apocalypse.

Our task is to make sure these actions do not come to pass.

NOTES AND REFERENCES

1. Meloy JR. The empirical basis and forensic application of affective and predatory violence. *Australian N Z J Psychiatry*. 2006;40:539–547.
2. McEllistrem J. Affective and predatory violence: A bimodal classification system of human aggression and violence. *Aggression Violent Behav*. 2004;10:1–30.
3. Siegel L, Victoroff J. Understanding human aggression: New insights from neuroscience. *Int J Law Psychiatry*. 2009;32: 209–215.
4. Siever L. Neurobiology of aggression and violence. *Am J Psychiatry*. 2008;165:429–442.

5. Douglas K, Hart S, Webster C, Belfrage H. *HCR-20 V3 Assessing Violence Risk User Guide.* Vancouver, BC: Simon Fraser University Mental Health, Law, and Policy Institute; 2013.

6. Meloy JR, Goodwill AM, Meloy MJ, Amat G, Martinez M, Morgan M. Some TRAP-18 indicators discriminate between terrorist attackers and other subjects of national security concern. *J Threat Assess Manage.* 2019;6(2):93–110. https://doi.org/10.1037/tam0000119

7. Gill P. *Lone-Actor Terrorists: A Behavioural Analysis.* London: Routledge; 2015.

8. Monahan, J. The individual risk assessment of terrorism. *Psychol Pub Pol Law.* 2012;18:167–205.

9. Monahan, J. The individual risk assessment of terrorism: Recent developments. In LaFree G, Freilich J, eds., *The Handbook of Criminology of Terrorism.* Hoboken, NJ: Wiley; 2016:520–534.

10. Fein R, Vossekuil B. Assassination in the United States: An operational study of recent assassins, attackers, and near lethal approachers. *J Forensic Sci.*1999;44:321–333.

11. Calhoun F, Weston S. *Contemporary Threat Management.* San Diego: Specialized Training Services; 2003.

12. Calhoun FS, Weston S. *Threat Assessment and Management Strategies.* 2nd edition. New York: CRC Press; 2016.

13. Meloy JR, Hoffmann J. *International Handbook of Threat Assessment.* New York: Oxford University Press; 2014.

14. Meloy JR, Hoffmann J. *International Handbook of Threat Assessment.* 2nd edition. New York: Oxford University Press;2020.

15. Gill P. Sequencing lone actor radicalization pathways. Research supported by the Office of University Programs Science and Technology Directorate of the U.S. Department of Homeland Security through the Center for the Study of Terrorism and Behavior (CSTAB – Center Lead). Grant made to the START Consortium (Grant # 2012-ST-61-CS0001); 2016.

16. Bouhana N, Corner E, Gill P, Schuurman B. Background and preparatory behaviours of right-wing extremist long actors: A comparative study. *Perspect Terrorism* 2018;12:150–162.

17. Meloy JR. *The TRAP-18 Manual Version 1.0.* Washington, DC: Global Institute of Forensic Research; 2017.

18. Lloyd M, Dean C. The development of structured guidelines for assessing risk in extremist offenders. *J Threat Assess Manage.* 2015;2(1):40–52. https://doi.org/10.1037/tam0000035

19. Pressman DE. *Risk Assessment Decisions for Violent Political Extremism (VERA).* Her Majesty the Queen in Right of Canada. Cat. No.: PS3-1/2009-2-1E-PDF ISBN No.: 978-1-100-13956-2, Ottawa; 2009.

20. Meloy JR, Hoffmann J, Guldimann A, James D. The role of warning behaviors in threat assessment: An exploration and suggested typology. *Behav Sci Law.* 2011:256–279. doi:10.1002/bsl.999.

21. Meloy JR, Yakeley J. The violent true believer as a "one wolf": Psychoanalytic perspectives on terrorism. *Behav Sci Law.* 2014;32(3):347–365. doi:10.1002/bsl.2109.

22. Meloy JR, Gill P. The lone actor terrorist and the TRAP-18. *J Threat Assess Manage.* 2016;3:37–52.

23. Monahan J, Steadman H. Violent storms and violent people: How meteorology can inform risk communications in mental health law. *Am Psychologist* 1996;51:931–938.

24. Koffka K. *Die Grundlagen der psychischen Entwicklung.* Osterwieck am Harz, Germany: A. W. Zickfeldt; 1921.

25. Kohler W. *Gestalt Psychology.* New York: Liveright; 1929.

26. Wertheimer, M. *Gestalt Theory: A Source Book of Gestalt Psychology.* London: Paul, Trench, Trubner; 1938. http://dx.doi.org/10.1037/11496- 001

27. Meloy JR, Pollard J. Lone actor terrorism and impulsivity. *J Forensic Sci.* 2017;62(6):1643–1646. doi:10.1111/1556-4029.13500.

28. Rahman T. Extreme overvalued beliefs: How violent extremist beliefs become "normalized." *Behav Sci.* 2018. doi:10.3390/bs8010010.

29. Rahman T, Meloy JR, Bauer R. Extreme overvalued beliefs: A tribute to Carl Wernicke. *J Am Acad Psychiatry Law.* 2019;47(2):180–187. doi:10.29158/JAAPL.003847-19.

30. Dietz PE. Mass, serial, and sensational homicides. *Bull NY Acad Med.* 1986;62:477–491.

31. Hempel A, Meloy JR, Richards T. Offender and offense characteristics of a nonrandom sample of mass murderers. *J Am Acad Psychiatry Law.* 1999;27:213–225.

32. Meloy JR, Mohandie K, Knoll J, Hoffmann J. The concept of identification in threat assessment. *Behav Sci Law.* 2015. doi:10.1002/bsl.2166.

33. Freud A. *The Ego and the Mechanisms of Defense.* New York: International Universities Press; 1937, 1966.

34. Erikson E. *Childhood and Society.* New York: Norton; 1950.

35. MacCulloch M, Snowden P, Wood P, Mills H. Sadistic fantasy, sadistic behavior and offending. *Br J Psychiatry.* 1983;143:20–29.

36. Hull C. *A Behavioral System.* New Haven, CT: Yale University Press; 1952.

37. Meloy JR, O'Toole ME. The concept of leakage in threat assessment. *Behav Sci Law.* 2011. doi:10.1002/bsl.986.

38. Horgan J, Gill P, Bouhana N, Silver J, Corner E. *Across the Universe? A Comparative Analysis of Violent Behavior and Radicalization Across Three*

Offender Types with Implications for Criminal Justice Training and Education. Washington, DC: US Dept. of Justice; 2016.

39. Darley JM, Latané B. Bystander intervention in emergencies: Diffusion of responsibility. *J Personality Soc Psychol*. 1968;8:377–383. doi:10.1037/h0025589.

40. Mohandie K, Duffy J. First responder and negotiation guidelines with the paranoid schizophrenic subject. *FBI Law Enforcement Bulletin*, Dec 1999:8–16. https://leb.fbi.gov/file-repository/archives/dec99leb.pdf/view

41. James D, MacKenzie R, Farnham F. *CTAP-25: Communicated Threat Assessment Protocol Manual*. Kent, UK: Theseus LLP; 2014.

42. Matsumoto D, Frank M, Hwang H. The role of intergroup emotions in political violence. *Curr Direct Psychol Sci*. 2015;24:369–373.

43. Meloy JR. Sexual desire, violent death, and the true believer. *Contemp Psychoanal*. 2018;54(1):64–83. doi:10.1080/00107530.2017.1414577.

44. Meloy JR, Roshdi K, Glaz-Ocik J, Hoffmann J. Investigating the individual terrorist in Europe. *J Threat Assess Manage*. 2015;2:140–152.

45. Gill P, Horgan J, Corner E, Silver J. Indicators of lone actor violent events: The problems of low base rates and long observational periods. *J Threat Assess Manage*. 2016;3:165–173.

46. Meloy JR, Hoffmann J, Roshdi K, Guldimann A. Some warning behaviors discriminate between school shooters and other students of concern. *J Threat Assess Manage*. 2014b;1:203–211.

47. Gill P, Horgan J, Deckert P. Bombing alone: Tracing the motivations and antecedent behaviors of lone-actor terrorists. *J Forensic Sci*. 2014;59(2):425–435. doi:10.1111/1556-4029.12312.

48. Doyle C. Terrorist material support: An overview of 18 U.S.C. §2339A and §2339B. Congressional Research Service, 8 Dec 2016. https://fas.org/sgp/crs/natsec/R41333.pdf

49. Challacombe DJ, Lucas PA. Postdicting violence with sovereign citizen actors: An exploratory test of the TRAP-18. *J Threat Assess Manage*. 2019;6(1):51–59. https://doi.org/10.1037/tam0000105

50. Goodwill A, Meloy JR. Visualizing the relationship among indicators for lone actor terrorist attacks: Multidimensional scaling and the TRAP-18. *Behav Sci Law*. 2019;37(5):522–539. doi:10.1002/bsl.2434.

51. Meloy JR, Habermeyer E, Guldimann A. The warning behaviors of Anders Breivik. *J Threat Assess Manage*. 2015;2:164–175.

52. Bockler N, Hoffmann J, Zick A. The Frankfurt Airport attack: A case study on the radicalization of a lone-actor terrorist. *J Threat Assess Manage*. 2015;2:153–163.

53. Meloy JR, Genzman J. The clinical threat assessment of the lone-actor terrorist. *Psychiatric Clin N Am*. 2016;39:649–662.

54. Bockler N, Hoffmann J, Meloy JR. "Jihad against the enemies of Allah": The Berlin Christmas market attack from a threat assessment perspective. *Violence Gender*. 2017;4(3):73–80. https://doi.org/10.1089/vio.2017.0040

55. Erlandsson A, Meloy JR. The Swedish school attack in Trollhattan. *J Forensic Sci*. 2018;63(6):1917–1927. doi:10.1111/1556-4029.13800.

56. Belew K. *Bring the War Home*. Cambridge, MA: Harvard University Press; 2018.

57. Serrano N. *One of Ours: Timothy McVeigh and the Oklahoma City Bombing*. New York: W.W. Norton; 1998.

58. Meloy JR. Professional notes.

59. Michel L, Herbeck D. *American Terrorist*. New York: Avon; 2002.

60. Meloy JR. Indirect personality assessment of the violent true believer. *J Personality Assess*. 2004;82:138–146.

61. Gabbard G. Two subtypes of narcissistic personality disorder. *Bull Menninger Clin*. 1989;53:527–532.

62. Meloy JR, Habermeyer E, Guldimann A. The warning behaviors of Anders Breivik. *J Threat Assess Manage*. 2015;2(3-4):164–175.

63. Hoffer E. *The True Believer*. New York: HarperCollins; 1951.

25

Use of Threat and Risk Assessment Tools in the Evaluation of Lone-Actor Terrorists

HY BLOOM, REEM ZAIA, AND ARYA SHAH

INTRODUCTION

Developing tools to identify and avert terrorist violence is "inherently complex and multifaceted."[1] It has generally been thought that terrorists do not present with the same characteristics and risk factors that most forensic mental health professionals are accustomed to dealing with. Decades ago, research by Russell and Miller[2] involving 18 terrorist groups (350 terrorists) from around the world showed that the terrorists—many of whom were well-educated middle to upper middle class—substantially differed in demographic and other features from typical criminals.

Any distinction between terrorism committed by affiliated terrorists and acts committed by lone-actor terrorists may be somewhat artificial; several authors classify both scenarios under the umbrella terms of "collective violence"[3] or "group-based violence,"[4] respectively. In this regard, Cook et al. explain that "much violence—if not most of it—is perpetrated by people whose decisions and behavior are influenced by one or more social groups to which they belong, with which they are affiliated, or with which they identify, and is often directed against people who do not belong to, are not affiliated with, or do not identify with the same groups."[4]

Because terrorist attacks do not constitute everyday criminal violence, they are anomalies on the risk assessment landscape for which no tool has established predictive ability.[5,6] For this reason, while they are not specifically designed for evaluating risk posed by affiliated and lone-actor terrorists, broad-range violence risk assessment tools are frequently utilized in threat and risk assessment in this population. Kebbell and Porter[7] point out that, apart from attempting to quantify risk, use of such tools also "provides an evidence base and audit trail for the decision-making process; it can be designed to ensure consistency of judgments, and therefore it is fair, thus reassuring vulnerable communities and complying with Human Rights legislation."

The following chapter, in addition to acknowledging the utility of basic principles of the psychiatric interview and assessment in these evaluations, outlines a variety of risk assessment tools that can be used in the evaluation of risk associated with terror. Broad-range violence risk assessment tools, while not developed specifically for evaluation of risk associated with individual and affiliated terror, are frequently utilized. They provide a structure and framework for the assessment and help in identifying historic, criminogenic, mental health, social, and environmental variables that assist—often with other tools that measure fundamentalism, radicalization, and preparedness to commit religious/ideological/politically based violence—in the calculating of a prospective or de facto terrorist's risk. Fewer tools and assessments measures have been studied with regards to risk associated with terror. The chapter includes some measures used to understand and characterize beliefs associated with extremism-related violence. We acknowledge that the Terrorist Radicalization Assessment Protocol (TRAP-18)[8] is the only tool that we are aware of that was specifically developed for risk assessment in the context of lone-actor terrorism; the TRAP-18 is discussed in detail in Chapter 24 of this volume.

VIOLENCE RISK ASSESSMENT

By its very nature, violence risk assessment is a prospective inquiry. It contemplates the potential for an adverse aggressive event to occur within a wide temporal range that includes the immediate (seconds, minutes, a few hours), the foreseeable (days, a few weeks, perhaps up to a year), and the distant (several years to indeterminate) future.[9]

Risk assessments identify which perpetrators will commit which actions by which means toward whom and within what timeframe. Although the subject is clearly the focus of the assessment, expert assessors appreciate that violence rarely occurs in a vacuum. It is interactional and almost invariably depends on the presence of or friction between two or more variables, including predisposed perpetrators and victims, environmental factors, and an event or stressor that serves as the accelerant for an outbreak of violence. In any violence risk assessment, examiners must develop a theory about from where and whence the violence derives.[9]

BASIC PRINCIPLES OF THE CLINICAL EVALUATION

Whether a threat assessment or risk assessment "the principle of data collection and analysis based on a framework of evidence about the nature of the outcome to be prevented remains the same."[10]

Some time ago, Stone[11] identified three categories for the assessment and prediction of violence risk. According to Stone, category two and three assessments, which contemplate timeframes for the occurrence of an adverse event of days to months or longer, are capable of being carried out in fairly settled circumstances (i.e., in a prison, forensic facility, hospitals, and at times, with the subject residing in the community). Assessments in these categories have some luxury of time and generally fall under the heading "risk assessment."

Category one assessments, which contemplate timeframes from seconds to a few weeks, on the other hand, are urgent or near-urgent situations that require close/constant surveillance and appraisal of multiple sources of potentially rapidly changing information and intervention to prevent the situation from spiraling into a calamity.[12] *Imminent risk*, which is in the domain of threat assessment, "is concerned with the dynamics and fluidity of the potential perpetrator's internal state and equally unstable elements in his environment."[12]

Key components of the psychiatric evaluation are reviewed separately in chapter 3 of this book. In brief, important baseline considerations in the performance of a threat or risk assessment include (1) determining assessor qualifications, (2) conducting the clinical interview, (3) reviewing existing documentation, (4) contacting collateral informants, and (5) performing a risk assessment.

Assessor Qualifications

Psychiatrists and psychologists who work in the forensic arena generally have various forms of violence risk assessment skills in their toolkits, but Logan and Lloyd[10] caution that, in contrast to more conventional risk assessment tasks, assessing risk of violence by extremists "is a complex undertaking, not least because the harmful outcomes to be prevented are many and diverse and what individuals are prepared to do to achieve their outcomes varies considerably." According to Dernevik and colleagues,[13] mental health professionals who engage in this work should be equipped with an understanding of the accused's ethnic, cultural, ideological, sociopolitical, psychiatric, and neurocognitive background and influences. Additional considerations unique to these assessments may also include an appreciation for the risk of countertransference and subjectivity in the assessor as well as an appreciation for early life grievances, conflicts, dynamics, and unresolved feelings that may impact beliefs, influence target selection, and motivate actions.

Conducting the Clinical Interview

Horgan[14] notes that ambivalence in the field, for example, about whether interviewing terrorists gives them a platform to espouse and publicize their cause has led to limitations in communication among mental health professionals concerning how to approach the task. Failure to go beyond "'talking to' [or] 'schmoozing' with or other ad hoc and largely unstructured" communication with terrorists has limited the creation and dissemination of research-based interviewing protocols.[13] "To understand the development of the terrorist," Taylor and Horgan[15] write, "we must ask questions about how decisions emerged, the meaning of those decisions, and their consequences for the person concerned." They suggest that the interview aim to understand the following in the accused individual[15]:

• Reasons for involvement in violence and terror
• Risk factors for involvement in terrorism

- Presence of characteristics associated with sustained terrorist membership
- Understanding how meaning is derived through affiliation with an ideology
- Understanding of ideological content and processes impinging on behavior

To do so, the assessor may wish to consider the following topics:

- Background of the evaluee's family of origin and key early life figures and influences
- Developmental history and, in particular, presence of early life trauma
- Personality structure and identity formation
- Medical and psychiatric health over life span
- Social and sexual development
- Emotional regulation and impulse control
- Nature of relationships and impact of others on the subject
- Capacity for intimacy
- Lifetime aspirations
- Potential disharmony between early life goals and actual trajectory
- The subject's worldview; philosophical, religious, political, and ideological beliefs, leanings, and affiliations

Documents and Materials

Clinicians should attempt to obtain the following materials:

- The examinee's medical, mental health, and substance use records
- School records
- Criminal and probation records
- Police/prosecution documents
- Military records, where applicable
- Employment records
- Individual's reading/media materials, writings, drawings, presentations
- Internet sites visited and social media communications
- Court documents referable to any civil actions

The assessor should conduct a World Wide Web search of the accused, his affiliates, and the organization(s) he has looked into.

Collateral Informants

Rahman et al.[16] note how difficult, if not impossible, it would be to identify the beliefs of any radicalized individual without collecting collateral information. Access to collateral informants is a tenet of forensic psychiatric assessment. Potential sources of collateral might include

- Parents, siblings, children, and relatives
- Peers, friends
- Current and former intimate partners
- Current and former co-workers, supervisors
- Religious leader(s)
- Teachers and school administration
- Probation/parole officer

General Risk Assessment

Risk factors are attributes that increase the likelihood that the outcome being measured occurs. Conversely, "protective factors . . . moderate (lessen) the salience of a risk factor."[17] In the terrorism context, protective factors are countervailing variables that bolster resilience to and shield the individual against extremist (or further extremist) indoctrination.[18]

As regards general risk factors, Smith[19] points out that many risk factors contained in extremist assessment tools are present in the general population; the co-occurrence of a number of factors, however, is less common and signals reason for concern. There is no clear boundary differentiating risk factors for affiliated versus lone-actor terrorism. Smith's[19] recent detailed review identified a number of potential risk factors common to both (in US perpetrators), including

- A history of criminal violence
- A criminal history
- Gang/delinquent peer involvement
- A friend who is a terrorist
- Extremist group membership over a protracted period of time
- A deep commitment to extremist ideology
- Psychological issues
- Unemployment
- Sporadic work history
- Less education
- Lower socioeconomic status
- Failure to achieve one's aspirations
- Troubled romantic relationships
- Troubled platonic relationships
- History of suffering abuse as an adult
- Estrangement from one's family

In contrast to such general risk factors, there exist a variety of specialized broad-range violence assessments tools, as well as newer tools developed to assess ideology, radicalization, and risk for affiliated or group-based violence. These are discussed in the sections to follow.

BROAD-RANGE VIOLENCE RISK ASSESSMENT TOOLS

Forensic mental health professionals are routinely called on to assess various types of violent or untoward behavior and risk for recurrence of same. This task, in fact, to a great extent defines the field. As Hart et al. note,

> There is now a well-developed evidence base concerning the use of decision support tools by threat assessment professionals. The evidence base indicates that a number of tools can be used by a wide range of professionals in many different countries to make decisions about the assessment and management of risk for diverse forms of violence—including general violence, sexual violence, intimate partner violence, stalking, workplace violence, honor-based violence, and so forth—with good reliability and validity.[20]

Existing broad-range violence tools do have limitations in terms of utility in predicting risk of affiliated and lone-actor terror. Pressman and Flockton[21] point out that instruments, such as the HCR-20, focus heavily on the issue of mental illness and psychopathology. Affiliated terrorists, however, are not for the most part known to suffer from serious mental illness, personality disorders, or other dysfunction. Other authors,[22,23] however, note that typical risk factors for general violence, like mental illness, substance abuse, and personality pathology, render some individuals susceptible to radicalization and recruitment and hence ought not to be dismissed outrightly as valueless. Past violence is also another common factor addressed in traditional risk assessment tools but is not always a factor in assessing extremists. Affiliated or group-based terrorists are generally not known to have prior criminal records, histories of violence, or serious mental health problems, whereas a larger percentage of lone actors have a history of personality disorder or mental illness and approximately half have a criminal history.[24]

Risk assessments can be divided into two categories: actuarial tools and structured professional judgment (SPJ) tools. While both types of methods utilize the weighing of known risk factors for violence, actuarial assessments leave little room for clinical interpretation and base risk on numeric algorithms; in contrast, tools in the category of SPJ assessments allow for a clinical decision on violence risk to be made by the evaluator who uses a combination of assessment scores, clinical history, and professional expertise to formulate overall risk.[25]

Some commonly utilized broad range violence risk SPJ tools include the Hare Psychopathy Checklist (PCL-R), the HCR-20, and the Structured Assessment of Risk of Violence in Youth (SAVRY). In comparison the Violence Risk Appraisal Guide (VRAG), discussed later, is an actuarial scale, which, as noted, leaves less room for professional judgment within the risk assessment process.

Hare Psychopathy Checklist—Revised (PCL-R)

Clinicians and researchers often rely on the Hare PCL-R[26] as a means of defining the extent to which an individual qualifies for the clinical construct "psychopath." High scores are consistently correlated to violence in both forensic patients and incarcerated offenders. The MacArthur Study confirms that the construct of psychopathy, as measured by the 12-item Hare Psychopathy Checklist: Screening Version,[26] has particularly robust capabilities compared to many of the other risk factors often considered.[27] Psychopathy is a core concept when it comes to assessing risk for violence to others. This may in part be due to the fact that each of the 20 items on the Hare PCL-R has been carefully defined.[28]

The PCL-R[29] is composed of a 20-item checklist to assess the extent to which the subject's score accords with the prototypical "psychopath." While not a risk assessment tool in its own right, it is considered one of the better studied and validated instruments for assessing risk for criminal behavior associated with psychopathology.[30] The PCL-R utilizes information gathered through a structured interview and review of collateral sources. This score is based on two factors: (1) interpersonal factors and (2) pattern of chronically antisocial lifestyle; each factor is further subdivided into two facets. Factor 1 assesses interpersonal (Facet one) and affective (Facet two) features that are central to the personality construct of psychopathy. Factor 2's focus is lifestyle (Facet three) and antisocial behavior patterns (Facet four)—the behavioral dimension of psychopathy that approaches diagnostic criteria of the *Diagnostic and Statistical Manual of Mental*

Disorders (DSM-5) for antisocial personality disorder. Further details with respect to Factors and Facets are described in Table 25.1.

There are two further Factors not associated with any of the preceding categories, namely promiscuous sexual behavior and history of multiple short marital relationships that comprise the two remaining items.

Each of the factors are scored as 0, 1, or 2. Scoring is based on lifetime history, not simply on presentation at time of evaluation. Total scores range from 0 to 40, with 30 generally being the cutoff that qualifies the individual for the characterological designation of "psychopath."[29] Of note, a version of the PCL has been studied for the evaluation of violence risk in youths and is known as the PCL-YV (Youth Version).[31]

Of note, the Violence Risk Appraisal Guide (VRAG)[32] is an actuarial tool that relies principally on the individual's PCL-R score and on a collection of other historic factors in order to predict the individual's risk for violent recidivism within a circumscribed period of time (i.e., 7–10 years). As one of the best known among the various actuarial tools, this instrument was created by drawing on data of mentally disordered offenders detained at the Oakridge/Penetanguishene maximum security psychiatric facility in Ontario, Canada, between 1965 and 1980. It is important to consider, however, that the actuarial nature of the VRAG renders it significantly limited in terms of the assessor's ability to utilize clinical judgment in the overall determination of risk.

Historical Clinical Risk–20–Revised

The HCR-20[33] and its newest edition, the HCR-20-V3,[34] is a violence assessment tool comprised of a 20-item checklist used to understand risk for future violence and create benchmark scores

for managing violence risk.[35] The tool has been utilized in both the criminal and psychiatric settings. The scale includes historical, clinical, and future management risk factors to consider in determining overall risk for violence. The HCR-20 has commonly been used in correctional, civil, psychiatric, and forensic settings; it has further been used to make decisions regarding release from institutions, transitioning to a different level of security, and continued risk management. With its focus on some point in the future, the HCR-20 is not likely to be useful in situations when decisions about threat must be made urgently.

The scale's checklist includes thee subscales: Historical, Clinical, and Risk Management.[36]

1. The *Historical Scale* considers 10 static factors from an individual's past that might contribute to future risk of violence, including previous violence, age at first violent incident, relationship instability, employment, substance use, mental illness, early life trauma, personality disorder, attitudes toward violence, and prior treatment response.

2. The *Clinical Scale* takes into account five psychological, behavioral, and mental health clinical characteristics that can affect risk of violence, including insight; violent ideation and/or intent; symptoms of mental illness; affective, behavioral, or cognitive instability; and outcomes of treatment.

3. The *Risk Management Scale* is speculative, considering five potential exacerbating and mitigating factors that may influence how an individual might respond to circumstances in the future. Such factors include possible future problems with professional services and plans, living situation, personal supports,

TABLE 25.1 SUMMARY OF HARE PSYCHOPATHY CHECKLIST (PCL-R) FACTORS AND FACETS

Factor 1	Facet one	Interpersonal factors include presence of superficial charm, grandiosity, pathological lying, and manipulative behavior.
	Facet two	Affective factors include lack of remorse, lack of emotional depth, lack of empathy, and lack of accountability for actions.
Factor 2	Facet three	Lifestyle factors include susceptibility to boredom, pattern of using others for own gain, lack of long-term goals, impulsivity, and irresponsibility.
	Facet four	Antisocial factors include pattern of poor behavioral control, history of early behavioral problems, history of juvenile delinquency, revocation of conditional release, and history of highly variable criminal behavior.

Adapted from Hare.[26]

treatment compliance and/or response, and stress.

Mossman characterizes the HCR-20 as an easy-to-understand device.[37] The HCR-20 and HCR-20-V3 manuals succinctly and clearly describe published research data that support the inclusion of the particular item.

In the HCR-20 scheme, each item was scored as either not present (0), possibly present (1), or definitely present (2) to yield a potential score of 40. The HCR-20-V3 scheme has replaced that scoring scheme with Y (factor is present), P (factor is possibly or partially present), and N (factor is not present).[35] Use of the scheme involves melding historical, dynamic, and future-oriented risk management factors in order to come up with a broad estimation of risk, expressed as low, moderate, or high risk for violent recidivism.

Most broad-range violence risk assessment tools recognize the importance of a past history of violence. As noted, group-based terrorists are often not known to have prior criminal records or histories of violence, nor do they typically have unstable education, employment, or childhood histories (with some variance seen when examining lone actors), factors which are routinely seen in most offender populations. As well, terrorists, according to Pressman and Flockton,[21] do not have emotional dysregulation or impulse control problems, which most broad-based violence risk assessment tools consider.

Structured Assessment of Violence Risk in Youth

The Structured Assessment of Violence Risk in youth (SAVRY)[38] is an assessment tool including 24 items categorized as either historical, social/contextual, individual, or protective factors. Its potential value in the limited armamentarium of tools available to assess risk of involvement in terrorism in youth is akin to the value of the HCR-20 V3 for similar purposes in adults. We earlier conceded that this tool, like essentially all broad-range violence risk assessment tools, is non-specific and arguably of limited value in assessing risk of terrorist involvement. The SAVRY items are described here:

1. *Historical*: History of violence, history of non-violent offending, young age at first violent episode, failure of prior interventions, history of self-injury or suicide attempts, history of exposure to violence in the home, history of abuse, criminality in parent or caregiver, disruption in caregiver at young age, poor achievement in school
2. *Social/contextual*: Peer delinquency, rejection by peers, stress and poor coping skills, poor parental supervision, lack of supports, disorganization in community environment
3. *Individual*: Negative attitudes, history of risk-taking and/or impulsivity, substance use, difficulties controlling anger, absence of empathy, difficulties with inattention or hyperactivity, poor treatment compliance, low interest in school work or goals
4. *Protective*: Prosocial activity, strong social support, strong attachments, positive view of authority or help, commitment to school or work, resilience

Each of the risk factors in the first three categories is scored as low, moderate or high, while protective items are scored as either absent or present.[39]

TOOLS TO MEASURE SCOPE AND INTENSITY OF RADICALIZATION/ EXTREMIST BELIEFS

Whether assessing affiliated or lone-actor terrorists to identify and eliminate a threat or evaluate risk for terrorist conduct or recidivism in the future, identifying beliefs—religious, political, ideological, etc.—is a core task. Several tools, described here, focus on evaluating the intensity and pervasiveness of the subject's belief system and the extent to which they can be considered fundamentalist. Liht et al.[40] define fundamentalism as "a personal orientation that asserts a suprahuman locus of moral authority, context unbound truth, and the appreciation of the sacred over the worldly components of experience." The assumption underpinning the importance of identifying beliefs is rather straightforward: beliefs animate the motivation(s) that drive planning and action.

The Religious Fundamentalism Scale

The Religious Fundamentalism Scale (RFS),[41] subsequently replaced by the Revised Religious Fundamentalism Scale (RRFS),[42] was designed to measure attitude about one's religious beliefs, regardless of the person's religious affiliation(s). The RFS/RRFS's 12 items allow an examiner to rate the scope and depth of the subject's religious convictions and worldview. Subjects reveal their reductionistic/fundamentalist views when, for example, they endorse Item 3, which reads, "The basic cause of evil in this world is Satan, who is still constantly and ferociously fighting against God."

Alternatively, a subject could expose a more moderate outlook on religion by endorsing Item 9, which covers similar subject matter from a markedly different perspective, for example, "Satan is just the name people give to their own bad impulses. There really is no such thing as a diabolical 'Prince of Darkness' who tempts us." Other items designed to tease out fundamentalist versus non-fundamentalist leanings are illustrated by Items 1 and 2:

1. "God has given humanity a complete unfailing guide to happiness and salvation, which must be totally followed."
Versus
2. "No single book of religious teachings contains all the intrinsic, fundamental truths about life."

The other eight items similarly allow assessors to gauge the degree of a subject's fundamentalist beliefs.

The authors[42] note that the scale's psychometric properties improved considerably after the RFS was revised and reduced to the 12-item version (RRFS), which has greater internal consistency.

Scales that measure religiosity and fundamentalism generally tap into three dimensions: external versus internal authority, fixed versus malleable religion, and affirmation versus rejection of worldliness.[40]

The Assessment and Treatment of Radicalization Scale

The Assessment and Treatment of Radicalization Scale (ATRS)[43] is a theoretically driven but empirically validated self-report instrument that was constructed to quantitatively measure Middle Eastern extremist ideologies on risk areas that are reported in the literature. The ATRS consists of six subscales and a total scale, with each subscale designed to tap into a prominent ideological theme promoted by Middle Eastern extremists. Subscales are categorized as follows:

1. Attitudes toward Israel
2. Political views
3. Attitudes toward women
4. Attitudes toward Western culture
5. Religiosity
6. Condoning fighting

A final, seventh subscale, is a validity scale that evaluates whether participants misunderstood the items, answered carelessly, or deliberately attempted to conceal their true answers. Items included in this subscale are additional to the ATRS. The total score consists of the answers to the items included in the first six subscales (i.e., items included in the validity subscale are not included in the total scale score). The ATRS is user-friendly.

Participants simply provide numeric responses indicating agreement or disagreement with the item, and the scale usually takes only a few minutes to complete. Scoring the scale is straightforward as the basic interpretation requires minimal professional time. The ATRS underwent four stages of development that have been described in detail elsewhere.[44] Practical reasons for the development of the ATRS include use by agencies that need risk assessments to identify individuals with extreme Middle Eastern ideologies or individuals who have beliefs supporting violence and to inform policies relating to the prevention of these violent acts or responses to terrorist threats and/or violence. It could also be used to guide and monitor therapeutic programs aimed at altering ideology and/or adherence to extremist views.

Militant-Extremist Mindset: 16 Themes

Saucier et al.,[45] like others, notes that some beliefs harbored by terrorists are also held by many members of the general population. As the authors point out, what distinguishes those who entertain a degree of extremist beliefs from those who envelop themselves in such beliefs, to an extent that they must necessarily be considered militant extremists (which they conceptualize as "an aggressive form of fanaticism"), is the scope and density of such beliefs. To develop their 16 themes characteristic of the militant-extremist mindset, Saucier at al. examined religious and secular extremist groups from across the world. "The key themes" they identified, "could be assembled to form a coherent and potentially compelling narrative, and this narrative may be the source of much of the appeal that salient militant-extremist groups generate."

Among other things, the 16 themes include items that examine beliefs about the person's/group's divinely derived justification for the use of violence to vanquish its enemies and cleanse the world of evil using any available means. A warrior mentality and reliance on Machiavellian methods to achieve the individual's/group's objectives is praised. Items also screen for values and attitudes that support dehumanization of the enemy, rejection of the authority and legitimacy of civil governments, disdain for Western culture, and support for the notion that a utopian destiny awaits those who fulfill their mission.

TOOLS DEVELOPED TO ASSESS RISK FOR AFFILIATED/GROUP-BASED EXTREMISM/TERRORISM

Kebbell and Porter's 22 Risk Factors for Extremist Violence

In Kebbell and Porter's[46] scheme, the 22 risk factors are organized under four levels of risk: standard risk factors, moderate risk factors, higher risk factor, and extreme risk factors. Standard risk factors occur sufficiently frequently in the population as to have weak predictive value. They principally describe younger disaffected Westerners who turn to belief systems they were not born into as their view of Western life, for one reason or another, sours over time. The significance of this stage is that it forms the foundational platform upon which higher order risk factors will be layered.

Moderate risk factors address the extent to which the subject is involved in the furtherance of his religious beliefs, both within the community and in his evolving mindset.

Higher risk factors rate the subject's movement toward action, sequestration within the world of radical ideology, and estrangement from the conventional (non-radical) world.

Extreme risk factors are indicators of seemingly irrevocable commitment to the cause, planning and training for an event, target selection, and evidence of credible preparedness to kill in the name of the cause.

The Extremist Risk Guidelines (ERG 22+)

The Extremist Risk Guidelines (ERG22+),[47] created for the UK National Offender Management Service, was designed to assist in formulating cases of individuals convicted of terrorist offenses and not to rate risk in would-be violent extremists. It draws on data derived from 50 convicted terrorists and from comparative data drawn from criminogenic profiles of mainstream criminal offenders compared to extremist offenders. Its intent and purpose is to inform risk management and risk decision-making, not to decide liability or predict whether a prisoner will reoffend.[48] There are 22 risk factors covering three domains: engagement, intent, and capability.

The 13 factors within the "Engagement" dimension deal with the subject's motivation(s) for involvement, the psychological meaning(s) of affiliations, ideological mindset, mental health, and the influence of others. The six factors on the "Intent" dimension rate the extent to which the subject has become indoctrinated in his views: for example, his preparedness to dehumanize the enemy, see himself in an "us versus them" battle, and justify violence to accomplish his/the group's objectives.

The three items on the "Capability" dimension look at practicalities; for example, the subject's skills and competencies, access to people and things needed to accomplish the goal, and whether he can draw on capability from his criminal history.

The "+" designation denotes that assessors need to consider a myriad of factors, not just treat the ERA as a definitive checklist.[49] Although there are similarities between the ERG22+ and the Violent Extremism Risk Assessment (VERA-2 R; discussed elsewhere in this section), the former tool's scope considers any criminal act in support of a cause or group promoting extremist views, while the latter tool's focus is on extremist violence alone.[50]

The RADAR

The RADAR was devised by Australian authorities principally to identify how far along the pathway to radicalization the individual is.[51] It contains 15 indicators drawn from three dimensions including (1) ideology, (2) social relations, and (3) action orientation, corresponding to the three phases of the individual's life during which he is likely to experience significant changes as the radicalization process progresses.[49] *Ideological shifts* are changes in beliefs toward radicalization. *Social relations shifts* refer to changes in dynamics with friends and family during the transition to radicalization, and *action orientation shifts* reflect the development of hateful feelings toward the enemy and the adoption of an "us versus them" mentality.[49]

Intensity-level indicators with ranges from "notable" (minor), "concerning" (moderate), to "attention required" (major) allow assessors to grade where the individual is along the radicalization continuum.[49]

The RADAR includes three protective factors: (1) presence of influential/supportive family members, (2) past (positive) example of societal engagement, and (3) generally not violent.

If the preceding initial screen discloses sufficient cause for concern, a second in-depth risk and needs assessment—involving 27 indicators clustered around the same three dimensions—is used to determine and design appropriate intervention(s).[52] The second phase requires that considerably more information be obtained.

The Violent Extremism Risk Assessment

The Violent Extremism Risk Assessment (VERA-2 R)[20] is an SPJ style tool designed to assess risk in individuals currently involved in criminal activity and who have a history of committing ideologically motivated violence. SPJs combine empirical knowledge derived from theoretically informed literature reviews, clinical experience, and professional judgment, drawing on information domains that often include historical, contextual, and personality or individual factors.[53]

Scarcella et al.[54] describe the VERA-2 R as "designed to be systematic, empirically grounded, developmentally informed, treatment-oriented, flexible and practical, and includes factors known to be relevant to the process of radicalization leading to violent extremism."[55]

The most recent iteration of the VERA[48]—the VERA-2 R—has 34 indicators over five domains as well as a further 11 indicators in three additional domains. The VERA-2 R considers the following domains:

1. The *Beliefs, Attitudes, and Ideology domain*, is of core importance and draws on indicators like grievances, perceived injustice, moral emotions, alienation, the relationship of the individual to the laws and norms governing the state, in-group affiliation, and identification with aggrieved persons or groups.
2. *Social Context and Intention*
3. The *History, Action, and Capacity domain* pertains to the individual's ability to conceive of, plan, and carry out a violent extremist attack. Areas focused on here include past criminality and violence, specialized training to a terrorist end, and access to people and resources.
4. The *Commitment and Motivation domain* looks at eight possible motivations considered drivers of terrorist violence. They may include an interest in adventure and excitement, a moral compunction to act, a need

to belong to a group, criminal and financial interests, or a conglomerate thereof.

5. The *Protective/Risk Mitigating domain* picks up on positive changes in the individual over the span of time as he or she disengages from terrorism. Factors in this domain may include psychological and emotional strengths and other supports that moderate and minimize problematic beliefs and affiliations.

A number of further indicators scattered across three domains (criminal history, personal history, and mental disorder) are also evaluated. These factors may be particularly important to youth. Of note, Herzog-Evans[56] recently compared the VERA and the ERG22+. Although she found that the two instruments had much in common, Herzog-Evans noted that the VERA's focus was on ideology, whereas the ERG22+'s focus was on identity as a core area of inquiry. Applying the two instruments to European extremist populations, the author found the ERG22+'s structure to be more straightforward and had less items that required access to classified data.

Structured Assessment of Violent Extremism

Unlike the VERA, ERG22+, and TRAP-18 (as regards lone actors, see later discussion), which have a significant behavioral focus, the Structured Assessment of Violent Extremism (SAVE) describes itself as taking a more "modest" approach in its focus on extremist perceptions and beliefs that contribute to risk.[42,57] The SAVE uses a two-tier approach consisting first of a 30-item checklist of cognitive risk indicators, and second, use of a "software program which functions as visualization application . . . [that] produces 3D 'risk surface' and 2D 'risk contour' plots which depict the extent of the 'risk potential' of a Person-of-Concern (PoC) who falls within the spectrum of the three slightly different violence extremism scales (terrorism scale—T1; militancy scale—M1; [and] shootings scale—S1)."[58]

Multi-Level Guidelines

Risk factors for the Multi-Level Guidelines–Version 2 (MLG 2)[59] were derived from a comprehensive and systematic review of the literature. Notably, the MLG 2 was not developed for the assessment or management of terrorists but is a generic tool that assesses risk for an individual engaging in any form of group-based violence, including terrorism. The MLG 2 draws on 16 risk factors organized under four categories.

The "Individual" domain screens for conduct, attitudinal, and social problems, as well as mental health issues. The "Individual-Group" domain evaluates the subject's group-based identity and commitment to the group, role in the group, and attitude toward outsiders.

The "Group" domain considers the group's cohesiveness, leadership structure, values, and its history of violence, and the "Group-Societal" domain draws on four items that examine how the group functions juxtaposed against conventional society. Logan and Sellers[60] describe the MLG as "a robust set of structured professional guidance for understanding violence within groups . . . [that] has obvious relevance to violent extremists." The authors note, however, that the tool's application to violent terrorist groups has yet to be substantially tested.

RISK ASSESSMENT SCALES FOR LONE-ACTOR TERRORISM

The Terrorist Radicalization Assessment Protocol

The TRAP-18,[8] is "an investigative template and organizing tool to help counterterrorism threat assessors prioritize cases for monitoring and risk assessment." Unlike the various tools to assess risk of extremism and terrorism in affiliated individuals discussed in the preceding sections, TRAP-18's focus is targeted threat by an individual. It was empirically developed drawing on a study of available literature on lone actors over 15 years and the author's practice and research. Meloy et al.,[61] in fact, disqualify the TRAP-18 as a risk assessment tool given limitations in its scientific foundation and instead characterize it as more of an investigative template to assist in the management of threats associated with lone actors. The TRAP-18 looks at 8 "proximal warning behaviors" to correlate patterns of behavior with the risk for violence as well as 10 dynamic "distal factors" associated with lone actors. To our knowledge, it is the first and only tool within the psychiatric toolbox that derives its actuarial composition from the attributes of lone actors as opposed to those who are part of, associated with, or act at the behest of a group. To increase the usefulness and acuity of the TRAP-18, its authors have recommended that use of the tool be combined with rating the individual on either the VERA-2 R or the MLG 2.[59] The TRAP-18 is discussed in more depth in chapter 24.

PRACTICAL APPLICATIONS

To avoid potentially leaving readers with a sense of disconnect—not knowing which process and tool(s) to use in what circumstances—we offer the following practical recommendations.

As a fundamental first step—perhaps an obvious one, dictated by circumstances alone—the situation itself will prescribe whether assessors are in a threat assessment or risk assessment mode. The latter category often presumes the availability of a subject of variable cooperation. In the threat assessment stream, antithetically, the subject likely does not even know that his every movement and interaction are under the watchful eyes of law enforcement or anti-terrorism experts, often with input of behavioral sciences expertise. Consequently, threat assessments tend to occur in the background, out of the subject's awareness. Perhaps the investigative team, drawing on documentary information obtained, observations made, and collateral information, has rated the degree of the subject's fundamentalist leanings using a tool like the ATRS[43] and then, to assess the extent of the subject's preparedness to migrate from thought to action, rated the level of threat he poses using the TRAP-18[8] combined with rating the individual on either the VERA-2 R[20] or the MLG 2,[59] as the TRAP-18 suggests.

The process and pathway are different if the task is a risk assessment for either sentencing or subsequent release from custody or parole purposes. In these cases, and again subject to the defendant's/inmate's cooperation, the larger clinical evaluation model described earlier is appropriate. Since threat has been contained, the TRAP-18 is of less benefit, even in the case of a lone actor to be sentenced or released.

The assessor should then—in their distillation of all the information gathered (which would include mental health and behavioral observations and tests carried out while the defendant has been in custody)—draw on a combination of both broad-based and terrorism-specific tools. It is common practice in Canada in any risk assessment scenario to score the subject on the PCL-R,[26] the implications of which were discussed earlier. PCL-R scores are, among other things and to variable degrees, drawn on a rating risk for violence in the short-term and longer-term using the HCR-20 V3[34] (or SAVRY,[38] in the case of youth) or the VRAG,[32] respectively. The next steps of inquiry that the risk assessment could include are measures of fundamentalist attitude (e.g., using the RRFS[42]), the degree of radicalized outlook (e.g., using the ATRS[43]), and finally, a measure of terrorism-specific risk using tools like the ERG22+[47] and/or the VERA-2 R.[20]

CONCLUSION

Although lone-actor terrorism is not a new phenomenon, there has unfortunately been relatively little research carried out on this type of offender. Assessing risk for violence in everyday criminals is well-established and there are, in fact, a number of tools available to appraise extent of extremist ideology and preparedness for action in affiliated terrorists. Lone-actor terrorists share many features in common with affiliated terrorists but appear to be a distinct group from a phenomenological, psychological, social, and demographic perspective. There are various degrees of "loneness." Some lone actors remain entirely disconnected from any individual or network and conceive of their hoped-for terrorist act as a function of their imagination, individual psychology, adverse life experiences, shortcomings in goal fulfillment, and the influences of a plethora of internet-based materials and inspirations. It appears that the internet is the ether within which many lone actors swim. Lone actors are difficult to detect and seem to be responsible for considerably more loss of life and other damage than are affiliated terrorists. As it stands at present, there are no scientifically validated tools to appraise risk in lone actors. The TRAP-18 does not define itself as a risk appraisal tool, and, in essence, it is more of a management template to identify and deal with real-time threats posed by lone actors of any kind. Notwithstanding shortcomings in available technology, assessors are encouraged to stay true to the forensic mental health model of thinking about and appraising risk. The approach is highly investigative and thorough, and it entails the gathering and minute consideration of an abundance of diverse information from multiple sources. Existing extremist/terrorist appraisal guides described in this chapter, although created principally for affiliated terrorists, provide guidance, wisdom, and a template for approaching the task and/or the distillation of the information gathered.

NOTES AND REFERENCES

1. Dugas M, Belanger, JJ, Moyano, M, et al. The quest for significance motivates self-sacrifice. *Motivation Science.* 2016;2(1):15–32.
2. Russell CA, Miller, BH. Profile of a terrorist. *Terrorism.* 1997;1(1): 17–34.
3. Hoffman JS. World report on violence and health. In Krug EG, Dahlberg LL, Mercy JA, Zvi AB, Lozano R, eds. Geneva: World Health Organization; 2002, 2003:93. https://injuryprevention.bmj.com/content/9/1/93.1.short
4. Cook AN, Hart SD, Krupp PR. Multi-level guidelines for the assessment and management of group-based violence, Version 1. Burnaby, CAN: Mental Health, Law, & Policy Institute, Simon Fraser University; 2013.
5. Hamilton M. A threat assessment framework for lone-actor terrorists. *Florida Law Rev.* 2018;70(6):1319–1356.
6. Singh J, Grann M, Fazel S. A comparative study of violence risk assessment tools: A systemic review and metaregression analysis of 68 studies involving 25,980 participants. *Clin Psychol Rev.* 2011;31(3):499–513.
7. Kebbell MR, Porter L. An intelligence assessment framework for identifying individuals at risk of committing acts of violent extremism against the west. *Security J.* 2011;1–17.
8. Meloy JR. Users' manual for the terrorist radicalization assessment protocol (TRAP-18). *Multihealth Systems.* 2017.
9. Bloom H, Schneider, R. *Mental Disorder and the Law: A Primer for Legal and Mental Health Professionals.* 2nd edition. Toronto: Irwin Law; 2017.
10. Logan C, Lloyd M. Violent extremism: A comparison of approaches to assessing and managing risk. *Legal Criminol Psychol.* 2019;24(1):141–161.
11. Stone AA. Psychiatry and the law. In Nicholi AM, ed., *The Harvard Guide to Psychiatry.* 3rd edition. Cambridge, MA: Harvard University Press; 1999.
12. Bloom H, Webster C. Assessing imminent risks for violence and threats. In Bloom H and Schneider RD, eds., *Law and Mental Disorder: A Comprehensive and Practical Approach.* Toronto: Irwin Law; 2013.
13. Dernevik M, Beck A, Grann M, et al. The use of psychiatric and psychological evidence in the assessment of terrorist offenders. *J Forensic Psychiatry Psychol.* 2009;20:508–515.
14. Horgan J. Interviewing the terrorists: Reflections on fieldwork and implications for psychological research. *Behav Sci Terrorism Political Aggression.* 2012;4(3):195–211.
15. Taylor M, Horgan J. A conceptual framework for addressing psychological processes in the development of the terrorist. *Terrorism Political Violence.* 2006;18:586–601.
16. Rahman T, Zhang L, Meloy JR. DSM-5 cultural and personality assessment of extreme overvalued beliefs (in press). *Aggression Violent Behav.* 2021. doi.org/10.1016/j.avb.2021.101552. https://www.sciencedirect.com/science/article/pii/S1359178921000069

17. Hamilton M. Risk assessment tools in the criminal legal system: Theory and practice: A resource guide. National Association of Criminal Defense Lawyers, Nov 2020. https://www.nacdl.org/Document/RiskAssessmentReport

18. Borum R. Assessing risk for terrorism involvement. *J Threat Assess Manage*. 2015;2:63–87.

19. Smith AG. Risk factors and indicators associated with radicalization to terrorism in the United States: What research sponsored by the National Institute of Justice tells us. National Institute of Justice: U.S. Department of Justice. 1 Jun 2018. https://nij.ojp.gov/library/publications/risk-factors-and-indicators-associated-radicalization-terrorism-united-states

20. Hart SD, Cook AN, Pressman DE, et al. *A Concurrent Evaluation of Threat Assessment Tools for the Individual Assessment of Terrorism*. Waterloo, ONT: Canadian Network for Research on Terrorism, Security, and Society; 2017:1–63.

21. Pressman DE, Flockton J. Calibrating risk for violent political extremism and terrorists: The VERA 2 structured assessment. *Br J Forensic Pract*. 2012;14:237–251.

22. Borum R. Psychological vulnerabilities and propensities for involvement in violent extremism. *Behav Sci Law*. 2014;32(3):286–305.

23. Corner E, Gill P. A false dichotomy? Mental illness and lone-actor terrorism. *Law Hum Behav*. 2015;39(1):23–34.

24. Gill P, Corner E, McKee A, et al. What do closed source data tell us about lone-actor terrorist behavior? A research note. *Terrorism Political Violence*. 2019. https://www.tandfonline.com/doi/abs/10.1080/09546553.2019.1668781?casa_token=9qFcYtMaje4AAAAA:CEPonEW0csg_v67sXBHH0tMoe-glZI-WZBFioiEx3ZF5O0AG-NqXZ0a9WALkt07D1n7DvIcoZ7lB9

25. Otto RK. Assessing and managing violence risk in outpatient settings. *J Clin Psychol*. 2000;56:1239–1262.

26. Hare RD. The *Psychopathy Checklist–Revised*. 2nd edition. Toronto: Multi-Health Systems; 2003.

27. Monahan J, Steadman H, Silver E, et al. *Rethinking Risk Assessment: The MacArthur Study of Mental Disorder and Violence*. New York: Oxford University Press; 2001.

28. Webster CD, Dassinger C, Bloom H. The systematic assessment of risk for aggressive and violent behavior against others. In Bloom H, Schneider RD, eds., *Law and Mental Disorder: A Comprehensive and Practical Approach*. Toronto: Irwin Law; 2013.

29. Hart SD, Cox, DN, Hare, RD. *Manual for the Hare Psychopathy Checklist: Screening Version*. Toronto: Multi-Health Systems, Inc.; 1995.

30. Hare RD, Harpur TJ, Hakstian, AR, et al. The revised psychopathy checklist: reliability and factor structure. *Psychol Assess*. 1990;2(3):338.

31. Forth AE, Kosson D, Hare, RD. *The Hare Psychopathy Checklist: Youth Version*. Toronto: Multi-Health Systems; 2003.

32. Quinsley VL, Harris GT, Rice ME, et al. *Violent Offenders: Appraising and Managing Risk*. Washington, DC: American Psychological Association; 1998.

33. Webster CD, Douglas KS, Eaves D, et al. *HCR-20 Assessing Risk for Violence Version 2*. Burnaby, BC: Simon Fraser University, Mental Health Law and Policy Institute; 1995.

34. Douglas KS, Hart SD, Webster CD et al. *HCR-20-V3: Assessing Risk for Violence: User Guide*. Burnaby, BC: Simon Fraser University, Mental Health Law and Policy Institute; 2013.

35. Douglas KS, Hart SD, Webster CD, et al. Historical-clinical-risk management-20, Version 3 (HCR-20-V3): Development and overview. *Intl J Forensic Mental Health*. 2014;13(2):93–108.

36. Douglas KS, Kropp, PR. A prevention-based paradigm for violence risk assessment: Clinical and research applications. *Crim Justice Behav*. 2002;29(5) 617–658.

37. Mossman D. Understanding prediction instruments. Textbook of forensic psychiatry. 2004: 501–523.

38. Borum R, Bartel P, Forth AE. *SAVRY, Structured Assessment of Violence Risk in Youth: Professional Manual*. Lutz, FL: Psychological Assessment Resources, Inc.; 2006.

39. Lodewijks HP, Doreleijers TA, de Ruiter C, et al. Predictive validity of the Structured Assessment of Violence Risk in Youth (SAVRY) during residential treatment. *Intl J Law Psychiatry*. 2008;31(3):263–271. https://doi.org/10.1016/j.ijlp.2008.04.009

40. Liht J, Conway LG, Savage S, et al. Religious fundamentalism: An empirically derived construct and measurement scale. *Arch Psychol Relig*. 2011;33:299–323.

41. Altemeyer B, Hunsberger B. Authoritarianism, religious fundamentalism, quest, and prejudice. *Intl J Psychol Religion*. 1992;2(2):113–133.

42. Altemeyer B, Hunsberger B. A Revised Religious Fundamentalism Scale: The short and sweet of it. *Intl J Psychol Religion*. 2004;14(1):47–54.

43. Loza W. *The Assessment and Treatment of Radicalization Scale*. Unpublished manuscript. 2007.

44. Loza W, Youssef A, Johan P, et al. The prevalence of extreme Middle Eastern ideologies around the world. *J Interpersonal Violence*. 2011;26(3):522–538.

45. Saucier G, Akers LG, Shen-Miller S, Kneževié, G, Stankov, L. Patterns of thinking in militant extremism. *Perspect Psychol Sci*. 2009;4(3):256–271.

46. Kebbell MR, Porter L. An intelligence assessment framework for identifying individuals at risk of committing acts of violent extremism against the west. *Security J*. 2011;1–17.

47. Lloyd M, Dean C. The development of structured guidelines for assessing risk in extremist offenders. *J Threat Assess Manage*. 2015;2(1):40–52.

48. Lloyd M. *Extremist Risk Assessment: A Directory*. Lancaster, UK: Centre for Research and Evidence on Security Threats; 2009.

49. RTI International. Countering violent extremism: The application of risk assessment tools in the criminal justice and rehabilitation process. Literature review. Prepared for First Responders Group, Department of Homeland Security, Science and Technology Directorate, 1 Feb 2018. https://www.google.com/url?sa=t&rct=j&q=&esrc=s&source=web&cd=&ved=2ahUKEwiqlOyJ2aruAhVwF1kFHdAzB04QFjABegQIAhAC&url=https%3A%2F%2Fwww.dhs.gov%2Fsites%2Fdefault%2Ffiles%2Fpublications%2FOPSR_TP_CVE-Application-Risk-Assessment-Tools-Criminal-Rehab-Process_2018Feb-508.pdf&usg=AOvVaw3YWEgjD4JJ-InNSEHF43tBH

50. Webster S, Kerr J, Tompkins C. A process evaluation of the structured risk guidance for extremist offenders. HM Prison and Probation Service, 2017. https://www.google.com/url?sa=t&rct=j&q=&esrc=s&source=web&cd=&ved=2ahUKEwiC8NiHmfTuAhUHEFkFHT3XC44QFjAAegQIAxAD&url=https%3A%2F%2Fassets.publishing.service.gov.uk%2Fgovernment%2Fuploads%2Fsystem%2Fuploads%2Fattachment_data%2Ffile%2F661787%2Fprocess-evaluation-srg-extremist-offender-report.pdf&usg=AOvVaw11mEMjUJNwE-vKjj5MOigl

51. Kuznar L, Jafri A, Kuznar E. Dealing with radicalization in IDP camps. NSI Reachback Report, Feb 2020. https://nsiteam.com/social/wp-content/uploads/2020/02/NSI-Reachback_B5_Dealing-with-Radicalization-in-IDP-Camps_Feb2020_Final.pdf

52. van der Heide L, van der Zwan M, van Leyenhorst M. The Practitioner's Guide to the Galaxy: A Comparison of Risk Assessment Tools for Violent Extremism. Amsterdam: International Centre for Counter-terrorism (ICCT); 2019:3.

53. Monahan J, Skeem JL. The evolution of violence risk assessment. *CNS Spectrums*. 2014;19(5):419–424.

54. Scarcella A, Page R, Furtado V. Terrorism, radicalization, extremism, authoritarianism and fundamentalism: A systemic review of the quality and psychometric properties of assessments. *PLoS ONE*. 2016;11(12):1–19.

55. Clemmow C, Schumann S, Salman NL, et al. The base rate study: Developing base rates for risk factors and indicators for engagement in violent extremism. *J Forensic Sci*. 2020;65(3):865–881.

56. Herzog-Evans M. A comparison of two structured professional judgment tools for violent extremism and their relevance in the French context. *Eur J Probation*. 2018;10(1):3–27.

57. Meloy RJ, Gill P. The lone-actor terrorist and the TRAP-18. *J Threat Assess Manage*. 2016;3(1):37–52.

58. Dean G, Pettit G. The 3 R's of risk assessment for violent extremism. *J Forensic Pract*. 2017;19(2):91–101.

59. Lee, V. Risk domains and factors of the Multi-Level Guidelines: An updated examination of their support in the literature. PhD diss., Arts & Social Sciences: Department of Psychology, 2019.

60. Logan C, Sellers R. Risk assessment and management in violent extremism: A primer for mental health practitioners. *J Forensic Psychiatry Psychol*. 2021;32(3):355–377. https://doi.org/10.1080/14789949.2020.1859591

61. Meloy JR, Roshdi K, Glaz-Ocik J et al. Investigating the individual terrorist in Europe. *J Threat Assess Manage*. 2015;2:140–152. doi:https://doi.org/10.1037/tam0000036.

26

Developing a Risk Assessment and Intervention Strategy

Future Directions in Research and Practice

JACOB C. HOLZER, ANDREA J. DEW,
*PATRICIA R. RECUPERO, AND PAUL GILL**

INTRODUCTION

This chapter reviews some of the salient topics discussed in this volume, along with two predominant events which occurred during its writing—the COVID pandemic and the Capitol insurrection in Washington, DC—as a basis from which to consider future directions in this area. A number of important foci in lone-actor terrorism, such as pre-attack behaviors, social media, weapons, laws addressing hate and domestic terrorism, prosocial measures, coordination between professions, insider-threat management, and the use of propaganda, all provide opportunity for proactive intervention and future research.

SALIENT ISSUES EXAMINED IN THIS BOOK

Defining Lone-Actor Terrorism

As noted in this text, one of the primary difficulties in studying and understanding lone-actor terrorism is the lack of an international scholarly consensus regarding its definition.[1-3] Many incidents which could be characterized as lone-actor terrorism in that they were perpetrated by an individual are nonetheless connected in some way to more organized hate groups or political groups through the internet. Furthermore, a perpetrator's motive is often complicated; attacks that seem at first to be ideologically motivated—for example, because the perpetrator had shared anti-government views online—may in fact be more disorganized violence, perhaps motivated by poorly controlled paranoia and delusional beliefs.

Describing someone as a "terrorist" or characterizing an incident as "terrorism" (as opposed to some other form of violence) is a decision that carries political and social implications. Defining terrorism—what it is and what it is not—can be, and often is, politically tinged, which carries ethical implications. For the purposes of this book, we have understood terrorism to be "linked to a radicalized or extremist cause or ideology" (i.e., distinct from mass killings without ideology, such as crimes thought to be due to mental illness, momentary rage without ideology, or acts of unknown etiology). The definition of a domestic "terrorist" used by Smith and colleagues in Chapter 17, reviewing US legal aspects is focused on the intended outcome, not the perpetrator's motivation: "whether a person is a terrorist depends not on the beliefs that motivate them to act, but rather whether they intend the action to intimidate or coerce the government or the civilian population." The line between terrorism and hate crimes is often blurred.

Complexity

Another chief difficulty in studying lone-actor terrorism is its complexity. The lone-actor terrorist's motives are often muddied, frequently

---

* The opinions in this chapter are those of the chapter authors and not that of the US Navy War College or the Department of Defense.

combining political or religious ideology with a personal grievance, particularly in recent years. Such grievances often lead the person to find "online sympathizers."[4] Often "lone" actors are not entirely *alone*[5]: as Hamm and Ayers note in Chapter 1, on historical aspects, many lone actors identify or sympathize with extremist groups. Other scholars have noted that "social ties play a crucial role throughout the process leading from ideological radicalization to the planning and preparation of terrorist attacks."[5] The complexity of many incidents of lone-actor terror warrants a multifaceted, multidisciplinary approach, underscoring the importance of involving experts from diverse professional backgrounds. Collaboration between professionals in different fields can help to improve our understanding of lone-actor terrorism and, ideally, improve our chances of intervening to lessen the risk of future attacks.

Lone-Actor Terrorism Offenders

There is no single unified profile of the lone-actor terrorist. Almost all perpetrators are male,[6] and many have a history of domestic violence. Lone actors are more likely than group-based terrorists to have mental health difficulties,[7] and many are self-recruited. Compared to other perpetrators of homicide, many perpetrators of lone-actor terrorism did not have a known prior history of violence and did not previously know their victims, although a subgroup of lone-actor terrorist offenders do have histories of violence and criminal convictions.[8] Target selection often involves subjects of ideological or symbolic significance,[8] such as military or police in the United States[4] and security forces in the European Union.[8] Weapons are often chosen on the basis of their availability, which partially explains the higher prevalence of firearms attacks in the United States and Canada than in other regions where firearms are less easily accessible. However, some offenders choose their weapons to emulate tactics deployed in previous attacks. Many lone-actor terrorists engage in long-term, detailed attack planning, potentially creating a large window of time during which threats might be detected, apprehended, and thwarted.[6,9]

Contagion

A desire to emulate or outdo previous lone-actor terror attack characterizes many incidents today. Hamm and Ayers, Drogin, and other authors in this text describe the phenomenon of copycat attacks, noting that many lone-actor terrorists are inspired by and act in imitation of previous offenders,[10] including in their choice of weapons, down to the specific *type* of firearm chosen for an attack.[11] Some lone actors today draw inspiration from numerous previous attacks, and each incident can have a long-term compounded effect on future attacks. Our knowledge of the phenomenon of copycat attacks raises some important ethical issues to consider. Chief among these is the role of media outlets and the potential for news coverage to increase or decrease the risk of future attacks. Clearly, reporting crimes is an important responsibility of the press, but excessive media coverage of an incident, particularly coverage that humanizes, glorifies, or sympathizes with the perpetrator, is likely to inspire future lone-actor terrorists, many of whom recognize the value of media coverage for amplifying whatever message they hope to send through their violent act.[12] As Kushner and Candilis note in Chapter 14, on ethical aspects, detailed media coverage of the Isla Vista rampage in 2014 led more isolated young men with grievances into incel communities online and may have played a role in inspiring subsequent terror incidents, such as the Toronto van attack in 2018.

The Internet and Technology

Although there are variables that differ considerably between different lone-actor terror attacks, one thread that runs through most such attacks in recent years is the vital role of the internet and communications technology. As several chapters in this volume have noted, technology and the internet are of vital importance to the phenomenon of lone-actor terrorism today. The use of the internet and social media by the Islamic State of Iraq and al-Sham (ISIS) has been so extensive that it was dubbed a "cyber caliphate." As Hassan and colleagues explain in Chapter 19, on online indoctrination, there are striking similarities in the ways which cults and extremist communities online attract and groom new members. Involvement in an extremist community, even if only online, can help to fulfill the vulnerable individual's basic social need to belong. The way in which extremist propaganda has evolved can be traced back through technological changes throughout history. Just as the films of Leni Riefenstahl played a major role in the twentieth century, today's advanced technology such as deepfakes stand to transform what we think of as propaganda.

With respect to extremist propaganda online, full eradication through censorship seems unlikely. Although some countries, such as China, have attempted to eliminate citizens' exposure to extremist materials in this way, such restrictions of individuals' rights run afoul of civil liberties protections in the United States and many other jurisdictions. Drogin, in Chapter 8, on propaganda, also notes the tendency of internet-based content to repopulate and reappear under other domain names and other accounts, a phenomenon that some have dubbed the "whack-a-mole" problem[13]: as soon as a video or other violent content is posted online, it is often shared and retweeted almost instantaneously again and again by third parties across the web and social media. In other words, "once it's out there, it's out there." Such is the case with the writings and videos of extremists like Anwar al-Awlaki, whose views repopulate and persist online to inspire future lone-actor terrorists.

The internet and social media today are frequently used as means to communicate terrorist intent. The social media accounts of lone-actor terrorists frequently contain leakage of violent fantasies and plans and other warning signs that can help to identify credible threats. The development of linguistic analysis—particularly linguistic inquiry and word count analysis software—and sophisticated tools like artificial intelligence and predictive analytics show promise for the possibility of identifying lone-actor terrorists prospectively through their language. The predominant complication and challenge for technology and law enforcement is sorting out the very small number of potential lone actors with intent from the much larger group of individuals who interact on social media with no intent to act.

Leakage of Intent

Many, if not most, lone-actor terrorists engage in some form of attack signaling, intent broadcasting, or other forms of leakage of violent intentions. Lone offenders often exhibit pre-attack behaviors that are observed by bystanders close to the person. Many lone-actor terrorists share a common trajectory toward violence, which can be helpful in developing intervention and counterterrorism strategies. Sinai, in Chapter 23 on countering terrorism during the pre-incident phase, describes a model containing eight stages in a pathway-to-violence trajectory: Triggers, Cognitive Opening, Violent Ideation/ Fantasy, Threshold into Violence, Planning, Preparation, Approach, and Attack. Leakage of violent intent or other warning sign behaviors may be noticeable to others during several phases of this trajectory. The lone-actor terrorist's intent is often known or suspected by those close to them, such as relatives, work colleagues, and close friends.

Difficulties for Investigation and Prevention

Despite these encouraging developments, lone-actor terrorism poses significant difficulties for investigation and prevention. The statistical rarity of lone-actor terror incidents makes prediction of these events nearly impossible, and variables associated with other forms of violence, such as substance abuse, are often absent in the lone-actor terrorist. The troubling finding that 75% of lone-actor terrorists between 2001 and early 2020 were successful in carrying out their attacks and evading detection illustrates the dire need for improved strategies for investigation and prevention. Some lone-actor terrorists, such as the "Mad Bomber" and Unabomber in the twentieth century, have been able to carry out multiple attacks before being apprehended despite the dedication of large investigative teams that had been assigned to their cases. By definition, lone-actor terrorists act alone, so detection through infiltration of terrorist organizations is unlikely to be effective against lone-actor incidents.

The finding that 40% of right-wing extremists were detected or apprehended by chance suggests that there is both need and room for improvement in detection methods.[14] Furthermore, some investigation tactics have come under criticism for their infringement on civil liberties or their other ethical implications. For example, widespread covert surveillance of civilian populations runs counter to human rights principles, and the use of informants to investigate potential suspects in religious organizations has raised concerns of entrapment as well as infringement of citizens' civil liberties, such as freedom of assembly and religious liberty. Several structured approaches show promise for improving investigation of potential lone-actor terrorists. Behavioral threat assessment and management (BTAM) or threat assessment and management (TAM), for example, can be helpful, and standardized tools such as the Terrorist Radicalization Assessment Protocol (TRAP-18) may help to identify missed opportunities for prevention when a future lone-actor terrorist's behavior changes in a way that is (or would be) noticeable to their coworkers and others close to them.

Legal Issues

This text discusses legal approaches to lone-actor terrorism, including its prosecution and laws governing the boundaries of appropriate investigative techniques. Prosecutions of lone-actor terrorists who have been apprehended have been successful at both the federal and state levels, and terrorist acts may be charged as murder, attempted murder, arson, or assault. Additional laws have been passed prohibiting the provision of financial or material support to terrorists. Other charges might include use of weapons of mass destruction, unauthorized possession of weapons, and interfering with citizens' access to services, such as abortion or voting. Following the terrorist attacks of September 11, 2001, the United States passed regulations that allowed for increased and potentially invasive surveillance of civilians in the hopes of deterring future attacks. Such laws have been controversial due to the risk of infringement on private citizens' civil rights, but many laws with sunset provisions have been repeatedly extended or reauthorized. Questions about what constitutes an unreasonable search and seizure in violation of the Fourth Amendment of the US Constitution have been complicated due to the importance of digital and electronic evidence. In general, US laws protecting civil liberties, such as the Bill of Rights and freedom-of-speech protections, have limited potential avenues for prosecuting lone-actor terrorists or would-be lone actors. In the United Kingdom, there are laws allowing for the prosecution and conviction for actions that may not be illegal in the United States. For example, mere acquisition or possession of a bomb-making manual or mere membership in an organization deemed to be "terrorist" would not, in itself, be illegal in the United States.

Trends Over Time

The book discusses trends over time in lone-actor terrorism cases. Hamm and Ayers in Chapter 1 the history of lone-actor terrorism back to the nineteenth Century, while Meloy et al. in the chapter reviewing the TRAP-18 argue that it dates to Biblical times,[15] with its more recent history commencing around the late 1800s. Smith and colleagues Chapter 17 on US legal aspects note that four US presidents have been assassinated by lone actors, and the actions of lone-actor terrorists have been lauded as martyrs among their supporters as far back as the early 1900s. One common thread over time is the way in which acts of lone-actor terror inspire future attacks. Although terrorism has existed for centuries, it was often prosecuted under general criminal statutes until the 1990s, when the United States began passing terrorism-specific legislation. Drogin (Chapter 8) discusses the history of propaganda and its role in lone-actor terrorism, including the notion of "propaganda by deed," which today has shifted toward expression on the internet and social media.

Finally, several chapters have noted recent trends, such as the important influence of ISIS in shaping lone-actor terrorism after 2013 and the growth in hate-driven violence against members of racial or religious minority groups. Conspiracy theories appear to be growing in importance as motivating factors for lone-actor terrorists in recent years, due in part to the ease and speed with which they are spread and shared through social media. Individual lone-actor terrorist attacks can significantly influence future attacks. To cite only one example, vehicle-ramming attacks were relatively rare until an incident in Canada in 2014 that garnered a great deal of attention, after which such attacks by vehicle grew more common. Another recent development to note is the shift of extremists toward encrypted internet communications channels. Where formerly extremists organized openly on Facebook and Twitter, many now rely on encrypted messaging apps such as Gab and Telegram, making it harder for law enforcement investigators to detect them and monitor their communications.[16,17]

Ethical Issues

Addressing lone-actor terrorism and its prevention is an exercise fraught with ethical dilemmas. Often, security risks must be balanced against individual civil liberties. Predictive analytics and preventive policing pose intriguing questions: If a risk-assessment algorithm identifies someone as "likely" to commit a violent crime, what can or should be done? Such a risk score is not sufficient; the police cannot arrest an individual on the basis of probable future behavior when a crime has not been committed. Attempts to prosecute individuals who were intercepted while in the process of preparing an attack often failed in the United Kingdom. With risk screening comes the potential for a large number of false positives; many individuals whose behaviors arouse concern in others are not, and do not become, violent. Limited resources are another factor that may generate ethical dilemmas: police departments do not always have sufficient personnel or time to follow through exhaustively on every potential threat.

A number of important ethical issues relate to the US Bill of Rights and citizens' civil liberties. For example, propaganda, including sophisticated deepfake videos, can be extremely effective online in terms of radicalizing a vulnerable person; however, removing such content runs into freedom-of-speech protections. The First Amendment also protects freedom of assembly, which may include assembly via social media and the internet, particularly during times of pandemic lockdowns. The government's use of the "Third-Party Doctrine" to gain access to personal communications and information represents another ethical issue that may arise.

CONTEMPORARY EVENTS AND IMPACT ON LONE-ACTOR TERRORISM

In January 2021, US Department of Homeland Defense (DHS) officials authorities published their assessment of extremism and violence in the United States, noting that "Throughout 2020, Domestic Violent Extremists (DVEs) targeted individuals with opposing views engaged in First Amendment-protected, non-violent protest activity. DVEs motivated by a range of issues, including anger over COVID-19 restrictions, the 2020 election results, and police use of force have plotted and on occasion carried out attacks against government facilities."[18,19]

Many of the chapters in this book consider the role of foreign terrorist movements, including the violent Salafist jihadi movements led by and inspired by the al-Qaeda and ISIS groups and their influence over what the DHS described as "Homegrown Violent Extremists (HVEs) inspired by foreign terrorist groups, who committed three attacks targeting government officials in 2020."[18] The emphasis by the DHS on the DVE threat, however, was in partial response to the Capitol Riot in Washington, DC, on January 6, 2021, which also reanimated a broader conversation in the United States about DVE movements. Five people died during the attack, including Capitol Police Officer Brian D. Sicknick; a US air force veteran who had entered the building with the rioters; and three other people who died from medical-related issues.[20]

Based on the FBI indictments and convictions to date, the people who stormed the US Capitol after listening to President Trump's speech, in order to disrupt or prevent Vice President Pence's confirmation of the 2020 election results, showed all the characteristics of twenty-first-century terrorist in terms of message, messenger, media, and organization. First, they were comprised of a spectrum of organization types: from highly organized groups—some wearing an identifying color or garment to signify their group identity—to lose affiliates, and unaffiliated individuals who were inspired by social media. Some of the key social media platforms that helped to organize and inspire

participants have been identified in other chapters as central to the propagation of extremist views: from QAnon's conspiracy theories, to extremist Facebook groups, to Reddit and 4Chan message boards. Participants used Twitter and recorded videos of themselves storming the Capitol, which they posted to social media sites.

The FBI took the jurisdictional lead in bringing charges against more than 100 people in the Capitol Riot for a range of charges that include unlawful entry of a federal building all the way to "assaulting, resisting, or impeding certain officers using a dangerous weapon."[21] In a press release from the 100th day after the riot, the FBI detailed the guilty plea of one of the rioters, which noted the linkages to an organization (the Oath Keepers) and assigned the press release topics as related to "Counter-terrorism" and "National Security."[22] Additional arrests also cited membership of another organized group (the Proud Boys) that Canada subsequently designated a terrorist organization and banned in February 2021.[23,24]

The Southern Poverty Law Center (SPLC) has a detailed examination of the linkages between the founder of the Proud Boys and alt-right (alternative right-wing) movements and publications. In particular, the SPLC emphasizes the role of social media, podcasting, and radio talk shows to connect the underlying ideology of the Proud Boys to a wider audience. One of the strategies used by the Proud Boys leaders is to claim a more innocuous identity based on grievances (the undermining of their version of white masculinity) that attracts a broader audience base, coupled with guest spots on radio talk shows that invite more outspoken alt-right figures to air their views. This bait-and-switch approach to recruitment and propagation is not without risks: at the "Unite the Right" rally in Charlottesville, Virginia, in August 2017, which was organized by a member of the Proud Boys group, a protestor, who identified with the boogaloo alt-right movement, drove his car into the crowds, killing one woman and injuring many other people in the crowds.[25] In the aftermath, the group attempted to distance themselves from the incident, but leaders continued to speak about the need for violence, particularly against the anti-fascist movements (antifa) from 2018 onward, that counter-protested rallies across the United States.[26]

In the aftermath of the 2021 Capitol Riot, new attention has been paid to the rise of far-right terrorism globally. As early as 2011, researchers using data from the SPLC and the Klan Watch argued that of the more than 6,000 far-right groups in the United States, the use of violence was not the norm (around 20% had members who had used violence) but that "Groups that had charismatic leaders, or advocated for leaderless resistance tactics or used leaderless resistance tactics were significantly more likely to be involved in violence."[27]

The DHS Bulletin also noted the role of COVID-19 restrictions in polarizing and inspiring violent actions.[18,28] In fall 2020, the US Attorney's Office for Western Michigan charged six people with conspiracy to kidnap Michigan Governor Gretchen Whitmer who had been vociferously criticized by Michigan Republican politicians and President Donald Trump for her COVID-19 restrictions.[29] The six defendants, whom the indictment described as "Wolverine Watchmen, a Michigan-based self-styled 'militia' group" trained in Wisconsin to carry out the kidnapping and were arrested on October 7, 2020, by an undercover FBI agent.[29]

The Network Contagion Research Institute (NCRI) noted in early 2021 the confluence between alt-right views and anti-vaccination views that was creating a new focus for domestic extremists. In their report, *A Contagion of Institutional Distrust: Viral Disinformation of the COVID Vaccine and the Road to Reconciliation*, they note that *deplatforming*—the removal of groups or individuals from social media such as Facebook and Twitter—was pushing these extremist views into private platforms such as Telegram and onto the DarkWeb.[30,31]

If tracing and tracking DVE groups has become more difficult, the NCRI report also notes the confluence of factors that may serve as proxies for understanding where and when the radicalization process is taking place. By running regression analysis overlaid on geographical maps of the United States, researchers identified 30 geographical hotspots of alt-right conspiracy theory activity. Those factors included the presence of aggressive and sometimes violent anti-Black Lives Matters protests; the perceived severity of public health COVID-19 restrictions, including mask-wearing laws; and Google searches for the term "New World Order." While this current overlap between different conspiracy theories may not persist, it is worth noting that DVE groups continue to evolve and refine their organizations, their social media strategies, and their messages to embrace new fissures and divides in our societies.

Finally, as we consider the future of terrorism and its ability to attract lone actors to its methods

and messages, it is important to note that this is not an American phenomena: The disruptive effects of COVID-19 restrictions were also noted by Interpol in December 2020, in a bulletin in which they warned that "Terrorists—like all criminals—have sought to profit from COVID-19, to make money, strengthen their base and to fuel division."[32] In particular, Interpol singled out "attempts by far-right violent extremists to radicalize social movements, such as clashing with far-left groups and/or provoking the use of force."[32]

AREAS FOR PROACTIVE INTERVENTION

As emphasized throughout this volume, lone-actor terrorism is a complex, multidimensional concept. In the world of radicalization and extremism, use of social media, clinical variables, maladjustment, and limited resources and choices, some individuals are prone to commit violence, potentially resulting in mass causalities. In many cases, a number of variables come together, providing law enforcement with a basis to investigate and intervene proactively, although unfortunately, some individuals slip through the cracks. This section, not meant to be all-inclusive, outlines some relevant major categories where opportunities for intervention at the "macro" level exist that could lead to lowering the lone-actor (and organized) terrorism risk.

Pre-Attack States, Behaviors, and Warnings

Research has shown a number of common pre-attack behavioral variables that may offer clues about some at-risk individuals. Gill et al. described a set of pre-event behaviors in some individuals, including a religious and/or ideological belief intensification, a change of address, a change in employment status, or an intensification in external stressors. Some individuals experienced being the target of prejudice, being disrespected, or victimized.[6] In many cases others knew something about the offender's grievance, intent, beliefs, or extremist ideology prior to the event or planned event.[6] Gill et al.'s research results point to a number of other findings that could lead to proactive interventions, including for those socially isolated or engaged in activities within a wider group or organization. Additionally, there were discernable differences between the subgroups lone-actors identified with (i.e., extremist right-wing, single-issue, Islamist).

As is reviewed in chapters of this volume, use of the internet and social media in contemporary lone-actor violence is pervasive. The internet empowers and facilitates individuals to find other individuals with similar interests and ideologies and create networks internationally.[33] Research from RAND Europe showed a number of findings: (a) the internet creates more opportunities to become radicalized, (b) the internet acts as an "echo chamber," (c) the internet accelerates the process of radicalization, (d) the internet allows radicalization to occur without physical contact, and (e) the internet increases opportunities for self-radicalization.[34] Numerous functions of the internet have been identified, including (a) belief reinforcement, (b) seeking legitimacy, (c) broadcasting propaganda, (d) recruitment, and (e) attack signaling.[35] Balancing these pro-terrorism roles of the internet, engaging with others through the internet and social media can create opportunities for intelligence collection and counterterrorism. One article examining strategies for countering online radicalization discusses different approaches, reasoning that attempting to restrict freedom of speech and remove content from the internet may be the least desirable or effective; more effective approaches may include reducing the demand for radicalization and extremism in the longer term by encouraging social challenges to extremist narratives and promoting awareness and education in young people, along with shorter term exploitation of online communications for intelligence and evidence collection.[36]

The clinical "sphere" is another important concept—the presence of psychiatric or psychological symptoms, behaviors, and mental illness in some lone actors. A principle is that this relationship—lone-actor terrorism and mental illness—can be viewed as unidirectional: mental illness does not cause lone-actor terrorism, and people with mental illness are not disposed to terrorism. As reviewed in an earlier chapter, the medical literature does show some association with specific psychiatric diagnoses, substance abuse, and violence, but that finding is not equivalent to engaging in terrorism. Rather, research has shown an increased rate of mental illness in lone-actor terrorists when compared to terrorists who belong to a group[37] and that no one etiology or narrative can explain a lone-actor terrorist's drive and behavior. Instead, it is accepted in the literature that a convergence of different variables and factors, including psychiatric or psychological factors, can result in lone-actor violence

in some individuals. As outlined in an earlier chapter, preliminary research by one author (JH) reviewing high-profile lone-actor cases found numerous diverse clinical mental health variables in the sample, although this was in the context of a larger array of non-clinical variables which may factor into an individual's potential to act violently. Family members, friends, colleagues, etc., may recognize some of these variables in an individual, raising concern for the potential for violence and a possible opportunity to intervene proactively. In addition, state laws provide a basis for individuals who pose a direct risk of harm to themselves or others based on mental illness to be held on an emergency basis for psychiatric evaluation, which could theoretically allow for an intervention in a narrow set of circumstances, although there is variability between states on issues like duration, who originates the emergency hold, details regarding etiology, and patient rights.[38]

Social Media

Use of social media, as reviewed in this volume, is pervasive in the domains where extremism, ideology, rhetoric, and violence intersect. Although lone-actor terrorism existed long before the internet and social media, these platforms have resulted in the advancement of terrorism; a refinement in the radicalization process; increased capacity for socialization and networking; a foundation for recruitment, organization and planning; and a means to broadcast goals and intent, raise funds, and build support. As reviewed earlier, although attempts to remove content that may be inciteful or hateful may have limited success, social media companies can play an increasingly important role in monitoring content for potential correlation with ideologically related violence and interceding to block content from being uploaded or removing content when identified. As the political drama in the United States played out in the weeks before the presidential inauguration in January 2021, culminating in the mob attack on the Capitol, restrictions in the use of social media platforms such as Twitter could have resulted in a reduced risk of incitement and violence. An obvious important discussion in the social media context is the balance between restriction of hateful prejudiced content targeted at individuals and groups that could result in violence and freedom of speech. It should be apparent that people cannot just say whatever they want without any restriction or limitation when violence is a potential outcome. There are numerous legal references examining this debate in detail; these go beyond the scope of this text. However, one review article addressing hateful speech and the First Amendment indicates that under contemporary freedom of speech doctrine, the government may not prohibit or punish hateful, offensive speech unless it proves incitement—that the speaker intended to incite immediate lawless violence before a volatile crowd in a situation that makes violence a likely outcome.[39] Although one individual may be prone to act (lone actor), a "volatile crowd" could be interpreted as a broader group communicating in a hateful, offensive context on social media, and it would not be a stretch for some of that content to be inciteful.

A complexity in monitoring and interceding in social media is the potential high false-positive rate—the low base rate of individuals who will go on to commit violence among a much larger group of those who espouse bigotry and violence but will not go on to act. Artificial intelligence can assist in this process and holds promise for improving the ability to identify potential lone actors from a wider group of non-actors. But even with extremely accurate instruments and capacity, there will never be 100% accuracy, with no false-positives. Research by Kleinberg et al. on large-scale security processes (e.g., airport security and passenger screening) discussed that when the base rate is very low (as would be the case with social media use), even a highly accurate screening system can result in a large number of false positives (i.e., classification of ordinary users into the potential lone-actor group) and that a cascading filtering system of independent screening tools may address this problem.[40] The high false-positive risk can result in individuals who are innocent being targeted as a potential terrorist. In most democracies, societies would lean toward preventing innocent people from being accused with the risk of allowing potential violent actors to go free, rather than the reverse, as demonstrated by the high US legal standard of "beyond a reasonable doubt" in a criminal proceeding, higher than that found in the civil standard.

Firearms

The topic of firearms—rights, controls, types of weapons, availability, legal versus illegal purchase—is complex when applied to lone-actor terrorism. In part, this is due to the availability and variability in types of weapons used in terrorism incidents. Although assault weapons have been used in a large number of shooting cases (such as the 2015 San Bernardino shooting and the 2016 Orlando nightclub shooting), lone-actor terrorism cases have also involved other firearms (2017 Quebec City mosque shooting, 2009 Fort Hood shooting, 2015 Charleston church shooting), and, as stressed in this book, lone-actor terrorism is not confined to firearms: a number of incidents have been carried out by other weapons—machetes and knives, cars and trucks, and explosives. The prevalence of firearms in the United States may translate into more firearm-related incidents, but strict gun control measures in other parts of the world have not eliminated the lone-actor terrorism risk. A unique focus in the United States has been the "bipolar" debate between the argument that (a) the lethality of events could be reduced by curtailing access to specific weapons and that (b) access to weapons could allow for better defense and disruption in the execution of lone-actor terrorism events. The policy implications land squarely in how different societies and interest groups in societies navigate the tension between individual rights and individual and collective responsibilities. In the case of the United States, this tends to focus on gun control. The logic behind this focus is that the lethality can be reduced and perhaps even the planning of terrorism events can be disrupted if guns were regulated in a different way or access to guns was changed. This immediately runs into the issue of individual rights and responsibilities, in particular well-trodden ground on the interpretation of the Second Amendment statement "A well-regulated Militia, being necessary to the security of a free State, the right of the people to keep and bear Arms, shall not be infringed."[41] The debate on gun control and the powerful interest groups involved further polarize discussion on whether lethality of lone-actor terrorism can be reduced using this policy tool and how to navigate changes in the law. This challenge of balancing rights and responsibilities is not limited to the United States. As reviewed throughout this volume, other countries have examined legal tools to identify possible lone-actor attackers and the challenge of balancing civil rights, the role of laws and courts in protecting those rights, and broader social issues of how to balance individual liberty and privacy issues against safety and security. An important subtopic in the firearm discussion is the availability of assault weapons in the United States. The Violent Crime Control and Law Enforcement Act 1994 (the federal assault weapons ban) was passed in September 1994 and expired 10 years later. It applied to the manufacture and civilian use of specific categories of semi-automatic weapons and high-capacity magazines that fell under the umbrella term of "assault weapons" after the legislation (including semi-automatic rifles, pistols, and shotguns meeting detailed criteria).[42] Although research showed the ban had limited impact on general crime and firearms-related deaths,[43,44] the ban did have a meaningful impact on reducing mass-shooting incidents (consistent with some lone-actor mass causality incidents). One study by DiMaggio et al. found a dramatic drop in mass-shooting fatalities during the ban period.[45] Another study showed a correlation in timing with a mass-casualty shooting increase after the ban ended.[46] Still, mass-shooting incidents have occurred under the ban, and an assault weapons ban would reduce but not eliminate the risk of mass shootings. The fact that these weapons are abundant in the United States, held legally by a majority of owners, and that an outright ban would not eliminate those already manufactured and owned but could prompt an underground market for these weapons, leads to the need for further research and discussion both within the government and society-wide regarding these weapons and terrorism.

Another topic in the discussion about firearms and lone-actor terrorism/mass causality risk is the concept of "red flag laws" applied in specific states. Red flag laws are state laws that allow, under judicial order, the police to temporarily remove firearms from a person deemed by a judge to be a danger to themselves or others—the request can come by way of relatives, friends, or the police. The removal is meant to be temporary, and continued removal may require another court hearing. As of 2019, 17 states had approved some version of this law, with many states approving following the 2018 mass shooting at the Marjory Stoneman Douglas High School in Florida.[47] A red flag bill at the federal level has tended to be impeded in Congress, although there has been increasing bipartisan support for passage of red flag laws in more states. Although it may be difficult to discern the impact on preventing a mass-shooting incident, studies have shown the laws have a substantial effect on reducing suicide risk.[47] These laws appear to have broad public support across the political spectrum (NPR, Poll 8/19).[48] Vice President Kamala Harris proposed measures aimed at reducing domestic terrorism following the El Paso Texas mass shooting in August 2019 as a Senator, specifically creating a federal red flag law and requiring background checks for online gun sales,[49] which at the time appeared backed by then Senate Majority Leader Mitch McConnell.

An observation by some in security, intelligence, and forensic mental health communities is the unique risk posed by individuals who "simulate" being a commando—carrying a firearm (assault or non-assault) in the context of being "battle ready" and wearing and utilizing tactical gear, including camouflage clothing, helmets, night-vision equipment, knives, communications equipment, etc. in the setting of public protest or demonstration or in other non-military/non-law enforcement contexts, which in some respects may parallel the "pseudocomando," defined in forensic mental health as a heavily armed individual who plans a mass murder in advance and arrives at the crime scene in camouflage or warrior gear.[50] Although there are little data examining this area of risk, a legitimate question exists on whether an individual prepared for combat "as if" in the military, in association with other risk factors outlined in this volume, poses a higher risk of violence (consistent with the definition of lone-actor terrorism).

Domestic Terrorism Laws

There has been an active examination in the United States on how domestic terrorism is managed within the broader definition of terrorism. Whereas international terrorism is viewed within the context of a criminal offense, there are no domestic terrorism laws in the United States as of this writing. The answer to why that is may be convoluted, based on social values and norms, freedoms, and preserving safety and security. After the synagogue attack in Pittsburgh, Daniel Byman[51] made a cogent argument for calling right-wing extremism that results in violence (or the threat of violence) domestic terrorism because it meets the technical definition of terrorism even if "home-grown" rather than originating from overseas. Essentially, one could view any "home-grown" terrorism as domestic terrorism (i.e., extreme right-wing, left-wing, based on a specific ethnicity, religion, etc., or single-issue cause). Calling these acts of terrorism what they are can result in three benefits to combating terrorism: (1) more resources (such as FBI resources) devoted to fighting domestic terrorism, (2) allow for a rapid response early to threats before they escalate to the point where violence erupts, and (3) clarity around what is and is not terrorism from the federal government, which could allow technology to act more definitively.[51] There is, however, an obvious tension between the "adjudication" of home-grown terrorism within the criminal justice system and preserving freedom of speech, with extreme-leaning individuals and groups who do not commit violence worried about infringement on their First Amendment rights. Although the latter is a legitimate argument, the creation of domestic terrorism laws should be able to focus on the preservation of legitimate rights while opening up criminal liability to those who threaten or commit violence. This tension is played out in a debate between two sets of references (a) the American Civil Liberties Union criticism of the definition of domestic terrorism in the USA PATRIOT Act, indicating that its broad character captures those who may protest as an act that could be viewed as dangerous to human life and that the definition should be narrowed to those acts that "cause serious physical injury or death,"[52] and (b) the US Justice Department arguing that the PATRIOT Act limits domestic terrorism to conduct that breaks criminal laws, endangering human life, that "peaceful groups that dissent from government policy" without breaking laws cannot be targeted, that the Act protects Americans' First Amendment rights, and that terrorism investigators have no interest in the library habits of ordinary Americans.[53]

A recent *Wall Street Journal* article following the US Capitol attack underscores the problem with the absence of a formal domestic terrorism law: the FBI can monitor and disrupt international terrorism potentially before it occurs, but its ability to investigate *solely* based on hateful speech or affiliation with known domestic extremists is strictly limited by the First and Second Amendments, among other provisions, protecting rights involving speech, organization, and firearms. "The law-enforcement response to domestic terrorism has been largely reactive—investigating and helping prosecute attacks after they occur."[54] Following the January 6, 2021 Capitol attack, a bipartisan bill has been introduced, the Domestic Terrorism Prevention Act, which would allow the Departments of Homeland Security and Justice to dedicate more resources to managing the domestic terrorism threat.[54,55]

The attack on the US Capitol put a spotlight on the pressing need for clearly delineated laws and resources to manage terrorism, whether it originates within the United States or internationally, by one or two people or within a group, in order to both protect freedoms salient to our democracy while simultaneously disrupting and combating those who would threaten and commit violence for some ideological or political goal.

Pro-Social Measures

An array of novel interventions are being tried in various countries in an effort to "divert" individuals who are at risk for violence (either individually or through affiliation with a group or gang) by way of proactively addressing an underlying need (potentially to avoid a violent group from addressing that same need). In a review of countering violent extremism (CVE),[56] the authors discuss the different approaches to countering and preventing violent extremism: (a) the "hard" CVE method, which emphasizes the role of the military, intelligence, and police to contain/disrupt terrorism and violent extremism; (b) the "soft" approach more traditionally identified with CVE, emphasizing cultural and social variables and proactive de-radicalization before violent extremism ensues; and (c) the "smart" approach, emphasizing a mix of the two depending on the context of the social and political dimensions of the extremism and risk of violence. This review paper provides an assessment of different CVE approaches in viewing and intervening in extremism.[56] For example, one approach involves viewing violent extremism as a social problem, emphasizing community and engagement in society. Another example is viewing violent extremism as an economic issue by way of addressing poverty and economic problems, noting that terrorism has most affected poor countries. A third example highlighted in this paper involves peace-building measures, such as conflict prevention, mediation, strengthening the rule of law, good governance, and resilience approaches.

In another excellent reference reviewing the Countering Violent Extremism Research Conference 2014, several categories of research effort were examined: (a) assessing local drivers that may lead some individuals toward extremism, including "push factors," such as poverty, unemployment, sectarianism, lack of opportunity, and "pull factors" that draw individuals toward extremism, such as money, incentives, protection, and sense of belonging; (b) countering the narrative of extremism "injustices happening, there is a need to act, violence is the only way"; (c) undertaking efforts at disengagement, de-radicalization, and reintegration of former combatants (which can extend to radicalized individuals); and (d) involving the community in efforts at countering violent extremism.[57] One innovative approach in this research review is work examining the role of family counseling in de-radicalization and counterterrorism, examining two models in Denmark and Germany.[58] The countering and preventing violent extremism literature reviews a range of novel interventions or approaches that can help reduce the risk of terrorism committed by radicalized individuals.

A range of pro-social programs and activities exist, focused in part on the geographic region and needs of its population; examples include "deprogramming" efforts, neighborhood protection, education aimed at healthy interpersonal behaviors, and resilience training.[59]

Coordination Between Law Enforcement and Mental Health Professionals

There has been an effort to embed mental health professionals in law enforcement settings, with an overall positive outcome for law enforcement efforts. Related to lone-actor terrorism, one broad focus in this type of consultation would be toward a subgroup of individuals with behavioral issues, possible psychiatric or psychological conditions, or cognitive symptoms who exhibit a pattern of behavior—radicalization, violence, isolation, preoccupation, etc. Identifying those individuals proactively may allow for interventions aimed at both helping the individual (clinically, socially, occupationally, etc.) and reducing the potential risk. Organized police–mental health collaboration has advanced at the local law enforcement level throughout the United States at model learning sites, in coordination with the Council of State Governments Justice Center and the US Department of Justice Bureau of Justice Assistance.[60] The focus of this collaboration includes training, jail diversion, elder abuse prevention, crisis stabilization and response, and homeless outreach. The Bureau of Justice Assistance has a resource site for police–mental health collaboration.[61] Although police–mental health collaboration at the local level has produced benefits, reports indicate the need for improvement at the federal level,[62] noting that the FBI needs to improve the ability to assess whether people with mental health problems pose legitimate threats to national security. This is underscored by a law enforcement study finding in the United Kingdom, where approximately half of people felt to be at risk for radicalization and terrorist sympathies may have mental health or psychological problems.[63] The Prevent Program is a multiagency program at the UK national level, in coordination with police agencies, which focuses on preventing vulnerable individuals from being drawn into terrorism and other criminal behavior.[64]

In the United States, "operational psychology" is one method to liaison psychology and security-law enforcement, intelligence, and the military,[65] although other mental health professionals including psychiatry, nursing, social work, and rehabilitation specialists function in operational roles. The FBI has the resources of the Behavioral Analysis Unit, which focuses on training and research in a number of areas relevant to the FBI mission, including terrorism. In discussion with law enforcement staff at the state and federal levels, there is increasing interest in collaboration with mental health professionals in the law enforcement mission, and the US military and State Department have units that use the mental health professional–investigator relationship to work on various targeted violence cases, including terrorism.[50]

Insider-Threat Management

Insider-threat risk is an important category to consider within lone-actor terrorism. The DHS defines "insider-threat" as a threat that an employee or a contractor will use his or her authorized access, wittingly or unwittingly, to do harm to the United States.[66] Unfortunately, there are numerous examples of insider-threat–driven lone-actor incidents, some outlined in this text. Definitive examples include Nidal Hasan and the November 2009 Fort Hood mass shooting,[67] and Aaron Alexis and the September 2013 Washington Navy Yard mass shooting.[68] A terrorist attack that was averted involved former Coast Guard Officer Christopher Paul Hasson, a self-described white nationalist who had amassed an arsenal of weapons, ammunition, and gear and who, according to court documents, planned a mass casualty assault to further his white extremist views. He pleaded guilty to federal drug and weapons crimes and was sentenced to 13 years in prison.[69]

An important resource to combat insider-threat risk is the National Insider Threat Task Force (NITTF),[70] run by the US Attorney General and the Director of National Intelligence in coordination with the FBI and the National Counterintelligence Executive, comprising representatives from numerous federal agencies. Cases can involve espionage, unauthorized disclosure, suicide, workplace violence, or sabotage. One focus of the NITTF is on insider-threat detection, but they emphasize that not all insider threats have malicious intent, and, in some cases, individuals may be vulnerable and need help from others or can be an unwitting insider at risk of being exploited by others.[70] The Center for Development of Security Excellence (CDSE) provides a comprehensive review of potential insider-threat risk indicators in the security setting. These include access characteristics (security clearance level, access to facilities, systems, and applications), performance (declining or poor ratings, reprimands, demotions), variables related to foreign connections, security and compliance incidents, and suspect technical activity, along with other areas such as criminal, violent, or abusive behaviors; financial issues; substance abuse; and possible judgment or character issues.[71]

Gelles and Mitchell of Deloitte LLP describe several steps to consider in developing a proactive approach to mitigating insider-threat risk. These include defining what insider threat is in relation to the organization and where the organization is in relation to risk tolerance, realizing that insider threat mitigation is not simply based on technology but is "people-centric," understanding that it is important to establish routine and random auditing of functions, and that, because insider threats are seldom impulsive, the importance of looking for precursors to threat behavior and setting behavioral expectations by way of clear and consistently enforced policies, among other variables.[72] The approach to mitigating terrorist insider threat can be complex and multifaceted. The reader is referred to an excellent resource site by the Cybersecurity and Infrastructure Security Agency (CISA) providing a large number of interagency resources focused on terrorism insider threat[73] and to a publication by Bunn and Sagan addressing insider threat with case examples and addressing biases that can lead to minimizing the threat at the organizational level.[74]

Propaganda, Rhetoric, and Message Amplification

As emphasized throughout this volume, propaganda and rhetoric can play an important role in propagating and reinforcing extremist beliefs that can lead to violence. There are numerous case examples of this relationship. Nidal Hasan was in contact with Anwar Al-Awlaki by email in the year before the Fort Hood shooting, and although some reports indicated the communications had to do with Hasan seeking spiritual guidance, other reports raised significant concern about why an Army major would be in communication with an extremist like al-Awlaki, who was preaching hate and inciting violence against the United Stated.[75] James Fields, who drove his car into a crowd, killing one and injuring dozens of others on August 12, 2017, acted in the context of the heated propaganda of the Unite the Right rally in Charlottesville, Virginia. Unfortunately, the inflammatory language in the rally was amplified by the then President[76] who announced there were "some very fine people on both sides." Cesar A. Sayoc Jr., who sent pipe bombs to those he considered to be President Trump's enemies, acted at a time of angry rhetoric regarding immigrants and political opponents. Sayoc, who drew inspiration from then President Trump, had covered his van in stickers that glorified Trump and placed President Obama and Secretary of State Clinton in red cross-hairs.[77] Juliette Kayyem, a former assistant secretary at the DHS, and others have described this phenomenon as *stochastic terrorism*—a pattern that cannot be predicted precisely but can be analyzed (statistically predictable but individually unpredictable) involving the demonization of groups through media and propaganda that can result in violence because listeners interpret it as promoting targeted violence.[78,79]

A critical and recent incident was the US Capitol attack on January 6, 2021, by a large mob of the then President's followers, who had assembled prior to the riot to listen to the President. In the months leading to the 2020 election, then President Trump and others angrily reinforced the belief that the election, which was won by Joe Biden, was fraudulent and had been "stolen," something disproved in numerous courts.[80,81] In that context, the Capitol was attacked in an effort to interrupt the Electoral College vote count and overturn the election. Although some level of premeditated organization was believed to have occurred, there also appeared to be some coordination between individuals, with one former FBI agent commenting that "historically . . . leadership has produced rhetoric to . . . increase radicalization and recruitment, and then stand[s] back and let[s] small cells or individual lone offenders follow through on that rhetoric with violent action."[82] Events leading to and taking place on January 6 highlight the critical role that heated propaganda and rhetoric play in spinning up emotions and the risk for violence from both individuals and groups, even in the face of concrete contradictory evidence.

FUTURE RESEARCH

Looking back over the chapters that make up this volume, it is that clear a lot of research has been done in a relatively small period of time. The number of academic papers cited almost outnumber the lone-actor terrorists themselves. This is not necessarily a bad thing. Replication, after all, is fundamental to the scientific process. Larger scale replication projects have shown mixed, and often worrying, results. The Reproducibility Project for Psychology, for example, showed that only 35 of the tested 97 original "significant" effects could be replicated.[83] These high rates of failed replications raise concerns about the quality of research output in the psychological sciences as well as the procedures and standards applied by its authors. The study of violent extremism is likely not immune.

Perhaps one of the least understood areas, however, relates to the onset of violent extremist beliefs and attitudes. In particular, what are the risk and protective factors that enable and destabilize the often slow mobilization to violence? This should be a priority for future research and will necessitate, on many occasions, zooming out from those who engaged in lone-actor terrorist violence and instead focusing on the wider categories of people who hold similar attitudes and belief systems.

Indeed, much recent research is trying to sample active exposure to violent extremists, their settings, and materials in general population samples.[84,85] But there is much more work to be done. For example, more research is needed on whether similar risk factors functionally apply across different ideological domains and risk specifications (e.g., vulnerability to radicalization, engagement with extremist materials, support for violent extremist intentions).

Equally, survey style designs in this space have yet to investigate dynamics longitudinally. Instead, cross-sectional designs are the norm. Properly designed longitudinal studies will provide sufficient power to detect meaningful change over time within sampled groups.

Additionally, methodological developments in the psychological sciences utilize intensive repeated measures. Whereas traditional longitudinal designs focus on a large sample and a large survey of 200+ items that is measured four times over 4 years, intensive repeat measure designs focus on a much smaller sample with approximately 20 items measured intensively (e.g., 30 times) over a small-temporal period (e.g., a month). This form of data collection is becoming more popular in the psychological sciences because it affords quantitative ideographic research designs that intensely monitor intra-individual change over a short period of time. The

widespread adoption of mobile technology has made it easier and cheaper for research projects to collect such intensive longitudinal data. Such designs have the capability of measuring very short-term shifts in violent extremist beliefs, attitudes, and intentions and their lagged relationship with daily experiences. Such analyses are highly valuable to real-world interventions and are becoming more popular in clinical practice generally to inform individualized care and treatment plans.

Speaking of interventions, there is still much work to be done on protective factors. There are major conceptual debates in the general violence literature. Protective factors have been conceptualized and operationalized across individual studies in three broad ways.[86] First, they have been viewed as the absence of a risk factor (e.g., the presence of informal social and personal controls).[87] Second, they have been viewed as the opposite of a risk factor on a single continuum[88] (e.g., some studies might depict excellent school performance as a protective factor and its inverse, poor school performance, as a risk factor). Third, they have been treated as a completely independent and conceptually distinct factor with no corresponding risk factor.[89]

Protective factors are increasingly coming to the fore of debates within risk assessment and management practice. Scientific research lags behind across a wide range of violent crimes. Protective factors research has been described as "extremely limited" for sexual violence,[90] the subject of "little attention" for interpersonal and youth violence,[91,92] "in its infancy" for gang violence,[93] and "limited" for physical abuse of children.[94] The lack of research on protective factors has been ascribed to numerous conceptual and methodological issues. Issues raised have included a historical overemphasis on risk factors compared to protective factors, inadequate research designs and analyses to evidence a protective factor, and a failure to consider that select factors can be a risk or protective factor depending on developmental period or individual circumstances.[95–97]

CONCLUSION

This chapter highlights the broad array of variables that need to be considered in the approach to understanding and intervening in lone-actor terrorism. A large number of variables reviewed provide opportunities for potential intervention aimed at reducing the risk to society. It is important that future research focus on measures that can expand our understanding of this complex public health threat and translate this into meaningful risk management.

NOTES AND REFERENCES

1. Hamm M, Spaaij R. *The Age of Lone-Wolf Terrorism*. New York: Columbia University Press; 2017.
2. Simon JD. *Lone Wolf Terrorism: Understanding the Growing Threat*. Amherst, NY: Prometheus Books; 2013.
3. United States Department of Justice, Federal Bureau of Investigation, Behavioral Analysis Unit. *Lone Offender: A Study of Lone Offender Terrorism in the United States (1972–2015)*. Quantico, VA: FBI National Center for the Analysis of Violent Crime, Nov 2019. https://www.fbi.gov/file-repository/lone-offender-terrorism-report-111319.pdf
4. Hamm M, Spaaij R. *Lone Wolf Terrorism in America: Using Knowledge of Radicalization Pathways to Forge Prevention Strategies*. Report to the US Department of Justice, No. 248691, Feb 2015. https://www.ncjrs.gov/pdffiles1/nij/grants/248691.pdf
5. Schuurman B, Lindekilde L, Malthaner S, O'Connor F, Gill P, Bouhana N. End of the lone wolf: The typology that should not have been. *Stud Conflict Terrorism* 2019;42(8): 771–778. doi:10.1080/1057610X.2017.1419554.
6. Gill P, Horgan J, Deckert P. Bombing alone: Tracing the motivations and antecedent behaviors of lone-actor terrorists. *J Forensic Sci*. 2014;59(2):425–435. doi:10.1111/1556-4029.12312.
7. Jensen M, LaFree G, James PA, et al., and National Consortium for the Study of Terrorism and Responses to Terrorism (START), University of Maryland. Final report: Empirical assessment of domestic radicalization (EADR). Report to the National Institute of Justice, Office of Justice Programs, US Department of Justice, Dec 2016. https://start.umd.edu/pubs/START_NIJ_EmpiricalAssessmentofDomesticRadicalizationFinalReport_Dec2016.pdf
8. Gill P, Corner E. Lone-actor terrorist target choice. *Behav Sci Law*. 2016;34(5): 693–705. doi:10.1002/bsl.2268.
9. Schuurman B, Bakker E, Gill P, Bouhana N. Lone actor terrorist attack planning and preparation: A data-driven analysis. *J Forensic Sci*. 2018;63(4):1191–1200. doi:10.1111/1556-4029.13676.
10. Parker D, Pearce JM, Lindekilde L, Rogers MB. Press coverage of lone-actor terrorism in the UK and Denmark: Shaping the reactions of the public, affected communities and copycat attackers. *Crit Stud Terrorism*. 2019;12(1):110–131. doi:10.1080/17539153.2018.1494792.
11. Miller V, Hayward KJ. "I did my bit": Terrorism, Tarde and the vehicle ramming attack as an imitative event. *Br J Criminol*. 2019;59(1):1–23. doi:10.1093/bjc/azy017.
12. Murray JL. Mass media reporting and enabling of mass shootings. *Cult Stud Crit Methodol*. 2017;17(2):114–124. doi:10.1177/1532708616679144.
13. Wright S, Denney D, Pinkerton A, Jansen VAA, Bryden J. Resurgent insurgents: Quantitative research into jihadists who get suspended but return on Twitter. *J Terrorism Res*.2016;7(2):1–13.
14. Ellis C, Pantucci R, van Zuijdewijn JdR, et al. Analysing the processes of lone-actor terrorism: Research findings. *Perspect Terror*. 2016;10(2): 33–41.
15. Meloy JR, Goodwill AM, Meloy MJ, Amat G, Martinez M, Morgan M. Some TRAP-18 indicators discriminate between terrorist attackers and other subjects of national security concern. *J Threat Assess Manage*. 2019;6(2):93–110, p.94; doi:10.1037/tam0000119.
16. Wray CA, Dir. Federal Bureau of Investigation. Statement before the Committee on Homeland Security, US House of Representatives, at a hearing entitled "Worldwide Threats." Testimony presented 17 Sep 2020. https://www.c-span.org/video/?475444-1/fbi-director-wray-foreign-interference-elections-not-tolerated
17. Shehabat A, Mitew T. Black-boxing the black flag: Anonymous sharing platforms and ISIS content distribution tactics. *Perspect Terrorism*. 2018;12(1):81–99.
18. Department of Homeland Security. National terrorism advisory system bulletin, 27 Jan 2021. https://www.dhs.gov/ntas/advisory/national-terrorism-advisory-system-bulletin-january-27-2021
19. MacFarquhar N, Gibbons-Neff T. Air Force sergeant with ties to extremist group charged in federal officer's death. *New York Times*, 16 Jun 2020. https://www.nytimes.com/2020/06/16/us/steven-carrillo-air-force-boogaloo.html
20. Healy J. These are the 5 people who died in the Capitol riot. *New York Times*, 22 Feb 2021. https://www.nytimes.com/2021/01/11/us/who-died-in-capitol-building-attack.html
21. United States District of Columbia Attorney's Office. Capitol Breach Cases. https://www.justice.gov/usao-dc/capitol-breach-cases
22. Department of Justice, Office of Public Affairs. Lifetime founding member of the Oath Keepers pleads guilty to breaching Capitol on Jan. 6 to obstruct Congressional proceeding. Department of Justice, 16 Apr 2021. https://www.justice.gov/opa/pr/lifetime-founding-member-oath-keepers-pleads-guilty-breaching-capitol-jan-6-obstruct

23. Southern Poverty Law Center. PROUD BOYS. https://www.splcenter.org/fighting-hate/extremist-files/group/proud-boys

24. Reuters. Proud Boys Canada dissolves itself, months after designation as terrorist entity. *The Guardian*, 2 May 2021. https://www.theguardian.com/world/2021/may/03/proud-boys-canada-dissolves-itself-months-after-designation-as-terrorist-entity

25. Southern Poverty Law Center. The people, groups and symbols at Charlottesville. 15 August 2017. https://www.splcenter.org/news/2017/08/15/people-groups-and-symbols-charlottesville

26. Romo V. Charlottesville jury convicts "Unite the Right" protester who killed woman. NPR, 7 Dec 2018. https://www.npr.org/2018/12/07/674672922/james-alex-fields-unite-the-right-protester-who-killed-heather-heyer-found-guilt

27. Chermak SM, Freilich JD, Suttmoeller M. The organizational dynamics of far-right hate groups in the United States: Comparing violent to nonviolent organizations. National Consortium for the Study of Terrorism and Responses to Terrorism, Dec 2011. https://www.dhs.gov/sites/default/files/publications/944_OPSR_TEVUS_Comparing-Violent-Nonviolent-Far-Right-Hate-Groups_Dec2011-508.pdf

28. MacFarquhar N, Gibbons-Neff T. *Air Force Sergeant With Ties to Extremist Group Charged in Federal Officer's Death*. New York Times, June 16, 2020. https://www.nytimes.com/2020/06/16/us/steven-carrillo-air-force-boogaloo.html

29. Katkov M. Suspect pleads guilty in plot to kidnap Michigan Governor, turns government witness. NPR, 27 Jan 2021. https://www.npr.org/2021/01/27/961215604/suspect-pleads-guilty-in-plot-to-kidnap-michigan-governor-turns-government-witne

30. Ross AR, Modi M, Paresky P, et al. A contagion of institutional distrust: Viral disinformation of the COVID vaccine and the road to reconciliation. Network Contagion Research Institute, 11 Mar 2021. https://networkcontagion.us/reports/a-contagion-of-institutional-distrust/

31. Dickson EJ. The QAnon Community Is in Crisis—But On Telegram, It's Also Growing. Rolling Stone. 22 January 2021; https://www.rollingstone.com/culture/culture-news/qanon-telegram-channels-increase-1117869/

32. INTERPOL. Terrorist groups using COVID-19 to reinforce power and influence. 22 Dec 2020. https://www.interpol.int/en/News-and-Events/News/2020/INTERPOL-Terrorist-groups-using-COVID-19-to-reinforce-power-and-influence

33. Stevens T, Neumann PR. *Countering Online Radicalisaiton: A Strategy for Action*. International Centre for the Study of Radicalisation and Political Violence, eds. London: King's College London; 2009.

34. von Behr I, Reding A, Edwards C, Gribbon L. *Radicalisation in the Digital Era: The Use of the Internet in 15 Cases of Terrorism and Extremism*. Cambridge: Rand; 2013. https://www.rand.org/content/dam/rand/pubs/research_reports/RR400/RR453/RAND_RR453.pdf

35. Gill P. *Lone-Actor Terrorists: A Behavioural Analysis*. Abingdon and New York: Routledge; 2016:ch. 5.

36. Neumann PR. Options and strategies for countering online radicalization in the United States. *Stud Conflict and Terrorism*. 2013;36:6,431–459. doi:10.1080/1057610X.2013.784568.

37. Corner E, Gill P. A false dichotomy? Mental illness and lone-actor terrorism. *Law Hum Behav*. 2015;39(1):23–34.

38. Leslie C, Hedman LC, Petrila J, Fisher WH, et al. State laws on emergency holds for mental health stabilization. Psychiatry OnLine, Psychiatric Services, 29 Feb 2016. https://doi.org/10.1176/appi.ps.201500205

39. Rotunda RD. The right to shout fire in a crowded theatre: Hateful speech and the First Amendment. *Chapman Law Rev*. 2019 Spring;22(2):319–368. Chapman University Dale E. Fowler School of Law. https://digitalcommons.chapman.edu/cgi/viewcontent.cgi?article=1443andcontext=chapman-law-review

40. Kleinberg B, Arntz A, Verschuere B. Detecting deceptive intentions: Possibilities for large-scale applications. In T. Docan-Morgan ed., *The Palgrave Handbook of Deceptive Communication*; 2019:ch. 21. https://doi.org/10.1007/978-3-319-96334-1_21

41. Congress.gov. Second Amendment: Doctrine and Practice. https://constitution.congress.gov/browse/essay/amdt2-1/ALDE_00000408/

42. Public Safety and Recreational Firearms Use Protection Act, H.R.3355, 103rd Congress (1993–1994).

43. Koper CS, Woods DJ, Roth JA. *An Updated Assessment of the Federal Assault Weapons Ban: Impacts on Gun Markets and Gun Violence, 1994–2003*. Report to the National Institute of Justice. Washington, DC: United States Department of Justice; Jun 2004.

44. Wellford CF, Pepper JV, Petrie CV. *Firearms and Violence: A Critical Review* (electronic ed.). Washington, DC: National Academies Press; 2005.

45. DiMaggio C, Avraham J, Berry C, et al. Changes in US mass shooting deaths associated with the 1994–2004 federal assault weapons ban: Analysis of open-source data. *J Trauma Acute Care Surg*. Jan 2019;86(1):11–19.

46. Lemieux F, Bricknell S, Prenzler T. Mass shootings in Australia and the United States, 1981–2013. *J Criminol Res Pol Pract*., 2015;1(3):131–142.

47. Williams T. What are "red flag" gun laws, and how do they work? *New York Times*, 6 Aug 2019.

48. Paterson L. Poll: Americans, including Republicans and gun owners, broadly support red flag laws. NPR, 20 Aug 2019. https://choice.npr.org/index.html?origin=https://www.npr.org/2019/08/20/752427922/poll-americans-including-republicans-and-gun-owners-broadly-support-red-flag-law

49. Lah K, Wright J. Kamala Harris proposes taking on domestic terrorism by limiting gun access. CNN, 14 Aug 2019. https://edition.cnn.com/2019/08/14/politics/kamala-harris-red-flag-law-proposal/index.html

50. Knoll JL. The "Pseudocommando" Mass Murderer: Part I, The Psychology of Revenge and Obliteration. J Am Acad Psychiatry Law. Online March 2010;38(1):87–94; http://jaapl.org/content/38/1/87.short

51. Byman D. When to call a terrorist a terrorist. *Foreign Policy*, 27 Oct 2018. https://foreignpolicy.com/2018/10/27/when-to-call-a-terrorist-a-terrorist/

52. ACLU. How the USA Patriot Act redefines "domestic terrorism." https://www.aclu.org/other/how-usa-patriot-act-redefines-domestic-terrorism

53. US Department of Justice. Dispelling some of the major myths about the USA PATRIOT Act. https://www.justice.gov/archive/ll/subs/u_myths.htm

54. Levy R. A domestic terrorism law is debated anew after capitol riot. *Wall Street Journal*, 13 Feb 2021.

55. Schneider B. Domestic Terrorism Prevention Act (DTPA) of 2021 Introduced in House 2021. https://schneider.house.gov/media/press-releases/domestic-terrorism-prevention-act-dtpa-2021-introduced-house

56. Schomerus M, El Taraboulsi-McCarthy S, Sandhar J. *Countering Violent Extremism* (Topic Guide). Birmingham, UK: GSDRC, University of Birmingham; 2017.

57. Zeiger S, Aly A. *Countering Violent Extremism: Developing an Evidence-base for Policy and Practice*. Perth, AUS: Curtin University; 2015.

58. Koehler D. Family counselling, de-radicalization and counter-terrorism: The Danish and German programs in context. In Zeiger S, Aly A, eds., *Countering Violent Extremism: Developing an Evidence-base for Policy and Practice*. Perth, AUS: Curtin University; 2015.

59. Organization for Security and Co-operation in Europe. Preventing Terrorism and Countering Violent Extremism and Radicalization that Lead to Terrorism: A Community-Policing Approach. © OSCE 2014, https://www.osce.org/files/f/documents/1/d/111438.pdf

60. Bureau of Justice Assistance. *Overview of Law Enforcement—Mental Health Resources*. 2020. https://www.ojp.gov/sites/g/files/xyckuh241/files/media/document/resourceoverviewpw.pdf

61. Police-Mental Health Collaboration Toolkit - https://bja.ojp.gov/program/pmhc

62. AP Washington. FBI lacks strategy for handling tips on people with mental health problems. *The Guardian*, 4 Mar 2020. https://www.theguardian.com/us-news/2020/mar/04/report-finds-weaknesses-inconsistencies-how-fbi-handles-terrorism-tips

63. Dodd V. Police study links radicalisation to mental health problems. *The Guardian*, 20 May 2016. https://www.theguardian.com/uk-news/2016/may/20/police-study-radicalisation-mental-health-problems

64. Counter Terrorism Advisory Network. PREVENT. https://www.counterterrorism.police.uk/what-we-do/prevent/

65. Palarea RE. Operational psychology: An emerging discipline. AP-LS News, Fall 2007:9–11.

66. https://www.dhs.gov/science-and-technology/cybersecurity-insider-threat

67. Poppe K. Nidal Hasan: A case study in lone-actor terrorism. GW Program on Extremism, Oct 2018. https://extremism.gwu.edu/sites/g/files/zaxdzs2191/f/Nidal%20Hasan.pdf

68. Center for Development of Security Excellence. Behavioral indicators of an active shooter. Defense Counterintelligence and Security Agency. https://www.cdse.edu/index.html

69. Williams P. White supremacist Coast Guard officer sentenced to 13 years in prison. NBC News, 31 Jan 2020. https://www.nbcnews.com/news/us-news/white-supremacist-coast-guard-officer-sentenced-13-years-prison-n1112763670.

70. NITTF. National insider threat task force mission fact sheet. https://www.dni.gov/files/NCSC/documents/products/National_Insider_Threat_Task_Force_Fact_Sheet.pdf

71. CDSE. Potential risk indicators: Insider threat. https://www.cdse.edu/Training/Insider-Threat/

72. Gelles MG, Mitchell K. Top 10 considerations for building an insider threat mitigation program. *J Threat Assess Manage*. 2016;2(3-4):1–4. https://www2.deloitte.com/us/en/pages/public-sector/articles/key-considerations-for-building-an-insider-threat-mitigation-program.html

73. Cybersecurity and Infrastructure Security Agency. Insider threat terrorism. https://www.cisa.gov/terrorism

74. Bunn M, Sagan SD. *Insider Threats*. Ithaca, NY: Cornell University Press; 2016.

75. Egerton B. Imam's e-mails to Fort Hood suspect Hasan tame compared to online rhetoric. *Dallas Morning News*, 29 Nov 2009.

76. Gray R. Trump defends white-nationalist protesters: "Some very fine people on both sides. *The Atlantic*, 17 Aug 2017. https://www.theatlantic.

com/politics/archive/2017/08/trump-defends-
white-nationalist-protesters-some-very-fine-
people-on-both-sides/537012/

77. Weiser B, Watkins A. Cesar Sayoc, who mailed
pipe bombs to Trump critics, is sentenced to
20 years. *New York Times*, 5 Aug 2019. https://
www.nytimes.com/2019/08/05/nyregion/cesar-
sayoc-sentencing-pipe-bombing.html

78. Kayyem J. There are no lone wolves. *Washington
Post*, 4 Aug 2019. https://www.washingtonpost.
com/opinions/2019/08/04/there-are-no-lone-
wolves/

79. Keats J. Jargon watch: The rising danger of stochastic terrorism. *Wired*, 21 Jan 2019. https://
www.wired.com/story/jargon-watch-rising-
danger-stochastic-terrorism/

80. Cummings W, Garrison J, Sergent J. By the numbers: President Donald Trump's failed efforts to
overturn the election. *USA Today*, 6 Jan 2021.
https://www.usatoday.com/in-depth/news/poli-
tics/elections/2021/01/06/trumps-failed-efforts-
overturn-election-numbers/4130307001/

81. Rutenberg J, Corsaniti N, Feuer A. Trump's
fraud claims died in court, but the myth of stolen
elections lives on. *New York Times*, 7 Jan 2021.
https://www.nytimes.com/2020/12/26/us/poli-
tics/republicans-voter-fraud.html

82. Barrett D, Hsu SS, David AC. "Be ready to
fight": FBI probe of US Capitol riot finds evidence
detailing coordination of an assault. *Washington
Post*, 30 Jan 2021.

83. Open Science Collaboration. Maximizing the
reproducibility of your research. In Lilienfeld
SO, Waldman ID, eds., *Psychological Science
Under Scrutiny: Recent Challenges and Proposed
Solutions*. New York: Wiley Blackwell; 2017:3–21.

84. Clemmow C, Schumann S, Salman NL, Gill P.
The base rate study: Developing base rates for
risk factors and indicators for engagement in
violent extremism. *J Forensic Sci*. 2020;65(3):
865-881.

85. Rottweiler B, Gill P, Bouhana N. Individual and
environmental explanations for violent extremist intentions: A German nationally representative survey study. *Justice Q.*, 2021:1–22.

86. Ttofi MM, Farrington DP, Piquero AR, Lösel F,
DeLisi M, Murray J. Intelligence as a protective
factor against offending: A meta-analytic review
of prospective longitudinal studies. *J Crim Justice*. 2016;45:4–18.

87. Dickens GL, O'Shea LE. (2018). Protective factors in risk assessment schemes for adolescents
in mental health and criminal justice populations: A systematic review and meta-analysis
of their predictive efficacy. *Adolesc Res Rev*.
2018;3(1):95–112.

88. O'Shea LE, Dickens GL. Performance of protective factors assessment in risk prediction for
adults: Systematic review and meta-analysis. *Clin
Psychol Sci Pract*. 2016;23(2):126–138.

89. Sameroff AJ, Fiese BH. Transactional regulation: The developmental ecology of early intervention. *Handbk Early Childhood Intervent*.
2000;2:135–159.

90. Tharp AT, DeGue S, Valle LA, Brookmeyer KA,
Massetti GM, Matjasko JL. A systematic qualitative review of risk and protective factors for
sexual violence perpetration. *Trauma Violence
Abuse*. 2013;14(2):133–167.

91. Walker K, Bowen E, Brown S. Psychological and
criminological factors associated with desistance
from violence: A review of the literature. *Aggression Violent Behav*. 2013;18(2):286–299.

92. van der Merwe A, Dawes A. Youth violence: A
review of risk factors, causal pathways and effective intervention. *J Child Adolesc Mental Health*.
2007;19(2):95–113.

93. O'Brien K, Daffern M, Chu CM, Thomas SD.
Youth gang affiliation, violence, and criminal
activities: A review of motivational, risk, and
protective factors. *Aggression Violent Behav*.
2013;18(4):417–425.

94. Meinck F, Cluver LD, Boyes ME, Mhlongo EL.
Risk and protective factors for physical and
sexual abuse of children and adolescents in
Africa: A review and implications for practice.
Trauma Violence Abuse. 2015;16(1):81–107.

95. Hall JE, Simon TR, Lee RD, Mercy JA. Implications of direct protective factors for public health research and prevention strategies
to reduce youth violence. *Am J Prevent Med*.
2012;43(2):S76–S83.

96. Lösel F, Farrington DP. Direct protective and
buffering protective factors in the development of youth violence. *Am J Prevent Med*.
2012;43(2):S8–S23.

97. Lösel F, Bender D. Protective factors against
crime and violence in adolescence. In Sturmey
P. (ed.), *The Wiley Handbook of Violence and
Aggression*, New York: Wiley; 2017:1–15.

INDEX

For the benefit of digital users, indexed terms that span two pages (e.g., 52–53) may, on occasion, appear on only one of those pages.

Figures and tables are indicated by *f* and *t* following the page numbers.